Dental
Radiography

Dental Radiography

PRINCIPLES AND TECHNIQUES

Joen Iannucci Haring, DDS, MS
Associate Professor of Clinical Dentistry
Section of Primary Care
Director, Sterilization Monitoring Service
The Ohio State University
College of Dentistry
Columbus, Ohio

Laura Jansen, RDH, MS
Clinical Associate Professor
Department of Dental Ecology
The University of North Carolina at Chapel Hill
School of Dentistry
Chapel Hill, North Carolina

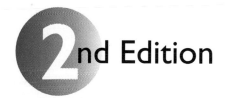

2nd Edition

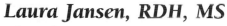

W.B. SAUNDERS COMPANY
An Imprint of Elsevier Science
Philadelphia   London   New York   St. Louis   Toronto   Sydney

W.B. SAUNDERS COMPANY
An Imprint of Elsevier Science

The Curtis Center
Independence Square West
Philadelphia, Pennsylvania 19106

Library of Congress Cataloging-in-Publication Data

Haring, Joen Iannucci.
Dental radiography: principles and techniques/Joen Iannucci Haring, Laura Jansen.—2nd ed.

p.; cm.

Includes bibliographical references and index.

ISBN 0–7216–8545–5

1. Teeth—Radiography. I. Jansen, Laura. II. Title.

[DNLM: 1. Radiography, Dental—methods. WN 230 H281d 2000]

RK309 .H36 2000   616.07′572—dc21

Acquisition Editor: Shirley A. Kuhn
Production Manager: Peter Faber
Project Manager: Agnes Hunt Byrne
Illustration Specialist: Francis Moriarty

DENTAL RADIOGRAPHY: PRINCIPLES AND TECHNIQUES   ISBN 0–7216–8545–5

Printed in the United States of America.

Last digit is the print number: 9   8   7   6   5

To my family and friends
who have encouraged me
throughout my career

and

To my guardian angels,
Angelo M. and Mary Lou Iannucci.

—*JIH*

To my family and friends who are the best part of my life,
and especially,
Jim, Tom, and Larry.

—*LJ*

Contributors

Cheryl H. DeVore, RDH, MS, JD
Director and Associate Professor
Dental Hygiene, Section of Primary Care
The Ohio State University
College of Dentistry
Columbus, Ohio

Private Practice of Law
Dublin, Ohio

Legal Issues and the Dental Radiographer

Robert M. Jaynes, DDS, MS
Assistant Professor
Section of Primary Care/Oral Radiology Group
The Ohio State University
College of Dentistry
Columbus, Ohio

Panoramic Radiography
Extraoral Radiography

Preface

As the title *DENTAL RADIOGRAPHY: PRINCIPLES AND TECHNIQUES* suggests, the purpose of this text is to present the basic principles of dental radiography and to provide detailed information concerning radiographic techniques. This text serves as both a reference source and a training manual; it provides the reader with basic theory as well as complete technique instruction.

A NOTE TO THE READER . . .

This text has been written exclusively for you, the dental hygiene or dental assistant student. It is an understandable dental radiography text that truly provides you, the reader, with a balance of theory and practice.

DENTAL RADIOGRAPHY: PRINCIPLES AND TECHNIQUES has been designed so that a dental auxiliary student without background in radiography, anatomy, or related topics can literally pick up the book and learn dental radiography, chapter by chapter.

A NOTE TO EDUCATORS . . .

Educators who use *DENTAL RADIOGRAPHY: PRINCIPLES AND TECHNIQUES* and the corresponding slide series will find both to be effective teaching tools.

DENTAL RADIOGRAPHY: PRINCIPLES AND TECHNIQUES is written so that it is easy to understand—simple, straightforward explanations are used throughout the text in order to foster comprehension and retention of the material presented. You will find that this text provides the reader with a logical, step-by-step approach to learning dental radiography. You will also find that this text is more heavily illustrated than the other texts on this topic. The purpose of including the numerous illustrations, photographs, and radiographs is to enhance learning.

ABOUT THE TEXT ORGANIZATION . . .

One of the strengths of this text is its organization. It is organized to facilitate learning. Each chapter begins with a list of objectives to focus the reader on the important aspects of the material presented. At the beginning of each chapter, key words are listed; each key word is highlighted in boldface as it is introduced in the text. Quiz questions are included at the completion of each chapter; answers to the quiz questions are provided at the end of the book. A glossary of over 600 terms is included at the end of the book. This text also includes numerous charts and helpful hints to further organize information.

ABOUT THE TEXT TOPICS . . .

The dental auxiliary student will find that this text contains just the right amount of basic information. As in the first edition, this second edition is divided into manageable parts (for both the reader and the educator) to facilitate learning:

- Radiation Basics
- Equipment, Film, and Processing Basics
- Dental Radiographer Basics
- Technique Basics
- Normal Anatomy and Film Mounting Basics
- Radiographic Interpretation Basics

ABOUT THE SECOND EDITION . . .

As technology and techniques change, a book revision is essential. Since the first edition was published in 1996, a dramatic increase in the use of digital radiography has occurred. As a result, a chapter on *Digital Radiography* has been added to this second edition. A chapter has also been added on *Normal Anatomy—Panoramic Films;* you will find that this topic is not covered in depth in other texts. Another addition to this second edition is the *Self-Study Examination,* a feature currently not included in the other radiography texts for dental auxiliary students. The purpose of including the practice examination is to prepare the dental auxiliary student for the dental radiography portion of the board examinations required for dental hygiene and dental assistant licensure.

ABOUT LEARNING DENTAL RADIOGRAPHY . . .

Are there any tricks to learning dental radiography? Most definitely. Attend class. Stay awake. Pay attention. Ask questions. Read the book. Learn the material. Do not cram. Prepare for tests. Do not give up.

Joen Iannucci Haring, DDS, MS
Laura Jansen, RDH, MS

Acknowledgments

The authors thank the following colleagues for their expertise in the preparation of this manuscript: contributing author Cheryl H. DeVore, RDH, MS, JD (Associate Professor, The Ohio State University), and manuscript reviewer Anna Layton, CDA (Radiology Technologist, The Ohio State University). We would also like to express our gratitude to photographer David Harrison (Dublin, Ohio) and models Susan Bauchmoyer, Kelly Eyer, and Mindy Jones. We would also like to acknowledge the work of the staff of the Learning Resource Center at the School of Dentistry at The University of North Carolina at Chapel Hill. In addition, we would like to extend our gratefulness to Shirley Kuhn, Acquisitions Editor at W.B. Saunders Company.

We also wish to express our deepest appreciation to our families and friends for their unending support during the preparation of this manuscript. Finally, a very special thanks to our husbands, Robert S. Haring, DDS, MS, and William L. Lind, DDS, for their patience, encouragement, and understanding.

Joen Iannucci Haring, DDS, MS
Laura Jansen, RDH, MS

Contents

Radiation Basics

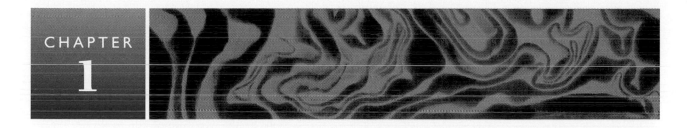

CHAPTER 1

Radiation History

OBJECTIVES

After completion of this chapter, the student will be able to:

- *Define the key words.*
- *Summarize the importance of dental radiographs.*
- *List the uses of dental radiographs.*
- *Summarize the discovery of x-radiation.*
- *Recognize the pioneers in dental x-radiation and their contributions and discoveries.*
- *List the highlights in the history of x-ray equipment and film.*
- *List the highlights in the history of dental radiographic techniques.*

INTRODUCTION

The dental radiographer cannot appreciate the x-ray technology of today without looking back to the discovery and history of x-radiation. A thorough knowledge of x-radiation begins with its discovery, a review of the pioneers in dental x-radiation, and the history of dental x-ray equipment, film, and radiographic techniques. In addition, before the dental radiographer can begin to understand x-radiation and its role in dentistry, an introduction to basic dental radiography terms and a discussion of the importance of dental radiographs are necessary. The purpose of this chapter is to introduce basic dental radiography terms, to detail the importance of dental radiographs, and to review the history of x-radiation.

DENTISTRY AND X-RADIATION

Basic Terminology

Prior to detailing the importance of dental radiographs and the discovery and history of x-rays, an understanding of a number of basic terms pertaining to dentistry and x-radiation is necessary.

Radiation: A form of energy carried by waves or a stream of particles.

X-radiation: A high-energy radiation produced by the collision of a beam of electrons with a metal target in an x-ray tube.

X-ray: A beam of energy that has the power to penetrate substances and record image shadows on photographic film.

Radiology: The science or study of radiation as used in medicine; a branch of medical science that deals with the use of x-rays, radioactive substances, and other forms of radiant energy in the diagnosis and treatment of disease.

Radiograph: A picture (visible photographic record) on film produced by the passage of x-rays

through an object or body. In practice, often called an x-ray; this is not correct. X-ray is a term that refers to a beam of energy.

Dental radiograph: A photographic image produced on film by the passage of x-rays through teeth and related structures.

Radiography: The art and science of making radiographs by the exposure of film to x-rays.

Dental radiography: The making of radiographs of the teeth and adjacent structures by the exposure of film to x-rays.

Dental radiographer: Any person who positions, exposes, and processes dental x-ray film.

Importance of Dental Radiographs

The dental radiographer must have a working knowledge of the value and uses of dental radiographs. Dental radiographs are a necessary component of comprehensive patient care. In dentistry, radiographs enable the dental professional to identify many conditions that may otherwise go undetected and to see conditions that cannot be identified clinically. An oral examination without dental radiographs limits the practitioner to what is seen clinically—the teeth and soft tissue. With the use of dental radiographs, the dental radiographer can obtain a wealth of information about the teeth and supporting bone.

Detection is one of the most important uses of dental radiographs. Through the use of dental radiographs, the dental radiographer can detect disease. Many dental diseases and conditions produce no clinical signs or symptoms and are typically discovered *only* through the use of dental radiographs. The objectives of dental radiograph examination are listed in the "Uses of Dental Radiographs" chart.

USES OF DENTAL RADIOGRAPHS

- To *detect* lesions, diseases and conditions of the teeth and surrounding structures that cannot be identified clinically.
- To *confirm* or *classify* suspected disease.
- To *localize* lesions or foreign objects.
- To *provide information* during dental procedures (e.g., root canal therapy).
- To *evaluate* growth and development.
- To *illustrate* changes secondary to caries, periodontal disease, and trauma.
- To *document* the condition of a patient at a specific point in time.

DISCOVERY OF X-RADIATION

Roentgen and the Discovery of X-rays

The history of dental radiography begins with the discovery of the x-ray. Wilhelm Conrad Roentgen (pronounced "ren ken"), a Bavarian physicist, discovered the x-ray on November 8, 1895 (Fig. 1–1). This monumental discovery revolutionized the diagnostic capabilities of the medical and dental professions and, as a result, forever changed the practice of medicine and dentistry.

Prior to the discovery of the x-ray, Roentgen had experimented with the production of cathode rays (streams of electrons). He used a vacuum tube, an electrical current, and special screens covered with a material that glowed (fluoresced) when exposed to radiation. He made the following observations about cathode rays: the rays appeared as streams of colored light passing from one end of the tube to the other, the rays did not travel far outside the tube, and the rays caused fluorescent screens to glow.

While experimenting in a darkened laboratory with a vacuum tube, Roentgen noticed a faint green glow

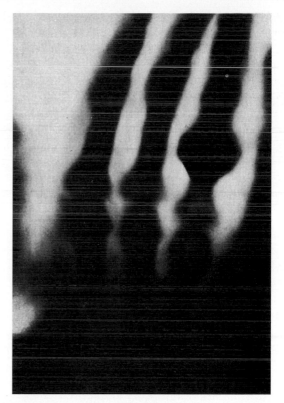

FIGURE 1–2. First radiograph of the human body, showing the hand of Roentgen's wife. (From Goaz PW, and White SC: Oral Radiology and Principles of Interpretation, 2nd ed. St. Louis; CV Mosby, 1987.)

coming from a nearby table. He discovered that the mysterious glow, or "fluorescence," was coming from screens located several feet away from the tube. Roentgen observed that the distance between the tube and the screens was much greater than the distance cathode rays could travel. He realized that something from the tube was striking the screens and causing the glow. Roentgen concluded that the fluorescence must be due to some powerful "unknown" ray.

In the following weeks, Roentgen continued experimenting with these unknown rays. He replaced the fluorescent screens with a photographic plate. He demonstrated that shadowed images could be permanently recorded on the photographic plates by placing objects between the tube and the plate. Roentgen proceeded to make the first radiograph of the human body; he placed his wife's hand on a photographic plate and exposed it to the unknown rays for 15 minutes. When Roentgen developed the photographic plate, the outline of the bones in her hand could be seen (Fig. 1–2).

Roentgen named his discovery x-rays, the "x" referring to the unknown nature and properties of such

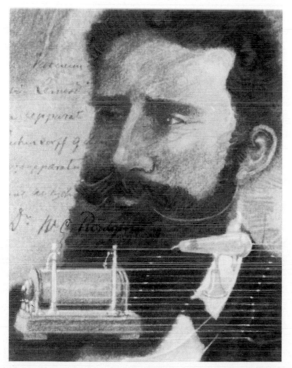

FIGURE 1–1. Roentgen, the father of x-rays, discovered the early potential of an x-ray beam in 1895. (Courtesy of Eastman Kodak Company, Rochester, NY.)

rays. (The symbol x is used in mathematics to represent the unknown.) He published a total of three scientific papers detailing the discovery, properties, and characteristics of x-rays. During his lifetime, Roentgen was awarded many honors and distinctions, including the first Nobel prize ever awarded in physics.

Following the publication of Roentgen's papers, scientists throughout the world duplicated his discovery and produced additional information on x-rays. For a number of years after his discovery, x-rays were referred to as roentgen rays, radiology was referred to as roentgenology, and radiographs were known as roentgenographs.

Experimentation Prior to X-ray Discovery

The primitive vacuum tube used by Roentgen in the discovery of the x-rays represented the collective findings of many investigators. Before the discovery of x-rays in 1895, a number of European scientists had experimented with fluorescence in sealed glass tubes.

In 1838 a German glass blower named Heinrich Geissler built the first **vacuum tube,** a sealed glass tube from which most of the air had been evacuated. This original vacuum tube, known as the Geissler tube, was modified by a number of investigators and became known by their respective names (e.g., the Hittorf-Crookes tube, the Lenard tube).

Johann Wilhelm Hittorf, a German physicist, used the vacuum tube to study **fluorescence** (a glow that results when a fluorescent substance is struck by light, cathode rays, or x-rays). In 1870, he observed that the discharges emitted from the negative electrode of the tube traveled in straight lines, produced heat, and resulted in a greenish fluorescence. He called these discharges **cathode rays.** In the late 1870s, William Crookes, an English chemist, redesigned the vacuum tube and discovered that cathode rays were streams of charged particles. The tube used in Roentgen's experiments incorporated the best features of the Hittorf and Crookes designs and was known as the Hittorf-Crookes tube (Fig. 1–3).

In 1894 Philip Lenard discovered that cathode rays could penetrate a thin window of aluminum foil built into the walls of the glass tubes and cause fluorescent screens to glow. He noticed that when the tube and screens were separated by at least 8 cm, the screens would not fluoresce. It has been postulated that Lenard might have discovered the x-ray if he had used more sensitive fluorescent screens.

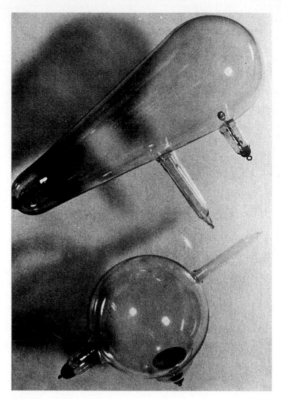

FIGURE 1–3. Hittorf-Crookes tubes used by Roentgen to discover x-rays. (From Goaz PW, and White SC: Oral Radiology and Principles of Interpretation, 2nd ed. St. Louis, CV Mosby, 1987.)

▓ PIONEERS IN DENTAL X-RADIATION

Following the discovery of x-rays in 1895, a number of pioneers helped to shape the history of dental radiography. The development of dental radiography can be attributed to the research of hundreds of investigators and practitioners. Many of the early pioneers in dental radiography died from overexposure to radiation. At the time x-rays were discovered, nothing was known about the hidden dangers that resulted from using these penetrating rays.

Shortly after the announcement of the discovery of x-rays in 1895, a German dentist, Otto Walkhoff, made the first dental radiograph. He placed a glass photographic plate wrapped in black paper and rubber in his mouth and submitted himself to 25 minutes of x-ray exposure. In that same year, W.J. Morton, a New York physician, made the first dental radiograph in the United States using a skull. He also lectured on the usefulness of x-rays in dental practice and made the first whole body radiograph using a 3- by 6-foot sheet of film.

C. Edmund Kells, a New Orleans dentist, is credited

with the first practical use of radiographs in dentistry in 1896. Kells exposed the first dental radiograph in the United States using a living person. During his many experiments, Kells exposed his hands to numerous x-rays every day for years. This overexposure to x-radiation caused the development of numerous cancers of his hand. Kells' dedication to the development of x-rays in dentistry ultimately cost him his fingers, later his hand, and then his arm.

Other pioneers in dental radiography include William H. Rollins, a Boston dentist who developed the first dental x-ray unit. While experimenting with radiation, Dr. Rollins suffered a burn to his hand. This initiated an interest in radiation protection and later the publication of the first paper on the dangers associated with radiation. Frank Van Woert, a dentist from New York City, was the first to use film in intraoral radiography and Howard Riley Raper, an Indiana University professor, established the first college course in radiography for dental students.

Highlights in the history of dental radiography are listed in Table 1–1. The development of dental radiography has moved forward from these early discoveries and continues to improve even today as new technologies become available.

HISTORY OF DENTAL X-RAY EQUIPMENT

In 1913, William D. Coolidge, an electrical engineer, developed the first hot cathode x-ray tube, a high

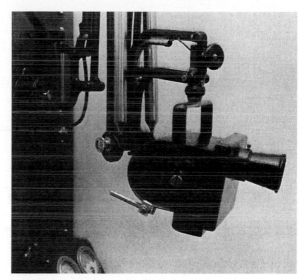

FIGURE 1–4. Victor CDX shockproof tube housing (1919). (From Goaz PW, and White SC: Oral Radiology and Principles of Interpretation, 2nd ed. St. Louis, CV Mosby, 1987.)

vacuum tube that contained a tungsten filament. Coolidge's x-ray tube became the prototype for all modern x-ray tubes and revolutionized the generation of x-rays.

In 1923, a miniature version of the x-ray tube was placed inside the head of an x-ray machine and immersed in oil; this served as the precursor for all modern dental x-ray machines and was manufactured by the Victor X-Ray Corporation of Chicago (Fig. 1–4). Later, in 1933, a new machine with improved features was introduced by General Electric. From that time on, the dental x-ray machine changed very little until a

TABLE 1–1. Highlights in the History of Dental Radiography

Year	Event	Person/Company
1895	Discovery of x-rays	W.C. Roentgen
1896	First dental radiograph	O. Walkhoff
1896	First dental radiograph in U.S. (skull)	W.J. Morton
1896	First dental radiograph in U.S. (live patient)	C.E. Kells
1901	First paper on dangers of x-radiation	W.H. Rollins
1904	Introduction of bisecting technique	W.A. Price
1913	First dental text	H.R. Raper
1913	First prewrapped dental films	Eastman Kodak Company
1913	First x-ray tube	W.D. Coolidge
1920	First machine-made film packets	Eastman Kodak Company
1923	First dental x-ray machine	Victor X-Ray Corporation of Chicago
1925	Introduction of bite-wing technique	H.R. Raper
1933	Concept of rotational panoramics proposed	
1947	Introduction of long-cone paralleling technique	F.G. Fitzgerald
1948	Introduction of panoramic radiography	
1955	Introduction of D-speed film	
1957	First variable kilovoltage dental x-ray machine	General Electric
1978	Introduction of dental xeroradiography	
1981	Introduction of E-speed film	
1987	Introduction of intraoral digital radiography	

variable kilovoltage machine was introduced in 1957. Later, in 1966, a recessed long-beam tubehead was introduced.

■ HISTORY OF DENTAL X-RAY FILM

From 1896 to 1913, dental x-ray packets consisted of glass photographic plates or film cut into small pieces and hand-wrapped in black paper and rubber. The hand-wrapping of intraoral dental x-ray packets was a time-consuming procedure. In 1913 the Eastman Kodak Company manufactured the first prewrapped intraoral films and consequently increased the acceptance and use of x-rays in dentistry. The first machine-made periapical film packets became available in 1920.

Today, the films used in dental radiography are greatly improved compared with the films of the past. Present-day fast film requires a very short exposure time, which in turn reduces the radiation exposure received by the patient. The fast film used today requires one-fifth of the amount of exposure required 25 years ago.

■ HISTORY OF DENTAL RADIOGRAPHIC TECHNIQUES

The intraoral techniques used in dentistry include the bisecting technique, the paralleling technique, and the bite-wing technique. The dental practitioners who developed these radiographic techniques include Weston Price, a Cleveland dentist, who introduced the bisecting technique in 1904, and Howard Riley Raper, who redefined the original bisecting technique and introduced the bite-wing technique in 1925. Raper also wrote one of the first dental radiography textbooks in 1913.

The paralleling technique was first introduced by C. Edmund Kells in 1896 and then later, in 1920, used by Franklin W. McCormack in practical dental radiography. F. Gordon Fitzgerald, the "father of modern dental radiography," revived interest in the paralleling technique with the introduction of the long-cone paralleling technique in 1947.

The extraoral technique used most commonly in dentistry is panoramic radiography. In 1933, Hisatugu Numata of Japan was the first to expose a panoramic radiograph; however, the film was placed lingually to the teeth. Yrjo Paatero of Finland is considered to be the father of panoramic radiography. He experimented with a slit beam of radiography, intensifying screens, and rotational techniques.

■ SUMMARY

- An x-ray is a beam of energy that has the power to penetrate substances and record image shadows on photographic film.
- A radiograph is a photographic image produced on film by the passage of x-rays through an object or body.
- Radiography is the art and science of making radiographs by the exposure of film to x-rays.
- A dental radiographer is any person who positions, exposes, and processes dental x-ray film.
- Disease detection is one of the most important uses for dental radiographs.
- Wilhelm Conrad Roentgen discovered the x-ray in 1895.
- Following the discovery of the x-ray, numerous investigators contributed to advancements in dental radiography.

BIBLIOGRAPHY

Barr JH, Stephens RG: Appendix II. *In* Dental Radiology: Pertinent Basic Concepts and Their Applications in Clinical Practice. Philadelphia, WB Saunders, 1980, p. 385.

DeLyre WR, Johnson ON: Radiography in dental practice. *In* Essentials of Dental Radiography for Dental Assistants and Hygienists, 5th edition. Norwalk, Appleton and Lange, 1995, pp. 1–4.

Frommer HH: Ionizing radiation and basic principles of x-ray generation. *In* Radiology for Dental Auxiliaries, 6th edition. St. Louis, Mosby-Year Book, 1996, pp. 1–29.

Goaz PW, White SC: Origins of dental radiology. *In* Oral Radiology and Principles of Interpretation, 2nd edition. St. Louis, CV Mosby, 1987, pp. 1–17.

Haring JI, Lind LJ: The importance of dental radiographs and interpretation. *In* Radiographic Interpretation for the Dental Hygienist. Philadelphia, WB Saunders, 1993, pp. 1–12.

Kasle MJ, Langlais RP: Historical notes. *In* Basic Principles of Oral Radiography: Exercises in Dental Radiology, Vol. 4. Philadelphia, WB Saunders, 1981, pp. 169–174.

Langland OE, Langlais RP, McDavid WD: History of panoramic radiography. *In* Panoramic Radiology, 2nd edition. Philadelphia, Lea & Febiger, 1989, pp. 3–37.

Langland OE, Langlais RP: Early pioneers of oral and maxillofacial radiology. Oral Surgery, Oral Medicine, Oral Pathology 80: 496–511, 1995.

Langland OE, Sippy FH, Langlais RP: Introduction and history of dental radiology. *In* Textbook of Dental Radiography, 2nd edition. Springfield, IL, Charles C Thomas, 1984, pp. 3–42.

Langland OE, Sippy FH, Langlais RP: X-rays, their production, and the x-ray beam. *In* Textbook of Dental Radiography, 2nd edition. Springfield, IL, Charles C Thomas, 1984, pp. 43–87.

Manson-Hing LR: Physical foundation of radiography. *In* Fundamentals of Dental Radiography, 3rd edition. Philadelphia, Lea & Febiger, 1990, pp. 1–15.

Mauriello SM, Overman VP, Platin E: Development of dental radiology. *In* Radiographic Imaging for the Dental Team. Philadelphia, JB Lippincott Company, 1995, pp. 2–10.

Miles DA, Van Dis ML, Jensen CW, Ferretti A: X-ray properties and the generation of x-rays. *In* Radiographic Imaging for Dental Auxiliaries, 3rd edition. Philadelphia, WB Saunders, 1999, pp. 73–85.

Quiz Questions

MATCHING

For questions 1 to 9, match each term with its corresponding definition.

a. radiation
b. radiograph
c. radiograph, dental
d. radiographer, dental
e. radiography
f. radiography, dental
g. radiology
h. radiation
i. x-ray

C   1. A photographic image produced on film by the passage of x-rays through teeth and related structures.

I   2. A beam of energy that has the power to penetrate substances and record image shadows on photographic film.

A   3. A form of energy carried by waves or a stream of particles.

D   4. Any person who positions, exposes, and processes x-ray film.

E   5. The making of radiographs by the exposure of film to x-rays.

H   6. A high-energy radiation produced by the collision of a beam of electrons with a metal target in an x-ray tube.

G   7. The science or study of radiations as used in medicine.

F   8. The making of radiographs of the teeth and adjacent structures by the exposure of film to x-rays.

b   9. A picture on film produced by the passage of x-rays through an object or body.

For questions 10 to 19, match the following dental pioneers with their contributions.

C   10. Coolidge

H   11. Fitzgerald

J   12. Kells

A   13. McCormack

G   14. Morton

D   15. Price

I   16. Raper

B   17. Roentgen

F   18. Rollins

E   19. Walkhoff

a. Used paralleling technique in practical dental radiography
b. Discovered x-rays
c. Developed first x-ray tube
d. Introduced bisecting technique
e. Exposed first dental radiograph
f. Wrote first paper on the danger of x-radiation
g. Exposed first dental radiograph in United States (skull)
h. Introduced long-cone paralleling technique
i. Wrote first dental text; introduced bite-wing technique
j. Exposed first dental radiograph in United States (live patient)

ESSAY

20. Discuss the importance of dental radiographs.

21. Summarize the discovery of x-radiation.

Answers are supplied at the end of this book.

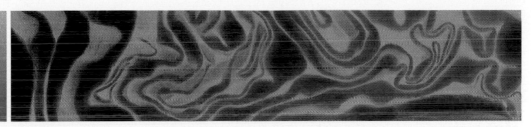

Radiation Physics

OBJECTIVES

After completion of this chapter, the student will be able to:

- *Define the key words.*
- *Identify the structure of the atom.*
- *Describe the process of ionization.*
- *Discuss the difference between radiation and radioactivity.*
- *List the two types of ionizing radiation and give examples of each.*
- *List the characteristics of electromagnetic radiation.*
- *List the properties of x-radiation.*
- *Identify the component parts of the x-ray machine.*
- *Label the parts of the dental x-ray tubehead and the dental x-ray tube.*
- *Describe in detail how dental x-rays are produced.*
- *List and describe the possible interactions of x-rays with matter.*

KEY WORDS

Absorption	Matter
Alpha particles	Metal housing
Aluminum disks	Milliamperage
Amperage	Milliampere (mA)
Ampere (A)	Molecule
Anode	Molybdenum cup
Atom	Nanometer
Atom, neutral	Neutron
Atomic number	Nucleon
Atomic weight	Nucleus
Autotransformer	Orbit
Beam, primary	Periodic table of the
Beam, useful	elements
Beta particles	Photoelectric effect
Binding energy	Photon
Cathode	Position-indicating
Cathode ray	device
Circuit	Proton
Circuit, filament	Quanta
Circuit, high-voltage	Radiation
Coherent scatter	Radiation,
Compton scatter	Bremsstrahlung
Control panel	Radiation, characteristic
Copper stem	Radiation,
Current, alternating (AC)	electromagnetic
Current, direct (DC)	Radiation, general
Electric current	Radiation, ionizing
Electricity	Radiation, particulate
Electromagnetic spec-	Radiation, primary
trum	Radiation, scatter
Electron	Radiation, secondary
Electron, Compton	Radioactivity
Electron, recoil	Rectification
Electron-volt (eV)	Scatter
Electrostatic force	Shell
Element	Thermionic emission
Energy	Transformer
Extension arm	Transformer, step-
Frequency	down
Insulating oil	Transformer, step-up
Ion	Tubehead
Ion pair	Tubehead seal
Ionization	Tungsten filament
Kilo-electron-volt (keV)	Tungsten target
Kilovoltage	Velocity
Kinetic energy	Voltage
Lead collimator	Wavelength
Leaded-glass housing	X-rays
Mass number	X-ray tube

INTRODUCTION

To understand how x-rays are produced, the dental radiographer must understand the nature and interactions of atoms. A complete understanding of x-radiation includes an understanding of the fundamental concepts of atomic and molecular structure as well as a working knowledge of ionization, ionizing radiation, and the properties of x-rays. An understanding of the dental x-ray machine, x-ray tube, and circuitry is also necessary. The purpose of this chapter is to present the fundamental concepts of atomic and molecular structure, to define and characterize x-radiation, to introduce the x-ray machine, and to describe in detail how x-rays are produced. This chapter also includes a discussion of the interactions of x-radiation with matter.

FUNDAMENTAL CONCEPTS

Atomic and Molecular Structure

The world is composed of matter and energy. **Matter** is anything that occupies space and has mass; when matter is altered, **energy** results. The fundamental unit of matter is the **atom**. All matter is composed of atoms, or tiny invisible particles. An understanding of the structure of the atom is necessary before the dental radiographer can understand the production of x-rays.

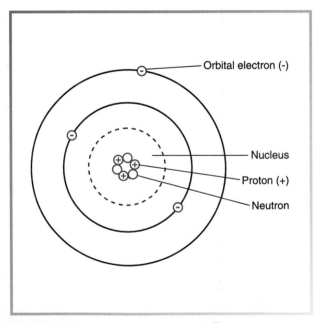

FIGURE 2–1. The atom consists of a central nucleus and orbiting electrons.

ATOMIC STRUCTURE

The atom consists of two parts: a central nucleus and orbiting electrons (Fig. 2–1). The identity of an atom is determined by the composition of its nucleus and the arrangement of its orbiting electrons; at present, 105 different atoms exist.

Nucleus. The **nucleus**, or dense core of the atom, is composed of particles known as **protons** and **neutrons** (also known as **nucleons**); protons carry positive electrical charges, whereas neutrons carry no electrical charge. The nucleus of an atom occupies very little space; in fact, most of the atom is empty space. For example, if an atom were imagined to be the size of a football stadium, the nucleus would be the size of a football.

Atoms differ from one another based on their nuclear composition. The number of protons and neutrons in the nucleus of an atom determines its **mass number** or **atomic weight.** The number of protons inside the nucleus equals the number of electrons outside the nucleus and determines the **atomic number** of the atom. Each atom has an atomic number ranging from that of hydrogen, the simplest atom, which has an atomic number of 1, to that of hahnium, the most complex atom, which has an atomic number of 105. Atoms are arranged in increasing atomic number on a chart known as the **periodic table of the elements** (Fig. 2–2). **Elements** are substances made up of only one type of atom.

Electrons. **Electrons** are tiny negatively charged particles that have very little mass; an electron weighs approximately 1/1800 as much as a proton or neutron. The arrangement of the electrons and neutrons in an atom resembles that of a miniature solar system. Just as the planets revolve around the sun, electrons travel around the nucleus in well-defined paths known as **orbits** or **shells.**

An atom contains a maximum of seven shells, each

	I A	II A	III B	IV B	V B	VI B	VII B	VIII	VIII	VIII	I B	II B	III A	IV A	V A	VI A	VII A	0
1	1 Hydrogen H																	2 Helium He
2	3 Lithium Li	4 Beryllium Be											5 Boron B	6 Carbon C	7 Nitrogen N	8 Oxygen O	9 Fluorine F	10 Neon Ne
3	11 Sodium Na	12 Magnesium Mg											13 Aluminum Al	14 Silicon Si	15 Phosphorous P	16 Sulfur S	17 Chlorine Cl	18 Argon Ar
4	19 Potassium K	20 Calcium Ca	21 Scandium Sc	22 Titanium Ti	23 Vanadium V	24 Chromium Cr	25 Mangenese Mn	26 Iron Fe	27 Cobalt Co	28 Nickel Ni	29 Copper Cu	30 Zinc Zn	31 Gallium Ga	32 Germanium Ge	33 Arsenic As	34 Selenium Se	35 Bromine Br	36 Krypton Kr
5	37 Rubidium Rb	38 Strontium Sr	39 Yttrium Y	40 Zirconium Zr	41 Niobium Nb	42 Molybdenum Mo	43 Technetium Tc	44 Ruthenium Ru	45 Rhodium Rh	46 Palladium Pd	47 Silver Ag	48 Cadmium Cd	49 Indium In	50 Tin Sn	51 Antimony Sb	52 Tellurium Te	53 Iodine I	54 Xenon Xe
6	55 Cesium Cs	56 Barium Ba	57-71 Series of Lanthanide Elements	72 Hafnium Hf	73 Tantalum Ta	74 Tungsten W	75 Rhenium Re	76 Osmium Os	77 Iridium Ir	78 Platinum Pt	79 Gold Au	80 Mercury Hg	81 Thallium Tl	82 Lead Pb	83 Bismuth Bi	84 Polonium Po	85 Astatine At	86 Radon Rn
7	87 Francium Fr	88 Radium Ra	89-103 Series of Actinide Elements	104	105 Hahnium Hn													

Series of Lanthanide Elements	57 Lanthanum La	58 Cerium Ce	59 Praseo dymium Pr	60 Neodymium Nd	61 Promethium Pm	62 Samarium Sm	63 Europium Eu	64 Gadolinium Gd	65 Terbium Tb	66 Dysprosium Dy	67 Holium Ho	68 Erbium Er	69 Thulium Tm	70 Ytterbium Yb	71 Lutetium Lu
Series of Actinide Elements	89 [illegible] Ac	90 [illegible] Th	91 [illegible] Pa	92 [illegible] U	93 [illegible] Np	94 [illegible] Pu	95 Americium Am	96 Curium Cm	97 Berkelium Bk	98 Californium Cf	99 Einsteinium Es	100 Fermium Fm	101 Mendelevium Md	102 Nobelium No	103 Lawrentium Lr

FIGURE 2–2. Periodic table of the elements.

located at a specific distance from the nucleus and representing different energy levels. The shells are designated with the letters K, L, M, N, O, P, and Q; the K shell is located closest to the nucleus and has the highest energy level (Fig. 2–3). Each shell has a maximum number of electrons it can hold (Fig. 2–4).

Electrons are maintained in their orbits by the **electrostatic force,** or attraction, between the positive nucleus and the negative electrons. This is known as the **binding energy** or binding force of an electron. The binding energy is determined by the distance between the nucleus and the orbiting electron and is different for each shell. The strongest binding energy is found closest to the nucleus in the K shell, whereas electrons located in the outer shells have a weak binding energy. The binding energies of orbital electrons are measured in **electron-volts** (eV) or **kilo-electron-volts** (keV). (One kilo-electron-volt equals 1000 electron-volts.)

The energy required to remove an electron from its orbital shell must exceed the binding energy of the electron in that shell. A great amount of energy is required to remove an inner shell electron, but electrons loosely held in the outer shells can be affected by lesser energies. For example, in the tungsten atom, the binding energies are as follows:

70 keV	K shell electrons
12 keV	L shell electrons
3 keV	M shell electrons

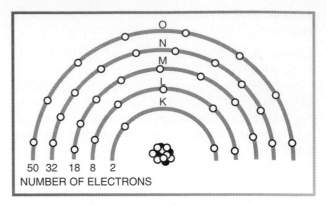

FIGURE 2–4. The maximum number of electrons that can exist in each shell of a tungsten atom. (Modified from Langland OE, Sippy FH, and Langlais RP: Textbook of Dental Radiography, 2nd ed. Springfield, IL, Charles C Thomas, 1984.)

Notice that the binding energy is greatest in the shell closest to the nucleus. To remove a K shell electron from a tungsten atom, 70 keV (70,000 eV) of energy would be required, whereas only 3 keV (3000 eV) of energy would be necessary to remove an electron from the M shell.

MOLECULAR STRUCTURE

Atoms are capable of combining with each other to form **molecules.** A molecule can be defined as two or more atoms joined by chemical bonds, or the smallest amount of a substance that possesses its characteristic properties. Like the atom, the molecule is also a tiny invisible particle. Molecules are formed in one of two ways—by the transfer of electrons, or by the sharing of electrons between the outermost shells of atoms. An example of a simple molecule is water (H_2O); the symbol H_2 represents two atoms of hydrogen, and the symbol O represents one atom of oxygen (Fig. 2–5).

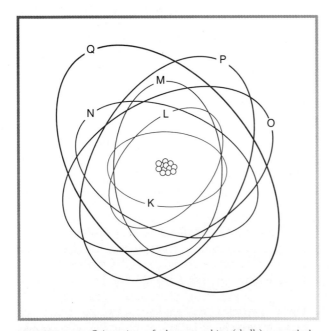

FIGURE 2–3. Orientation of electron orbits (shells) around the nucleus.

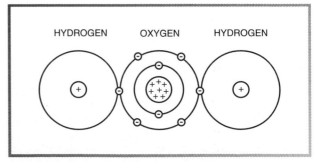

FIGURE 2–5. A molecule of water (H_2O) consists of two atoms of hydrogen connected to one atom of oxygen.

Ionization, Radiation, and Radioactivity

Now that the fundamental concepts of atomic and molecular structure have been reviewed, an understanding of ionization, radiation, and radioactivity is possible. Before the dental radiographer can understand how x-rays are produced, a working knowledge of ionization and the difference between radiation and radioactivity is necessary.

IONIZATION

Atoms can exist in a neutral or in an electrically unbalanced state. Normally, most atoms are neutral. A **neutral atom** contains an equal number of protons (positive charges) and electrons (negative charges). An atom with an incompletely filled outer shell is electrically unbalanced and attempts to capture an electron from an adjacent atom. If the atom gains an electron, it has more electrons than protons and neutrons and therefore a negative charge. Similarly, the atom that loses an electron has more protons and neutrons and thus has a positive charge. An atom that gains or loses an electron and becomes electrically unbalanced is known as an **ion.**

Ionization is the production of ions, or the process of converting an atom into ions. Ionization deals with electrons only and requires sufficient energy to overcome the electrostatic force that binds the electron to the nucleus. When an electron is removed from an atom in the ionization process, an **ion pair** results. The atom becomes the positive ion, and the ejected electron becomes the negative ion (Fig. 2–6). This ion pair reacts with other ions until electrically stable, neutral atoms are formed.

RADIATION AND RADIOACTIVITY

Radiation, as previously defined in Chapter 1, is the emission and propagation of energy through space or a substance in the form of waves or particles. The terms radioactivity and radiation are sometimes confused; it is important to note that they do *not* mean the same thing. An understanding of these terms is required before the concept of ionizing radiation is presented.

Radioactivity can be defined as the process by which certain unstable atoms or elements undergo spontaneous disintegration, or decay, in an effort to attain a more balanced nuclear state. A substance is considered radioactive if it gives off energy in the form of particles or rays as a result of the disintegration of

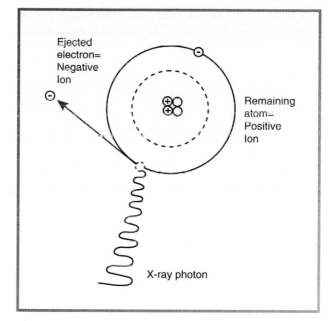

FIGURE 2–6. An ion pair is formed when an electron is removed from an atom; the atom is the positive ion, and the ejected electron is the negative ion.

atomic nuclei. In dentistry, radiation (specifically x-radiation) is used, *not* radioactivity.

Ionizing Radiation

Ionizing radiation can be defined as radiation that is capable of producing ions by removing or adding an electron to an atom. Ionizing radiation can be classified into two groups: particulate radiation and electromagnetic radiation.

PARTICULATE RADIATION

Particulate radiations are tiny particles of matter that possess mass and travel in straight lines and at high speeds. Particulate radiations transmit kinetic energy by means of their extremely fast-moving, small masses. Four types of particulate radiation are recognized (Table 2–1).

- **Electrons** can be classified as beta particles or cathode rays. They differ in origin only. **Beta particles** are fast-moving electrons emitted from the nucleus of radioactive atoms. **Cathode rays** are streams of high-speed electrons that originate in an x-ray tube.
- **Alpha particles** are emitted from the nuclei of heavy metals and exist as two protons and neutrons, without electrons.

TABLE 2–1. Particulate Radiations

Particle	Mass Units	Charge	Origin
Alpha particle	4.003000	+2	Nucleus
Electron beta particle	0.000548	−1	Nucleus
Electron cathode rays	0.000548	−1	X-ray tube
Protons	1.007597	+1	Nucleus
Neutrons	1.008986	0	Nucleus

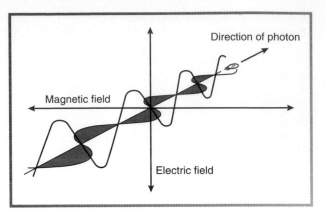

FIGURE 2–7. Oscillating electric and magnetic fields are characteristic of electromagnetic radiations.

- **Protons** are accelerated particles, specifically hydrogen nuclei, with a mass of 1 and a charge of +1.
- **Neutrons** are accelerated particles with a mass of 1 and no electrical charge.

ELECTROMAGNETIC RADIATION

Electromagnetic radiation can be defined as the propagation of wave-like energy (without mass) through space or matter. The energy that is propagated is accompanied by oscillating electric and magnetic fields positioned at right angles to one another—hence the term electromagnetic (Fig. 2–7).

Electromagnetic radiations are manmade or occur naturally; examples include cosmic rays, gamma rays, x-rays, ultraviolet rays, visible light, infrared light, radar waves, microwaves, and radio waves. Electromagnetic radiations are arranged according to their energies in what is termed the **electromagnetic spectrum** (Fig. 2–8). All energies of the electromagnetic spectrum share common characteristics (see the "Properties of Electromagnetic Radiations" chart). Depending on their energy levels, electromagnetic radiations can be classified as ionizing or non-ionizing. In the electromagnetic spectrum, only high-energy radiations (cosmic rays, gamma rays, and x-rays) are capable of ionization.

Electromagnetic radiations are believed to move through space as *both* a particle and a wave; hence, two concepts, the particle concept and the wave concept, must be considered.

PARTICLE CONCEPT

The particle concept characterizes electromagnetic radiations as discrete bundles of energy called **photons**

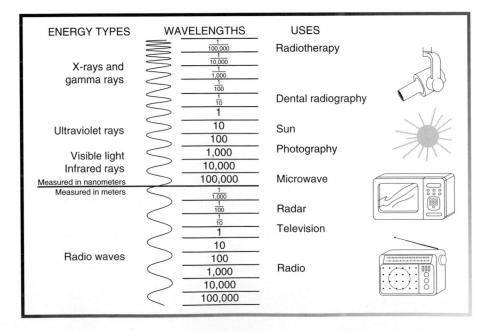

FIGURE 2–8. The electromagnetic energy spectrum.

PROPERTIES OF ELECTROMAGNETIC RADIATIONS

- Have no mass or weight
- Have no electrical charge
- Travel at the speed of light (3×10^8 meters/second; 186,000 miles/second)
- Travel as both a particle and a wave
- Propagate an electric field at right angles to path of travel
- Propagate a magnetic field at right angles to the electric field
- Have different measurable energies (frequencies and wavelengths)

or **quanta**. Photons are bundles of energy with no mass or weight that travel as waves at the speed of light and move through space in a straight line, "carrying the energy" of electromagnetic radiation.

WAVE CONCEPT

The wave concept characterizes electromagnetic radiations as waves and focuses on the properties of velocity, wavelength, and frequency.

- **Velocity** refers to the speed of the wave. All electromagnetic radiations travel as waves or a continuous sequence of crests at the speed of light (3×10^8 meters per second [186,000 miles per second]) in a vacuum.
- **Wavelength** can be defined as the distance between the crest of one wave and the crest of the next (Fig. 2–9). Wavelength determines the energy and penetrating power of the radiation; the shorter the distance between the crests, the shorter the wavelength and the higher the energy and ability to penetrate matter. Wavelength is measured in **nanometers**

(1×10^{-9} meters or one-billionth of a meter) for short waves and in meters for longer waves.

- **Frequency** refers to the number of wavelengths that pass a given point in a certain amount of time (Fig. 2–10). Frequency and wavelength are inversely related; if the frequency of the wave is high, the wavelength will be short, and if the frequency is low, the wavelength will be long.

The amount of energy an electromagnetic radiation possesses depends on the wavelength and frequency.

Low-frequency electromagnetic radiations have a long wavelength and less energy, and, conversely, high-frequency electromagnetic radiations have a short wavelength and more energy.

For example, communications media use the low-frequency, longer waves of the electromagnetic spectrum; the wavelength of a radio wave can be as long as 100 meters, whereas the wavelength of a television wave is approximately 1 meter. In contrast, diagnostic radiography uses the high-frequency, shorter waves in the electromagnetic spectrum; x-rays used in dentistry have a wavelength of 0.1 nanometers or 0.00000000001 meters.

◼ X-RADIATION

Definition

X-radiation is a high-energy, ionizing electromagnetic radiation. Like all electromagnetic radiations, x-rays have properties of *both* waves and particles. **X-rays** can be defined as weightless bundles of energy (photons) without an electrical charge that travel in waves with a specific frequency at the speed of light. X-ray photons interact with the materials they penetrate and cause ionization.

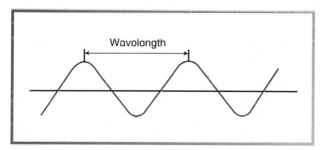

FIGURE 2–9. Wavelength is the distance between the crest (peak) of one wave and the crest of the next.

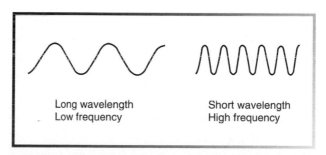

Long wavelength
Low frequency

Short wavelength
High frequency

FIGURE 2–10. Frequency is the number of wavelengths that pass a given point in a certain amount of time. The shorter the wavelength, the higher the frequency will be, and vice versa.

PROPERTIES OF X-RAYS

• *Appearance:* X-rays are invisible and cannot be detected by any of the senses.
• *Mass:* X-rays have no mass or weight.
• *Charge:* X-rays have no charge.
• *Speed:* X-rays travel at the speed of light.
• *Wavelength:* X-rays travel in waves and have short wavelengths with a high frequency.
• *Path of travel:* X-rays travel in straight lines and can be deflected, or scattered.
• *Focusing capability:* X-rays cannot be focused to a point and always diverge from a point.
• *Penetrating power:* X-rays can penetrate liquids, solids, and gases. The composition of the substance determines whether x-rays penetrate or pass through, or are absorbed.
• *Absorption:* X-rays are absorbed by matter; the absorption depends on the atomic structure of matter and the wavelength of the x-ray.
• *Ionization capability:* X-rays interact with materials they penetrate and cause ionization.
• *Fluorescence capability:* X-rays can cause certain substances to fluoresce or emit radiation in longer wavelengths (e.g., visible light and ultraviolet light).
• *Effect on film:* X-rays can produce an image on photographic film.
• *Effect on living tissues:* X-rays cause biologic changes in living cells.

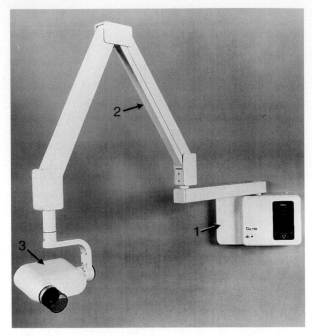

FIGURE 2–11. Three component parts of the dental x-ray machine: (1) control panel, (2) extension arm, (3) tubehead. (Courtesy of Gendex Corporation, Des Plaines, IL.)

Properties

X-rays have certain unique properties or characteristics. The dental radiographer must be familiar with the properties of x-rays (see "Properties of X-rays" chart).

▉▉▉ THE X-RAY MACHINE

X-rays are produced in the dental x-ray machine. For learning purposes, the dental x-ray machine can be divided into three study areas: the component parts, the x-ray tube, and the x-ray generating apparatus.

Component Parts

The dental x-ray machine consists of three visible component parts: the control panel, the extension arm, and the tubehead (Fig. 2–11).

CONTROL PANEL

The **control panel** of the dental x-ray machine contains an on-off switch and an indicator light, an exposure button and indicator light, and control devices (time, kilovoltage, and milliamperage selectors) to regulate the x-ray beam. The control panel is plugged into an electrical outlet and appears as a panel or cabinet mounted on the wall outside the dental operatory.

EXTENSION ARM

The wall-mounted **extension arm** suspends the x-ray tubehead and houses the electrical wires that extend from the control panel to the tubehead. The extension arm allows for movement and positioning of the tubehead.

TUBEHEAD

The x-ray **tubehead** is a tightly sealed, heavy metal housing that contains the x-ray tube that produces dental x-rays. The component parts of the tubehead include the following (Fig. 2–12):

• **Metal housing,** or the metal body of the tubehead that surrounds the x-ray tube and transformers and is filled with oil; it protects the x-ray tube and grounds the high-voltage components.
• **Insulating oil,** or the oil that surrounds the x-ray tube and transformers inside the tubehead; it prevents overheating by absorbing the heat created by the production of x-rays.

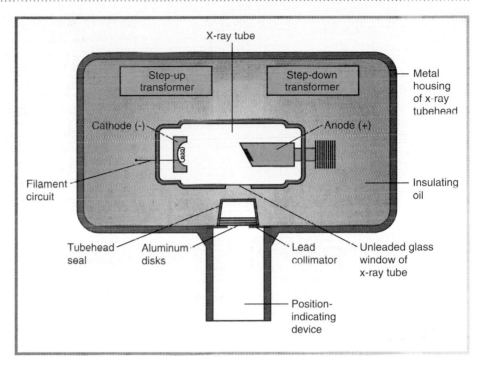

FIGURE 2–12. Diagram of the dental x-ray tubehead.

- **Tubehead seal,** or the aluminum or leaded-glass covering of the tubehead that permits the exit of x-rays from the tubehead; it seals the oil in the tubehead and acts as a filter to the x-ray beam.
- **X-ray tube,** or the heart of the x-ray generating system, is discussed later in this chapter (Fig. 2–13).
- **Transformer,** or a device that alters the voltage of incoming electricity, is discussed later in this chapter.
- **Aluminum disks,** or sheets of 0.5-mm thick aluminum placed in the path of the x-ray beam; they

filter out the non-penetrating, longer wavelength x-rays (Fig. 2–14). Aluminum filtration is discussed in greater detail in Chapter 5.
- **Lead collimator,** or a lead plate with a central hole that fits directly over the opening of the metal housing where the x-rays exit; it restricts the size of the x-ray beam (Fig. 2–15). Collimation is also discussed in greater detail in Chapter 5.
- **Position-indicating device (PID),** or open-ended,

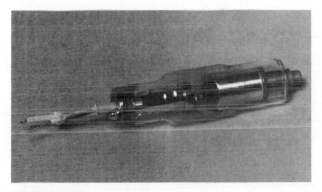

FIGURE 2–13. Actual dental x-ray tube. (From Matteson SR, Whaley C, and Secrist VC: Dental Radiology, 4th ed. Copyright © 1988 by The University of North Carolina Press. Used by permission of the publisher.)

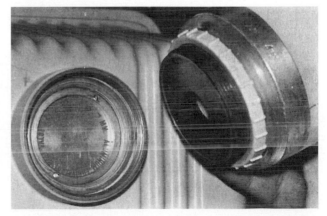

FIGURE 2–14 Aluminum filtration disk in the x-ray tubehead. (From Kasle MJ, and Langlais RP: Basic Principles of Oral Radiography: Exercises in Dental Radiography, Vol. 4. Philadelphia, WB Saunders, 1981.)

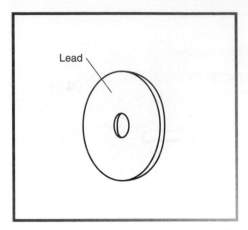

FIGURE 2–15. The lead collimator, or lead plate with a central opening, restricts the size of the x-ray beam.

lead-lined cylinder that extends from the opening of the metal housing of the tubehead; it aims and shapes the x-ray beam (Fig. 2–16). The PID is sometimes referred to as the cone.

X-ray Tube

The x-ray tube is the heart of the x-ray generating system; it is critical to the production of x-rays and warrants a separate discussion from the rest of the x-ray machine. The x-ray tube is a glass vacuum tube

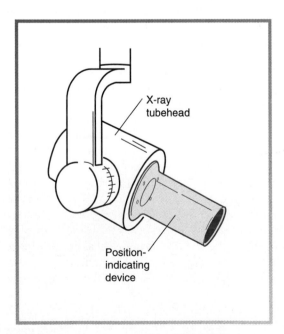

FIGURE 2–16. The position-indicating device (PID) or cone.

from which all of the air has been removed. The x-ray tube used in dentistry measures approximately several inches long by 1 inch in diameter. The component parts of the x-ray tube include a leaded-glass housing, a negative cathode, and a positive anode (Fig. 2–17).

LEADED-GLASS HOUSING

The **leaded-glass housing** is a leaded-glass vacuum tube that prevents x-rays from escaping in all directions. One central area of the leaded-glass tube has a "window" that permits the x-ray beam to exit the tube and directs the x-ray beam toward the aluminum disks, lead collimator, and PID.

CATHODE

The **cathode,** or negative electrode, consists of a tungsten wire filament in a cup-shaped holder made of molybdenum. The purpose of the cathode is to supply the electrons necessary to generate x-rays. In the x-ray tube, the electrons produced in the negative cathode are accelerated toward the positive anode. The cathode includes the following:

- The **tungsten filament,** or coiled wire made of tungsten, which produces electrons when heated.
- The **molybdenum cup,** which focuses the electrons into a narrow beam and directs the beam across the tube toward the tungsten target of the anode.

ANODE

The **anode,** or positive electrode, consists of a wafer-thin tungsten plate embedded in a solid copper rod. The purpose of the anode is to convert electrons into x-ray photons. The anode includes the following:

- A **tungsten target,** or plate of tungsten, which serves as a focal spot and converts bombarding electrons into x-ray photons.
- The **copper stem,** which functions to dissipate the heat away from the tungsten target.

X-ray Generating Apparatus

To understand how the x-ray tube functions and how x-rays are produced, the dental radiographer must understand electricity and electric currents, electrical circuits, and transformers.

ELECTRICITY AND ELECTRIC CURRENTS

Electricity is the energy that is used to make x-rays. Electrical energy consists of a flow of electrons through a conductor; this flow is known as the **electric cur-**

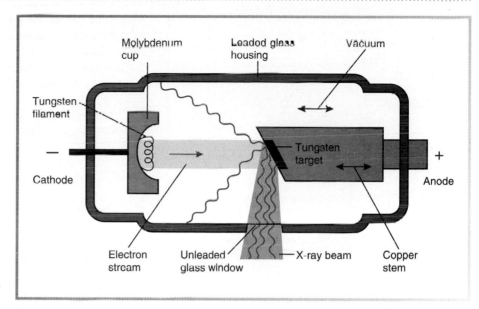

FIGURE 2-17. Diagram of the x-ray tube.

rent. The electrical current is termed **direct current (DC)** when the electrons flow in one direction through the conductor. The term **alternating current (AC)** describes a current in which the electrons flow in two opposite directions. **Rectification** is the conversion of alternating current to direct current; the dental x-ray tube acts as a self-rectifier in that it changes AC into DC while producing x-rays. This ensures that the current is always flowing in the same direction, more specifically, from cathode to anode. Generators on older machines produced an x-ray beam with a wavelike pattern, whereas newer constant potential x-ray machines produce a homogenous beam of consistent wavelengths during radiation exposure. Constant potential machines also reduce patient exposure to radiation by 20%, an important consideration for patient protection. **Amperage** is the measurement of the number of electrons moving through a conductor. Current is measured in **amperes** or **milliamperes** (mA). **Voltage** is the measurement of electrical force that causes electrons to move from a negative pole to a positive one. Voltage is measured in **volts** or **kilovolts** (kV).

In the production of x-rays, both the amperage and the voltage can be adjusted. In the x-ray tube, the amperage, or number of electrons passing through the cathode filament, can be increased or decreased by the **milliamperage** (mA) adjustment on the control panel of the x-ray machine. The voltage of the x-ray tube current, the current passing from the cathode to the anode, is controlled by the **kilovoltage** peak (kVp) adjustment on the control panel.

CIRCUITS

A **circuit** is a path of electrical current. Two electrical circuits are used in the production of x-rays: a low-voltage or filament circuit and a high-voltage circuit.

The **filament circuit** uses 3 to 5 volts, regulates the flow of electrical current to the filament of the x-ray tube, and is controlled by the milliampere settings. The **high-voltage circuit** uses 65,000 to 100,000 volts, provides the high voltage required to accelerate electrons and to generate x-rays in the x-ray tube, and is controlled by the kilovoltage settings.

TRANSFORMERS

A **transformer** is a device that is used to either increase or decrease the voltage in an electrical circuit (Fig. 2–18). Transformers alter the voltage of the incoming electrical current and then route the electrical energy to the x-ray tube. In the production of dental x-rays, three transformers are used to adjust the electrical circuits: the step-down transformer, the step-up transformer, and the autotransformer.

The filament circuit uses 3 to 5 volts. A **step-down transformer** is used to decrease the voltage from the incoming 110 or 220 line voltage to the 3 to 5 volts required. A step-down transformer has more wire coils in the primary coil than in the secondary coil (see Fig. 2–18). The coil that receives the alternating electrical current is the primary or input coil; the secondary coil is the output coil. The electrical current that energizes the primary coil induces a current in the secondary coil.

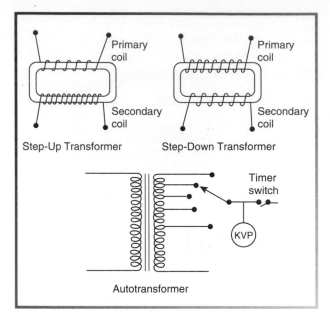

FIGURE 2–18. Three different transformers are used in the production of dental x-rays.

The high-voltage circuit requires 65,000 to 100,000 volts and uses both a step-up transformer and an auto-transformer. A **step-up transformer** is used to increase the voltage from the incoming 110 or 220 line voltage to the 65,000 to 100,000 volts required. A step-up transformer has more wire coils in the secondary coil than in the primary coil (see Fig. 2–18). An **auto-transformer** serves as a voltage compensator that corrects for minor fluctuations in the current.

▉ PRODUCTION OF X-RADIATION

Production of Dental X-rays

Now that the component parts of the x-ray machine, the x-ray tube, and the x-ray generating apparatus have been reviewed, a discussion of the production of dental x-rays is possible. A step-by-step explanation of x-ray production follows (Fig. 2–19).

1. Electricity from the wall outlet supplies the power to generate x-rays. When the x-ray machine is turned on, the electric current enters the control panel via the cord plugged into the wall outlet. The current travels from the control panel to the tubehead via the electrical wires in the extension arm.
2. The current is directed to the filament circuit

and step-down transformer in the tubehead. The transformer reduces the 110 or 220 entering line voltage to 3 to 5 volts.

3. The filament circuit uses the 3 to 5 volts to heat the tungsten filament in the cathode portion of the x-ray tube. **Thermionic emission** occurs; thermionic emission is the release of electrons from the tungsten filament when the electric current passes through it and heats it up. The outer shell electrons of the tungsten atom acquire enough energy to move away from the filament surface, and an electron cloud forms around the filament. The electrons stay in an electron cloud until the high-voltage circuit is activated.
4. When the exposure button is pushed, the high-voltage circuit is activated. The electrons produced at the cathode are accelerated across the x-ray tube to the anode. The molybdenum cup in the cathode directs the electrons to the tungsten target in the anode.
5. The electrons travel from the cathode to the anode. When the electrons strike the tungsten target, their energy of motion (**kinetic energy**) is converted to x-ray energy and heat. Less than 1% of the energy is converted to x-rays; the remaining 99% is lost as heat.

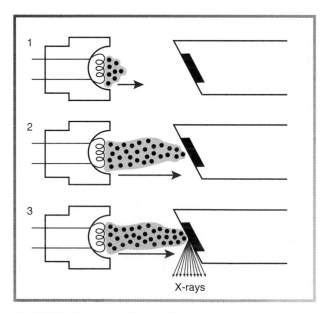

FIGURE 2–19. The production of dental x-rays occurs in the x-ray tube. 1. When the filament circuit is activated, the filament heats up, and thermionic emission occurs. 2. When the exposure button is activated, the electrons are accelerated from the cathode to the anode. 3. The electrons strike the tungsten target, and their kinetic energy is converted to x-rays and heat.

6. The heat produced during the production of x-rays is carried away from the copper stem and absorbed by the insulating oil in the tubehead. The x-rays produced are emitted from the target in all directions; however, the leaded-glass housing prevents the x-rays from escaping from the x-ray tube. A small number of x-rays are able to exit from the x-ray tube via the unleaded glass window portion of the tube.

7. The x-rays travel through the unleaded glass window, the tubehead seal, and the aluminum disks. The aluminum disks remove or filter the longer wavelength x-rays from the beam.

8. Next, the size of the x-ray beam is restricted by the lead collimator. The x-ray beam then travels down the lead-lined PID and exits the tubehead at the opening of the PID.

Types of X-rays Produced

Not all x-rays produced in the x-ray tube are the same; x-rays differ in energy and wavelength. The energy and wavelength of x-rays varies based on how the electrons interact with the tungsten atoms in the anode. The kinetic energy of the electrons is converted to x-ray photons via one of two mechanisms: **general (Bremsstrahlung) radiation** or **characteristic radiation**.

GENERAL RADIATION

Speeding electrons slow down because of their interactions with the tungsten target in the anode. Many electrons that interact with the tungsten atoms undergo not one but many interactions within the target. The radiation produced in this manner is known as general (Bremsstrahlung), or **braking radiation**. The term braking refers to the sudden stopping, or "braking," of high-speed electrons when they hit the tungsten target in the anode. Most x-rays are produced in this manner; approximately 70% of the x-ray energy produced at the anode can be classified as general radiation.

General radiation is produced when an electron hits the nucleus of a tungsten atom or when an electron passes very close to the nucleus of a tungsten atom (Fig. 2–20). An electron rarely hits the nucleus of the tungsten atom. However, when it does, all of its kinetic energy is converted into a high-energy x-ray photon. Instead of hitting the nucleus, most electrons nearly miss the nucleus of the tungsten atom. When the electron comes close to the nucleus, it is attracted to the nucleus and slows down. Consequently, an x-ray photon of lower energy results. The electron that

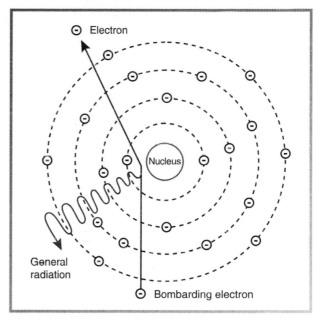

FIGURE 2–20. When an electron that passes close to the nucleus of a tungsten atom is slowed down, an x-ray photon of lower energy known as general radiation results.

misses the nucleus continues to penetrate many atoms, producing lower-energy x-rays before it imparts all of its kinetic energy. As a result, general radiation consists of x-rays of many different energies and wavelengths.

CHARACTERISTIC RADIATION

Characteristic radiation is produced when a high-speed electron dislodges an inner shell electron from the tungsten atom and causes ionization of that atom (Fig. 2–21). Once the electron is dislodged, the remaining orbiting electrons are rearranged to fill the vacancy. This rearrangement produces a loss of energy that results in the production of an x-ray photon. The x-rays produced by this interaction are known as characteristic x-rays.

Characteristic radiation accounts for a very small part of x-rays produced in the dental x-ray machine and occurs only at 70 kVp and above because the binding energy of the K shell electron is approximately 70 keV.

X-radiation Definitions

Terms such as primary, secondary, and scatter are often used to describe x-radiation. A knowledge of these terms is required before the interactions of x-radiation with matter can be discussed.

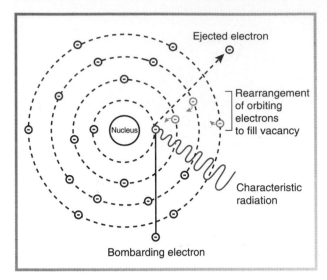

FIGURE 2–21. An electron that dislodges an inner shell electron from the tungsten atom results in the arrangement of the remaining orbiting electrons and the production of an x-ray photon known as characteristic radiation.

PRIMARY RADIATION

Primary radiation refers to the penetrating x-ray beam that is produced at the target of the anode and exits the tubehead. This x-ray beam is often referred to as the **primary beam** or **useful beam.**

SECONDARY RADIATION

Secondary radiation refers to x-radiation that is created when the primary beam interacts with matter. (In dental radiography, matter includes the soft tissues of the head, the bones of the skull, and the teeth.) Secondary radiation is less penetrating than primary radiation.

SCATTER RADIATION

Scatter radiation is a form of secondary radiation and is the result of an x-ray that has been deflected from its path by the interaction with matter. Scatter radiation is deflected in all directions by patient tissues and travels to all parts of the patient's body and to all areas of the dental operatory. Scatter radiation is detrimental to both the patient and the radiographer.

■ INTERACTIONS OF X-RADIATION

Now that the production of dental x-rays has been reviewed, a discussion of x-radiation interactions is

necessary. What happens after an x-ray exits the tube-head? When x-ray photons arrive at the patient with energies produced by the dental x-ray machine, one of several events may occur.

- X-rays can pass through the patient without any interaction
- X-ray photons can be completely absorbed by the patient
- X-ray photons can be scattered (Fig. 2–22)

A knowledge of atomic and molecular structure is required to understand such interactions and effects. At the atomic level, four possibilities can occur when an x-ray photon interacts with matter: (1) no interaction, (2) absorption or photoelectric effect, (3) Compton scatter, and (4) coherent scatter.

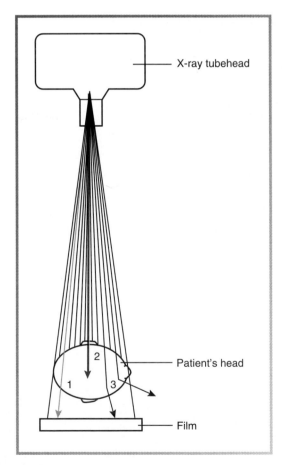

FIGURE 2–22. Three types of radiation interactions with the patient may occur. 1. The x-ray photon may pass through the patient without interaction and reach the film. 2. The x-ray photon may be absorbed by the patient. 3. The x-ray photon may be scattered onto the film or away from the film.

No Interaction

It is possible for an x-ray photon to pass through matter or the tissues of a patient without any interaction (Fig. 2–23). The x-ray photon passes through the atom unchanged and leaves the atom unchanged. The x-ray photons that pass through a patient without interaction are responsible for producing densities on film and make dental radiography possible.

Absorption of Energy and Photoelectric Effect

It is possible for an x-ray photon to be completely absorbed within matter or the tissues of a patient. **Absorption** refers to the total transfer of energy from the x-ray photon to the atoms of matter through which the x-ray beam passes. Absorption depends upon the energy of the x-ray beam and the composition of the absorbing matter or tissues.

At the atomic level, absorption occurs as a result of the photoelectric effect. In the **photoelectric effect**, ionization takes place. An x-ray photon collides with a tightly bound, inner shell electron and gives up all of its energy to eject the electron from its orbit (Fig. 2–24). The x-ray photon imparts *all* of its kinetic energy to the orbital electron, is absorbed, and ceases to exist.

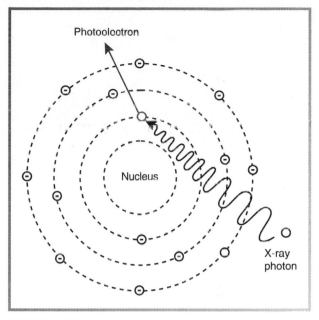

FIGURE 2–24. When an x-ray photon collides with an inner shell electron, a photoelectric effect occurs: the photon is absorbed and ceases to exist, and a photoelectron with a negative charge is produced.

The ejected electron is termed a photoelectron and has a negative charge; it is readily absorbed by other atoms because it has very little penetrating power. The atom that remains has a positive charge. The photoelectric effect accounts for 30% of the interactions of matter with the dental x-ray beam.

Compton Scatter

It is possible for an x-ray photon to be deflected from its path during its passage through matter. The term **scatter** refers to this type of radiation. At the atomic level, the Compton effect accounts for most of the scatter radiation that takes place.

In **Compton scatter**, ionization takes place. An x-ray photon collides with a loosely bound, outer shell electron and gives up part of its energy to eject the electron from its orbit (Fig. 2–25). The x-ray photon loses energy and continues in a different direction (scatters) at a lower energy level. The new, weaker x-ray photon interacts with other atoms until all of its energy is gone. The ejected electron is termed a **Compton** or **recoil electron** and has a negative charge. The remaining atom is positively charged. Compton scatter accounts for 62% of the scatter that occurs in diagnostic radiography.

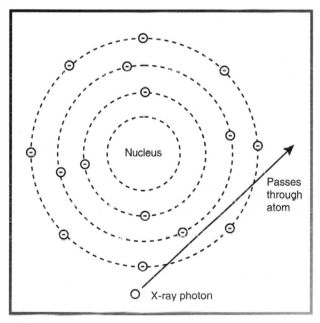

FIGURE 2–23. When an x-ray photon passes through an atom unchanged, no interaction has taken place.

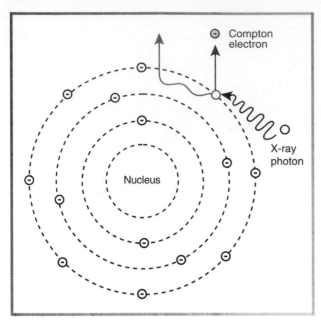

FIGURE 2–25. When an x-ray photon collides with an outer shell electron and ejects the electron from its orbit, Compton scatter results: the photon is scattered in a different direction at a lower energy, and the ejected electron is referred to as a Compton or recoil electron.

Coherent Scatter

Another type of scatter radiation that may take place when x-rays interact with matter is known as **coherent** or unmodified **scatter.** Coherent scatter involves an

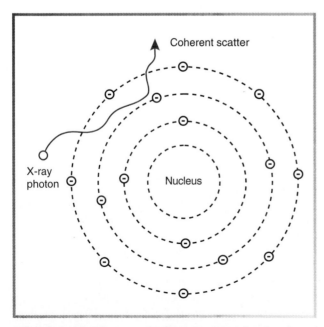

FIGURE 2–26. When an x-ray photon is scattered and no loss of energy occurs, the scatter is termed coherent.

x-ray photon that has its path altered by matter (Fig. 2–26). Coherent scatter occurs when a low-energy x-ray photon interacts with an outer shell electron. No change in the atom occurs, and an x-ray photon of scattered radiation is produced. The x-ray photon is scattered in a different direction than the incident photon; no loss of energy and no ionization occurs. Essentially, the x-ray photon is "unmodified" and simply undergoes a change in direction without a change in energy. Coherent scatter accounts for 8% of the interactions of matter with the dental x-ray beam.

◼ SUMMARY

- An atom consists of a central nucleus composed of protons, neutrons, and orbiting electrons.
- Most atoms exist in a neutral state and contain equal numbers of protons and neutrons.
- When unequal numbers of protons and electrons exist, the atom is electrically unbalanced and is termed an ion.
- The production of ions is termed ionization; an ion pair (a positive ion and a negative ion) is produced. The atom is the positive ion, and the ejected electron is the negative ion.
- Ionizing radiation is capable of producing ions and can be classified as particulate or electromagnetic.
- Electromagnetic radiations (e.g., x-rays) exhibit characteristics of both particles and waves and are arranged according to their energies.
- The energy of an electromagnetic radiation depends on the wavelength and frequency.
- A low-energy radiation has a low frequency and a long wavelength; a high-energy radiation has a high frequency and a short wavelength.
- X-rays are weightless, neutral bundles of energy (photons) that travel in waves with a specific frequency at the speed of light.
- X-rays are generated in an x-ray tube located in the x-ray tubehead.
- The x-ray tube consists of a leaded-glass housing, a negative cathode, and a positive anode. Electrons are produced in the cathode and accelerated toward the anode; the anode converts the electrons into x-rays.
- After the x-rays exit the tubehead, several interactions are possible: x-rays can pass through the patient (no interaction), be completely absorbed by the patient (photoelectric effect), or be scattered (Compton scatter and coherent scatter).

BIBLIOGRAPHY

Barr JH, Stephens RG: The physics of x-rays. *In* Dental Radiology. Pertinent Basic Concepts and Their Applications in Clinical Practice, Philadelphia, WB Saunders, 1980, pp. 1–8.

Frommer HH: Ionizing radiation and basic principles of x-ray generation. *In* Radiology for Dental Auxiliaries, 6th edition. St. Louis, Mosby-Year Book, 1996, pp. 1–29.

Goaz PW, White SC: Radiation physics. *In* Oral Radiology and Principles of Interpretation, 3rd edition. St. Louis, Mosby-Year Book, 1994, pp. 1–23.

Johnson ON, McNally MA, Essay CE: Characteristics of radiation. *In* Essentials of Dental Radiography for Dental Assistants and Hygienists, 6th edition. Norwalk, CT, Appleton and Lange, 1999, pp. 15–35.

Johnson ON, McNally MA, Essay CE: The dental x-ray machine—components and functions. *In* Essentials of Dental Radiography for Dental Assistants and Hygienists, 6th edition. Norwalk, CT, Appleton and Lange, 1999, pp. 37–60.

Kasle MJ, Langlais RP: Basic Principles of Oral Radiography Exercises in Dental Radiology, Vol. 1. Philadelphia, WB Saunders, 1981, pp. 2–4, 9–15, 25–27, 34–36.

Kelsey CA: Atomic and molecular structure. *In* Essentials of Radiology Physics. St. Louis, Warren H. Green, 1985, pp. 34–42.

Langland OE, Sippy FH, Langlais RP: X-rays, their production and the x-ray beam. *In* Textbook of Dental Radiography, 2nd edition. Springfield, Charles C Thomas, 1984, pp. 44–53, 56–68, 79.

Manson-Hing LR: Physical foundation of radiography. *In* Fundamentals of Dental Radiography, 3rd edition. Philadelphia, Lea & Febiger, 1990, pp. 1–13.

Mauriello SM, Overman VP, Platin F: Radiologic physics. *In* Radiographic Imaging for the Dental Team. Philadelphia, JB Lippincott Company, 1995, pp. 50–67.

Miles DA, Van Dis ML, Razmus TF: Radiation physics. *In* Basic Principles of Oral and Maxillofacial Radiology. Philadelphia, WB Saunders, 1992, pp. 1–17.

O'Brien RC: The nature and generation of x-rays. *In* Dental Radiography: An Introduction for Dental Hygienists and Assistants, 4th edition. Philadelphia, WB Saunders, 1982, pp. 1–12.

Quiz Questions ·

MULTIPLE CHOICE

_D_   1. Which of the following electrons has the greatest binding energy?

      a. N shell electrons
      b. M shell electrons
      c. L shell electrons
      d. K shell electrons

_B_   2. What type of electrical charge does the electron carry?

      a. positive charge
      b. negative charge
      c. no charge
      d. positive or negative charge

_C_   3. Which term describes two or more atoms that are joined by chemical bonds?

      a. ion
      b. ion pair
      c. molecule
      d. proton

_B_   4. Which of the following describes ionization?

      a. an atom without a nucleus
      b. an atom that loses an electron
      c. an atom with equal numbers of protons and electrons
      d. none of the above

_B_   5. Which term describes the process by which unstable atoms undergo a spontaneous disintegration in an effort to attain a more balance nuclear state?

      a. radiation
      b. radioactivity
      c. ionization
      d. ionizing radiation

_D_   6. Which of the following is NOT a type of particulate radiation?

      a. alpha particles
      b. beta particles
      c. protons
      d. nucleons

_A_   7. Which of the following is NOT a type of electromagnetic radiation?

      a. electrons
      b. radar waves
      c. microwaves
      d. x-rays

_____ B 8. Which of the following is INCORRECT?

   a. velocity—the speed of a wave
   b. wavelength—distance between waves
   c. frequency—number of wavelengths that pass a given point in a certain amount of time
   d. frequency and wavelength are inversely related

_____ A 9. Which of the following is INCORRECT?

   a. x-rays travel at the speed of sound
   b. x-rays have no charge
   c. x-rays cannot be focused to a point
   d. x rays cause ionization

_____ B 10. Which of the following is a CORRECT statement?

   a. x-rays are a form of electromagnetic radiation; visible light is not
   b. x-rays have more energy than visible light
   c. x-rays have a longer wavelength than visible light
   d. x-rays travel more slowly than visible light

IDENTIFICATION

For questions 11 to 18, identify each of the labeled structures in Figure 2–27.

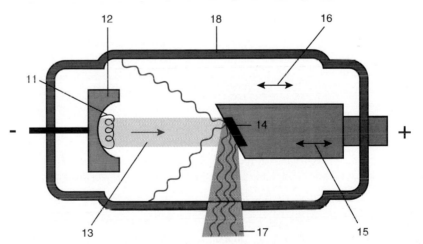

FIGURE 2–27. The dental x-ray tube.

For questions 19 to 26, identify each of the labeled structures in Figure 2–28.

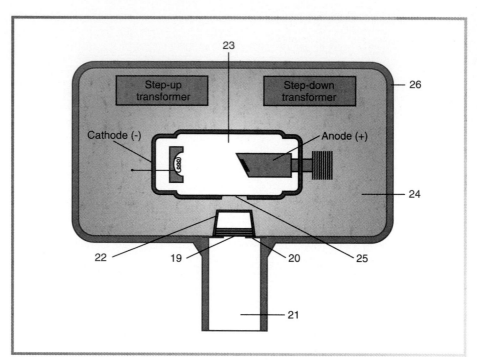

FIGURE 2–28. The dental x-ray tubehead.

MULTIPLE CHOICE

___*B*___ **27.** Which of the following regulates the flow of electrical current to the filament of the x-ray tube?

    a. high-voltage circuit
    b. low-voltage circuit
    c. high-voltage transformer
    d. low-voltage transformer

___*A*___ **28.** Which of the following is used to increase the voltage in the high-voltage circuit?

    a. step-up transformer
    b. step-down transformer
    c. autotransformer
    d. step-up circuit

___*C*___ **29.** Which of the following does NOT occur when the high-voltage circuit is activated?

    a. the unit produces an audible and visible signal
    b. electrons produced at the cathode are accelerated across the tube to the anode
    c. x-rays travel from the filament to the target
    d. heat is produced

_B_ 30. Which of the following is the location in which x-rays are produced?

    a. positive cathode
    b. positive anode
    c. negative cathode
    d. negative anode

_C_ 31. Which of the following is the location in which thermionic emission occurs?

    a. positive cathode
    b. negative anode
    c. negative cathode
    d. negative anode

_A_ 32. Which of the following accounts for 70% of all the x ray energy produced at the anode?

    a. general radiation
    b. characteristic radiation
    c. Compton scatter
    d. coherent scatter

_B_ 33. Which of the following occurs only at 70 kVp or higher and accounts for a very small part of the x-rays produced in the dental x-ray machine?

    a. general radiation
    b. characteristic radiation
    c. Compton scatter
    d. coherent scatter

_A_ 34. Which of the following describes primary radiation?

    a. radiation that exits the tubehead
    b. radiation that is created when x-rays come in contact with matter
    c. radiation that has been deflected from its path by the interaction with matter
    d. none of the above

_C_ 35. Which of the following describes scatter radiation?

    a. radiation that exits the tubehead
    b. radiation that is more penetrating than primary radiation
    c. radiation that has been deflected from its path by interaction with matter
    d. none of the above

_A_ 36. Which of the following type of scatter occurs most often with dental x-rays?

    a. Compton
    b. coherent
    c. photoelectric
    d. none of the above

IDENTIFICATION

For questions 37 to 40 identify the x-radiation interaction with matter in Figures 2–29, 2–30, 2–31, and 2–32.

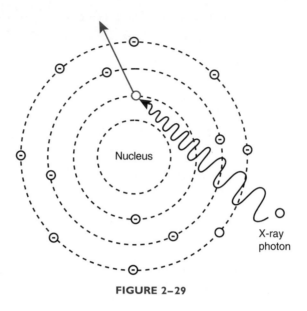

FIGURE 2–29

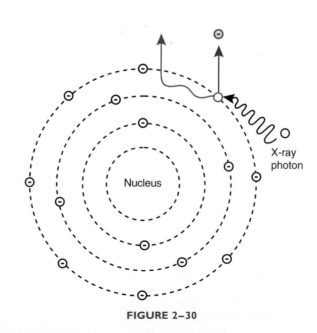

FIGURE 2–30

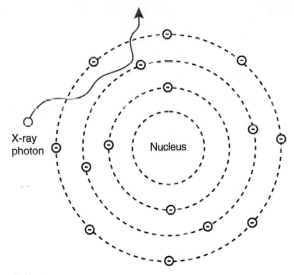

FIGURE 2-31

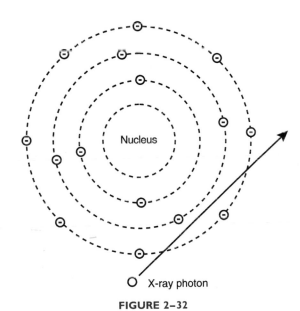

FIGURE 2-32

MULTIPLE CHOICE

For questions 41 to 44, refer to Figures 2–29, 2–30, 2–31, and 2–32.

_____ **41.** The interaction of x-radiation with matter illustrated in Figure 2–29 demonstrates:

   a. no scatter, no ionization
   b. no scatter, ionization
   c. scatter, no ionization
   d. scatter, ionization

_____ **42.** The interaction of x-radiation with matter illustrated in Figure 2–30 demonstrates:

  a. no scatter, no ionization
  b. no scatter, ionization
  c. scatter, no ionization
  d. scatter, ionization

_____ **43.** The interaction of x-radiation with matter illustrated in Figure 2–31 demonstrates:

  a. no scatter, no ionization
  b. no scatter, ionization
  c. scatter, no ionization
  d. scatter, ionization

_____ **44.** The interaction of x-radiation with matter illustrated in Figure 2–32 demonstrates

  a. no scatter, no ionization
  b. no scatter, ionization
  c. scatter, no ionization
  d. scatter, ionization

_____

Answers are supplied at the end of this book.

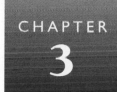

CHAPTER 3

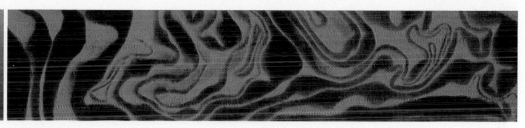

Radiation Characteristics

OBJECTIVES

After completion of this chapter, the student will be able to:

- *Define the key words.*
- *Describe the effect that the kilovoltage peak has on the quality of the x-ray beam.*
- *Describe how milliamperage influences the quantity of the x-ray beam.*
- *Identify the range of kilovoltage and milliamperage required for dental radiography.*
- *Describe how increasing and decreasing exposure factors affect the density and contrast of the film.*
- *State the rules governing kilovoltage, milliamperage, distance, and exposure time that are used when changing exposure variables.*
- *Describe how kilovoltage, milliamperage, exposure time, and source-to-film distance influences the intensity of the x-ray beam*
- *Calculate an example of radiation intensity using the Inverse Square Law.*
- *Explain how the half-value layer determines the penetrating quality of the x-ray beam.*

KEY WORDS

Ampere (A)	Milliamperage
Contrast	Milliampere (mA)
Density	Milliampere-seconds
Exposure time	(mAs)
Half-value layer (HVL)	Polychromatic x-ray
Impulse	beam
Intensity (of x-ray	Quality (of x-ray
beam)	beam)
Inverse Square Law	Quantity (of x-ray
Kilovolt (kV)	beam)
Kilovoltage	Volt (V)
Kilovoltage peak (kVp)	Voltage

INTRODUCTION

Radiation characteristics include x-ray beam quality, quantity, and intensity. Variations in the character of the x-ray beam have an influence on the quality of the resulting radiographs.

The dental radiographer must have a working knowledge of radiation characteristics. The purpose of this chapter is to detail the concepts of x-ray beam quality and quantity, to define the concept of beam intensity, and, to discuss how exposure factors influence these radiation characteristics.

X-RAY BEAM QUALITY AND QUANTITY

X-ray Beam Quality and Voltage

Wavelength determines the energy and penetrating power of radiation. X-rays with shorter wavelengths have more penetrating power, whereas those with longer wavelengths are less penetrating and more likely to be absorbed by matter. In dental radiography, the term **quality** is used to describe the mean energy or penetrating ability of the x-ray beam. The quality, or wavelength and energy of the x-ray beam, is controlled by kilovoltage.

KILOVOLTAGE AND KILOVOLT (kV)

Voltage is a measurement of force that refers to the potential difference between two electrical charges. Inside the dental x-ray tubehead, voltage is the measure-

ment of electrical force that causes electrons to move from the negative cathode to the positive anode. Voltage determines the speed of electrons that travel from cathode to anode. When voltage is increased, the speed of the electrons is increased. When the speed of the electrons is increased, the electrons strike the target with greater force and energy, resulting in a penetrating x-ray beam with a short wavelength.

Voltage is measured in volts or kilovolts. The **volt (V)** is the unit of measurement used to describe the potential that drives an electrical current through a circuit. Dental x-ray equipment requires the use of high voltages. Most radiographic units operate using kilovolts; 1 **kilovolt (kV)** is equal to 1000 volts.

Dental radiography requires the use of 65 to 100 kV. The use of less than 65 kV does not allow adequate penetration, whereas the use of more than 100 kV results in overpenetration.

Kilovoltage can be adjusted according to the individual diagnostic needs of the patients. The use of 85 to 100 kV produces more penetrating dental x-rays with greater energy and shorter wavelengths, whereas the use of 65 to 75 kV produces less penetrating dental x-rays with less energy and longer wavelengths. A higher kilovoltage should be used when the area to be examined is dense or thick.

KILOVOLTAGE PEAK (kVp)

Kilovoltage is controlled by the kilovoltage peak adjustment on the x-ray control panel (Fig. 3–1). **Kilovoltage peak (kVp)** can be defined as the maximum or peak voltage. The voltage meter on the control panel measures the x-ray tube voltage, which is actually the peak voltage of an alternating current (abbreviated AC) (Fig. 3–2). This peak voltage is measured in kilovolts, thus, the term kilovoltage peak, or kVp, is used. For example, when 90 kVp is used to expose a film, the peak voltage of the tube current is 90,000 volts. As a result of varying kilovoltages occurring in the tube current, a **polychromatic x-ray beam**, or a beam that contains many different wavelengths of varying intensities, is produced.

QUALITY AND KILOVOLTAGE PEAK

The quality, or wavelength and energy of the x-ray beam, is controlled by the kilovoltage peak. The kilovoltage peak regulates the speed and energy of the electrons and determines the penetrating ability of the x-ray beam. When kilovoltage peak is increased, a higher energy x-ray beam with increased penetrating ability results.

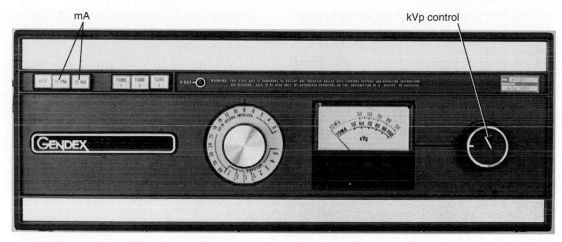

FIGURE 3–1. The kilovoltage peak (kVp) and milliamperage (mA) controls are located on the x-ray machine. (Courtesy of Gendex Corporation, Des Plaines, IL.)

DENSITY AND KILOVOLTAGE PEAK

Density is the overall darkness or blackness of a film. An adjustment in kilovoltage peak results in a change in the density of a dental radiograph. When the kilovoltage peak is increased while other exposure factors (milliamperage, exposure time) remain constant, the resultant film exhibits an increased density and appears darker (Fig. 3–3A and B); if kilovoltage peak is decreased, the resultant film exhibits a decreased density and appears lighter (Fig. 3–4A and B). Table 3–1 summarizes the effect of kilovoltage peak on density. A complete discussion of density is found in Chapter 8.

CONTRAST AND KILOVOLTAGE PEAK

Contrast refers to how sharply dark and light areas are differentiated or separated on a film. An adjust-

ment in kilovoltage peak results in a change in the contrast of a dental radiograph. With low kilovoltage peak settings (65 to 70 kVp), a high contrast film results. A film with "high" contrast has many black and white areas and few shades of gray (Fig. 3–5). A film with high contrast is useful for the detection and progression of dental caries.

With high kilovoltage peak settings (≥90 kVp), low contrast results. A film with "low" contrast has many shades of gray instead of black and white. A film with low contrast is useful for the detection of periodontal or periapical disease (Fig. 3–6). Mounted radiographs that demonstrate low contrast and are viewed properly on an illuminated surface with masked extraneous light are preferred in dental radiography. A compromise between high contrast and low contrast is desirable. Table 3–1 summarizes the effect of kilovoltage peak on contrast. A complete discussion of contrast is found in Chapter 8.

EXPOSURE TIME AND KILOVOLTAGE PEAK

Exposure time refers to the interval of time during which x-rays are produced. Exposure time is measured

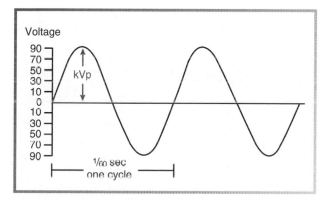

FIGURE 3–2. Kilovoltage peak (kVp) controls the quality of the x-ray beam and measures the peak voltage of the current.

TABLE 3–1. Effect of Kilovoltage Peak on Film Density and Contrast		
Adjustment	**Density**	**Contrast**
↑ kVp	↑ (darker)	low
↓ kVp	↓ (lighter)	high

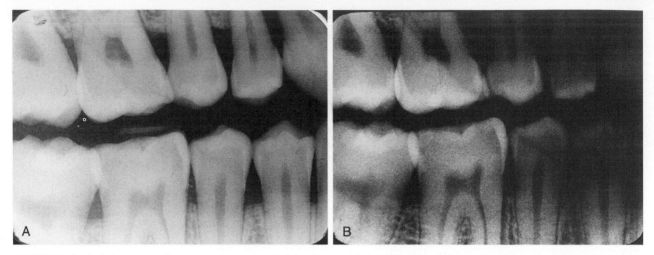

FIGURE 3–3. *A,* A diagnostic radiograph. *B,* An increase in kilovoltage results in a film that exhibits increased density; the film appears darker.

in **impulses** because x-rays are created in a series of bursts or pulses rather than in a continuous stream. One impulse occurs every 1/60 of a second; therefore, 60 impulses occur in 1 second.

To compensate for the penetrating power of the x-ray beam, an adjustment in exposure time is necessary when kilovoltage peak is increased (see "Kilovoltage Peak Rule").

For example, a film is exposed using 90 kVp and 0.5 seconds. If the kilovoltage peak setting is decreased from 90 to 75, the exposure time must be increased from 0.5 to 1.0 second to maintain proper film density and contrast.

X-ray Beam Quantity and Amperage

Quantity refers to the number of x-rays produced. Amperage determines the amount of electrons passing through the cathode filament. An increase in the number of electrons available to travel from the cathode to the anode results in production of an increased number of x-rays. The quantity of the x-rays produced is controlled by milliamperage.

MILLIAMPERAGE AND MILLIAMPERES (mA)

The **ampere (A)** is the unit of measure used to describe the number of electrons, or current flowing

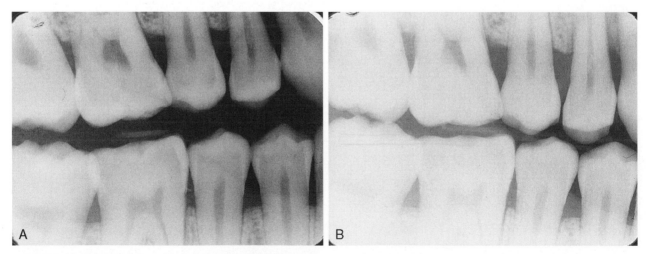

FIGURE 3–4. *A,* A diagnostic radiograph. *B,* A decrease in kilovoltage results in a film that exhibits decreased density; the film appears lighter.

FIGURE 3–5. A film produced with lower kilovoltage exhibits high contrast; many light and dark areas are seen as demonstrated by the use of the stepwedge.

through the cathode filament. The number of amperes needed to operate a dental x-ray unit is small; therefore, amperage is measured in milliamperes. One **milliampere (mA)** is equal to 1/1000 of an ampere. Some dental x-ray units have a fixed milliampere setting, whereas others have a milliampere adjustment on the control panel (see Fig. 3–1). In dental radiography, the use of 7 to 15 mA is required; a setting above 15 mA is not recommended because of the excessive heat production in the x-ray tube that results.

Milliamperage regulates the temperature of the cathode filament. A higher milliampere setting increases the temperature of the cathode filament and

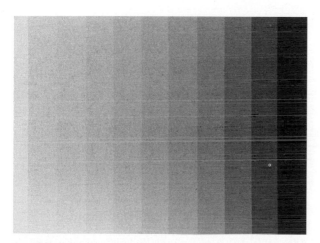

FIGURE 3–6. A film produced with higher kilovoltage exhibits low contrast; many shades of gray are seen instead of black and white.

KILOVOLTAGE PEAK RULE

When kilovoltage peak is increased by 15, exposure time should be decreased by one-half. Conversely, when kilovoltage peak is decreased by 15, the exposure time should be doubled.

---

consequently increases the number of electrons produced. An increase in the number of electrons that strike the anode increases the number of x-rays emitted from the tube.

MILLIAMPERE-SECONDS (mAs)

Both milliamperes and exposure time have a direct influence on the number of electrons produced by the cathode filament, and when combined, they form a common factor called milliampere-seconds. A combination of milliamperes and exposure time is termed **milliampere-seconds (mAs)**.

Milliamperes × exposure time (seconds) =

milliampere-seconds

When milliamperage is increased, the exposure time must be decreased and vice versa if the density of the exposed radiograph is to remain the same.

EXAMPLE

Using 10 mA with an exposure time of 1.5 seconds would result in 15 mAs (10 mA × 1.5 seconds = 15 mAs). If the milliamperage is increased to 15, the time must be decreased to 1.0 seconds (15 mA × 1.0 second = 15 mAs). Notice that both of these exposures result in the same number of milliampere-seconds, which produces the same density on a dental radiograph.

For example, if a patient has difficulty holding still during the exposure, the dental radiographer can increase the milliamperage and decrease the exposure time to compensate for movement of the patient.

QUANTITY AND MILLIAMPERAGE

The quantity, or number of x-rays emitted from the tubehead, is controlled by milliamperage. Milliamper-

TABLE 3–2. Effect of Milliamperage on Film Density

Adjustment	Density
↑ mA	↑ (darker)
↓ mA	↓ (lighter)

age controls the amperage of the filament current and the amount of electrons that pass through the filament. As the milliamperage is increased, more electrons pass through the filament and more x-rays are produced. For example, if the milliamperage is increased from 5 to 10, twice as many electrons travel from the cathode to the anode, and twice as many x-rays are produced.

DENSITY AND MILLIAMPERAGE

Milliamperage, like kilovoltage peak, has an effect on the density of a dental radiograph. An increase in milliamperage increases the overall density of the radiograph and results in a darker image. Conversely, a decrease in milliamperage decreases the overall density of the film and results in a lighter image. Table 3–2 summarizes the effect of milliamperage on film density.

EXPOSURE TIME AND MILLIAMPERAGE

Milliamperage and exposure time are inversely related. When altering milliamperage, the exposure time must be adjusted to maintain the diagnostic density of a film. When milliamperage is increased, the exposure time must be decreased and conversely, when milliamperage is decreased, the exposure time must be increased.

Guidelines for adjusting kilovoltage peak, milliamperage, and exposure time are given in Table 3–3.

TABLE 3–3. Guidelines for Altering Kilovoltage Peak, Milliamperage, and Exposure Time

↑ kVp by 15	↓ exposure time by 1/2
↓ kVp by 15	↑ exposure time by 2
↑ mA	↓ exposure time
↓ mA	↑ exposure time

X-RAY BEAM INTENSITY

Quality refers to the energy or penetrating ability of the x-ray beam; quantity refers to the number of x-ray photons in the beam. Quality and quantity are described together in a concept known as intensity. **Intensity** is defined as the product of the quantity (number of x-ray photons) and quality (energy of each photon) per unit of area per unit of time of exposure.

$$\text{Intensity} = \frac{(\text{no. photons}) \times (\text{energy of each photon})}{(\text{area}) \times (\text{exposure rate})}$$

Intensity of the x-ray beam is affected by a number of factors, including kilovoltage peak, milliamperage, exposure time, and distance.

Intensity and Kilovoltage Peak

Kilovoltage peak regulates the penetrating power of the x-ray beam by controlling the speed of the electrons traveling between the cathode and the anode. Higher kilovoltage peak settings produce an x-ray beam with more energy and shorter wavelengths; higher kilovoltage levels increase the intensity of the x-ray beam.

Intensity and Milliamperage

Milliamperage controls the penetrating power of the x-ray beam by controlling the number of electrons produced in the x-ray tube and the number of x-rays produced. Higher milliampere settings produce a beam with more energy and increase the intensity of the x-ray beam.

Intensity and Exposure Time

Exposure time, like milliamperage, affects the number of x-rays produced. A longer exposure time produces more x-rays. As with milliamperage, an increase in exposure time produces a more intense x-ray beam.

Intensity and Distance

The distance the x-ray beam travels affects the intensity of the beam. Several distances must be considered when exposing a dental radiograph. These distances include

- the distance from the source of radiation to the patient's skin (target-surface distance)
- the distance from the source of radiation to the tooth (target-object distance)
- the distance from the source of radiation to the film (target-film distance) (Fig 3–7).

The distance between the source of radiation and the film has a marked effect on the intensity of the x-ray beam. As x-rays travel from their point of origin, or away from the target anode, they diverge like waves of light and spread out to cover a larger surface area. As x-rays travel away from their source of origin, the intensity of the beam lessens. Unless a corresponding change is made in one of the other exposure factors (kilovoltage peak, milliamperage), the intensity of the x-ray beam is reduced as the distance increases.

The x-ray beam that exits from an 8-inch position-indicating device (PID) is more intense than one that exits from a 16-inch PID. The Inverse Square Law is used to explain how distance affects the intensity of the x-ray beam.

Inverse Square Law

The **Inverse Square Law** is stated as follows:

> The intensity of radiation is inversely proportional to the square of the distance from the source of radiation.

"Inversely proportional" means that as one variable increases, the other decreases. When the source-to-film distance is increased, the intensity of the beam is decreased.

For example, when the PID length is changed from 8 to 16 inches, the source-to-film distance is doubled. According to the Inverse Square Law, the resultant beam is *one-fourth* as intense (Fig. 3–8). When the PID length is changed from 16 to 8 inches, the source-to-film distance is reduced by one-half. According to the Inverse Square Law, the resultant beam is *four times* as intense.

The following mathematical formula is used to calculate the Inverse Square Law.

$$\frac{\text{original intensity}}{\text{new intensity}} = \frac{\text{new distance}^2}{\text{original distance}^2}$$

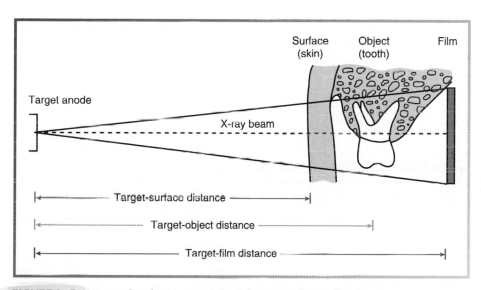

FIGURE 3–7. Target-surface distance, target-object distance, and target-film distance.

EXAMPLE

If the PID length is changed from 8 inches to 16 inches, how does this increase in source-to-film distance affect the intensity of the beam?

$$\frac{I}{x} = \frac{16^2}{8^2}$$

$$\frac{I}{x} = \frac{256}{64}$$

$$\frac{I}{x} = \frac{4}{1}$$

$$\frac{I}{x} = 1/4$$

This mathematical formula reveals that the intensity of the beam will be 1/4 as intense if the source-to-film distance is changed from 8 to 16 inches (assuming that kilovoltage peak and milliamperage remain constant). In this example, the Inverse Square Law reveals that doubling the distance from the source of radiation to the film (from an 8-inch to a 16-inch PID) results in a beam that is one-fourth as intense. Remember, the intensity of the radiation is inversely proportional to the *square* of the distance.

Half-Value Layer

To reduce the intensity of the x-ray beam, aluminum filters are placed in the path of the beam inside the dental x-ray tubehead. Aluminum filters are used to remove the low-energy, less penetrating, longer wavelength x-rays. Aluminum filters increase the mean penetrating capability of the x-ray beam while reducing the intensity. The thickness of a specified material, such as aluminum, that when placed in the path of the x-ray beam reduces the intensity by one-half is termed the **half-value layer (HVL)**.

For example, if an x-ray beam is said to have a half-value layer of 4 mm, a thickness of 4 mm of aluminum would be necessary to decrease its intensity by one-half. Measuring the half-value layer determines the penetrating quality of the beam. The higher the half-value layer, the more penetrating the beam. More information about filtration of the x-ray beam is found in Chapter 5.

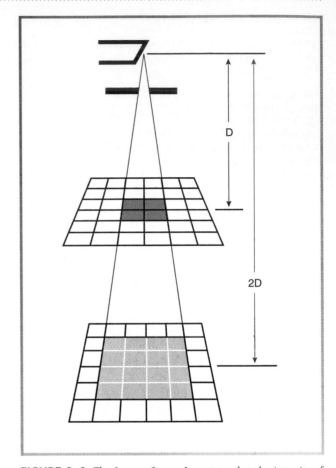

FIGURE 3–8. The Inverse Square Law states that the intensity of radiation is inversely proportional to the square of the distance from the source. Notice on the diagram that as the source-to-film distance is doubled, the intensity of radiation is one-fourth as intense. (From *X-rays in Dentistry*. Rochester, NY, Eastman Kodak Company, 1985.)

SUMMARY

- Radiation characteristics include x-ray beam quality, quantity, and intensity.
- Quality refers to the mean (average) energy or penetrating ability of the x-ray beam and is controlled by the kilovoltage peak (kVp).
- Increased kilovoltage peak produces x-rays with increased energy, shorter wavelengths, and increased penetrating power; kilovoltage peak affects film density and contrast.
- Quantity refers to the number of x-rays produced and is controlled by the milliamperage (mA).
- Increased milliamperage produces an increased number of x-rays; milliamperage affects film density.
- Exposure time also influences the number of x-rays produced.
- Intensity is the total energy contained in the x-ray beam in a specific area at a given time; intensity is affected by

kilovoltage peak, milliamperage, exposure time, and distance.

- Increased kilovoltage peak, milliamperage, or exposure time results in increased intensity of the x-ray beam.
- Intensity of the x-ray beam is reduced with increased distance. The Inverse Square Law is used to explain how distance affects the intensity of the x-ray beam.
- An aluminum filter is placed in the path of the x-ray beam to reduce the intensity and remove the low-energy x-rays from the beam.
- The thickness of aluminum placed in the path of the x-ray beam that reduces the intensity by one-half is termed the half-value layer.

BIBLIOGRAPHY

Barr JH, Stephens RG: Radiographic objectives. *In* Dental Radiology: Pertinent Basic Concepts and Their Applications in Clinical Practice. Philadelphia, WB Saunders, 1980, pp 118–157.

Frommer HH: Ionizing radiation and basic principles of x-ray generation. *In* Radiology for Dental Auxiliaries, 6th edition. St. Louis, Mosby-Year Book, 1996, pp. 1–29.

Frommer HH: Image formation, image receptors. *In* Radiology for Dental Auxiliaries, 6th edition. St. Louis, Mosby-Year Book, 1996, pp. 31–47.

Goaz PW, White SC: Radiation physics. *In* Oral Radiology and Principles of Interpretation, 3rd edition. St. Louis, Mosby-Year Book, 1994, pp. 1–23.

Johnson ON, McNally MA, Essay CE: The Dental x-ray machine—components and functions. *In* Essentials of Dental Radiography for Dental Assistants and Hygienists, 6th edition. Norwalk, CT, Appleton and Lange, 1999, pp. 37–60.

Johnson ON, McNally MA, Essay CE: Producing quality radiographs. *In* Essentials of Dental Radiography for Dental Assistants and Hygienists, 6th edition. Norwalk, CT, Appleton and Lange, 1999, pp. 61–85.

Kasle MJ, Langlais RP: The components and function of the dental x-ray machine. *In* Basic Principles of Oral Radiography: Exercises in Dental Radiology, Vol. 4. Philadelphia, WB Saunders, 1981, pp. 9–22.

Langland OE, Sippy FH, Langlais RP: X-rays, their production, and the x-ray beam. *In* Textbook of Dental Radiography, 2nd edition. Springfield, IL, Charles C Thomas, 1984, pp. 43–87.

Langland OE, Sippy FH, Langlais RP: Diagnostic quality of dental radiographs. *In* Textbook of Dental Radiography, 2nd edition. Springfield, IL, Charles C Thomas, 1984, pp. 130–152.

Manson-Hing LR: Physical foundation of radiography. *In* Fundamentals of Dental Radiography, 3rd edition. Philadelphia, Lea & Febiger, 1990, pp. 1–15.

Miles DA, Van Dis ML, Jensen CW et al: X-ray properties and the generation of x-rays. *In* Radiographic Imaging for Dental Auxiliaries, 3rd edition. Philadelphia, WB Saunders, 1999, pp. 73–85.

Miles DA, Van Dis ML, Jensen CW, et al: Image characteristics. *In* Radiographic Imaging for Dental Auxiliaries, 3rd edition. Philadelphia, WB Saunders, 1999, 87–99.

Miles DA, Van Dis ML, Razmus TF. Radiation physics. *In* Basic Principles of Oral and Maxillofacial Radiology. Philadelphia, WB Saunders, 1992, pp 1–19.

O'Brien RC: The nature and generation of x-rays. *In* Dental Radiography: An Introduction for Dental Hygienists and Assistants, 4th edition. Philadelphia, WB Saunders, 1982, pp. 1–25.

Quiz Questions

MULTIPLE CHOICE

_A_   1. In dental radiography, the quality of the x-ray beam is controlled by:

    a. kVp
    b. mA
    c. exposure time
    d. source-to-film distance

_C_   2. Identify the kilovoltage range for most dental x-ray machines:

    a. 50–60 kV
    b. 60–70 kV
    c. 65–100 kV
    d. >100 kV

_D_   3. A higher kilovoltage produces x-rays with:

    a. greater energy levels
    b. shorter wavelengths
    c. more penetrating ability
    d. all of the above

_B_   4. Identify the unit of measurement used to describe the amount of electric current flowing through the x-ray tube:

    a. volt
    b. ampere
    c. kilovoltage peak
    d. force

_A_   5. Radiation produced with high kilovoltage results in:

    a. short wavelengths
    b. long wavelengths
    c. less penetrating radiation
    d. lower energy levels

_D_   6. In dental radiography, the quantity of radiation produced is controlled by:

    a. kVp
    b. mA
    c. exposure time
    d. b and c

_D_   7. Increasing milliamperage results in an increase in:

    a. temperature of the filament
    b. mean energy of the beam
    c. number of x-rays produced
    d. a and c

_C_   8. Identify the milliamperage range for dental radiography:

    a. 1–5 mA
    b. 4–10 mA
    c. 7–15 mA
    d. >15 mA

B.

9. The overall blackness or darkness of a film is termed:

  a. contrast
  b. density
  c. overexposure
  d. polychromatic

A

10. If kilovoltage is decreased with no other variations in exposure factors, the resultant film will:

  a. appear lighter
  b. appear darker
  c. remain the same
  d. either a or b

A

11. Identify the term that describes how dark and light areas are differentiated on a film:

  a. contrast
  b. density
  c. intensity
  d. polychromatic

C

12. A radiograph that has many light and dark areas with few shades of gray is said to have:

  a. high density
  b. low density
  c. high contrast
  d. low contrast

A

13. The radiograph described in question 12 was produced with:

  a. low kilovoltage
  b. high kilovoltage
  c. low milliamperage
  d. high milliamperage

C

14. Increasing milliamperage alone results in a film with:

  a. high contrast
  b. low contrast
  c. increased density
  d. decreased density

A

15. A diagnostic film is produced using 90 kVp and 0.25 second. What exposure time is needed to produce the same film at 75 kVp?

  a. 0.50 second
  b. 0.75 second
  c. 1.00 second
  d. 1.25 second

B

16. A diagnostic film is produced using 10 mA and 0.45 second. What exposure time is needed to produce the same film at 15 mA?

  a. 0.25 second
  b. 0.30 second
  c. 0.45 second
  d. 0.50 second

_____C_____   17. The total energy contained in the x-ray beam in a specific area at a given time is termed:

   a. kilovoltage peak
   b. beam quality
   c. intensity
   d. milliampere-second

_____C_____   18. Increasing which of the following exposure controls will increase the intensity of the x-ray beam? (1) kilovoltage, (2) milliamperage, (3) exposure time, (4) source-to-film distance

   a. 1 and 2
   b. 2 and 3
   c. 1, 2, and 3
   d. all of the above

_____A_____   19. The length of the PID is changed from 16 inches to 8 inches. The resultant intensity of the beam will be:

   a. four times as intense
   b. twice as intense
   c. one-half as intense
   d. one-fourth as intense

_____D_____   20. The half-value layer is:

   a. the amount of lead that restricts the diameter of the beam by one-half
   b. the amount of the copper needed to cool the anode
   c. the amount of aluminum needed to reduce scatter radiation by one-half
   d. the amount of aluminum needed to reduce x-ray beam intensity by one-half

_____

Answers are supplied at the end of this book.

CHAPTER

4

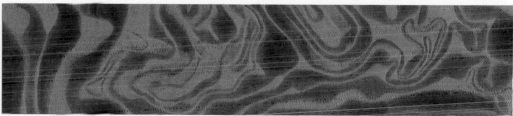

Radiation Biology

OBJECTIVES

After completion of this chapter, the student will be able to:

- *Define the key words.*
- *Describe the mechanisms, theories, and sequence of radiation injury.*
- *Define and discuss the dose-response curve and radiation injury.*
- *List the determining factors for radiation injury.*
- *Discuss the short-term and long-term effects, and the somatic and genetic effects of radiation exposure.*
- *Describe the effects of radiation exposure on cells, tissues, and organs.*
- *Identify the relative sensitivity of a given tissue to x-radiation.*
- *Define the units of measurement used in radiation exposure.*
- *List common sources of radiation exposure.*
- *Discuss risk and risk estimates for radiation exposure.*
- *Discuss dental radiation and exposure risks.*
- *Discuss the risk versus benefit of dental radiographs.*

KEY WORDS

Cell	Long-term effects
Cell differentiation	Mitotic activity
Cell metabolism	Nonstochastic effects
Coulomb (C)	Quality factor (QF)
Critical organ	Radiation, background
Cumulative effects	Radiation absorbed
Direct theory	dose (rad)
Dose	Radiation biology
Dose, total	Radioresistant
Dose equivalent	Radiosensitive
Dose rate	Recovery period
Dose-response curve	Risk
Exposure	Roentgen (R)
Free radical	Roentgen equivalent
Genetic cells	(in) man (rem)
Genetic effects	Short-term effects
Gray (Gy)	Sievert (Sv)
Indirect theory	Somatic cells
Injury, period of	Somatic effects
Ionization	Stochastic effects
Latent period	

INTRODUCTION

All ionizing radiations are harmful and produce biologic changes in living tissue. The damaging biologic effects of x-radiation were first documented shortly after the discovery of x-rays. Since that time, information about the harmful effects of high-level exposure to x-radiation has increased based on studies of atomic bomb survivors, workers exposed to radioactive materials, and patients undergoing radiation therapy. The amount of x-radiation used in dental radiography is small, however, biologic damage does occur.

The dental radiographer must have a working knowledge of **radiation biology,** the study of the effects of ionizing radiation on living tissue, to understand the harmful effects of x-radiation. The purpose of this chapter is to describe the mechanisms and theories of radiation injury, to define the basic concepts and effects of radiation exposure, to detail radiation measurements, and to discuss the risks of radiation exposure.

RADIATION INJURY

Mechanisms of Radiation Injury

In diagnostic radiography not all x-rays pass through the patient and reach the dental x-ray film; some are absorbed by patient tissues. Absorption, as defined in Chapter 2, refers to the total transfer of energy from the x-ray photon to patient tissues. What happens when x-ray energy is absorbed by patient tissues? Chemical changes occur that result in biologic damage. Two specific mechanisms of radiation injury are possible: ionization and free radical formation.

IONIZATION

X-rays are a form of ionizing radiation; when x-rays strike patient tissues, **ionization** results. As described in Chapter 2, ionization is produced through the photoelectric effect or Compton scatter and results in the formation of a positive atom and a dislodged negative electron. The ejected high-speed electron is set into motion and interacts with other atoms within the absorbing tissues. The kinetic energy of such electrons results in further ionization, excitation, or breaking of molecular bonds, all of which cause chemical changes within the cell that results in biologic damage (Fig. 4–1). Ionization may have little effect on cells if the chemical changes do not alter sensitive molecules, or such changes may have a profound effect on structures of great importance to cell function (e.g., DNA).

FREE RADICAL FORMATION

X-radiation causes cell damage primarily through free radical* formation. Free radical formation occurs when an x-ray photon ionizes water, the primary component of living cells. Ionization of water results in the production of hydrogen and hydroxyl free radicals (Fig. 4–2). A **free radical** is an uncharged (neutral) atom or molecule that exists with a single, unpaired electron in its outermost shell. It is highly reactive and unstable; the lifetime of a free radical is approximately 10^{-10} seconds. To achieve stability, free radicals (1) may recombine without causing changes in the molecule, (2) may combine with other free radicals and cause changes, or (3) may combine with ordinary molecules to form a toxin (e.g., hydrogen peroxide) capable of producing widespread cellular changes (Fig. 4–3).

---

* A free radical with no charge is denoted by a dot following the chemical symbol (e.g., H·). A free radical with a charge is an ion.

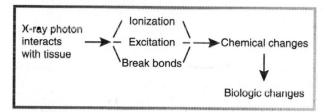

FIGURE 4–1. The x-ray photon interacts with tissues and results in ionization, excitation, or breaking of molecular bonds, all of which cause chemical changes that result in biologic damage.

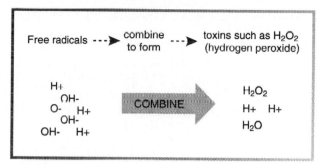

FIGURE 4–3. Free radicals can combine with each other to form toxins such as hydrogen peroxide.

Theories of Radiation Injury

Damage to living tissues due to exposure to ionizing radiation may result from a direct hit and absorption of an x-ray photon within a cell or from absorption of an x-ray photon by water within a cell accompanied by free radical formation. There are two theories about how radiation damages biologic tissues: the direct theory and the indirect theory.

THE DIRECT THEORY

The **direct theory** suggests that cell damage results when ionizing radiation directly hits critical areas, or targets, within the cell. For example, if x-ray photons directly strike the DNA of a cell, critical damage occurs, causing injury to the irradiated organism. Direct injuries from exposure to ionizing radiation occur infrequently; most x-ray photons pass through the cell and cause little or no damage.

THE INDIRECT THEORY

The **indirect theory** suggests that x-ray photons are absorbed within the cell and cause the formation of

toxins, which in turn damage the cell. For example, when x-ray photons are absorbed by water within a cell, free radical formation results. The free radicals combine to form toxins (e.g., H_2O_2), which cause cellular dysfunction and biologic damage. An indirect injury results because the free radicals combine and form toxins, *not* because of a direct hit by x-ray photons. Indirect injuries from exposure to ionizing radiation occur frequently because of the high water content of cells. The chances of free radical formation and indirect injury are great because cells are composed of 70 to 80% water.

Dose-Response Curve and Radiation Injury

If all ionizing radiations are harmful and produce biologic damage, what level of exposure is considered acceptable? To establish acceptable levels of radiation exposure, it is useful to plot the dose administered and the damage produced. With radiation exposure, a **dose-response curve** can be used to correlate the "response," or damage, of tissues with the "dose," or amount, of radiation received.

When dose and damage are plotted on a graph, a linear, nonthreshold relationship is seen. A linear relationship indicates that the response of the tissues is directly proportional to the dose. A nonthreshold relationship indicates that a threshold dose level for damage does not exist. A nonthreshold dose-response curve suggests that no matter how small the amount of radiation received, some biologic damage occurs (Fig. 4–4). Consequently, there is no *safe* amount of radiation exposure. In dental radiography, although the doses received by the patient are low, damage does occur.

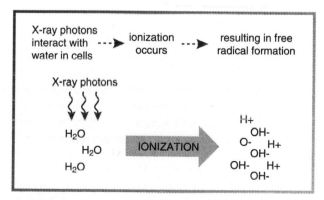

FIGURE 4–2. Examples of free radicals created when water is irradiated.

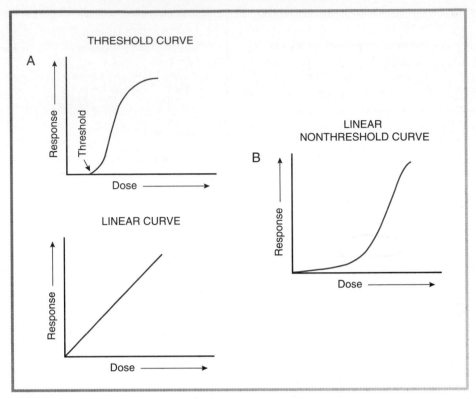

FIGURE 4–4. *A, Threshold curve:* This curve indicates that below a certain level (threshold), no response is seen. *Linear curve:* This curve indicates that response is proportional to dose. *B, Linear nonthreshold curve:* This dose-response curve indicates that a response is seen at any dose.

Most of the information used to produce dose-response curves for radiation exposure comes from studying the effects of large doses of radiation on populations, such as atomic bomb survivors. In the low-dose range, however, very little information has been documented; instead, the curve has been extrapolated based on animal and cellular experiments.

Stochastic and Nonstochastic Radiation Effects

Biologic effects from radiation can be classified as stochastic or nonstochastic. **Stochastic effects** occur as a direct function of dose. The probability of occurrence increases with increasing absorbed dose; however, the severity of effects does not depend on the magnitude of the absorbed dose. Like nonthreshold radiation effects, stochastic effects *do not* have a dose threshold. Examples of stochastic effects include cancer (i.e., tumor) induction and genetic mutations. **Nonstochastic effects** (deterministic effects) are somatic effects that have a threshold and increase in severity with increas-

ing absorbed dose. Examples of nonstochastic effects include erythema, loss of hair, cataract formation, and decreased fertility. When compared with stochastic effects, nonstochastic effects require larger radiation doses to seriously impair health.

Radiation Injury Sequence, Repair, and Accumulation

Chemical reactions (e.g., ionization, free radical formation) that follow the absorption of radiation occur rapidly at the molecular level. However, varying amounts of time are required for these changes to alter cells and cellular functions. As a result, the observable effects of radiation are not visible immediately after exposure. Instead, following exposure, a **latent period** occurs. A latent period can be defined as the time that elapses between exposure to ionizing radiation and the appearance of observable clinical signs. The latent period may be short or long depending on the total dose of radiation received and the amount of time, or rate, it took to receive the dose. The more radiation re-

exposure to radiation
and clinical signs, or redness of skin

ceived and the faster the dose rate, the shorter the latent period.

Following the latent period, a **period of injury** results. A variety of cellular injuries may result including cell death, changes in cell function, breaking or clumping of chromosomes, formation of giant cells, cessation of mitotic activity, or abnormal mitotic activity.

The last event in the sequence of radiation injury is the **recovery period**. Not all cellular radiation injuries are permanent. With each radiation exposure, cellular damage is followed by repair. Depending on a number of factors, cells can repair the damage caused by radiation. Most of the damage caused by low-level radiation is repaired within the cells of the body.

The effects of radiation exposure are additive and damage that remains unrepaired accumulates in the tissues. The **cumulative effects** of repeated radiation exposure can lead to health problems (e.g., cancer, cataract formation, birth defects). Table 4–1 lists organs and disorders that may result from the cumulative effects of repeated radiation exposure.

Determining Factors for Radiation Injury

In addition to understanding the mechanisms, theories, and sequence of radiation injury, it is important to recognize that certain factors influence radiation injury. A number of factors contribute to radiation injury including the total dose, dose rate, amount of tissue irradiated, cell sensitivity, and age of the person receiving the radiation.

- **Total dose** refers to the quantity of radiation received or the total amount of radiation energy absorbed. More damage occurs when large quantities of radiation are absorbed by a tissue.
- **Dose rate** is the rate at which exposure to radiation occurs and absorption takes place (dose rate =

dose/time). More radiation damage takes place with high dose rates because a rapid delivery of radiation does not allow time for the cellular damage to be repaired.

- **Amount of tissue irradiated** refers to the areas of the body exposed. Total body irradiation produces more adverse systemic effects than if small, localized areas of the body are exposed. An example of total body irradiation is a person exposed to a nuclear energy disaster. Extensive radiation injury occurs when large areas of the body are exposed because of the damage that occurs to the blood-forming tissues.
- **Cell sensitivity** also affects radiation injury. More damage occurs in cells that are most sensitive to radiation (e.g., rapidly dividing cells, young cells). Cell sensitivity is discussed in detail later in this chapter.
- **Age** is another determining factor for radiation injury. Children are more susceptible to radiation damage than adults.

RADIATION EFFECTS

Short-Term and Long-Term Effects

Radiation effects can be classified as either short-term or long-term. Following the latent period, effects that are seen within minutes, days, or weeks are termed **short-term effects**. Short-term effects are associated with large amounts of radiation absorbed in a short period of time (e.g., exposure to a nuclear accident or the atomic bomb). Acute radiation syndrome (ARS) is a short-term effect and includes nausea, vomiting, diarrhea, hair loss, and hemorrhage. Short-term effects are not applicable to dentistry.

Effects that appear after years, decades, or generations are termed **long-term effects**. Long-term effects are associated with small amounts of radiation absorbed repeatedly over a long period of time. Repeated low levels of radiation exposure are linked to the induction of cancer, birth abnormalities, and genetic defects.

Somatic and Genetic Effects

All the cells in the body can be classified as either somatic or genetic. **Somatic cells** are all the cells in the body *except* the reproductive cells. The reproductive cells (e.g., ova, sperm) are termed **genetic cells**. Depending on the type of cell that is injured by radia-

TABLE 4–1. Tissue and Radiation Effect	
Tissue or Organ	**Radiation Effect**
Hematopoietic (blood-forming)	Leukemia
Reproductive (ova, sperm)	Mutations
Thyroid	Carcinoma
Skin	Carcinoma
Eyes	Cataracts

tion, the biologic effects of radiation can be classified as either somatic or genetic.

Somatic effects are seen in the person irradiated. Radiation injuries that produce changes in somatic cells produce poor health in the irradiated individual. Major somatic effects of radiation exposure include the induction of cancer, leukemia, and cataracts. These changes, however, are not transmitted to future generations (Fig. 4–5).

Genetic effects are not seen in the person irradiated but are passed on to future generations. Radiation injuries that produce changes in genetic cells do not affect the health of the exposed individual. Instead, the radiation-induced mutations affect the health of the

offspring (see Fig. 4–5). Genetic damage cannot be repaired.

Radiation Effects on Cells

The **cell,** or basic structural unit of all living organisms, is composed of a central nucleus and surrounding cytoplasm. Ionizing radiation may affect the nucleus, the cytoplasm, or the entire cell. The cell nucleus is more sensitive to radiation than the cytoplasm. Damage to the nucleus affects the chromosomes containing DNA and results in disruption of cell division, which in turn may lead to disruption of cell function or cell death.

Not all cells respond to radiation in the same manner. A cell that is sensitive to radiation is termed **radiosensitive;** one that is resistant is termed **radioresistant.** The response of a cell to radiation exposure is determined by the following:

- **Mitotic activity:** Cells that divide frequently or undergo many divisions over time are more sensitive to radiation.
- **Cell differentiation:** Cells that are immature or are not highly specialized are more sensitive to radiation.
- **Cell metabolism:** Cells that have a higher metabolism are more sensitive to radiation.

Cells that are radiosensitive include blood cells, immature reproductive cells, and young bone cells. The cell that is most sensitive to radiation is the small lymphocyte. Radioresistant cells include cells of bone, muscle, and nerve. Table 4–2 lists cell types and their respective sensitivities to radiation.

Radiation Effects on Tissues and Organs

Cells are organized into larger functioning units termed tissues and organs. Just as cells vary in their sensitivity

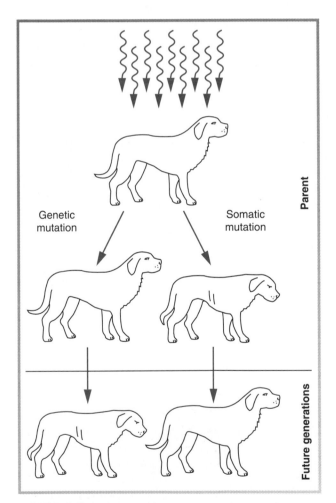

FIGURE 4–5. In this example, a somatic mutation produces poor health in the exposed animal but does not produce mutations in subsequent generations. In contrast, a genetic mutation does not affect the exposed animal but instead produces mutations in future generations.

TABLE 4–2. Tissue and Organ Sensitivity	
Radiosensitive Cells	**Radioresistant Cells**
Small lymphocyte	Mature bone
Bone marrow	Muscle
Reproductive cells	Nerve
Immature bone	

to radiation, so do tissues and organs. Radiosensitive organs are composed of radiosensitive cells and include lymphoid tissues, bone marrow, testes, and intestines. Examples of radioresistant tissues include the salivary glands, kidney, and liver.

In dentistry, some tissues and organs are designated as critical because they are exposed to more radiation than others during radiographic procedures. A **critical organ** is an organ that if damaged diminishes the quality of a person's life. Critical organs exposed during dental radiographic procedures in the head and neck region include:

- skin
- thyroid gland
- lens of the eye
- bone marrow

■ RADIATION MEASUREMENTS

Units of Measurement

Radiation can be measured in the same manner as other physical concepts, such as time, distance, and weight. Just as the unit of measurement for time is minutes, for distance miles or kilometers, and for weight pounds or kilograms, the International Commission on Radiation Units and Measurement (ICRU) has established special units for the measurement of radiation. Such units are used to define three quantities of radiation:

- exposure
- dose
- dose equivalent

The dental radiographer must command a knowledge of radiation measurements to be able to discuss exposure and dose concepts with the dental patient.

At present two systems are used to define radiation measurements. The older system is referred to as the *traditional* or *standard system*. The newer system is the metric equivalent known as the *SI* or *Systeme Internationale*.

The traditional units of radiation measurement include:

- the roentgen (R)
- the radiation absorbed dose (rad)
- the roentgen equivalent (in) man (rem)

The SI units include:

- coulombs/kilogram (C/kg)
- the gray (Gy)
- the sievert (Sv)

This text uses both the traditional and SI units of measurement; the dental radiographer should be familiar with both systems and know how to convert from one system to the other (Table 4–3). In addition, the dental radiographer must be familiar with a number of physics terms used in the definitions of both the traditional and SI units of radiation measurement (Table 4–4).

Exposure Measurement

The term **exposure** refers to the measurement of ionization in air produced by x-rays. The traditional unit of exposure for x-rays is the **roentgen (R)**. The roentgen is a way of measuring radiation exposure by determining the amount of ionization that occurs in air. A definition follows:

Roentgen: the quantity of x-radiation or gamma radiation that produces an electrical charge of 2.58×10^{-4} coulombs in a kilogram of air at standard temperature and pressure (STP) conditions.

In measuring the roentgen, a known volume of air is irradiated. The interaction of x-ray photons with air molecules results in ionization, or the formation of ions. The ions (electrical charges) that are produced are collected and measured. One roentgen is equal to the amount of radiation that produces approximately 2 billion, or 2.08×10^9 ion pairs in 1 cubic centimeter (cc) of air.

The roentgen has limitations as a unit of measure. The roentgen measures the amount of energy that reaches the surface of an organism, but it does not describe the amount of radiation absorbed. The roentgen is essentially limited to measurements in air. By definition, it is only used for x-rays and gamma rays and does not include other types of radiation.

There is no SI unit for exposure equivalent to the roentgen. Instead, exposure is simply stated in coulombs per kilograms (C/kg). The **coulomb (C)** is a unit of electrical charge. The unit coulombs per kilogram measures the number of electrical charges, or the number of ion pairs, in 1 kilogram of air. The conver-

TABLE 4–3. Units of Radiation Measurement

Traditional Unit	Symbol	Definition	Conversion	SI Unit	Symbol	Definition	Conversion
Roentgen	R	1 R = 87 erg/g	1 R = 2.58 × 10⁻⁴ C	Coulombs per kilogram	C/kg	—	1 C/kg = 3880 R
Radiation absorbed dose	rad	1 rad = 100 erg/g	1 rad = 0.01 Gy	Gray	Gy	1 Gy = 0.01 J/kg	1 Gy = 100 rad
Roentgen equivalent (in) man	rem	1 rem = rad × QF	1 rem = 0.01 Sv	Sievert	Sv	1 Sv = Gy × QF	1 Sv = 100 rem

TABLE 4-4. Radiation Measurement Terms

Term	Abbreviation	Definition
Coulomb	C	Unit of electrical charge, the quantity of electrical charge transferred by 1 ampere in 1 second
Ampere	A	Unit of electrical current strength, current yielded by 1 volt against 1 ohm of resistance
Erg	erg	Unit of energy equivalent to 1.0×10^{-7} joules or to 2.4×10^{-8} calories
Joule	J	SI unit of energy equivalent to the work done by the force of 1 newton acting over the distance of 1 meter
Newton	N	SI unit of force; the force that when acting continuously upon a mass of 1 kilogram, will impart to it an acceleration of 1 meter per second squared
Kilogram	kg	A unit of mass equivalent to 1000 grams or 2.205 pounds

sions for roentgen and coulombs per kilogram can be expressed as follows:

$$1 \text{ R} = 2.58 \times 10^{-4} \text{ C/kg}$$
$$1 \text{ C/kg} = 3.88 \times 10^{3} \text{ R}$$

Dose Measurement

Dose can be defined as the amount of energy absorbed by a tissue. The **radiation absorbed dose**, or **rad**, is the traditional unit of dose. Unlike the roentgen, the rad is not restricted to air and can be applied to all kinds of radiations. A definition follows:

Rad: a special unit of absorbed dose that is equal to the deposition of 100 ergs of energy per gram of tissue (100 erg/g).

Using SI units, one rad is equivalent to 0.01 joule per kilogram (0.01 J/kg). The SI unit equivalent to the rad is the **gray (Gy)**, or 1 J/kg. The conversions for rad and Gy can be expressed as follows:

$$1 \text{ rad} = 0.01 \text{ Gy}$$
$$1 \text{ Gy} = 100 \text{ rads}$$

Dose Equivalent Measurement

Different types of radiation have different effects on tissues. The **dose equivalent** measurement is used to compare the biologic effects of different types of radiation. The traditional unit of the dose equivalent is the **roentgen equivalent (in) man**, or **rem**. A definition follows:

Rem: the product of absorbed dose (rads) and a quality factor specific for the type of radiation.

To place the exposure effects of different types of radiation on a common scale, a **quality factor (QF)**, or dimensionless multiplier is used. Each type of radiation has a specific quality factor based on the fact that different types of radiation produce different types of biologic damage. For example, the QF for x-rays is equal to 1.

The SI unit equivalent of the rem is the **sievert (Sv)**. Conversions for the rem and sievert can be expressed as follows:

$$1 \text{ rem} = 0.01 \text{ Sv}$$
$$1 \text{ Sv} = 100 \text{ rems}$$

Measurements Used in Dental Radiography

In dental radiography, the gray and sievert are equal, and the roentgen, rad, and rem are considered approximately equal. Smaller multiples of these radiation units are commonly used in dentistry because of the small quantities of radiation used during radiographic procedures. The prefix *milli*, meaning 1/1000, allows the dental radiographer to express small quantities of exposure, dose, and dose equivalent.

RADIATION RISKS

Sources of Radiation Exposure

To understand radiation risks, the dental radiographer must be familiar with the potential sources of radiation exposure that exist. Knowledge of the potential sources of radiation exposure can then be used to better understand the radiation risks associated with dentistry.

On a daily basis, humans are exposed to **back-**

ground radiation, a form of ionizing radiation that is ubiquitous in the environment. Naturally occurring background radiation includes cosmic radiation and terrestrial radiation. Cosmic radiation originates from the stars and sun. A person's exposure to cosmic radiation depends on altitude: the higher the altitude, the greater the exposure to cosmic radiation. Terrestrial radiation also occurs naturally and is emitted from radioactive materials present in the earth and air. Examples of terrestrial radiation include potassium-40 and uranium.

In the United States, the average dose of background radiation received by an individual ranges from 150 to 300 mrads (0.0015 Gy to 0.003 Gy) per year. This exposure may vary according to geographic location. For example, geographic areas that contain more radioactive materials are associated with increased amounts of terrestrial radiation, whereas geographic areas at higher elevations (e.g., Denver, Colorado) are associated with increased amounts of cosmic radiation.

In addition to naturally occurring background radiation, modern technology has created artificial, or man-made, sources of radiation. Consumer products (e.g., luminous wristwatches, television), fallout from atomic weapons, weapons production, and the nuclear fuel cycle are all sources of radiation exposure.

Medical radiation, another source of radiation exposure, is the single largest contributor to artificial radiation exposure. Medical radiation includes medical radiographic procedures, dental radiography, fluoroscopy, nuclear medicine, and radiation therapy. Medical radiation exposure equals the average yearly dose from all other exposures combined and typically accounts for half of the total exposure received. Table 4–5 summarizes the sources of low-level radiation discussed in this section of Chapter 4.

Risk and Risk Estimates

A **risk** can be defined as the likelihood of adverse effects or death resulting from exposure to a hazard. In dental radiography, risk is the likelihood of an adverse effect, specifically cancer induction, occurring from exposure to ionizing radiation.

The potential risk of dental radiography inducing a fatal cancer in an individual has been estimated to be approximately 3 in 1,000,000. The risk of a person developing cancer spontaneously is much higher, or 3300 in 1,000,000. To keep the concept of risk in perspective, the risk of incurring a fatal cancer from

TABLE 4–5. Radiation Sources and Exposure

Radiation Source	Whole Body (mrem/year)	Whole Body (Sv/year)
Natural		
Radon	200.00	0.002
Cosmic	27.00	0.00027
Terrestrial	28.00	0.00028
Internal	39.00	0.00039
Artificial		
Medical or dental	53.00	0.00053
Consumer products	9.00	0.00009
Other		
Occupational	<1.00	<0.00001
Nuclear fuel cycle	<1.00	<0.00001
Fallout	<1.00	<0.00001

dental radiographs should be compared to commonplace risks. For example, a 1 in 1,000,000 risk of a fatal outcome is associated with each of the following activities: riding 10 miles on a bike, 300 miles in an auto or 1000 miles in an airplane, or smoking 1.4 cigarettes per day. These risk estimates suggest that death is more likely to occur from common activities than from dental radiographic procedures and that cancer is far more likely to be unrelated to radiation exposure. In other words, the risks from dental radiography are not significantly greater than the risks of other everyday activities in modern life.

Dental Radiation and Exposure Risks

To calculate the risk from dental radiographic procedures, doses to critical organs must be measured. As previously defined, a critical organ, if damaged, diminishes the quality of an individual's life. With dental radiographic procedures, the critical organs at risk include the thyroid gland and active bone marrow. The skin and eyes may also be considered critical organs.

RISK ESTIMATES

Thyroid Gland. Although the thyroid gland is not irradiated by the primary beam in dental radiographic procedures, thyroid radiation exposure does occur. An estimated dose of 6000 mrad (0.06 Gy) is necessary to produce cancer in the thyroid gland; such a large dose is not incurred in dental radiography. Instead, the average dose to the thyroid gland (rectangular collimation, D-speed film, long PID, 20-film series) is 6 mrads (0.00006 Gy), or 1/1000 of the dose necessary to induce thyroid cancer.

Bone Marrow. The areas of the maxilla and mandible exposed during dental radiography account for a very small percentage of active bone marrow. The risk of cancer induction (leukemia) is directly associated with the amount of blood-producing tissues irradiated and the dose. Leukemia induction is most likely at doses of 5000 mrad (0.05 Gy) or more; a dose of such magnitude does not occur in dental radiography. The average bone marrow dose from periapical radiography is approximately 1 to 3 mrads (0.00001 to 0.00003 Gy) per film. Consequently, between 2000 and 5000 films would have to be exposed to induce leukemia.

Skin. A total of 250 rads (2.5 Gy) in a 14-day period causes erythema, or reddening, of the skin. To produce such changes, more than 500 dental films (E-speed film, exposure rate 0.7 R/second) in a 14-day period would have to be exposed. This is not a likely scenario in dental radiography.

Eyes. More than 200,000 mrads (2 Gy) are necessary to induce cataract formation (a cloudiness of the lens) in the eyes. Again, such high doses are not a consideration in dental radiography. Instead, the average surface dose to the cornea of the eye (D-speed film, long PID, 20-film series) is approximately 60 mrads (0.0006 Gy). In dental radiography, the chance of cataracts occurring is so unlikely that some scientists no longer consider the eyes a critical organ.

Patient Exposure and Dose

Dental patients must be protected from excess exposure to radiation. In Chapter 5, patient protection is discussed in detail. How much radiation exposure results from dental radiography? The amount of exposure varies depending on the following:

- **Film speed:** Radiation exposure can be limited by using the fastest film available. The use of E-speed film instead of D-speed reduces the absorbed dose by 50%.
- **Collimation:** Radiation exposure can be limited by using rectangular collimation. The use of rectangular collimation instead of round collimation reduces the absorbed dose by 60 to 70%.
- **Technique:** Radiation exposure can be limited by using a longer source-to-film distance. The use of the long cone paralleling technique and longer source-to-film distance reduces the skin dose.

- **Exposure factors:** Radiation exposure can be limited by using a higher kilovoltage peak. The use of higher kilovoltage peak reduces the skin dose.

Surface exposure, or the measure of the intensity of radiation at the patient's skin surface in coulombs per kilogram or roentgens, is commonly used when referring to patient exposure. A single intraoral radiograph (D-speed film, 70 kVp, long PID) results in a mean surface exposure of 250 mR. With E-speed film, a single intraoral radiograph results in a mean surface exposure of 125 mR.

The concept of absorbed dose may also be used when referring to patient exposure and dose. The absorbed dose from a 20-film series of dental radiographs (round collimation, E-speed film, long PID) is estimated to be 51 mrads (0.00051 Gy). If rectangular collimation is used, the absorbed dose decreases to approximately 16 mrads (0.00016 Gy) (Table 4–6).

Risk Versus Benefit of Dental Radiographs

X-radiation is harmful to living tissues. Because biologic damage results from x-ray exposure, dental radiographs should be prescribed for a patient *only* when the benefit of disease detection outweighs the risk of biologic damage. When dental radiographs are properly prescribed and exposed, the benefit of disease detection far outweighs the risk of damage due to x-radiation. The prescribing of dental radiographs is discussed in Chapter 5.

TABLE 4–6. Absorbed Doses from Intraoral Radiographs

Film	Absorbed Dose (mrad)
Bite-wing	
E-speed, 4 films, 16-inch PID, round	19.5
E-speed, 4 films, 16-inch PID, rectangular	3.1
Full Mouth Survey	
E-speed, 20 films, 16-inch PID, round	51.4
E-speed, 20 films, 16-inch PID, rectangular	16.1

Modified from Underhill TE, Chilvarquer I, Kazuyuki K, et al: Radiobiologic risk estimation from dental radiology. Oral Surg Oral Med Oral Pathol 66: 111–120, 1988.

◼️ SUMMARY

- All ionizing radiation is harmful and produces biologic changes in living tissue.
- Radiation injury occurs as a result of ionization or free radical formation.
- A dose-response curve is used to demonstrate the response (damage) of tissues to the dose (amount) of radiation received.
- A threshold dose for damage does not exist and the response of tissues is directly proportional to the dose received.
- Radiation injury follows a sequence of events: latent period, period of injury, and period of recovery.
- Radiation injury is affected by total dose, dose rate, amount of tissue irradiated, cell sensitivity, and age.
- Short-term radiation effects occur when large amounts of radiation are absorbed in a short period of time; long-term radiation effects occur when small amounts of radiation are absorbed over a long time period.
- Radiation effects are classified as somatic (seen in the person irradiated) or genetic (passed on to future generations).
- Cellular response to radiation depends on mitotic activity, cell differentiation, and cell metabolism.
- Radiosensitive cells include blood cells, immature reproductive cells, young bone cells, and epithelial cells. Radioresistant cells include the cells of bones, muscle, and nerve.
- Exposure is the measurement of ionization in air produced by x-rays, the units for exposure are the roentgen (R) and coulombs per kilogram (C/kg).
- Dose is the amount of energy absorbed by a tissue; the units for dose are the radiation absorbed dose (rad) and the gray (Gy).
- Dose equivalent measurement is used to compare the biologic effects of different types of radiation; the units for dose equivalent are the roentgen equivalent (in) man (rem) and the sievert (Sv).
- The risks of radiation exposure involved in dental radiography are not significantly greater than other everyday risks in life.
- The amount of exposure a patient receives from dental radiographs depends on the film speed, collimation, technique, and exposure factors used.
- Dental radiographs should be prescribed only for a patient when the benefit of disease detection outweighs the risk of damage from x-radiation.

BIBLIOGRAPHY

Frommer HH: Biologic effects of radiation. *In* Radiology for Dental Auxiliaries, 6th edition. St. Louis, Mosby-Year Book, 1996, pp. 49–65.

Goaz PW, White SC: Radiation biology. *In* Oral Radiology and Principles of Interpretation, 3rd edition. St. Louis, Mosby-Year Book, 1994, pp. 24–46.

Goaz PW, White SC: Health physics. *In* Oral Radiology and Principles of Interpretation, 3rd edition. St. Louis, Mosby-Year Book, 1994, pp. 47–68.

Johnson ON, McNally MA, Essay CE: Effects of radiation exposure. *In* Essentials of Dental Radiography for Dental Assistants and Hygienists, 6th edition. Norwalk, CT, Appleton and Lange, 1999, pp. 87–104.

Kasle MJ, Langlais RP: X-radiation measurement. *In* Basic Principles of Oral Radiography: Exercises in Dental Radiography, Vol. 4. Philadelphia, WB Saunders, 1981, pp. 134–139.

Kasle MJ, Langlais RP: Radiation biology. *In* Basic Principles of Oral Radiography: Exercises in Dental Radiography, Vol. 4. Philadelphia, WB Saunders, 1981, pp. 50–62.

Kelsey CA: Risk factors in diagnostic radiology. *In* Essentials of Radiology Physics. St. Louis, Warren H. Green, 1985, pp. 413–420.

Langland OE, Sippy FH, Langlais RP: Radiation biology. *In* Textbook of Dental Radiography, 2nd edition. Springfield, Charles C Thomas, 1984, pp. 153–160.

Langland OE, Sippy FH, Langlais RP: Radiation hazards and protection. *In* Textbook of Dental Radiography, 2nd edition. Springfield, Charles C Thomas, 1984, pp. 181–191.

Miles DA, Van Dis ML, Jensen CW, et al: Radiation biology and protection. *In* Radiographic Imaging for Dental Auxiliaries, 3rd edition. Philadelphia, WB Saunders, 1999, pp. 281–295.

Miles DA, Van Dis ML, Razmus TF: Radiation biology. *In* Basic Principles of Oral and Maxillofacial Radiology. Philadelphia, WB Saunders, 1992, pp. 22–29.

Miles DA, Van Dis ML, Razmus TF: Radiation protection. *In* Basic Principles of Oral and Maxillofacial Radiology. Philadelphia, WB Saunders, 1992, pp. 36–42.

Underhill TE, Chilvarquer I, Kazuyuki K, et al: Radiobiologic risk estimation from dental radiology. Oral Surgery Oral Medicine Oral Pathology 66:111–120, 1988.

Wilkins SR: Sources of low-level radiation exposure to the public. *In* Health Effects of Low-Level Radiation. Norwalk, CT, Appleton-Century-Crofts, 1984, pp. 4–45.

Quiz Questions

MULTIPLE CHOICE

___D___ 1. The latent period in radiation biology is the period of time between:

    a. exposure of film and development
    b. subsequent doses of radiation
    c. cell rest and cell mitosis
    d. exposure to x-radiation and clinical symptoms
    e. none of the above

___E___ 2. A free radical:

    a. is an uncharged molecule
    b. has an unpaired electron in the outer shell
    c. is highly reactive and unstable
    d. combines with molecules to form toxins
    e. all of the above

___A___ 3. Direct radiation injury occurs when:

    a. x-ray photons hit critical targets within a cell
    b. x-ray photons pass through the cell
    c. x-ray photons are absorbed and form toxins
    d. free radicals combine to form toxins
    e. none of the above

___C___ 4. Indirect radiation injury occurs when:

    a. x-ray photons hit critical targets within a cell
    b. x-ray photons pass through the cell
    c. x-ray photons are absorbed and form toxins
    d. x-ray photons hit the DNA of a cell
    e. none of the above

___C___ 5. Which of the following relationships describe the response of tissues to radiation?

    a. linear
    b. linear, threshold
    c. linear, nonthreshold
    d. nonlinear, nonthreshold
    e. none of the above

___E___ 6. Which of the following factors contribute to radiation injury?

    a. total dose
    b. dose rate
    c. cell sensitivity
    d. age
    e. all of the above

___D___ 7. Identify the correct statement.

    a. short-term effects are seen with small amounts of radiation absorbed in a short period
    b. short-term effects are seen with small amounts of radiation absorbed in a long period
    c. long-term effects are seen with small amounts of radiation absorbed in a short period
    d. long-term effects are seen with small amounts of radiation absorbed in a long period
    e. none of the above

_B_ 8. Radiation injuries that are not seen in the person irradiated but occur in future generations are termed:

  a. somatic effects
  b. genetic effects
  c. cumulative effects
  d. short-term effects
  e. long-term effects

_B_ 9. Which of the following is *most* susceptible to ionizing radiation?

  a. bone tissue
  b. small lymphocyte
  c. muscle tissue
  d. nerve tissue
  e. epithelial tissue

_D_ 10. The sensitivity of tissues to radiation is determined by:

  a. mitotic activity
  b. cell differentiation
  c. cell metabolism
  d. all of the above
  e. none of the above

_C_ 11. Which of the following is considered radioresistant?

  a. immature reproductive cells
  b. young bone cells
  c. mature bone cells
  d. epithelial cells
  e. none of the above

_A_ 12. An organ that if damaged diminishes the quality of an individual's life is termed a:

  a. critical organ
  b. somatic organ
  c. cumulative organ
  d. radioresistant organ
  e. none of the above

_E_ 13. The traditional unit for measuring x-ray exposure in air is termed:

  a. gray
  b. coulombs per kilogram
  c. rem
  d. rad
  e. roentgen

_C_ 14. The QF is used to determine which of the following radiation units:

  a. roentgen
  b. rad
  c. rem
  d. gray
  e. coulombs per kilogram

_____ B 15. The unit for measuring the absorption of x-rays is termed:

    a. roentgen
    b. rad
    c. rem
    d. QF
    e. sievert

_____ A 16. Identify the correct conversion.

    a. $1 R = 2.58 \times 10^{-4} C$
    b. $1 rad = 0.1 Gy$
    c. $1 rem = 0.1 Sv$
    d. $1 Gy = 10 rads$
    e. $1 Sv = 10 rem$

_____ A 17. Which of the following traditional units does not have an SI equivalent?

    a. roentgen
    b. rad
    c. rem
    d. QF
    e. none of the above

_____ E 18. Which of the following is used only for x-rays?

    a. sievert
    b. gray
    c. rem
    d. rad
    e. roentgen

_____ E 19. Identify the correct conversion(s).

    a. $1 R = 2.58 \times 10^{-4} C$
    b. $1 Gy = 100 rads$
    c. $1 Sv = 100 rem$
    d. $1 rem = rad \times QF$
    e. all of the above

_____ C 20. Identify the average dose of background radiation received by an individual in the United States.

    a. 0–100 mrads (0–0.001 Gy)
    b. 50–100 mrads (0.0005–0.001 Gy)
    c. 150–300 mrads (0.0015–0.003 Gy)
    d. 200–500 mrads (0.002–0.005 Gy)
    e. 500–1000 mrads (0.005–0.01 Gy)

_____ B 21. Identify the single largest contributor to artificial radiation exposure.

    a. radioactive materials
    b. medical radiation
    c. consumer products
    d. weapons production
    e. nuclear fuel cycle

_____ E   22. The amount of radiation exposure an individual receives varies depending on which of the following factors:

    a. film speed
    b. collimation
    c. technique
    d. exposure factors
    e. all of the above

_____ B   23. A single intraoral radiograph (D-speed film, 70 kVp, long PID) results in a mean surface exposure of:

    a. 50 mR
    b. 250 mR
    c. 500 mR
    d. 1 R
    e. 5 R

_____ D   24. Identify the dose at which leukemia induction is most likely to occur.

    a. 500 mrads (0.005 Gy)
    b. 1000 mrads (0.01 Gy)
    c. 2000 mrads (0.02 Gy)
    d. 5000 mrads (0.05 Gy)
    e. none of the above

_____ A   25. Identify the incorrect statement.

    a. x-radiation is not harmful to living tissues
    b. dental radiographs benefit the patient
    c. in dental radiography, the benefit of disease detection outweighs the risk of damage due to radiation
    d. radiographs should be prescribed only when the benefit outweighs the risk
    e. biologic damage results from x-ray exposure

Answers are supplied at the end of this book.

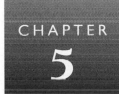

CHAPTER

5

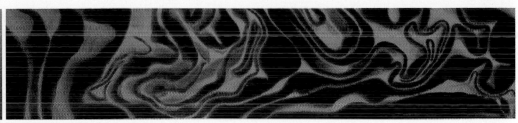

Radiation Protection

OBJECTIVES

After completion of this chapter, the student will be able to:

- *Define the key words.*
- *Describe in detail the basics of patient protection prior to x-ray exposure.*
- *Discuss the different types of filtration and state the recommended total filtration for dental x-ray machines operating above and below 70 kVp.*
- *Describe the collimator used in dental x-ray machines and state the recommended diameter of the useful beam at the patient's skin.*
- *List six ways to protect the patient from excess radiation during x-ray exposure.*
- *Describe the importance of film handling and processing after patient exposure to x-rays.*
- *Discuss operator protection in terms of adequate distance, shielding, and avoidance of the useful beam.*
- *Describe personnel and equipment monitoring devices used to detect radiation.*
- *Discuss radiation exposure guidelines, including radiation safety legislation, MPD, MAD, and ALARA.*
- *Discuss with the dental patient what radiation protection steps will be used before, during, and after x-ray exposure.*

INTRODUCTION

Many of the early pioneers in dental radiography suffered from the adverse effects of radiation. As discussed in Chapter 1, some of these pioneers lost fingers, limbs, and ultimately their lives to excessive doses of radiation. Today, the hazards of radiation are well documented, and radiation protection measures can be used to minimize radiation exposure to both the dental patient and the dental radiographer.

The purpose of this chapter is to discuss patient protection before, during, and after exposure to x-rays, to detail operator protection methods, and to present radiation exposure and safety guidelines. In addition, this chapter also includes a discussion of patient education about radiation protection.

PATIENT PROTECTION

X-radiation causes biologic changes in living cells and adversely affects all living tissue. With the use of proper patient protection techniques, the amount of x-radiation received by a dental patient can be minimized. Patient protection techniques can be used prior to, during, and after x-ray exposure.

Prior to Exposure

Patient protection measures can be used prior to any x-radiation exposure. Proper prescribing of dental radiographs and the use of equipment that complies with state and federal radiation guidelines can minimize the amount of x-radiation that a dental patient receives.

PRESCRIBING DENTAL RADIOGRAPHS

The first important step in limiting the amount of x-radiation a dental patient receives is the proper prescribing, or ordering, of dental radiographs. The person responsible for prescribing dental radiographs is the dentist. The professional judgment of the dentist is used to make decisions about the number, type, and frequency of dental radiographs.

Every patient's dental condition is different, and consequently, every patient should be evaluated for dental radiographs on an individual basis. A radiographic examination should never include a predetermined number of radiographs, nor should radiographs be taken at predetermined time intervals. For example, the dentist who prescribes a set number of radiographs (e.g., four bite-wings) at a set time interval (e.g., every 6 months) for every patient is not taking the individual needs of that patient into consideration.

The American Dental Association, in conjunction with the Food and Drug Administration (FDA), has adopted guidelines for prescribing the number, type, and frequency of dental radiographs. These guidelines summarize the recommendations that promote patient protection in diagnostic radiography (Table 5–1).

PROPER EQUIPMENT

Another important step in limiting the amount of x-radiation a dental patient receives is the use of proper equipment. The dental x-ray tubehead must be equipped with appropriate aluminum filters, lead collimator, and position-indicating device.

FILTRATION

There are two types of **filtration** used in the dental x-ray tubehead: inherent filtration and added filtration.

Inherent Filtration. **Inherent filtration** takes place when the primary beam passes through the glass window of the x-ray tube, the insulating oil, and the tubehead seal. The inherent filtration of the dental x-ray machine is equivalent to approximately 0.5 to 1.0 millimeter (mm) of aluminum. Inherent filtration alone does not meet the standards regulated by state and federal law. Therefore, added filtration is required.

Added Filtration. **Added filtration** refers to the placement of aluminum disks in the path of the x-ray beam between the collimator and the tubehead seal in the dental x-ray machine (Fig. 5–1). Aluminum disks can be added to the tubehead in 0.5-mm increments. The purpose of the aluminum disks is to filter out the longer wavelength, low-energy x-rays from the x-ray beam (Fig. 5–2). The low-energy, longer wavelength x-rays are harmful to the patient and are not useful in diagnostic radiography. Filtration of the x-ray beam results in a higher energy and more penetrating useful beam.

Total Filtration. The required thickness of **total filtration** (inherent plus added filtration) is regulated by state and federal law: dental x-ray machines operating at or below 70 kVp require a minimum total of 1.5 mm aluminum filtration, and machines operating above 70 kVp require a minimum total of 2.5 mm aluminum filtration.

COLLIMATION

Collimation is used to restrict the size and shape of the x-ray beam and to reduce patient exposure. A **collimator,** or lead plate with a hole in the middle, is fitted directly over the opening of the machine housing where the x-ray beam exits the tubehead (Fig. 5–3).

A collimator may have either a round or rectangular opening (Fig. 5–4). A rectangular collimator restricts the size of the x-ray beam to an area slightly larger than a size 2 intraoral film and significantly reduces patient exposure. A circular collimator produces a cone-shaped beam that is 2.75 inches in diameter, considerably larger than a size 2 intraoral film (Fig. 5–5). When using a circular collimator, federal regulations require that the x-ray beam be collimated to a

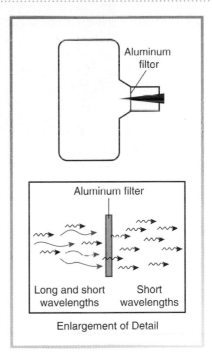

FIGURE 5–2. The purpose of placing aluminum disks in the path of the beam is to filter out the low-energy, long wavelengths that are harmful to the patient.

diameter of no more than 2.75 inches as it exits from the position-indicating device and reaches the skin of the patient (Fig. 5–6).

POSITION-INDICATING DEVICE

The **position-indicating device (PID),** or cone, appears as an extension of the x-ray tubehead and is used to direct the x-ray beam. There are three basic types of PIDs:

- conical
- rectangular
- round

The conical PID appears as a closed, pointed plastic cone. When x-rays exit from the pointed cone, they penetrate the plastic and produce scatter radiation (Fig. 5–7). To eliminate cone-produced scatter radiation, the conical PID is no longer used in dentistry. Instead, open-ended and lead-lined rectangular or round PIDs are used that do not produce scatter radiation (Fig. 5–8).

Both rectangular and round PIDs are commonly available in two lengths:

- short (8-inch)
- long (16-inch)

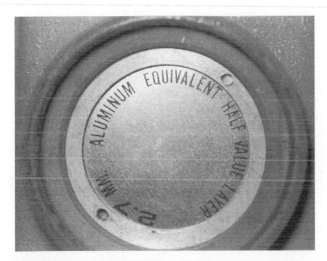

FIGURE 5–1. Aluminum disks are placed between the collimator and tubehead seal for added filtration. (From Miles DA, Van Dis ML, Jensen CW, Ferretti A: Radiographic Imaging for Dental Auxiliaries, 2nd ed. Philadelphia, WB Saunders, 1993.)

TABLE 5–1. Guidelines for Prescribing Dental Radiographs

The recommendations in this chart are subject to clinical judgment and may not apply to every patient. They are to be used by dentists only after reviewing the patient's health history and completing a clinical examination. The recommendations do not need to be altered because of pregnancy.

Patient Category	Child — Primary Dentition (prior to eruption of first permanent tooth)	Child — Transitional Dentition (following eruption of first permanent tooth)	Adolescent — Permanent Dentition (prior to eruption of third molars)	Adult — Dentulous	Adult — Edentulous
New Patient* All new patients to assess dental diseases and growth and development	Posterior bite-wing examination if proximal surfaces of primary teeth cannot be visualized or probed	Individualized radiographic examination consisting of periapical/occlusal views and posterior bite-wings or panoramic examination and posterior bitewings	Individualized radiographic examination consisting of posterior bite-wings and selected periapicals. A full mouth intraoral radiographic examination is appropriate when the patient presents with clinical evidence of generalized dental disease or a history of extensive dental treatment.		Full mouth intraoral radiographic examination or panoramic examination
Recall Patient* Clinical caries or high-risk factors for caries**	Posterior bite-wing examination at 6-month intervals or until no carious lesions are evident		Posterior bite-wing examination at 6- to 12-month intervals or until no carious lesions are evident	Posterior bite-wing examination at 12- to 18-month intervals	Not applicable
No clinical caries and no high-risk factors for caries**	Posterior bite-wing examination at 12- to 24-month intervals if proximal surfaces of primary teeth cannot be visualized or probed	Posterior bite-wing examination at 12- to 24-month intervals	Posterior bite-wing examination at 18- to 36-month intervals	Posterior bite-wing examination at 24- to 36-month intervals	Not applicable
Periodontal disease or a history of periodontal treatment	Individualized radiographic examination consisting of selected periapical and/or bite-wing radiographs for areas where periodontal disease (other than nonspecific gingivitis) can be demonstrated clinically		Individualized radiographic examination consisting of selected periapical and/or bite-wing radiographs for areas where periodontal disease (other than nonspecific gingivitis) can be demonstrated clinically		Not applicable

* Clinical situations for which radiographs may be indicated include:

A. Positive Historical Findings
1. Previous periodontal or endodontic therapy
2. History of pain or trauma
3. Familial history of dental anomalies
4. Postoperative evaluation of healing
5. Presence of implants

B. Positive Clinical Signs/Symptoms
1. Clinical evidence of periodontal disease
2. Large or deep restorations
3. Deep carious lesions
4. Malposed or clinically impacted teeth
5. Swelling
6. Evidence of facial trauma
7. Mobility of teeth
8. Fistula or sinus tract infection
9. Clinically suspected sinus pathology
10. Growth abnormalities
11. Oral involvement in known or suspected systemic disease
12. Positive neurologic findings in the head and neck
13. Evidence of foreign objects
14. Pain and/or dysfunction of the temporomandibular joint
15. Facial asymmetry
16. Abutment teeth for fixed or removable partial prosthesis
17. Unexplained bleeding
18. Unexplained sensitivity of teeth

Growth and development assessment	Usually not indicated	Individualized radiographic examination consisting of a periapical/occlusal or panoramic examination	Periapical or panoramic examination to assess developing third molars	Usually not indicated	Usually not indicated

19. Unusual eruption, spacing or migration of teeth
20. Unusual tooth morphology, calcification or color
21. Missing teeth with unknown reason

**

Patients at high risk for caries may demonstrate any of the following:

1. High level of caries experience
2. History of recurrent caries
3. Existing restoration of poor quality
4. Poor oral hygiene
5. Inadequate fluoride exposure
6. Prolonged nursing (bottle or breast)
7. Diet with high sucrose frequency
8. Poor family dental health
9. Developmental enamel defects
10. Developmental disability
11. Xerostomia
12. Genetic abnormality of teeth
13. Many multisurface restorations
14. Chemo/radiation therapy.

The recommendations contained in this table have been developed by an expert panel composed of representatives from the Academy of General Dentistry, American Academy of Dental Radiology, American Academy of Oral Medicine, American Academy of Pediatric Dentistry, American Academy of Periodontology and the American Dental Association under the sponsorship of the Food and Drug Administration (FDA). This chart has been reproduced and distributed to the dental community by Eastman Kodak Company in cooperation with the FDA. (Reprinted courtesy of Eastman Kodak Company.)

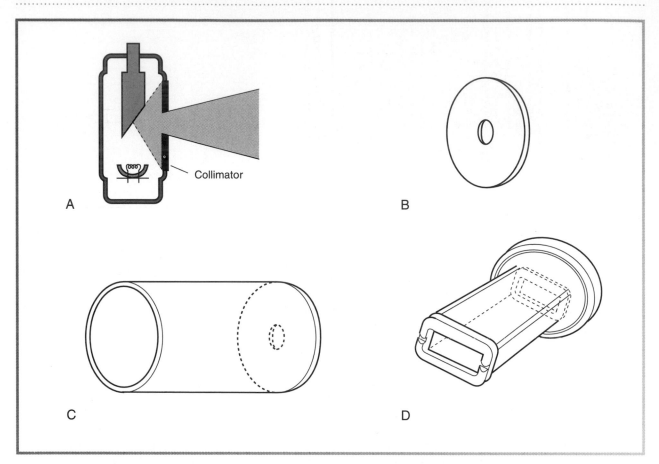

FIGURE 5–3. *A,* Collimation of an x-ray beam (shown in color) is achieved by restricting its useful size. *B,* Diaphragm collimator. *C,* Tubular collimator. *D,* Rectangular collimator. (From Goaz PW, White SC: Oral Radiology: Principles and Interpretation, 3rd ed. St. Louis, Mosby-Year Book, 1994.)

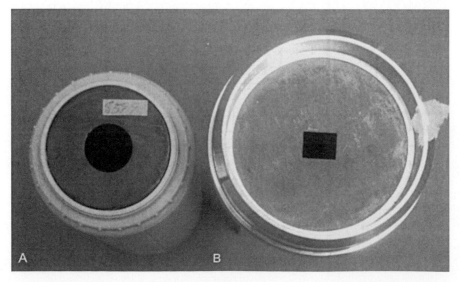

FIGURE 5–4. The hole in the collimator may be either round or rectangular. (From Miles DA, Van Dis ML, Jensen CS, Ferretti A: Radiographic Imaging for Dental Auxiliaries, 2nd ed. Philadelphia, WB Saunders, 1993.)

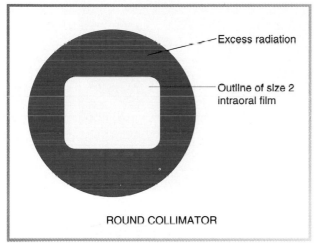

A

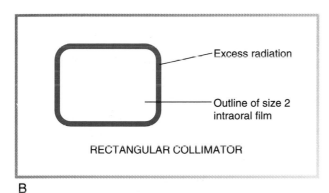

B

FIGURE 5-5. *A,* The beam produced by a circular collimator is 2.75 inches in diameter, which is much larger than a size 2 intraoral film. *B,* The beam produced by a rectangular collimator is just slightly larger than a size 2 intraoral film.

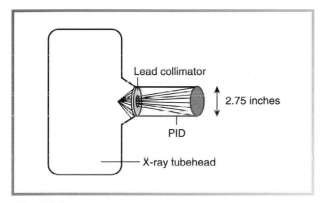

FIGURE 5-6. Federal regulations require that the diameter of a collimated x-ray beam be restricted to 2.75 inches at the patient's skin. PID, position indicating device.

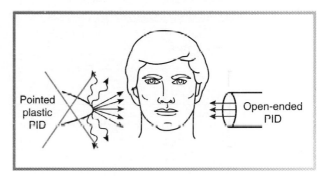

FIGURE 5-7. A plastic, pointed position-indicating device (PID) produces scatter radiation and is no longer used in dentistry.

The long PID is preferred because less divergence of the x-ray beam occurs (Fig. 5-9). Of the three types of PID, the rectangular type is most effective in reducing patient exposure.

During Exposure

Patient protection measures are used not only prior to x-ray exposure but also during exposure. A thyroid collar, lead apron, fast film, and film-holding devices are all used during x-ray exposure to limit the amount of radiation received by the patient. Proper selection of exposure factors and good technique further protect the patient from excess exposure to x-radiation.

THYROID COLLAR

The **thyroid collar** is a flexible lead shield that is placed securely around the patient's neck to protect the thyroid gland from scatter radiation (Fig. 5-10). The lead prevents radiation from reaching the gland and protects the highly radiosensitive tissues of the thyroid. The thyroid collar may exist as a separate shield or as part of the lead apron.

The thyroid gland is exposed to x-radiation during oral radiographic procedures because of its location. The use of the thyroid collar is recommended for all intraoral films (films that are placed inside the mouth). However, use of the thyroid collar is not recommended with extraoral films (films placed outside the mouth) because it obscures information on the film and results in a nondiagnostic radiograph.

LEAD APRON

The **lead apron** is a flexible shield that is placed over the patient's chest and lap to protect the reproductive and blood-forming tissues from scatter radiation: the

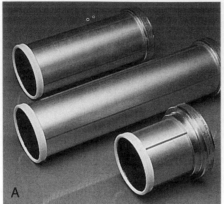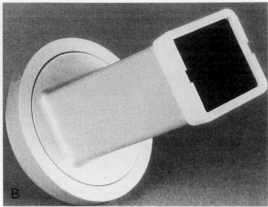

FIGURE 5–8. *A,* Open-ended, lead-lined position-indicating devices (PIDs) do not produce scatter radiation. Examples of round PIDs. *B,* Open-ended, lead-lined rectangular PID. (*A* and *B* courtesy of Rinn Corporation, Elgin, IL.)

lead prevents the radiation from reaching these radiosensitive organs (Fig. 5–11). Use of a lead apron is recommended for all intraoral and extraoral films. Many state laws mandate the use of a lead apron on all patients.

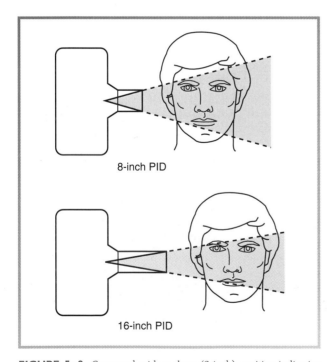

8-inch PID

16-inch PID

FIGURE 5–9. Compared with a short (8-inch) position-indicating device [PID], the longer (16-inch) PID is preferred because it produces less divergence of the x-ray beam.

FAST FILM

Fast film is the single most effective method of reducing a patient's exposure to x-radiation. Fast film is available for both intraoral and extraoral radiography. **E-speed,** or **Ektaspeed,** is the fastest intraoral film available. Prior to the introduction of E-speed film, **D-speed,** or **Ultra-Speed,** was the fastest film available. E-speed film is twice as fast as D-speed film and requires only one-half the exposure time.

FILM-HOLDING DEVICES

Film-holding devices are also effective in reducing a patient's exposure to x-radiation. A film-holding device helps to stabilize the film position in the mouth and reduces the chances of movement (Fig. 5–12). In addition, it eliminates the need for the patient to hold the film in place, and therefore, the patient's finger is not exposed to unnecessary radiation.

EXPOSURE FACTOR SELECTION

Exposure factor selection also limits the amount of x-radiation exposure received by a patient. The dental radiographer can control the exposure factors by adjusting the kilovoltage peak, milliamperage, and time settings on the control panel of the dental x-ray machine. A setting of 70 to 90 kVp keeps patient exposure to a minimum. On some dental x-ray units, the kilovoltage peak and milliamperage settings are preset by the manufacturer and cannot be adjusted. Exposure factors and their effect on the resultant radiographs are discussed in Chapter 3.

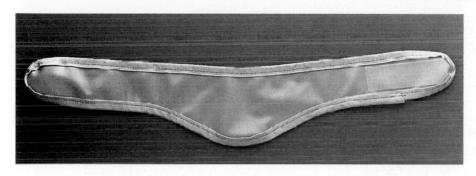

FIGURE 5–10. A thyroid collar. (Courtesy of Rinn Corporation, Elgin, IL.)

PROPER TECHNIQUE

Proper technique helps to ensure the diagnostic quality of films and reduce the amount of exposure a patient receives. Films that are nondiagnostic must be retaken; this results in additional radiation exposure to the patient. *All retakes must be avoided.*

To produce diagnostic films, one must have a thorough knowledge of the techniques commonly used in dental radiography. Techniques used most often include the paralleling technique, the bisecting technique, and the bite-wing technique. In addition to knowing how each film is exposed using these techniques, good technique requires an organized routine for taking the films. (Intraoral techniques are discussed in detail in Chapters 17, 18, and 19.)

After Exposure

The radiographer's role in limiting the amount of x-radiation a patient receives does not end during exposure. After the films have been exposed, they must be handled and processed. Meticulous film handling and proper processing techniques are critical for the production of high-quality diagnostic radiographs.

PROPER FILM HANDLING

Proper film handling is necessary to produce diagnostic radiographs and to limit patient exposure to x-radiation. From the time the films are exposed until they are processed, careful handling is of the utmost

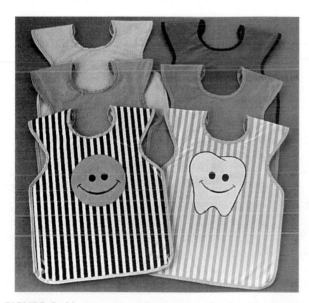

FIGURE 5–11. Examples of lead aprons. The thyroid collar may be attached to the lead apron or may exist as a separate shield. (Courtesy of Rinn Corporation, Elgin, IL.)

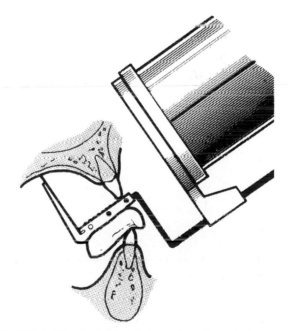

FIGURE 5–12. Film-holding devices reduce the patient's exposure to radiation by stabilizing the film in the mouth. (Courtesy of Rinn Corporation, Elgin, IL.)

importance. Artifacts due to improper film handling (see Chapter 9) result in nondiagnostic films. A nondiagnostic film must be retaken and consequently exposes the patient to excess radiation.

PROPER FILM PROCESSING

Proper film processing (developing) is also necessary to produce diagnostic radiographs and to limit patient exposure to x-radiation. Improper film processing (see Chapter 9) can render films nondiagnostic, thereby requiring retakes and needlessly exposing the patient to excess x-radiation.

OPERATOR PROTECTION

The dental radiographer must use proper protection measures to avoid occupational exposure to x-radiation (e.g., primary radiation, leakage radiation, and scatter radiation). The use of proper operator protection techniques can minimize the amount of radiation that a dental radiographer receives. Operator protection measures include following operator protection guidelines and using radiation-monitoring devices.

Operator Protection Guidelines

The purpose of operator protection guidelines is to provide the dental radiographer with basic safety information that is needed when working with x-radiation. Such guidelines are based on the following rule: *The dental radiographer must avoid the primary beam.* Operator protection guidelines include recommendations on distance, position, and shielding.

DISTANCE RECOMMENDATIONS

One of the most effective ways for the operator to avoid the primary beam and limit x-radiation exposure is to maintain an adequate distance during exposure. The dental radiographer must stand at least 6 feet away from the x-ray tubehead during x-ray exposure. When this distance is not possible, a protective barrier must be used.

POSITION RECOMMENDATIONS

Another important way for the operator to avoid the primary beam is to maintain proper positioning during x-ray exposure. To avoid the primary beam (which travels in a straight line) the dental radiographer must

be positioned perpendicular to the primary beam or at a 90- to 135-degree angle to the beam (Fig. 5–13).

Proper operator position also includes the following:

- The dental radiographer must *never* hold a film in place for a patient during x-ray exposure
- The dental radiographer must *never* hold the tubehead during x-ray exposure

SHIELDING RECOMMENDATIONS

Adequate shielding can greatly reduce the occupational exposure of the dental radiographer. **Protective barriers** that absorb the primary beam can be incorporated into the office design, thus protecting the operator from primary and scatter radiation. Whenever possible, the dental radiographer should stand behind a protective barrier such as a wall during x-ray exposure. Most dental offices incorporate adequate shielding in walls through the use of several thicknesses of common construction materials, such as dry wall.

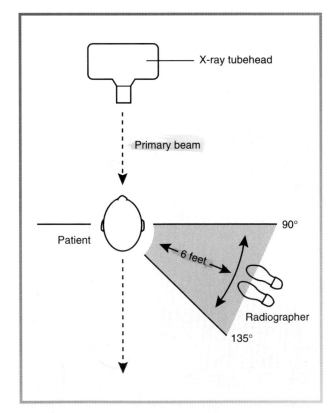

FIGURE 5–13. Operator protection guidelines suggest that the dental radiographer stand at an angle of 90 to 135 degrees to the primary beam.

Radiation Monitoring

Radiation monitoring can also be used to protect the dental radiographer and includes the monitoring of both equipment and personnel. The use of radiation monitoring can identify excess occupational exposure.

EQUIPMENT MONITORING

Dental x-ray machines must be monitored for leakage radiation. **Leakage radiation** is any radiation, with the exception of the primary beam, that is emitted from the dental tubehead. For example, if a dental x-ray tubehead has a faulty tubehead seal, leakage radiation results. Dental x-ray equipment can be monitored for leakage radiation through the use of a film device that can be obtained through the State Health Department or from manufacturers of dental x-ray equipment.

PERSONNEL MONITORING

The amount of x-radiation that reaches the body of the dental radiographer can be measured through the use of a personnel monitoring device known as a **film badge.** A film badge can be obtained from a film badge service company.

The film badge consists of a piece of radiographic film in a plastic holder (Fig. 5–14). Each radiographer should have his or her own film badge; the film badge

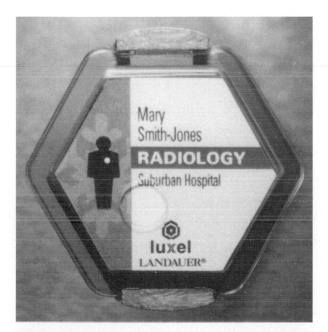

FIGURE 5–14. A film badge is used to measure the radiation exposure received by the dental radiographer. (Courtesy of Landauer, Glenwood, IL.)

should be worn at waist level whenever the dental radiographer is exposing x-ray films. When film badges are not worn, they should be stored in a radiation-safe area. A film badge should *never* be worn when the radiographer is undergoing x-ray exposure.

After the dental radiographer has worn the film badge for a specific time interval (e.g., one week, one month), the badge is returned to the service company. The film badge service company then processes and evaluates the film for exposure and provides the dental office with an exposure report for each radiographer.

RADIATION EXPOSURE GUIDELINES

All x-radiation is harmful. To protect the patient and operator from excess radiation exposure, radiation exposure guidelines have been established. Radiation exposure guidelines include radiation safety legislation and exposure limits for the general public and for persons who are occupationally exposed to radiation. Strict adherence to such guidelines is a must for all dental radiographers.

Radiation Safety Legislation

Radiation safety legislation has been established at both the state and federal levels to protect the patient, operator, and general public from radiation hazards. At the federal level, the Radiation Control for Health and Safety Act was enacted in 1968 to standardize the performance of x-ray equipment. Also at the federal level, the Consumer-Patient Radiation Health and Safety Act was enacted in 1981 to address the issues of the education and certification of persons using radiographic equipment.

Radiation legislation varies greatly from state to state; the dental radiographer must be familiar with the laws that apply to his or her work place. For example, in some states, before a dental radiographer can expose dental x-rays, he or she must successfully complete a radiation safety examination.

Maximum Permissible Dose

Radiation protection standards dictate the maximum dose of radiation that an individual can receive. The **maximum permissible dose (MPD)** is defined by the National Council on Radiation Protection and Measurements (NCRP) as the maximum dose equivalent that a body is permitted to receive in a specific period of time. The MPD is the dose of radiation that the body can endure with little or no injury.

The NCRP published the complete set of basic recommendations specifying dose limits for exposure to ionizing radiation in 1987, 1991, and 1993. This most recent report states the current MPD for occupationally exposed persons, or persons who work with radiation (e.g., dental radiographers), is 5.0 rem/year (0.05 Sv/year). For nonoccupationally exposed persons, the current MPD is 0.1 rem/year (0.001 Sv/year). The MPD for an occupationally exposed pregnant woman is the same as that for a nonoccupationally exposed person, or 0.1 rem/year (0.001 Sv/year).

Maximum Accumulated Dose

Occupationally exposed workers must not exceed an accumulated lifetime radiation dose. This is referred to as the **maximum accumulated dose (MAD).** MAD is determined by a formula based on the worker's age. To determine the MAD for an occupationally exposed person, the following formula is used:

$$MAD = (N - 18) \times 5 \text{ rem/year}$$
$$MAD = (N - 18) \times 0.05 \text{ Sv/year}$$

where N refers to the person's age in years. (Note that the number 18 refers to the minimum required age of a person who works with radiation.)

ALARA Concept

The **ALARA concept** states that all exposure to radiation must be kept to a minimum, or "*as low as reasonably achievable.*" To provide protection for both patients and operators, every possible method of reducing exposure to radiation should be employed to minimize risk. The radiation protection measures detailed in this chapter can be used to minimize patient and operator exposure, thus keeping radiation exposure "as low as reasonably achievable."

RADIATION PROTECTION AND PATIENT EDUCATION

Patients often have questions about radiation exposure. The dental radiographer must be prepared to answer such questions and to educate the dental patient about radiation protection topics. Patient education about radiation protection may take the form of an informal conversation or printed literature.

The dental radiographer must be prepared to explain exactly how patients are protected before, during, and after x-ray exposure. An informal discussion can take place as the dental radiographer prepares the patient for x-ray exposure. For example, as the dental radiographer places the lead apron and thyroid collar on the patient, he or she can make the following comments:

"Before we get started, let me tell you just how our office does all that is possible to protect you from unnecessary radiation."

"Before we expose you to any x-rays, the dentist custom orders your x-rays based on your individual needs. The x-ray equipment we use is frequently tested to ensure that state and federal radiation safety guidelines are met."

"During x-ray exposure we use a thyroid collar and a lead apron to protect your body from excess radiation. We use the fastest film available and a device to hold the film so that your fingers are not exposed to radiation. We also use good technique so we avoid making mistakes that require further exposure."

"Even after your dental x-ray films have been taken, we take steps to process the films carefully so that we don't have to take them over again. Hopefully, this quick review of radiation protection techniques has answered some of the questions you may have about dental x-rays. Do you have any questions before we begin?"

In addition to such an informal discussion, printed handouts or pamphlets outlining the steps used to protect patients from excess radiation can also be made available to the patient. Radiation protection pamphlets can be placed in the reception area or in the room where dental x-rays are taken.

SUMMARY

- Prior to x-ray exposure, the proper prescribing of dental radiographs and the use of proper equipment can minimize the amount of radiation that a patient receives.
- Radiographs must be prescribed by the dentist based on the individual needs of the patient.
- In the x-ray tubehead, aluminum disks are used to filter out the longer wavelength, low-energy x-rays from the x-ray beam.

- In the x-ray tubehead a collimator (lead plate with a hole in the middle) is used to restrict the size and shape of the x-ray beam.
- The PID is used to direct the x-ray beam; the rectangular PID is most effective in reducing patient exposure to x-rays.
- During x-ray exposure, a thyroid collar, a lead apron, fast film, and film-holding devices can be used to protect the patient from excess exposure to radiation. Proper selection of exposure factors and good technique can also be used to protect the patient.
- After x-ray exposure, careful film handling and film processing techniques are critical for the production of diagnostic radiographs.
- During x-ray exposure, the dental radiographer must always follow operator protection guidelines and avoid the **primary beam** (maintain an adequate distance) and use proper positioning and shielding.
- The dental radiographer must *never* hold a film or the tubehead in place for a patient during x-ray exposure.
- Radiation monitoring must include the monitoring of equipment and personnel.
- Federal and state legislation has been established that protects the patient, the operator, and the general public from radiation hazards.
- Exposure limits have been established for the general public and persons who work with radiation; the maximum permissible dose (MPD) for persons who work with radiation (e.g., dental radiographers) is 5.0 rem/year (0.05 Sv/year), the MPD for persons who do not work with radiation is 0.1 rem/year (0.001 Sv/year).
- ALARA (*as low as reasonably achievable*) is a concept that states that all exposure to radiation must be kept to a minimum.
- The dental radiographer must be prepared to explain how patients are protected before, during, and after x-ray exposure.

BIBLIOGRAPHY

Barr JH, Stephens RG: Radiological health. *In* Dental Radiology: Pertinent Basic Concepts and Their Application in Clinical Practice. Philadelphia, WB Saunders, 1980, pp. 66–80.

Frommer HH: Radiation protection. *In* Radiology for Dental Auxiliaries, 6th edition. St. Louis, Mosby-Year Book, 1996, pp. 67–87.

Goaz PW, White SC: Health physics. *In* Oral Radiology: Principles of Interpretation, 3rd edition. St. Louis, Mosby Year Book, 1994, pp. 47–68.

Haring JI, Lind LJ: The importance of dental radiographs and interpretation. *In* Radiographic Interpretation for the Dental Hygienist. Philadelphia, WB Saunders, 1993, pp. 1–12.

Johnson ON, McNally MA, Essay CE: Radiation protection. *In* Essentials of Dental Radiography for Dental Assistants and Hygienists, 6th edition. Norwalk, CT, Appleton and Lange, 1999, pp. 105–130.

Johnson ON, McNally MA, Essay CE: Patient relations and education. *In* Essentials of Dental Radiography for Dental Assistants and Hygienists, 6th edition. Norwalk, CT, Appleton and Lange, 1999, pp. 493–505.

Kasle MJ, Langlais RP: Basic Principles of Oral Radiography. Exercises in Dental Radiology, vol. 4. Philadelphia, WB Saunders, 1981, pp. 41–48.

Kasle MJ, Langlais RP: Basic Principles of Oral Radiography. Exercises in Dental Radiology, vol. 4. Philadelphia, WB Saunders, 1981, pp. 144–158.

Langland OE, Langlais RP: Radiologic health and protection. *In* Principles of Dental Imaging. Baltimore, Williams & Wilkins, 1997, pp. 311–328.

Langland OE, Sippy FH, Langlais RP: Radiation hazards and prevention. *In* Textbook of Dental Radiography, 2nd edition. Springfield, IL, Charles C Thomas, 1984, pp. 181–205.

Manson-Hing LR: Biologic effects, x-ray production, and radiologic health. *In* Fundamentals of Dental Radiography, 3rd edition. Philadelphia, Lea & Febiger, 1990, pp. 108–130.

Manson-Hing LR: Patient relations. *In* Fundamentals of Dental Radiography, 3rd edition. Philadelphia, Lea & Febiger, 1990, pp. 221–229.

Matteson SR, Whaley C, Secrist VC: Radiation biology and protection. *In* Dental Radiology, 4th edition. Chapel Hill, University of North Carolina Press, 1988, pp. 21–30.

Miles DA, Van Dis ML, Razmus TF: Radiation protection. *In* Basic Principles of Oral and Maxillofacial Radiology. Philadelphia, WB Saunders, 1992, pp. 37–48.

Miles DA, Van Dis ML, Jensen CW, Ferretti A: Intraoral radiographic technique. *In* Radiographic Imaging for Dental Auxiliaries, 3rd edition. Philadelphia, WB Saunders, 1999, pp. 1–47.

Miles DA, Van Dis ML, Jensen CW, Ferretti A: Radiation biology and protection. *In* Radiographic Imaging for Dental Auxiliaries, 3rd edition. Philadelphia, WB Saunders, 1999, pp. 281–295.

NCRP Report No. 116: Limitation of exposure to ionizing radiation. National Council on Radiation Protection and Measurements, 1993.

O'Brien RC: Biological effects of ionizing radiation. *In* Dental Radiography: An Introduction for Dental Hygienists and Assistants, 4th edition. Philadelphia, WB Saunders, 1982, pp. 26–41.

Quiz Questions ···

TRUE OR FALSE

_T_   1. Every patient should be evaluated for dental radiographs on an individual basis.

_F_   2. The 8-inch PID is more effective in reducing radiation exposure to the patient than the 16-inch PID.

_T_   3. Pointed cones should not be used because they increase scatter radiation.

_F_   4. The thyroid collar must be worn for all intraoral and extraoral films.

_F_   5. If necessary, the dental radiographer may hold a film in the patient's mouth to ensure a diagnostic image.

MULTIPLE CHOICE

_B_   6. Which of the following describes the use of a filter in a dental x-ray tubehead?

         a. a filter reduces the size and shape of the beam
         b. a filter removes low-energy x-rays
         c. a filter removes the dose of radiation to the thyroid gland
         d. a filter decreases the mean energy of the beam

_C_   7. Which of the following is *not* a component of inherent filtration?

         a. oil
         b. unleaded glass window
         c. a leaded cone
         d. tubehead seal

_B_   8. Which of the following is the single most effective method of reducing patient exposure to radiation?

         a. lead apron
         b. fast films
         c. round PID
         d. film-holding devices

_B_   9. Which of the following position-indicating devices is *most* effective in reducing patient exposure?

         a. conical PID
         b. rectangular PID
         c. round PID
         d. all are equally effective in reducing patient exposure

_B_   10. Which of the following is the device that restricts the size and shape of the x-ray beam?

         a. filter
         b. collimator
         c. barrier
         d. film badge

_A_ 11. Which of the following is used as a collimator?

    a. lead plate
    b. aluminum plate
    c. copper plate
    d. all of the above

_D_ 12. Which of the following describes the function of filtration?

    a. increases scatter radiation
    b. increases divergent rays
    c. increases long wavelengths
    d. reduces low-energy waves

_A_ 13. Which of the following is the recommended size of the beam at the patient's face?

    a. 2.75 inches
    b. 3.25 inches
    c. 3.50 inches
    d. 4.00 inches

_B_ 14. Which of the following terms describes the dose of radiation that the body can endure with little or no chance of injury?

    a. radiation limit
    b. maximum permissible dose
    c. occupationally exposed dose
    d. ALARA

_C_ 15. Which of the following is TRUE of film badges?

    a. film badges should be worn when the radiographer is undergoing x-ray exposure
    b. film badges can be shared between employees
    c. film badges should be worn at waist level when exposing x-ray films
    d. all of the above are true

FILL IN THE BLANK

16. State the requirements for proper filtration:

    machines operating ≤70 kVp require   _____ mm aluminum
    machines operating >70 kVp require   _____ mm aluminum

17. State the angle that the dental radiographer should stand to the primary beam: _____ degrees

18. State the formula for MAD:

19. State the maximum permissible dose for occupationally exposed persons:

    _____ rem/year   _____ Sv/year

20. State the maximum permissible dose for nonoccupationally exposed persons:

    _____ rem/year   _____ Sv/year

Answers are supplied at the end of this book.

Equipment, Film, and Processing Basics

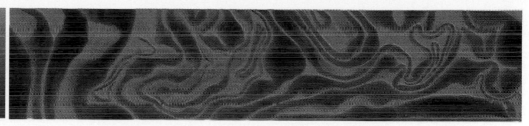

Dental X-ray Equipment

OBJECTIVES

After completion of this chapter, the student will be able to:

- *Define the key words.*
- *Discuss the regulation of dental x-ray machines at the federal, state, and local levels.*
- *Recognize dental x-ray machines used for intraoral and extraoral films.*
- *Identify the component parts of the x-ray machine.*
- *Describe the purpose and use of dental x-ray film holders and devices.*
- *Identify commonly used dental x-ray film holders and devices.*

INTRODUCTION

The dental radiographer must be familiar with dental x-ray equipment and dental x-ray film holders and devices. The purpose of this chapter is to introduce the dental radiographer to a variety of intraoral and extraoral dental x-ray machines, to detail the component parts of such machines, and to describe the more common dental x-ray film holders and devices.

DENTAL X-RAY MACHINES

A variety of intraoral and extraoral dental x-ray machines are available for diagnostic purposes. Dental x-ray equipment varies in both design and operation. The dental radiographer must have a clear understanding of the operating procedures for the specific equipment that is used in the dental office, otherwise, improper exposure of patients and dental personnel may occur.

Performance Standards

Before 1974, no federal standards existed for the manufacture of dental x-ray machines. All dental x-ray machines manufactured after 1974 must meet specific federal guidelines regulating diagnostic equipment performance standards. The federal government regulates the manufacture and installation of dental x-ray equipment. State and local governments regulate how dental x-ray equipment is used and dictate codes that pertain to the use of x-radiation. Depending on state and local radiation safety codes, dental equipment must be inspected and monitored periodically. A fee is typically charged for such an inspection.

Types of Machines

Dental x-ray machines may be used to expose **intraoral films** (films placed *inside* the mouth) or **extraoral films** (films placed *outside* the mouth). Some machines are used only for intraoral films, whereas others are limited to extraoral films. A variety of dental x-ray machines are available from a number of different manufacturers. Examples of dental x-ray units used for intraoral films are seen in Figure 6–1. Examples of dental x-ray units used for extraoral films are seen in Figure 6–2. Some examples of digital radiography units are illustrated in Chapter 24.

Component Parts

As detailed in Chapter 2, the typical intraoral dental x-ray machines features three component parts: the tubehead, the extension arm, and the control panel (see Fig. 2–11).

TUBEHEAD

The **tubehead,** or tube housing, contains the x-ray tube that produces dental x-rays (Fig. 6–3). Extending from the tubehead opening is the position-indicating device, or PID. The PID, sometimes referred to as the cone, may be circular or rectangular in shape and restricts the size of the x-ray beam.

EXTENSION ARM

The **extension arm** suspends the x-ray tubehead, houses the electrical wires, and allows for movement and positioning of the tubehead.

CONTROL PANEL

The **control panel** allows the dental radiographer to regulate the x-ray beam. The control panel is plugged into an electrical outlet and appears as a console or cabinet. A control panel may be mounted on a floor pedestal, a wall support, or a remote wall location outside the dental operatory. A single control panel may be used to operate more than one x-ray unit located in adjacent rooms. The control panel consists of (1) an on-off switch and indicator light, (2) an exposure button and indicator light, and (3) control devices (time, kilovoltage peak, and milliamperage selectors) (Fig. 6–4).

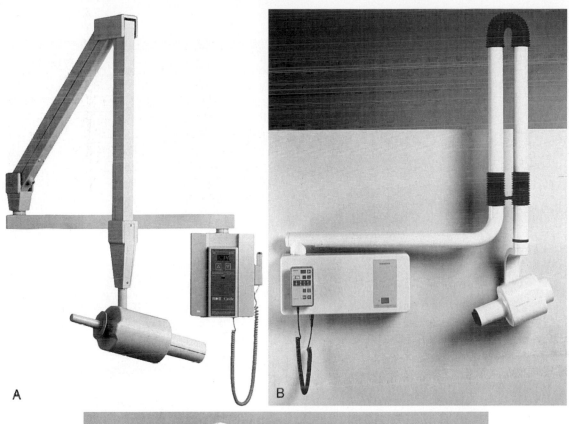

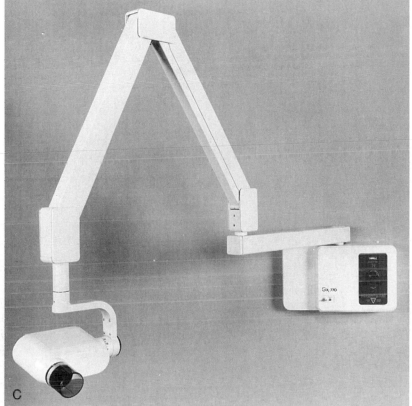

FIGURE 6–1. *A,* The Castle HDX intraoral x-ray machine. (Courtesy of MDT Diagnostic Company, North Charleston, SC.) *B,* The Heliodent MD intraoral x-ray machine. (Courtesy of Pelton and Crane, A Siemens Company, Charlotte, NC.) *C,* The Gendex 770 intraoral x-ray machine. (Courtesy of Gendex Corporation, Des Plaines, IL.)

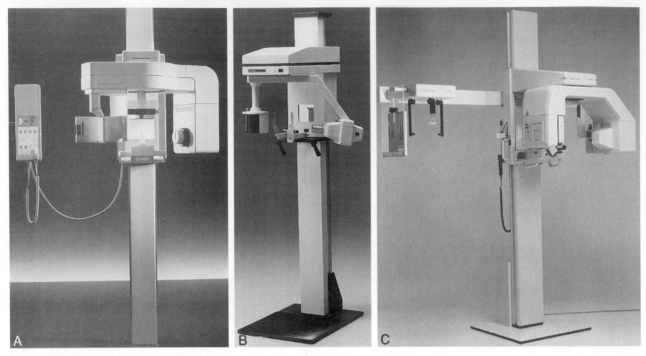

FIGURE 6–2. *A*, The Orthopantomograph 10E extraoral x-ray machine. (Courtesy of Pelton and Crane, A Siemens Company, Charlotte, NC.) *B*, The GX-Pan extraoral machine. (Courtesy of Gendex Corporation, Des Plaines, IL.) *C*, The Cranex 3+ Ceph extraoral machine. (Courtesy of Soredex Medical Systems, Conroe, TX.)

ON-OFF SWITCH

The **on-off switch** must be placed in the "on" position to operate the dental x-ray equipment. An **indicator light** is illuminated when the equipment is turned on.

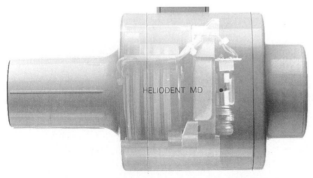

FIGURE 6–3. The tubehead contains the x-ray tube. (Courtesy of Pelton and Crane, A Siemens Company, Charlotte, NC.)

EXPOSURE BUTTON

The **exposure button** activates the machine to produce x-rays. The dental radiographer must firmly depress the exposure button until the preset exposure time is completed. As a visible sign that x-rays are being produced, an **exposure light** on the control panel is illuminated during x-ray exposure. In addition, a beep sounds during x-ray exposure as an audible signal that x-rays are being produced. The exposure light turns off and the beep stops when the x-ray exposure is completed.

CONTROL DEVICES

The **control devices** that regulate the x-ray beam include the timer and the kilovoltage peak and milliamperage selectors. The timer determines the length of exposure time in seconds or impulses. The kilovoltage peak and milliamperage selectors permit the dental radiographer to adjust and set the correct kilovoltage peak and milliamperage. Some dental x-ray units do

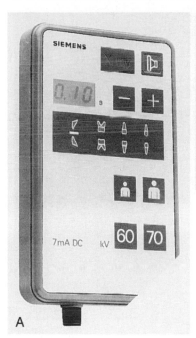

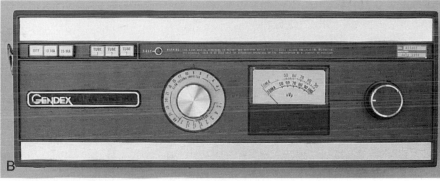

FIGURE 6–4. *A,* The Heliodent MD control panel. (Courtesy of Pelton and Crane, A Siemens Company, Charlotte, NC.) *B,* The Gendex-1000 control. (Courtesy of Gendex Corporation, Des Plaines, IL.)

not have adjustable kilovoltage peak or milliamperage selectors.

▰ DENTAL X-RAY FILM HOLDERS AND BEAM ALIGNMENT DEVICES

A **film holder** is a device used to hold and align intraoral dental x-ray films in the mouth. Film holders eliminate the need for the patient to stabilize the film. With certain intraoral techniques (e.g., paralleling technique), the use of a film-holding device is required. Specific intraoral techniques and film-holding devices are discussed in Chapters 17, 18, and 19.

A **beam alignment device** is an instrument used to help the dental radiographer position the PID in relation to the tooth and film. (Beam alignment devices are detailed in Chapters 17, 18, and 19.) For use in conjunction with a beam alignment device, a **collimating device,** or metal plate with an opening, can be used to restrict the size of the beam.

Types of Film Holders

Intraoral film holders are commercially available from a number of manufacturers. The simplest film holder is a disposable styrofoam bite-block with a backing plate and a slot for film retention; examples include the XCP Bite-Block or Stabe Bite-Block manufactured by the Rinn Corporation (Fig. 6–5). Sturdy molded plastic devices than can be sterilized are also available. An example of such a device is the EEZEE-Grip, formerly the Snap-A-Ray, also manufactured by the Rinn Corporation. The EEZEE-Grip is a double ended instrument that holds the film between two serrated plastic grips that can be locked in place (Fig. 6–6). Other Rinn film-holding products include the EndoRay and the Uni bite devices (Fig. 6–7).

Types of Beam Alignment Devices

Beam alignment devices and collimating devices are available from a number of manufacturers and are used to indicate the PID position in relation to the tooth and film. Examples of metal beam alignment and

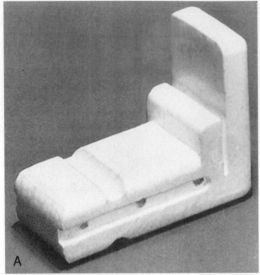

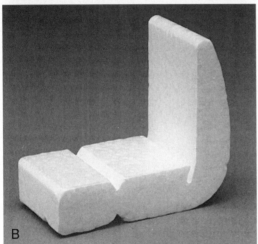

FIGURE 6–5. *A,* The XCP Bite-Block. *B,* The Stabe Bite-Block. (Courtesy of Rinn Corporation, Elgin, IL.)

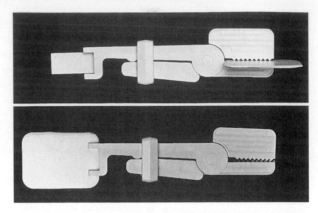

FIGURE 6–6. The EEZEE-Grip film holder. The film can be positioned for (*top*) anterior areas, and (*bottom*) most posterior areas. (Courtesy of Rinn Corporation, Elgin, IL.)

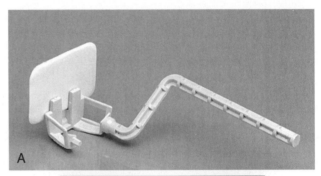

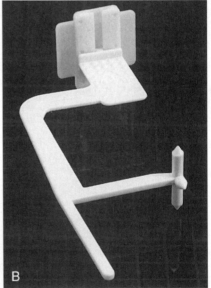

FIGURE 6–7. *A,* The EndoRay film holder is used during root canal procedures. It fits around rubber dam clamps and allows space for files to protrude from the tooth. (Courtesy of Rinn Corporation, Elgin, IL.) *B,* The Uni-bite is a universal film holder that can be used with the bite-wing technique or the long cone paralleling technique. (Courtesy of Rinn Corporation, Elgin, IL.)

collimating devices are Precision Film Holders manufactured by Masel Orthodontics. Precision Film Holders feature four metal collimating shields and film-holding devices that restrict the size of the x-ray beam to the size of the film (Fig. 6–8). Rinn XCP and BAI Instruments are other examples of beam alignment devices. Plastic bite-blocks, plastic aiming rings, and metal indicator arms are features of the Rinn XCP and BAI Instruments (Fig. 6–9). To reduce the amount of radiation a patient receives, a snap-on metal collimating device can be added to the plastic XCP and BAI rings (Fig. 6–10).

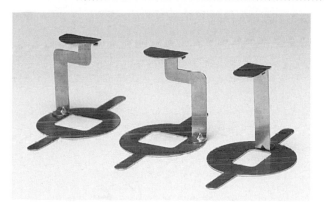

FIGURE 6–8. Precision film holders restrict the size of the x-ray beam to the size of the film.

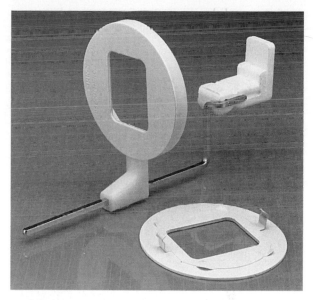

FIGURE 6–10. The Rinn Snap-on Ring Collimator can be used to reduce the amount of radiation a patient receives. (Courtesy of Rinn Corporation, Elgin, IL.)

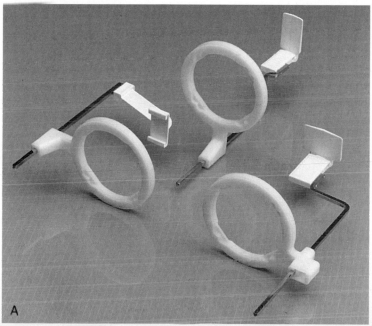

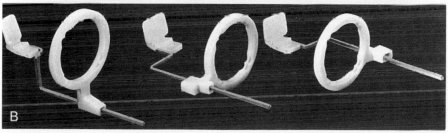

FIGURE 6–9. *A,* The Rinn XCP instruments. (Courtesy of Rinn Corporation, Elgin, IL.) *B,* The Rinn BAI instruments are used with the bisecting technique. (Courtesy of Rinn Corporation, Elgin, IL.)

SUMMARY

- The dental radiographer must be familiar with the x-ray equipment, film holders, and beam alignment devices used in dentistry.
- The typical intraoral dental x-ray machine consists of three component parts: the tubehead, the extension arm, and the control panel.
- A film holder can be used to stabilize an intraoral film.
- A beam alignment device can be used to help the dental radiographer position the PID in relation to the tooth and film.
- A collimating device can be used in conjunction with the beam alignment device to further restrict the size of the x-ray beam.

BIBLIOGRAPHY

Barr JH, Stephens RG: Radiographic facilities. *In* Dental Radiology: Pertinent Basic Concepts and Their Applications in Clinical Practice. Philadelphia, WB Saunders, 1980, pp. 82–90.

Frommer HH: Radiation protection. *In* Radiology for Dental Auxiliaries, 6th edition. St. Louis, Mosby-Year Book, 1996, pp. 67–87.

Johnson ON, McNally MA, Essay CE: The periapical examination. *In* Essentials of Dental Radiography for Dental Assistants and Hygienists, 6th edition. Norwalk, CT, Appleton and Lange, 1999, pp. 339–375.

Matteson SR, Whaley C, Secrist VC: Dental radiology practice and equipment. *In* Dental Radiology, 4th edition. Chapel Hill, University of North Carolina Press, 1988, pp. 14–16.

Miles DA, Van Dis ML, Razmus TF: Intraoral radiographic techniques. *In* Basic Principles of Oral and Maxillofacial Radiology. Philadelphia, WB Saunders, 1992, p. 80.

Quiz Questions ••

MULTIPLE CHOICE

_C_ 1. No federal standards existed for dental x-ray machines manufactured before the year:

    a. 1954
    b. 1964
    c. 1974
    d. 1984

_A_ 2. Dental films placed inside the mouth are termed:

    a. intraoral films
    b. extraoral films
    c. occlusal films
    d. all of the above

_B_ 3. The component part of the dental x-ray machine that contains the x-ray tube is termed the:

    a. control panel
    b. tubehead
    c. extension arm
    d. console

_B_ 4. The component part of the dental x-ray machine that allows movement and positioning of the tubehead is termed the:

    a. control panel
    b. extension arm
    c. console
    d. PID

_A_ 5. The dental radiographer can regulate the x-ray beam (kilovoltage peak, milliamperage, time) through the use of the:

    a. control panel
    b. extension arm
    c. tubehead
    d. PID

_B_ 6. An instrument that is used to help the dental radiographer position the PID in relation to the tooth and film is the:

    a. film holder
    b. beam alignment device
    c. collimating device
    d. none of the above

_C_ 7. A device that is used to stabilize an intraoral film is a:

    a. beam alignment device
    b. collimating device
    c. film holder
    d. none of the above

A

8. A metal instrument that is used to restrict the size of the x-ray beam to the size of an intraoral film is the:

    a. collimating device
    b. film holder
    c. beam alignment device
    d. none of the above

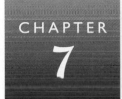

CHAPTER 7

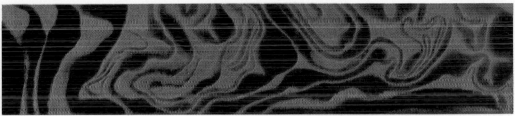

Dental X-ray Film

OBJECTIVES

After completion of this chapter, the student will be able to:

- *Define the key words.*
- *Describe in detail film composition and latent image formation.*
- *List and describe the different types of x-ray film used in dentistry.*
- *Define intraoral film and describe intraoral film packaging.*
- *Identify the types and sizes of intraoral film available.*
- *Discuss film speed.*
- *Discuss the differences between intraoral film and extraoral film.*
- *Describe the difference between screen and nonscreen films.*
- *Describe the use of intensifying screens and cassettes.*
- *Describe duplicating film.*
- *Discuss proper film storage and protection.*

INTRODUCTION

The dental radiographer must have a working knowledge of dental x-ray film. The film used in dental radiography is photographic film that has been adapted for dental use. A photographic image is produced on dental x-ray film when it is exposed to x-rays that have passed through teeth and adjacent structures. To avoid film-related errors that result in increased patient exposure to x-radiation, the dental radiographer must understand the composition of x-ray film and latent image formation. In addition, the dental radiographer must be familiar with the types of film used in dental radiography as well as film storage and protection.

The purpose of this chapter is to define film composition, to detail latent image formation, to describe the types of intraoral, extraoral, and duplicating film used in dentistry, and to discuss film storage and protection.

DENTAL X-RAY FILM COMPOSITION AND LATENT IMAGE

In dental radiography, after the x-ray beam passes through the teeth and adjacent structures, it reaches the x-ray film. The dental x-ray film serves as a recording medium or **image receptor**: the term **image** refers to a picture or likeness of an object, and the term **receptor** refers to something that responds to a stimulus. Images are recorded on the dental x-ray film when the film is exposed to a stimulus—specifically, energy in the form of x-radiation or light. To understand how these images result, an understanding of film composition and latent image formation is necessary.

Film Composition

The x-ray film used in dentistry has four basic components (Fig. 7–1).

FILM BASE

The **film base** is a flexible piece of polyester plastic that measures 0.2 mm thick and is constructed to withstand heat, moisture, and chemical exposure. The film base is transparent and exhibits a slight blue tint that is used to emphasize contrast and enhance image quality. The primary purpose of the film base is to provide a stable support for the delicate emulsion; it also provides strength.

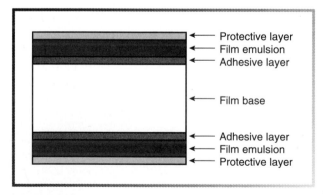

FIGURE 7–1. Schematic diagram of the construction of a typical dental x-ray film. The film emulsion is coated on both the top and bottom surfaces of the polyethylene base; this allows for reduced exposure time and therefore a "faster" film. (From Miles DA, Van Dis ML, Razmus TF: Basic Principles of Oral and Maxillofacial Radiology. Philadelphia, WB Saunders, 1992.)

ADHESIVE LAYER

The **adhesive layer** is a thin layer of adhesive material that covers both sides of the film base. The adhesive layer is added to the film base before the emulsion is applied and serves to attach the emulsion to the base.

FILM EMULSION

The **film emulsion** is a coating attached to both sides of the film base by the adhesive layer to give the film greater sensitivity to x-radiation. The emulsion is a homogeneous mixture of gelatin and silver halide crystals.

GELATIN

The **gelatin** is used to suspend and evenly disperse millions of microscopic silver halide crystals over the film base. During film processing, the gelatin serves to absorb the processing solutions and allows the chemicals to react with the silver halide crystals.

HALIDE CRYSTALS

A **halide** is a chemical compound that is sensitive to radiation or light. The halides used in dental x-ray film are made up of the element silver plus a halogen, either bromine or iodine. Silver bromide ($AgBr$) and silver iodide (AgI) are two types of **silver halide crystals** found in the film emulsion; the typical emulsion is 80 to 99% silver bromide and 1 to 10% silver iodide. The silver halide crystals absorb radiation during x-ray exposure and store energy from the radiation (Fig. 7-2).

PROTECTIVE LAYER

The **protective layer** is a thin, transparent coating placed over the emulsion. It serves to protect the emulsion surface from manipulation as well as mechanical and processing damage.

Latent Image Formation

Silver halide crystals absorb x-radiation during x-ray exposure and store the energy from the radiation; depending on the density of the objects in the area exposed, silver halide crystals contain various levels of stored energy. For example, the silver halide crystals on the film that are positioned behind an amalgam filling receive almost no radiation. The amalgam filling is dense and absorbs the x-ray energy. As a result, the silver halide crystals are not energized. In contrast, the silver halide crystals that correspond to airspace (no density) receive more radiation and are highly energized.

The stored energy within the silver halide crystals forms a pattern and creates an invisible image within the emulsion on the exposed film. This pattern of stored energy on the exposed film cannot be seen and is referred to as a **latent image**. The latent image remains invisible within the emulsion until it undergoes chemical processing procedures. When the exposed film with latent image is processed, a visible image results. Film processing procedures are discussed in Chapter 9.

How does the stored energy of the silver halide crystals result in a latent image? When the x-ray pho-

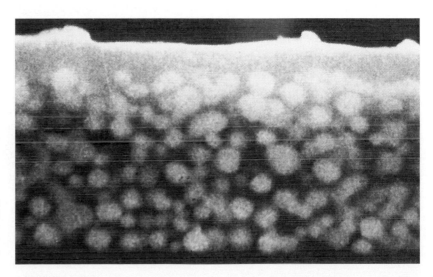

FIGURE 7-2. Scanning electron micrograph of unprocessed emulsion of Kodak Ultra-Speed dental x-ray film (5000×). Note white-appearing, unexposed silver bromide grains. (Reprinted courtesy of Eastman Kodak Company, Rochester, NY.)

tons hit the surface of the film emulsion, some silver bromide crystals are exposed and energized while others are not. The silver bromide crystals that are exposed to x-ray photons are ionized, and the silver and bromine atoms are separated. Irregularities in the lattice structure of the exposed crystal, known as **sensitivity specks,** attract the silver atoms (Fig. 7–3); these aggregates of neutral silver atoms are known as **latent image centers** (Fig. 7–4). Collectively, the crystals with aggregates of silver at the latent image centers become the latent image on the film.

TYPES OF DENTAL X-RAY FILM

Three types of x-ray film may be used in dental radiography:

- intraoral film
- extraoral film
- duplicating film

Intraoral Film

An **intraoral film,** as defined in Chapter 6, is one that is placed *inside* the mouth during x-ray exposure. An intraoral film is used to examine the teeth and supporting structures.

INTRAORAL FILM PACKAGING

Each intraoral film is packaged to protect it from light and moisture; the film and its surrounding packaging are referred to as a **film packet.** In dentistry, the terms film packet and film are often used interchangeably.

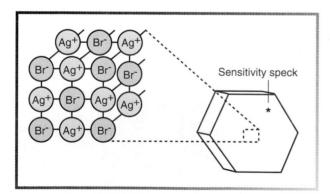

FIGURE 7–3. Each crystal in the radiographic emulsion consists of silver (Ag^+) and primarily bromide (Br^-) ions. Irregularities in the lattice structure form the sensitivity speck. (From Miles DA, Van Dis ML, Razmus TF: Basic Principles of Oral and Maxillofacial Radiology. Philadelphia, WB Saunders, 1992.)

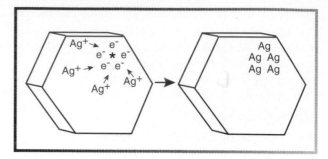

FIGURE 7–4. The sensitivity speck tends to attract free electrons (e^-), which in turn attract positively charged silver ions (Ag^+). The aggregate of neural silver atoms (Ag) makes up the latent image center in the crystal. (From Miles DS, Van Dis ML, Razmus TF: Basic Principles of Oral and Maxillofacial Radiology. Philadelphia, WB Saunders, 1992.)

Intraoral film packets are typically available in quantities of 25, 100, or 150 films per container. Film packets are packaged in convenient plastic trays or cardboard boxes that can be recycled (Fig. 7–5). Boxes of intraoral film are labeled with the type of film, film speed, film size, number of films per individual packet, total number of films enclosed, and the film expiration date.

Dental x-ray film packets have four basic components (Fig. 7–6).

X-RAY FILM

The intraoral **x-ray film** is a double-emulsion (emulsion on both sides) type of film; double-emulsion

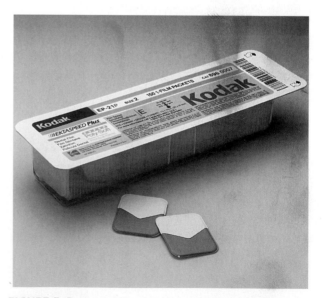

FIGURE 7–5. Intraoral film packets in recyclable plastic trays. (Reprinted courtesy of Eastman Kodak Company, Rochester, NY.)

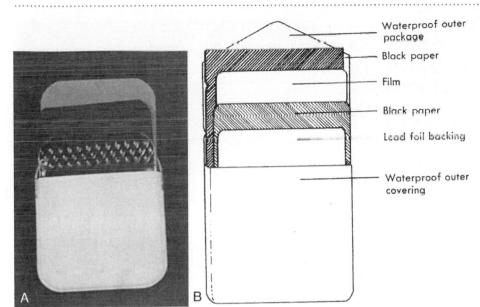

— Waterproof outer package

— Black paper

— Film

— Black paper

— Lead foil backing

— Waterproof outer covering

A B

FIGURE 7–6. A, Back of an opened dental film packet. B, Diagram of A. (A and B from Frommer HH: Radiology for Dental Auxiliaries, 5th ed. St. Louis, Mosby-Year Book, 1992.)

film is used instead of single-emulsion (emulsion on one side) film because it requires less radiation exposure to produce an image. A film packet may contain one film (**one-film packet**) or two films (**two-film packet**). A two-film packet produces two identical radiographs with the same amount of exposure necessary to produce a single radiograph. The two-film packet is used when a duplicate record of a radiographic examination is needed (e.g., for insurance claims, patient referrals).

In one corner of the intraoral x-ray film, a small raised bump known as the **identification dot** is found (Fig. 7–7). The raised bump is used to determine film orientation. After the film is processed, the raised identification dot is used to distinguish between the left and right sides of the patient. The dot is significant in film mounting and interpretation and is discussed further in Chapter 27.

PAPER FILM WRAPPER

The **paper film wrapper** within the film packet is a black paper protective sheet that covers the film and shields the film from light.

LEAD FOIL SHEET

The **lead foil sheet** is a single piece of lead foil that is found within the film packet and is located behind the film wrapped in black protective paper. The thin lead foil sheet is positioned *behind* the film to shield the film from back-scattered (secondary) radiation that results in film fog.

An embossed pattern is placed on the lead foil sheet by the film manufacturer; the pattern is visible on a processed radiograph if the film packet is inadvertently positioned in the mouth backward and then exposed (Fig. 7–8).

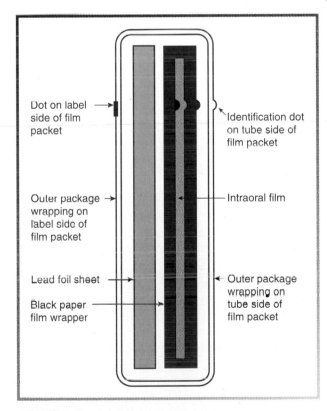

Dot on label side of film packet

Identification dot on tube side of film packet

Outer package wrapping on label side of film packet

Intraoral film

Lead foil sheet

Outer package wrapping on tube side of film packet

Black paper film wrapper

FIGURE 7–7. Labeled film packet.

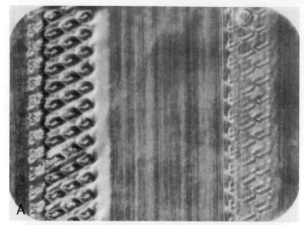

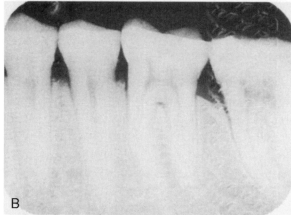

FIGURE 7–8. *A,* The lead foil insert in this packet has a raised diamond pattern across both ends. *B,* Radiograph showing the raised diamond pattern from the lead backing when the film is positioned backwards. (*A* and *B* reprinted courtesy of Eastman Kodak Company, Rochester, NY.)

OUTER PACKAGE WRAPPING

The **outer package wrapping** is a soft vinyl or paper wrapper that hermetically seals the film packet, protective black paper, and lead foil sheet. This outer wrapper serves to protect the film from exposure to light and saliva.

The outer wrapper of the film packet has two sides: tube side and label side.

Tube Side. The **tube side** is solid white and has a raised bump in one corner that corresponds to the identification dot on the x-ray film. When placed in the mouth, the white side (tube side) of the film packet must face the teeth and the tubehead.

Label Side. The **label side** of the film packet has a flap that is used to open the film packet to remove the film prior to processing. The label side is color-coded to identify films outside of the plastic packaging con-

TABLE 7–1. Kodak Film Packet Color Codes		
	One-Film Packets	Two-Film Packets
Kodak Ultra-Speed (D-Speed)	green	gray
Kodak Ektaspeed (E-Speed)	blue	mauve

tainer; color codes are used to distinguish between one-film and two-film packets and between film speeds (Table 7–1). When placed in the mouth, the color-coded side (label side) of the packet must face the tongue.

The following information is printed on the label side of the film packet (Fig. 7–9):

- a circle or dot that corresponds with the raised identification dot on the film
- the statement "opposite side toward tube"
- the manufacturer's name
- the film speed
- the number of films enclosed

INTRAORAL FILM TYPES

Three types of intraoral films are available.

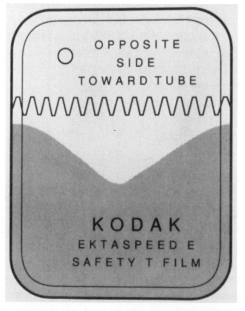

FIGURE 7–9. The label side of a film packet. (Reprinted courtesy of Eastman Kodak Company, Rochester, NY.)

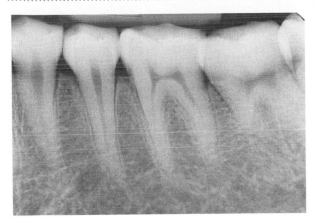

FIGURE 7–10. A periapical film. (Reprinted courtesy of Eastman Kodak Company, Rochester, NY.)

PERIAPICAL FILM PA

The **periapical film** is used to examine the entire tooth (crown and root) and supporting bone (Fig. 7–10). The term periapical is derived from the Greek word *peri,* meaning around, and the Latin word *apex,* meaning the terminal end of a tooth root. As the term suggests, this type of film shows the tip of the tooth root and surrounding structures as well as the crown.

BITE-WING FILM BW

The **bite-wing film** is used to examine the crowns of both the maxillary (upper) and mandibular (lower) teeth on one film (Fig. 7–11). The bite-wing film is particularly useful in examining the **interproximal,** or adjacent, tooth surfaces. The bite-wing film has a "wing," or tab, attached to the tube side of the film

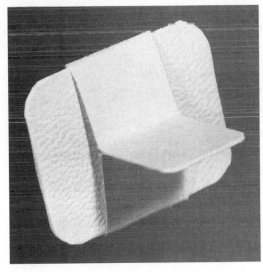

FIGURE 7–12. The bite-wing tab attached to the film. (From Goaz PW, White SC: Oral Radiology, Principles and Interpretation, 2nd ed. St. Louis, CV Mosby, 1987.)

(Fig. 7–12). The patient "bites" on the "wing" to stabilize the film, hence the term bite-wing. Bite-wing films may be purchased with tabs attached to the film or may be constructed from a periapical film and bite-wing loop.

OCCLUSAL FILM

The **occlusal film** is used for examination of large areas of the maxilla (upper jaw) or mandible (lower jaw) (Fig. 7–13). The occlusal film is so named because the patient "occludes" or bites on the entire film. The occlusal film is larger than periapical or bite-wing films.

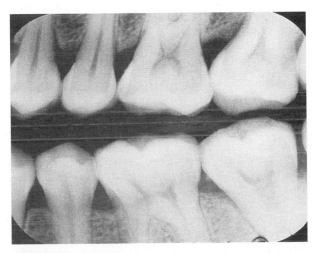

FIGURE 7–11. A bite-wing film. (Reprinted courtesy of Eastman Kodak Company, Rochester, NY.)

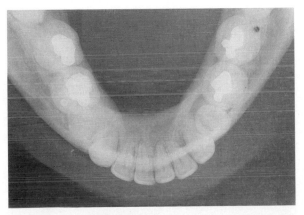

FIGURE 7–13. An occlusal film. (Reprinted courtesy of Eastman Kodak Company, Rochester, NY.)

INTRAORAL FILM SIZES

Intraoral film is manufactured in five sizes to accommodate the varying mouth sizes of children, adolescents, and adults. The larger the number, the larger the size of the film. Different sizes of film are used with periapical, bite-wing, and occlusal exposures (Fig. 7–14).

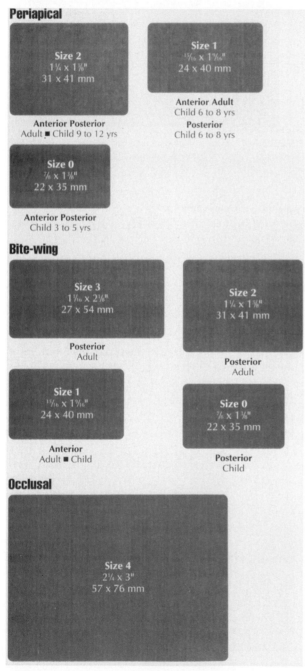

Periapical

Size 2
1¼ x 1⅜"
31 x 41 mm

Anterior Posterior
Adult ■ Child 9 to 12 yrs

Size 1
¹⁵⁄₁₆ x 1⁹⁄₁₆"
24 x 40 mm

Anterior Adult
Child 6 to 8 yrs
Posterior
Child 6 to 8 yrs

Size 0
⅞ x 1⅜"
22 x 35 mm

Anterior Posterior
Child 3 to 5 yrs

Bite-wing

Size 3
1¹⁄₁₆ x 2⅛"
27 x 54 mm

Posterior
Adult

Size 2
1¼ x 1⅜"
31 x 41 mm

Posterior
Adult

Size 1
¹⁵⁄₁₆ x 1⁹⁄₁₆"
24 x 40 mm

Anterior
Adult ■ Child

Size 0
⅞ x 1⅜"
22 x 35 mm

Posterior
Child

Occlusal

Size 4
2¼ x 3"
57 x 76 mm

FIGURE 7–14. These drawings indicate film sizes. (Reprinted courtesy of Eastman Kodak Company, Rochester, NY.)

Periapical Film. Three sizes of periapical film (0, 1, and 2) are available. Table 7–2 summarizes the measurements and uses of these films.

Size 0. This periapical film is the smallest intraoral film available and is used for very small children.

Size 1. This periapical film is used primarily to examine the anterior teeth in adults.

Size 2. This periapical film, also known as the **standard film,** is used to examine the anterior and posterior teeth in adults.

Bite-wing Film. Four sizes of bite-wing film (0, 1, 2, and 3) are available (Table 7–2). With the exception of the Size 3 film, the size and shape of the bite-wing film are identical to the size and shape of the periapical film.

Size 0. This bite-wing film is used to examine the posterior teeth in very small children.

Size 1. This bite-wing film is used to examine the posterior teeth in children. When positioned vertically, it can be used to examine the anterior teeth in adults.

Size 2. This bite-wing film is used to examine the posterior teeth in adults. This is the most frequently used bite-wing film.

Size 3. This film is longer and narrower than the standard Size 2 film and is used *only* for bite-wings. This bite-wing film shows all of the posterior teeth on one side of the arch in one radiograph.

Occlusal Film. The occlusal film is the largest intraoral film and is almost four times as large as a standard Size 2 periapical film (see Table 7–2).

Size 4. This occlusal film is used to show large areas of the upper or lower jaw.

INTRAORAL FILM SPEED

Film speed refers to the amount of radiation required to produce a radiograph of standard density. Film speed, or sensitivity, is determined by the following:

- the size of the silver halide crystals
- the thickness of the emulsion
- the presence of special radiosensitive dyes

Film speed determines how much radiation and how much exposure time are necessary to produce an image on a film. For example, a fast film requires less radiation exposure because the film responds more quickly; a fast film responds more quickly because the

TABLE 7–2. Size, Measurements, and Uses for Intraoral Film

Film Type	Size	Measurements	Adult	Children	Anterior	Posterior
Periapical	0	7/8 × 1 3/8 inch (22 × 35 mm)		X	X	X
	1	15/16 × 19/16 inch (24 × 40 mm)	X	X	X	X
	2	1 1/4 × 1 5/8 inch (31 × 41 mm)	X	X	X	X
Bite-wing	0	7/8 × 1 3/8 inch (22 × 35 mm)		X		X
	1	15/16 × 19/16 inch (24 × 40 mm)	X	X	X	X
	2	1 1/4 × 1 5/8 inch (31 × 41 mm)	X			X
	3	1 1/16 × 2 1/8 inch (27 × 54 mm)	X			X
Occlusal	4	2 1/4 × 3 inch (57 × 76 mm)	X	X		

silver halide crystals in the emulsion are larger. The larger the crystals, the faster the film speed.

An alphabetical classification system is used to identify film speed. X-ray films are given speed ratings ranging from A speed (the slowest) to F speed (the fastest). Only **D-speed film** and **E-speed film** are used for intraoral radiography. The American Dental Association (ADA) and the American Academy of Oral and Maxillofacial Radiology (AAOMR) currently recommend the use of E-speed film. E-speed film requires one-half the exposure time of D-speed film and has comparable image contrast and resolution. The use of E-speed film results in less radiation exposure for the patient. E-speed film is a faster film than D-speed because of the larger crystals and the increased amount of silver bromide in the emulsion. The E-speed films currently manufactured are extremely stable and forgiving and actually exhibit less contrast loss during processing than E-speed films produced in the past. The speed of a film is clearly indicated on the label side of the intraoral film packet as well as on the outside of the film box or container.

Extraoral Film

An **extraoral film**, as defined in Chapter 6, is one that is placed *outside* of the mouth during x-ray exposure. Extraoral films are used to examine large areas of the skull or jaws. Examples of common extraoral films include panoramic and cephalometric films; a **panoramic film** shows a panoramic (wide) view of the upper and lower jaws on a single radiograph (Fig. 7–15), whereas a **cephalometric film** exhibits the bony and soft tissue areas of the facial profile (Fig. 7–16).

EXTRAORAL FILM PACKAGING

Unlike intraoral films, extraoral films are designed to be used outside of the mouth and therefore are not enclosed in moisture-proof packets. Extraoral film used in dental radiography is available in 5 × 7-inch and 8 × 10-inch sizes, as well as the panoramic 5 × 12-inch and 6 × 12-inch sizes. Extraoral film is boxed in quantities of 50 or 100 films. Some manufacturers separate each piece of film with protective paper. Boxes of extraoral film are labeled with the type of film, film size, the total number of films enclosed, and the expiration date (Fig. 7–17).

EXTRAORAL FILM TYPES

Two types of film may be used in extraoral radiography: screen film and nonscreen film.

Screen Film. The majority of extraoral films are screen films. A **screen film** is a film that requires the use of a screen for exposure. (Screens are discussed later in this chapter.) A screen film is placed between two special intensifying screens in a cassette (Fig. 7–18). When the cassette is exposed to x-rays, the screens convert the x-ray energy into light, which in turn exposes the screen film. Screen film is sensitive to

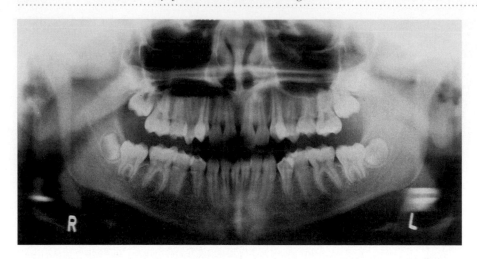

FIGURE 7–15. A panoramic film. (Reprinted courtesy of Eastman Kodak Company, Rochester, NY.)

fluorescent light rather than direct exposure to x-radiation.

Films used in a screen-film combination are sensitive to specific colors of fluorescent light. Some screen films are sensitive to blue light (Kodak X-Omat and Ektamat films), whereas others are sensitive to green light (Kodak Ortho and T-Mat films). **Blue-sensitive film** must be paired with screens that produce blue light, and **green-sensitive film** must be paired with screens that produce green light. Properly matched film-screen combinations are imperative to obtain high-quality images and minimize exposure to the patient.

Nonscreen Film. A **nonscreen film** is an extraoral film that does not require the use of screens for exposure. A nonscreen extraoral film is exposed directly to x-rays; the emulsion is sensitive to direct x-ray exposure rather than to fluorescent light. A nonscreen extraoral film requires more exposure time than a screen film and is not recommended for use in dental radiography.

EXTRAORAL FILM EQUIPMENT

In extraoral radiography, screen films are used in combination with two special equipment items: intensifying screens and cassettes.

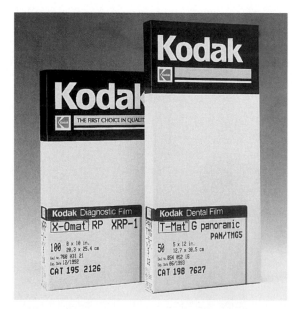

FIGURE 7–16. A cephalometric film. (Reprinted courtesy of Eastman Kodak Company, Rochester, NY.)

FIGURE 7–17. Extraoral film boxes are labeled with the type of film, film size, number of films enclosed and expiration date. (Reprinted courtesy of Eastman Kodak, Rochester, NY.)

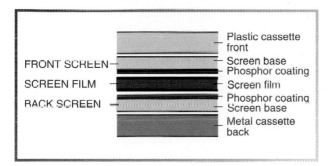

FIGURE 7–18. Inside the cassette, the screen film is placed between two intensifying screens.

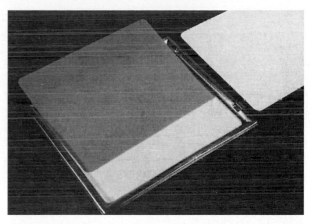

FIGURE 7–19. Cassette in open position, showing front and back intensifying screens and piece of film. (From Frommer HH: Radiology for Dental Auxiliaries, 5th ed. St. Louis, Mosby-Year Book, 1992.)

INTENSIFYING SCREENS

An **intensifying screen** is a device that transfers x-ray energy into visible light; the visible light, in turn, exposes the screen film. As the word intensifying suggests, these screens intensify the effect of x-rays on the film. With the use of intensifying screens, less radiation is required to expose a screen film, and the patient is exposed to less radiation.

In extraoral radiography, a screen film is sandwiched between two intensifying screens of matching size and secured in a cassette (Fig. 7–19). An intensifying screen is a smooth plastic sheet coated with minute fluorescent crystals known as **phosphors.** When exposed to x-rays, the phosphors **fluoresce** and emit visible light in the blue or green spectrum; the emitted light then exposes the film (Fig. 7–20). You may recall from Chapter 2 that one of the properties of x-rays is that they cause certain materials, like phosphors, to fluoresce.

Conventional **calcium tungstate screens** have phosphors that emit blue light. The newer **rare earth screens** have phosphors that are not commonly found in the earth (hence the name rare earth) and emit green light. Rare earth intensifying screens are more efficient than calcium tungstate intensifying screens at converting x-rays into light. As a result, rare earth screens require less x-ray exposure than calcium tungstate screens and are considered faster. The use of rare earth screens means less exposure to x-radiation for the patient. Rare earth intensifying screens (Kodak Lanex Regular and Medium screens) are designed for use with green-sensitive films (Kodak Ortho and T-Mat films), whereas conventional screens (Kodak X-Omatic Regular screens) are used with blue-sensitive films (Kodak X-Omat and Ektamat films).

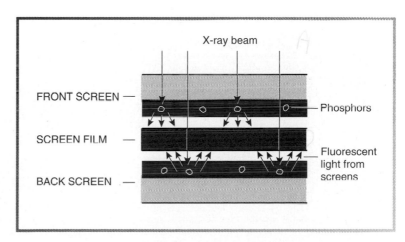

FIGURE 7–20. Phosphors in the intensifying screen emit visible light when hit by x-ray photons. Multiple visible light photons then strike and expose the film.

CASSETTE

A **cassette** is a special device that is used to hold the extraoral film and the intensifying screens. Cassettes are available in a variety of sizes that correspond to film and screen sizes. A cassette may be flexible or rigid; most cassettes are rigid with the exception of the panoramic cassette, which may be flexible (Fig. 7–21).

A rigid cassette is more expensive than a flexible one but usually lasts longer. A rigid cassette protects screens from damage better than a flexible one. The film fits the rigid cassette exactly and cannot be loaded incorrectly; however, to load the flexible cassette properly, the film must be placed between the two screens and pushed to the end of the cassette.

Both rigid and flexible cassettes must be light-tight not only to protect the extraoral film from exposure but also to hold the intensifying screens in perfect contact with the extraoral film. Contact between the screen and the film is critical; lack of contact between screen and film results in a loss of image sharpness.

A rigid cassette has a front and a back cover. The front cover is placed so that it faces the tubehead and is usually constructed of plastic to permit the passage of the x-ray beam. The back cover is constructed of heavy metal and serves to reduce scatter radiation. Intensifying screens are installed inside the front and back covers of the cassette. The film is positioned between the two intensifying screens. Each screen exposes one side of the film.

The cassette must be marked to orient the finished radiograph; a metal letter L is attached to the front cover of the cassette to indicate the patient's left side, and a metal letter R is used to indicate the patient's right side.

Duplicating Film

A **duplicate radiograph** is one that is identical to the original. In dentistry, there are several uses for duplicate radiographs. A duplicate radiograph is useful when a patient is referred to a specialist, for insurance claims, and as teaching aids. A special film, duplicating film, is required to make a duplicate radiograph.

DUPLICATING FILM DESCRIPTION

In dental radiography, **duplicating film** is a type of photographic film that is used to make an identical copy of an intraoral or extraoral radiograph. Unlike intraoral and extraoral films, duplicating film is used only in a darkroom setting and is not exposed to x-rays.

When examined in the darkroom under safelight conditions, duplicating film has an emulsion on one side only. The emulsion side of the film appears dull, whereas the side without the emulsion appears shiny. The emulsion side of the film must contact the radiograph during the duplication process. The equipment necessary for film duplication and the duplication process are described in Chapter 9.

DUPLICATING FILM PACKAGING

Radiographic duplicating film is available in periapical sizes as well as in 5 × 12-inch and 8 × 10-inch sheets. Duplicating film is boxed in quantities of 50, 100, or 150 sheets.

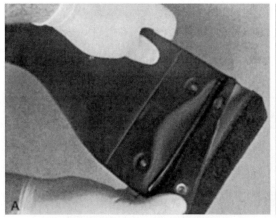 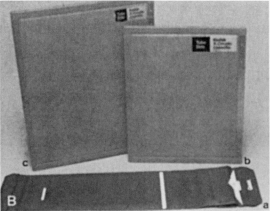

FIGURE 7–21. *A,* Close-up view of flexible 5 × 12-inch panoramic cassette. *B,* Flexible 5 × 12-inch panoramic cassette (a); 8 × 10-inch cassette for lateral cephalometric and other head and neck views (b); 10 × 14-inch cassette (c). (From Miles DA, Van Dis ML, Jensen CW, Ferretti A: Radiographic Imaging for Dental Auxiliaries, 2nd ed. Philadelphia, WB Saunders, 1993.)

FIGURE 7–22. The expiration date is clearly labeled on the package.

FILM STORAGE AND PROTECTION

Film is adversely affected by heat, humidity, and radiation. To prevent film fog (see Chapter 9), unexposed, unprocessed film must be kept in a cool, dry place. The optimum temperature for film storage ranges from 50 to 70 degrees Fahrenheit, and the optimum relative humidity level ranges from 30 to 50%. Film must be stored in areas that are adequately shielded from sources of radiation and should not be stored in areas where patients are exposed to x-radiation. To prevent film fog, lead-lined or radiation-resistant film dispensers and storage boxes are ideal.

All dental x-ray film has a limited shelf life. Each box or container of film is clearly labeled with an expiration date (Fig. 7–22). Film must be used before the labeled expiration date. The "first in, first out" rule of thumb should be applied to film use; the oldest film in stock should always be used before any new film.

use oldest film first

SUMMARY

- Dental x-ray film is an image receptor that has four basic components: film base, adhesive layer, film emulsion, and protective layer.
- Images are recorded on dental x-ray film when the film is exposed to x-radiation.
- The silver halide crystals in the film emulsion absorb the x-radiation during x-ray exposure and store the energy from the radiation; the stored energy forms an invisible pattern on the emulsion known as the latent image.
- When the exposed film with the latent image undergoes chemical processing procedures, a visible image results.
- Three types of film are used in dental radiography: intraoral film, extraoral film, and duplicating film.
- Intraoral film is placed inside the mouth and exposed, extraoral film is placed outside the mouth and exposed, and duplicating film is used to copy dental radiographs.

- Intraoral film packets have four components: x-ray film, paper film wrapper, lead foil sheet, and outer package wrapping.
- Intraoral films are manufactured in five sizes (0, 1, 2, 3, 4); the larger the number, the larger the size of the film.
- Intraoral film is available in D speed and E speed; E-speed film requires one half the exposure time of D-speed film and exhibits comparable image contrast and resolution.
- Extraoral films are typically screen films and require the use of intensifying screens and a cassette for exposure.
- Intensifying screens transform x-ray energy into visible light, which in turn exposes the screen film.
- The use of intensifying screens requires less radiation to expose a screen film and results in less radiation exposure for the patient.
- Duplicating film is a special type of photographic film used to make an identical copy of an intraoral or extraoral radiograph.
- Duplicating film is used in a darkroom setting and is not exposed to x-radiation.
- Film is adversely affected by heat, humidity, and radiation and must be stored away from sources of radiation in temperatures of 50 to 70 degrees Fahrenheit and with a relative humidity level of 30 to 50%.
- Dental film should always be used before the expiration date on the label.

BIBLIOGRAPHY

Eastman Kodak Company: Fundamentals of dental radiography. *In* X-Rays in Dentistry. Rochester, Eastman Kodak Company, 1985, pp. 9–10.

Eastman Kodak Company: Kodak Dental Products, 1993/94 Catalog and Reference Guide Rochester, Eastman Kodak Company, 1993, pp. 5, 24–28.

Frommer HH: Image formation, image receptors. *In* Radiology for Dental Auxiliaries, 6th edition. St. Louis, Mosby-Year Book, 1996, pp. 31–47.

Goaz PW, White SC: X-ray film, intensifying screens, and grids. *In* Oral Radiology: Principles and Interpretation, 3rd edition. St. Louis, Mosby-Year Book, 1994, pp. 79–97.

Johnson ON, McNally MA, Essay CE: Dental x-ray films. *In* Essentials of Dental Radiography for Dental Assistants and Hygienists, 6th edition. Norwalk, CT, Appleton and Lange, 1999, pp. 157–177.

Kasle MJ, Langlais RP: Film, cassettes and intensifying screens. *In* Basic Principles of Oral Radiography: Exercises in Dental Radiology, vol. 4. Philadelphia, WB Saunders, 1981, pp. 92–96.

Langland OE, Sippy FH, Langlais RP: Attenuation and recording the radiographic image. *In* Textbook of Dental Radiography, 2nd edition. Springfield, IL, Charles C Thomas, 1984, pp. 93–103.

Manson-Hing LR: Films, processing, darkroom, and duplicating. *In* Fundamentals of Dental Radiography, 3rd edition. Philadelphia, Lea & Febiger, 1990, pp. 16–21.

Matteson SR, Whaley C, Secrist VC: The film and the darkroom. *In* Dental Radiology, 4th edition. Chapel Hill, University of North Carolina Press, 1988, pp. 53–58.

Miles DA, Van Dis ML, Jensen CW, Ferretti A: Film processing and quality assurance. *In* Radiographic Imaging for Dental Auxiliaries, 3rd edition. Philadelphia, WB Saunders, 1999, pp. 49–71.

Miles DA, Van Dis ML, Razmus TF: Radiographic image production and film characteristics. *In* Basic Principles of Oral and Maxillofacial Radiology. Philadelphia, WB Saunders, 1992, pp. 50–54, 66, 74, 156.

Quiz Questions ••

FILL IN THE BLANK

1. The component part of an x-ray film described as a thin transparent coating that is placed over the emulsion is termed:

   _____

2. The component part of the x-ray film described as a flexible piece of plastic that withstands heat, moisture, and chemical heat is termed:

   _____

3. The chemical compounds that change when exposed to radiation or light are termed:

   _____

4. The invisible pattern of stored energy on the exposed film is termed:

   _____

For questions 5 to 11, identify the components that make up the intraoral film packet in Figure 7–23.

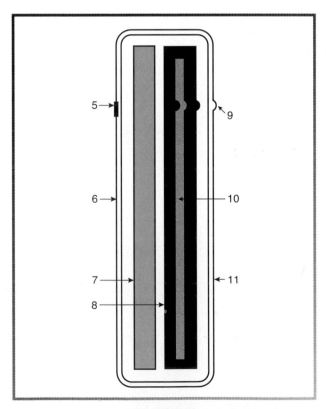

FIGURE 7–23

MULTIPLE CHOICE

_____C_____ 12. Dental x-ray film that is placed inside the mouth and used to examine the teeth and supporting structures is termed:

  a. duplicating film
  b. extraoral film
  c. intraoral film
  d. none of the above

_____D_____ 13. The identification dot on the intraoral film is significant because:

  a. the dot indicates the patient's right or left side
  b. the dot determines film orientation
  c. the dot is important in film mounting
  d. all of the above

_____A_____ 14. One advantage of a film with an emulsion coating on both sides (double-emulsion film) is that:

  a. the film requires less radiation exposure to make an image
  b. the image produced is less distorted
  c. the film has less sensitivity to radiation
  d. processing solutions are absorbed more easily

_____C_____ 15. The purpose of a lead foil sheet in the film packet is:

  a. to protect the film from primary radiation
  b. to protect the film from saliva
  c. to protect the film from back-scattered radiation
  d. to distinguish between the patient's right and left side

_____B_____ 16. Which of the following is NOT found on the label side of the film packet?

  a. the film speed
  b. the expiration date
  c. the phrase "opposite side toward tube"
  d. the number of films enclosed

_____C_____ 17. Which of the following film sizes is known as the standard film?

  a. size 0
  b. size 1
  c. size 2
  d. size 3

_____A_____ 18. Which of the following is the largest intraoral film size?
  a. size 4
  b. size 3
  c. size 2
  d. size 1

_____B_____ 19. The film characteristic that is "the amount of radiation needed to produce a radiograph of standard density" is:

  a. contrast
  b. speed
  c. image resolution
  d. size

_____ *A*   **20.** The speed of a film is determined by the size of the silver halide crystals in the emulsion. Identify the true statement:

   a. the larger the crystals, the faster the film speed
   b. the larger the crystals, the slower the film speed
   c. the smaller the crystals, the faster the film speed
   d. none of the above are correct

_____ *A*   **21.** A film that is placed outside of the mouth during x-ray exposure is termed:

   a. extraoral film
   b. intraoral film
   c. duplicating film
   d. periapical film

_____ *A*   **22.** A screen film is more sensitive to fluorescent light than to direct exposure to x-rays.

   a. true
   b. false

_____ *B*   **23.** Nonscreen extraoral film is commonly used in extraoral radiography.

   a. true
   b. false

_____ *D*   **24.** The device that transfers x-ray energy into visible light is termed a:

   a. cassette
   b. nonscreen film
   c. screen film
   d. intensifying screen

_____ *B*   **25.** The intensifying screen that emits green light and must be used with green-sensitive film is a:

   a. calcium tungstate screen
   b. rare earth screen
   c. phosphor screen
   d. rare tungstate screen

_____ *C*   **26.** The device used to hold the extraoral film and intensifying screens is termed a:

   a. screen holder
   b. film holder
   c. cassette
   d. any of the above

_____ *A*   **27.** Which of the following is TRUE?

   a. cassettes are available in sizes that correspond to film and screen sizes
   b. a flexible cassette is more expensive than a rigid cassette
   c. film can be loaded incorrectly in the rigid cassette
   d. film cannot be loaded incorrectly in the flexible cassette

_____ *C*   **28.** If the intensifying screens are not in perfect contact with the screen film, which of the following results?

   a. the screen may be damaged
   b. the film may be damaged
   c. a loss of image sharpness occurs
   d. none of the above

_____ C 29. Identify the FALSE statement.

    a. duplicating film is not exposed to x-rays
    b. duplicating film is used in the darkroom
    c. duplicating film may be placed intraorally or extraorally
    d. duplicating film is used to make copies of radiographs

_____ A 30. Identify the ideal temperature and humidity levels for film storage.

    a. 50 to 70°F, 30 to 50%
    b. 60 to 80°F, 50 to 60%
    c. 70 to 90°F, 60 to 70%
    d. below 50°F, 0 to 30%

Answers are supplied at the end of this book.

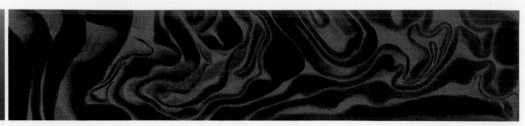

CHAPTER 8

Dental X-ray Image Characteristics

OBJECTIVES

After completion of this chapter, the student will be able to:

- *Define the key words.*
- *Differentiate between radiolucent and radiopaque areas on a dental radiograph.*
- *Describe a diagnostic dental radiograph.*
- *List the two visual characteristics of the radiographic image.*
- *List the factors that influence film density and contrast.*
- *Discuss the difference between high and low contrast.*
- *Describe film contrast and subject contrast.*
- *Describe the difference between short-scale and long-scale contrast.*
- *Identify images of high contrast, low contrast, no contrast, short-scale contrast, and long-scale contrast.*
- *Describe a stepwedge.*
- *List the three geometric characteristics of the radiographic image.*
- *List the factors that influence sharpness, magnification, and distortion.*

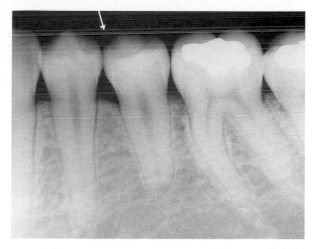

FIGURE 8–1. Air space (*arrow*) appears radiolucent, or dark, because the dental x-rays pass through freely.

INTRODUCTION

Dental x-ray image characteristics include both visual characteristics and geometric characteristics. A variety of influencing factors affect the visual image characteristics of film density and contrast as well as the geometric image characteristics of sharpness, magnification, and distortion.

The dental radiographer must have a working knowledge of dental x-ray image characteristics. The purpose of this chapter is to describe in detail the visual image characteristics of film density and contrast, to define the geometric image characteristics of sharpness, magnification, and distortion, and to discuss how influencing factors alter these image characteristics.

DENTAL X-RAY IMAGE CHARACTERISTICS

A dental radiograph appears as a black and white image or picture that includes varying shades of gray. When viewed on a light source, the darkest area of a radiograph appears black and the lightest area appears white. Two terms are used to describe the black and white areas viewed on a dental radiograph: radiolucent and radiopaque.

Radiolucent: Radiolucent refers to that portion of a processed radiograph that is *dark* or *black*. A structure that appears radiolucent on a radio-graph lacks density and permits the passage of the x-ray beam with little or no resistance. For example, air space freely permits the passage of dental x-rays and appears mostly radiolucent on a dental radiograph (Fig. 8–1).

Radiopaque: Radiopaque refers to that portion of a processed radiograph that appears *light* or *white*. Radiopaque structures are dense and absorb or resist the passage of the x-ray beam. For example, structures that resist the passage of the x-ray beam include enamel, dentin, and bone, and appear radiopaque on a dental radiograph (Fig. 8–2).

pulp is radiolucent
compact bone *amalgam*

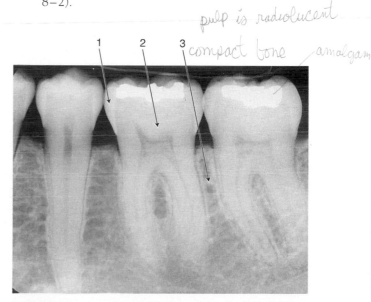

FIGURE 8–2. Dense structures, such as (1) enamel, (2) dentin, and (3) bone, resist the passage of x-rays and appear radiopaque, or white.

The ideal dental radiograph is not too light and not too dark. The quality of a dental radiograph is determined by its image characteristics. The image characteristics of a dental radiograph include the visual characteristics of proper film density and contrast as well as the geometric characteristics of sharpness with minimal magnification and distortion. The ideal dental radiograph is a diagnostic one. A **diagnostic radiograph** provides a great deal of information; the images exhibit proper density and contrast, have sharp outlines, and are of the same shape and size as the object radiographed.

VISUAL CHARACTERISTICS

Two visual characteristics of the radiographic image—density and contrast—directly influence the diagnostic quality of a dental radiograph.

Density

The overall blackness or darkness of a dental radiograph is termed **density**.

DESCRIPTION

When a dental radiograph is viewed against a light source, the relative transparency of areas on the radiograph depends on the distribution of black silver particles in the emulsion. Darker areas represent heavier deposits of black silver particles. Density is this degree of silver blackening.

Images of teeth and supporting structures must have enough density to be viewed on a light source; however, if the density of a film is too great, the film appears too dark, resulting in images that cannot be visually separated from each other. A radiograph with the correct density enables the radiographer to view black areas (air spaces), white areas (enamel, dentin, and bone), and gray areas (soft tissue) (Fig. 8–3).

INFLUENCING FACTORS

A number of factors have a direct influence on the density of a dental radiograph. As previously discussed in Chapter 3, three **exposure factors** control the density of a dental radiograph:

- milliamperage (mA)
- operating kilovoltage peak (kVp)
- exposure time

Any increase in such exposure factors, separately or combined, increases the density of a dental radiograph.

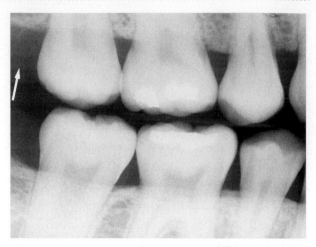

FIGURE 8–3. Notice the grayish area behind the last molar teeth (*arrow*); this represents the gingival tissues.

In addition, the subject thickness also influences film density (Table 8–1).

Milliamperage (mA): An increase in milliamperage produces more x-rays that expose the film and, as a result, increases film density. If the milliamperage is increased, the film density increases and the radiograph appears darker. Conversely, if the milliamperage is decreased, the film density decreases and the radiograph appears lighter.

Operating kilovoltage peak (kVp): An increase in operating kilovoltage increases film density by increasing the mean or average energy of the x-rays and by producing x-rays of higher energy. If the operating kilovoltage is increased, the film density increases and the radiograph appears darker. Conversely, if kilovoltage is decreased, the film density decreases and the radiograph appears lighter.

Exposure time: An increase in exposure time increases film density by increasing the total number of x-rays that reach the film surface. If the exposure time is increased, more x-rays reach the film, the film density increases, and the radiograph appears darker. Conversely, if the exposure time is decreased, the film density decreases and the radiograph appears lighter.

Subject thickness: Fewer x-rays reach the film in a patient with an increased amount of soft tissue or thick, dense bones. As a result, the radiograph has less density and appears lighter. Adjustments in operating kilovoltage peak, milliamperage, or

TABLE 8–1. Visual Characteristics and Influencing Factors

Visual Characteristics	Influencing Factors	Effect of Influencing Factors		
Density	mA	↑ mA	=	↑ density
		↓ mA	=	↓ density
	kVp	↑ kVp	=	↑ density
		↓ kVp	=	↓ density
	Time	↑ time	=	↑ density
		↓ time	=	↓ density
	Subject thickness	↑ thickness	=	↓ density
		↓ thickness	=	↑ density
Contrast	kVp	↑ kVp	=	long-scale contrast; low contrast
		↓ kVp	=	short-scale contrast; high contrast

mA, milliamperage; kVp, kilovoltage peaks

exposure time can be made to compensate for variations in the size of patients and subject thickness.

Contrast

The difference in the degrees of blackness (densities) between adjacent areas on a dental radiograph is termed **contrast**.

DESCRIPTION

The differences in the amount of light transmitted through adjacent areas of a dental radiograph can also be described as contrast. When viewed on a light source, a dental radiograph that has very dark areas and very light areas is said to have **high contrast**; the dark and light areas are strikingly different. A radiograph that does not have very dark and very light areas but instead has many shades of gray is said to have **low contrast**. In dental radiography, a film that is a compromise between low contrast and high contrast is preferred. The overall contrast of a dental radiograph is determined by the film properties, or film contrast, and by the object radiographed, or subject contrast.

Film contrast: Film contrast refers to the characteristics of the film that influence radiographic contrast. The characteristics of the film that influence contrast include the inherent qualities of the film and film processing. The inherent qualities of the film are under the control of the film manufacturer and cannot be changed by the den-

tal radiographer. Film processing, however, is under the control of the dental radiographer. Development time or the temperature of the developer solution affects the contrast of a dental radiograph. An increase in development time or developer temperature results in a film with increased contrast.

Subject contrast: Subject contrast refers to the characteristics of the subject that influence radiographic contrast. Subject contrast is determined by the thickness, density, and composition (atomic number) of the subject. Subject contrast can be altered by increasing or decreasing the kilovoltage. When a high operating kilovoltage peak (>90 kVp) is used, low subject contrast results, and many shades of gray are seen on the dental radiograph. Conversely, when a low operating kilovoltage peak (65 to 70 kVp) is used, high subject contrast results, and areas of black and white are seen.

INFLUENCING FACTORS

Only one exposure factor has a direct influence on the contrast of a dental radiograph. As previously discussed in Chapter 3, the operating kilovoltage peak (kVp) affects film contrast.

Operating kilovoltage peak: Increasing the kilovoltage affects film contrast by increasing the mean or average energy of the x-rays and by producing higher energy x-rays. X-rays with higher energy are better able to penetrate tissue.

As a result, more variations in tissue density are recorded on the film and appear as varying shades of gray. A higher kilovoltage produces a film with decreased or low contrast; the radiograph exhibits many shades of gray. Conversely, a lower kilovoltage produces a film with increased or high contrast; the radiograph has many black and white areas.

The effects of kilovoltage on contrast are summarized in Table 8–1. A series of dental radiographs showing the influence of kilovoltage on both density and contrast is illustrated in Figure 8–4.

SCALES OF CONTRAST

The range of useful densities seen on a dental radiograph is termed the **scale of contrast**. In dental radi-ography, the terms short-scale contrast and long-scale contrast may be used to describe the appearance of a radiograph.

Short-scale contrast: A dental radiograph that shows only two densities, areas of black and white, has a short contrast scale. A lower kilovoltage range results in a radiograph with a short-scale contrast; many areas of black and white are seen rather than shades of gray. A radiograph that exhibits a short contrast scale can also be described as having *high* contrast, in which areas of black and white are easily distinguished from each other (Table 8–2).

Long-scale contrast: A dental radiograph that exhibits many densities, or many shades of gray, has a long contrast scale. A higher kilovoltage range results in a radiograph with a long-scale

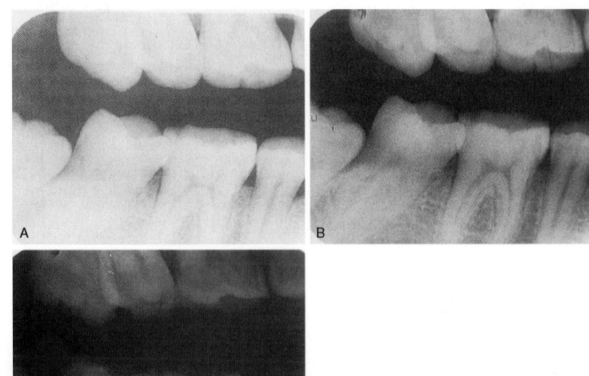

FIGURE 8–4. *A,* Exposure series showing the influence of kVp. When kVp is low, the result is low density (the degree of blackness created by developed silver) and high contrast (the relative difference between the lightest and darkest elements in a radiograph). *B,* The optimal image is created when a proper balance between kVp and mA is obtained. This image is considered optimal because it provides a full range of tones from white to black. *C,* When kVp is high, the result is very high density with very little contrast. (*A* to *C* reprinted courtesy of Eastman Kodak Company, Rochester, NY.)

TABLE 8–2. The Effect of Kilovoltage on Contrast

Kilovoltage	Contrast	Scale of Contrast	Example
High (>90 kVp)	Low	Long-scale	See Fig. 8–16A
Low (<70 kVp)	High	Short-scale	See Fig. 8–16B

kVp, kilovoltage peaks

contrast; many shades of gray are present rather than areas of black and white. A radiograph that exhibits a long contrast scale can also be described as having *low* contrast, in which areas of gray are not easily distinguished from each other (see Table 8–2).

A device known as a **stepwedge** can be used to demonstrate short-scale and long-scale contrast. A stepwedge consists of uniform layered thicknesses of an x-ray absorbing material, usually aluminum. The typical stepwedge is constructed of aluminum steps in 2-mm increments (Fig. 8–5). When a stepwedge is placed on top of a film and exposed to x-rays, the different steps absorb varying amounts of x-rays. As a result, different film densities appear on the dental radiograph.

The use of a stepwedge to demonstrate corresponding film densities and contrast scales is illustrated in Figure 8–6. The stepwedge can be used to monitor the quality of the film and film processing; quality control tests using the stepwedge are further discussed in Chapter 10.

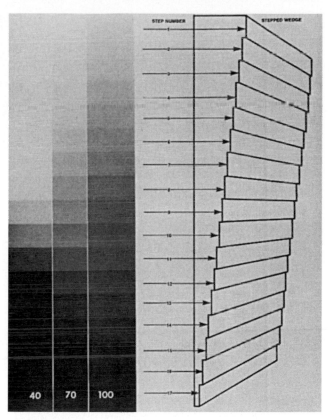

FIGURE 8–6. Radiographs taken at 40 kVp are predominantly black and white—that is, they have high contrast (a short contrast scale). Those taken at 100 kVp show many shades of gray (a long contrast scale). (From Miles DA, Van Dis ML, Jensen CW, Ferretti A: Radiographic Imaging for Dental Auxiliaries, 2nd ed. Philadelphia, WB Saunders, 1993.)

GEOMETRIC CHARACTERISTICS

Three geometric characteristics of the radiographic image—sharpness, magnification, and distortion—influence the diagnostic quality of a dental radiograph. These geometric characteristics must be minimized to produce an accurate radiographic image.

Sharpness

Sharpness (also known as detail, resolution, or definition) refers to the capability of the x-ray film to reproduce the distinct outlines of an object, or, in other words, to how well the smallest details of an object are reproduced on a dental radiograph.

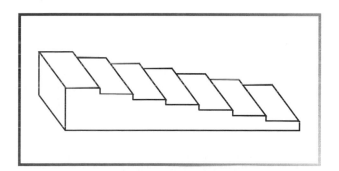

FIGURE 8–5. A stepwedge is made of uniform layered thicknesses.

DESCRIPTION

A certain lack of image sharpness, or unsharpness, is present in every dental radiograph. The fuzzy, unclear area that surrounds a radiographic image is termed the **penumbra.** The term penumbra is derived from two Latin words, *pene,* meaning almost, and *umbra,* meaning shadow. Penumbra can be defined as the unsharpness, or blurring, of the edges of a radiographic image.

INFLUENCING FACTORS

The sharpness of a film is influenced by three factors (Table 8–3):

- focal spot size
- film composition
- movement

Focal spot size: As described in Chapter 2, the tungsten target of the anode serves as a focal spot; this small area converts bombarding electrons into x-ray photons. The focal spot concentrates the electrons and creates an enormous amount of heat. To limit the amount of heat produced and to prevent damage to the x-ray tube, the size of the focal spot is limited. The size of the focal spot ranges from 0.6 mm² to 1.0 mm² and is determined by the manufacturer of the x-ray equipment; most manufacturers use the smallest focal spot area possible based on heat production restrictions.

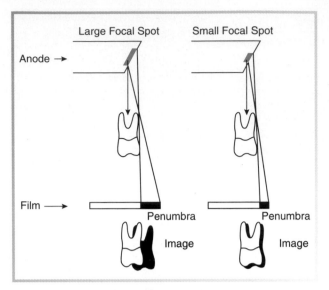

FIGURE 8–7. The smaller the focal spot area, the sharper the image appears; the larger the focal spot area, the greater the amount of penumbra and loss of image sharpness.

The smaller the focal spot area, the sharper the image appears; the larger the focal spot area, the greater the loss of image sharpness (Fig. 8–7). If x-rays were produced from one spot or a single "point source," no unsharpness would be present (Fig. 8–8). However, a single point source of x-ray production is impossible because of the limited capacity of the x-ray tube.

TABLE 8–3. Geometric Characteristics and Influencing Factors

Geometric Characteristics	Influencing Factors	Effect of Influencing Factors	
Sharpness	Focal spot size	↓ focal spot size	= ↑ sharpness
		↑ focal spot size	= ↓ sharpness
	Film composition	↓ crystal size	= ↑ sharpness
		↑ crystal size	= ↓ sharpness
	Movement	↓ movement	= ↑ sharpness
		↑ movement	= ↓ sharpness
Magnification	Target-film distance (TFD)	↑ TFD	= ↓ magnification
		↓ TFD	= ↑ magnification
	Object-film distance (OFD)	↑ OFD	= ↑ magnification
		↓ OFD	= ↓ magnification
Distortion	Object-film alignment	Object and film parallel	= ↓ distortion
		Object and film not parallel	= ↑ distortion
	X-ray beam alignment	Beam perpendicular to object and film	= ↓ distortion
		Beam not perpendicular to object and film	= ↑ distortion

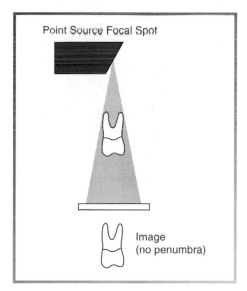

FIGURE 8-8. Theoretical "point source" of x-rays would produce a sharp image without penumbra.

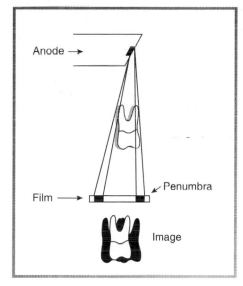

FIGURE 8-9. Diagram illustrating the influence of motion on film sharpness. Notice that the image outline is blurred owing to penumbra formation.

Film composition: The composition of the film emulsion influences sharpness. Sharpness is relative to the size of the crystals found in the film emulsion. The emulsion of faster film contains larger crystals that produce less image sharpness, whereas slower film contains smaller crystals that produce more image sharpness. Unsharpness occurs because the larger crystals do not produce object outlines as well as smaller crystals.

Movement: Movement influences film sharpness. A loss of image sharpness occurs if either the film or the patient moves during x-ray exposure (Fig. 8-9). Even slight amounts of film or patient movement result in unsharpness (Fig. 8-10).

Magnification

Image **magnification** refers to a radiographic image that appears larger than the actual size of the object it represents.

DESCRIPTION

Magnification, or enlargement of a radiographic image, results from the divergent paths of the x-ray beam. As you may recall from Chapter 2, x-rays travel in diverging straight lines as they radiate from the focal spot. Because of these diverging paths, some degree of image magnification is present in every dental radiograph (Fig. 8-11).

INFLUENCING FACTORS

The image magnification on a dental radiograph is influenced by the target-film distance and the object-film distance (see Table 8-3).

Target-film distance: As defined in Chapter 3, the target-film distance (also known as the source-to-film distance) is the distance between the source of x-rays (focal spot on the tungsten target) and the film. The target-film distance is determined by the length of the position-indicating device (PID). When a longer PID is used, more parallel

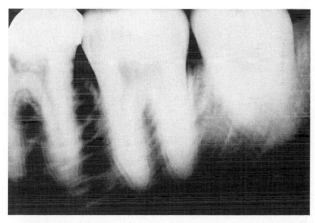

FIGURE 8-10. Radiograph of a patient who moved during x-ray exposure. Notice the blurred image outline.

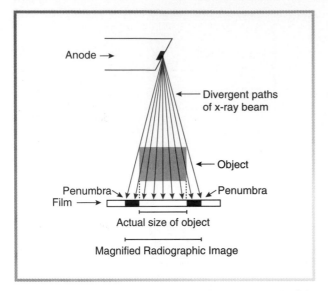

FIGURE 8–11. Diagram illustrating magnification as a result of the divergent paths of the x-ray beam.

rays from the middle of the x-ray beam strike the object rather than the diverging x-rays from the periphery of the beam. As a result, a longer PID and target-film distance result in less image magnification, and a shorter PID and target-film distance result in more image magnification (Fig. 8–12).

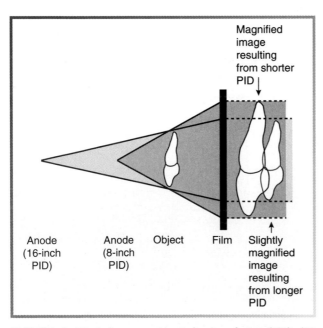

FIGURE 8–12. A longer position-indicating device (PID) (16 inches) and target-film distance results in less image magnification.

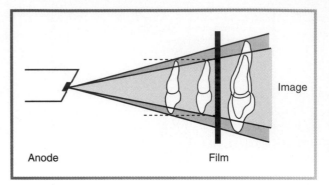

FIGURE 8–13. Diagram illustrating object-film distance. Notice that the closer the proximity of the tooth to the film, the less image enlargement is seen on the film.

Object-film distance: As defined in Chapter 3, the object-film distance is the distance between the object being radiographed (the tooth) and the dental x-ray film. The tooth and the x-ray film should always be placed as close together as possible. The closer the proximity of the tooth to the film, the less image enlargement there will be on the film. A decrease in object-film distance results in a decrease in magnification, and an increase in object-film distance results in an increase in image magnification (Fig. 8–13).

Distortion

Dimensional **distortion** of a radiographic image is a variation in the true size and shape of the object

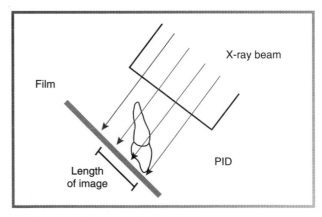

FIGURE 8–14. If the tooth and film are not parallel, an angular relationship is formed and a distorted image results. In this example, the length of the image that appears on the film is shorter than the actual tooth.

being radiographed. A distorted image does not have the same size and shape as the object being radiographed.

DESCRIPTION

A distorted image results from the unequal magnification of different parts of the same object. Distortion results from improper film alignment or angulation of the x-ray beam.

INFLUENCING FACTORS

The dimensional distortion of a radiographic image is influenced by object-film alignment and x-ray beam angulation (see Table 8–3).

Object-film alignment: To minimize dimensional distortion, the object and film must be parallel to each other. If the object (tooth) and film are not parallel, an angular relationship results. An angular relationship produces a variation of distances between the tooth and the film that result in a distorted image. A distorted image may appear too long or too short (Fig. 8–14). Such distortions are discussed in the later chapters on technique.

X-ray beam angulation: To minimize dimensional distortion, the x-ray beam must be directed perpendicular to the tooth and the film. The central ray of the x-ray beam must be as nearly perpendicular to the tooth and film as possible to record the adjacent structures in their true spatial relationships (Fig. 8–15).

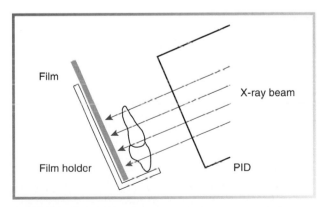

FIGURE 8–15. To limit distortion, the central ray of the x-ray beam must be perpendicular to the tooth and film.

▓▓ SUMMARY

- A number of influencing factors affect the visual image characteristics of film density and contrast as well as the geometric characteristics of sharpness, magnification, and distortion.
- The milliamperage, operating kilovoltage peak, and exposure time can be used to adjust the density of a dental radiograph. Subject thickness also influences the density of a film.
- Only the operating kilovoltage peak has a direct influence on film contrast.
- A radiograph that exhibits areas of black and white is termed *high* contrast and is said to have a *short* contrast scale; a radiograph that exhibits many shades of gray is termed *low* contrast and is said to have a *long* contrast scale.
- A stepwedge can be used to demonstrate short-scale and long-scale contrast patterns.
- The influencing factors that affect the geometric characteristics of sharpness, magnification, and distortion are reviewed in Table 8–3.
- To create a sharp image, the dental radiographer uses the smallest focal spot possible, chooses a film with small crystals in the emulsion, and limits patient and film movement.
- To limit image magnification, the longest target-film distance and the shortest object-film distance are used.
- To limit image distortion, the film and the tooth are positioned parallel to each other, and the x-ray beam is directed perpendicular to the tooth and film.

BIBLIOGRAPHY

Barr JH, Stephens RG: Image production with x-rays. *In* Dental Radiology: Pertinent Basic Concepts and Their Applications in Clinical Practice. Philadelphia, WB Saunders, 1980, pp. 53–65.

Eastman Kodak Company: Fundamentals of dental radiography. *In* X-Rays in Dentistry. Rochester, Eastman Kodak Company, 1985, p. 8.

Eastman Kodak Company: Successful Intraoral Radiography. Rochester, Eastman Kodak Company, 1993, pp. 3–5.

Frommer HH: Image formation, image receptors. *In* Radiology for Dental Auxiliaries, 6th edition. St. Louis, Mosby-Year Book, 1996, pp. 31–47.

Goaz PW, White SC: X-ray film, intensifying screens, and grids. *In* Oral Radiology: Principles and Interpretation, 3rd edition. St. Louis, Mosby-Year Book, 1994, pp. 79–97.

Johnson ON, McNally MA, Essay CE: Producing quality radiographs. *In* Essentials of Dental Radiography for Dental Assistants and Hygienists, 6th edition. Norwalk, Appleton and Lange, 1999, pp. 61–85.

Kasle MJ, Langlais RP: The quality image: Geometric factors, density, and contrast. *In* Basic Principles of Oral Radiography: Exercises in Dental Radiology, vol. 1. Philadelphia, WB Saunders, 1981, pp. 56–72.

Langland OE, Sippy FH, Langlais RP: Diagnostic quality of dental radiographs. *In* Textbook of Dental Radiography, 2nd edition. Springfield, IL, Charles C Thomas, 1984, pp. 130–151.

Manson-Hing LR: Radiographic quality and artifacts. *In* Fundamentals of Dental Radiography, 3rd edition. Philadelphia, Lea & Febiger, 1990, pp. 40–45.

Matteson SR, Whaley C, Secrist VC: The film and the darkroom. *In* Dental Radiology, 4th edition. Chapel Hill, University of North Carolina Press, 1988, pp. 55–58.

Miles DA, Van Dis ML, Jensen CW, Ferretti A: Image characteristics. *In* Radiographic Imaging for Dental Auxiliaries, 3rd edition. Philadelphia, WB Saunders, 1999, pp. 87–99.

Miles DA, Van Dis ML, Razmus TF: Radiographic image production and film characteristics. *In* Basic Principles of Oral and Maxillofacial Radiology. Philadelphia, WB Saunders, 1992, pp. 51–66.

O'Brien RC: Dental x-ray film and dark room processing. *In* Dental Radiography: An Introduction for Dental Hygienists and Assistants, 4th edition. Philadelphia, WB Saunders, 1982, pp. 48–51.

Quiz Questions ···

MULTIPLE CHOICE

_B_ 1. The portion of a processed radiograph that appears dark or black is termed:

    a. dense
    b. radiolucent
    c. radiopaque
    d. transparent

_B_ 2. The portion of a processed radiograph that appears light or white is termed:

    a. radiolucent
    b. radiopaque
    c. dense
    d. high density

_D_ 3. Which of the following appears most radiolucent on a dental radiograph?

    a. bone
    b. enamel
    c. dentin
    d. air space

_D_ 4. An example of a radiopaque structure seen on dental x-rays is:

    a. bone
    b. enamel
    c. dentin
    d. all of the above

_A_ 5. The overall blackness or darkness of a dental radiograph is termed:

    a. density
    b. contrast
    c. subject thickness
    d. diagnostic quality

_A_ 6. Increasing the milliamperage (mA) will cause:

    a. an increase in density; the film appears darker
    b. an increase in density; the film appears lighter
    c. a decrease in density; the film appears darker
    d. a decrease in density; the film appears lighter

_A_ 7. Increasing the operating kilovoltage peak (kVp) will cause:

    a. an increase in density; the film appears darker
    b. an increase in density; the film appears lighter
    c. a decrease in density; the film appears darker
    d. a decrease in density; the film appears lighter

_A_ 8. Increasing the exposure time will cause:

    a. an increase in density; the film appears darker
    b. an increase in density; the film appears lighter
    c. a decrease in density; the film appears darker
    d. a decrease in density; the film appears lighter

_D_   9. A dental patient has thick soft tissues and dense bones. To compensate for this increase in subject thickness and provide a film of diagnostic density, the dental radiographer may:

    a. increase the exposure time
    b. increase the milliamperage
    c. increase the operating kilovoltage peak
    d. any of the above

_B_   10. The difference in the degrees of blackness between adjacent areas on a dental radiograph is termed:

    a. density
    b. contrast
    c. subject thickness
    d. diagnostic quality

_B_   11. When viewed on a light source, a dental radiograph that demonstrates many shades of gray is said to have:

    a. high contrast
    b. low contrast
    c. high density
    d. low density

_A_   12. When viewed on a light source, a dental radiograph that demonstrates very dark areas and very light areas is said to have:

    a. high contrast
    b. low contrast
    c. high density
    d. low density

For questions 13 to 17, refer to Figure 8–16.

_____   13. In Figure 8–16, which diagram exhibits *high* contrast?

    a. A
    b. B
    c. C

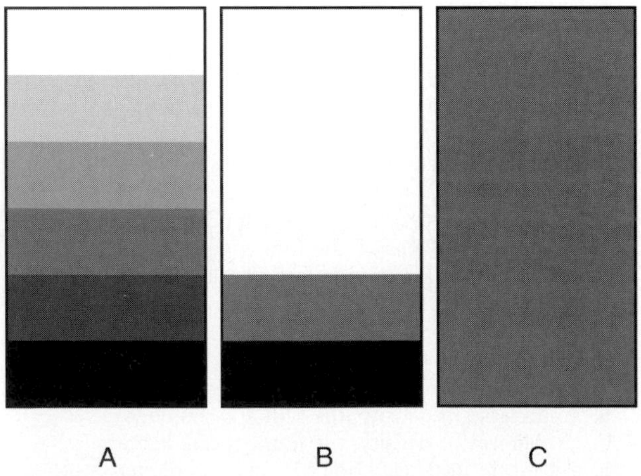

FIGURE 8–16

_____ 14. In Figure 8–16, which diagram exhibits *low* contrast?

    a. A
    b. B
    c. C

_____ 15. In Figure 8–16, which diagram exhibits *long-scale* contrast?

    a. A
    b. B
    c. C

_____ 16. In Figure 8–16, which diagram exhibits *short-scale* contrast?

    a. A
    b. B
    c. C

_____ 17. In Figure 8–16, which diagram exhibits *no* contrast?

    a. A
    b. B
    c. C

___A___ 18. The one exposure factor that has a direct influence on the contrast of a dental radiograph is:

    a. operating kilovoltage peak
    b. milliamperage
    c. exposure time
    d. subject thickness

___D___ 19. The type of contrast preferred in dental radiography is:

    a. low contrast
    b. long-scale contrast only
    c. short-scale contrast only
    d. a compromise between short-scale contrast and long-scale contrast

___C___ 20. The stepwedge is used for all of the following *except:*

    a. to demonstrate short-scale and long-scale contrast
    b. to monitor quality control of film processing
    c. to increase the penetrating quality of the x-ray beam
    d. to demonstrate film densities

___A___ 21. The capability of the x-ray film to reproduce distinct outlines of an object is termed:

    a. sharpness
    b. magnification
    c. distortion
    d. diagnostic quality

___C___ 22. The unsharpness or blurred edges seen on a radiographic image is termed:

    a. distortion
    b. umbra
    c. penumbra
    d. contrast

___D___   **23.** The geometric characteristic that refers to a radiographic image that appears larger than its actual size is termed:

    a. distortion
    b. detail
    c. definition
    d. magnification

___B___   **24.** A variation in the true size and shape of the object being radiographed is termed:

    a. magnification
    b. distortion
    c. sharpness
    d. resolution

FILL IN THE BLANK

For questions 25 to 35, fill in the blank with the words *increase* or *decrease*.

25. Decrease focal spot size   =   _____   sharpness

26. Increase crystal size   =   _____   sharpness

27. Decrease crystal size   =   _____   sharpness

28. Decrease movement   =   _____   sharpness

29. Increase movement   =   _____   sharpness

30. Increase target-film distance   =   _____   magnification

31. Increase object-film distance   =   _____   magnification

32. Decrease object-film distance   =   _____   magnification

33. Object and film are parallel   =   _____   distortion

34. Beam perpendicular to object and film   =   _____   distortion

35. Beam not perpendicular to object and film   =   _____   distortion

Answers are supplied at the end of this book.

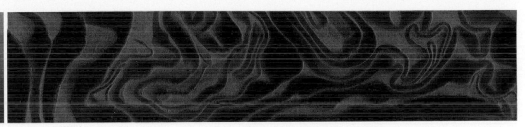

Dental X-ray Film Processing

OBJECTIVES

After completion of this chapter, the student will be able to:

- *Define the key words.*
- *Describe in detail how a latent image becomes a visible image.*
- *List and discuss the five steps of film processing.*
- *List and describe the four basic ingredients of the developer solution.*
- *List and describe the four basic ingredients of the fixer solution.*
- *Discuss the location, size, lighting, and equipment requirements necessary for the darkroom.*
- *Discuss safelighting.*
- *Discuss the parts of the processing tank: insert tanks, master tank, and lid.*
- *List and describe the equipment needed for manual film processing.*
- *List and discuss the step-by-step procedures for manual film processing.*
- *Describe the care and maintenance of the processing solutions, equipment, and equipment accessories used in manual film processing.*

- *Discuss the advantages of automatic film processing.*
- *List and identify the component parts of the automatic film processor.*
- *Describe the mechanism of automatic film processing.*
- *List and discuss the step-by-step procedures used for automatic film processing.*
- *Describe the care and maintenance of the automatic film processor and automatic processing solutions.*
- *Discuss the equipment requirements and step-by-step procedures used for film duplication.*
- *Describe film processing problems that result from time and temperature errors.*
- *Describe film processing problems that result from chemical contamination errors.*
- *Describe film processing problems that result from film handling errors.*
- *Describe film processing problems that result from lighting errors.*

KEY WORDS

Accelerator	Film recovery slot
Acetic acid	Fingernail artifact
Acidifier	Fingerprint artifact
Air bubbles	Fixation
Ammonium thiosulfate	Fixer cut-off
Compartment, developer	Fixer solution
Compartment, fixer	Fixer spots
Compartment, water	Fixing agent
Darkroom	Hardening agent
Darkroom plumbing	Humidity level
Darkroom storage space	Hydroquinone
Darkroom work space	Hypo
Daylight loader	Latent image
Developer cut-off	Light-tight
Developer solution	Light leak
Developer spots	Oxidation
Developing agent	Potassium alum
Development	Potassium bromide
Drying chamber	Preservative
Elon	Processing, automatic
Film, cleaning	Processing, manual
Film, duplicating	Processor, automatic
Film, fogged	Processor housing
Film, overdeveloped	Radiolucent
Film, overlapped	Radiopaque
Film, scratched	Reduction
Film, underdeveloped	Reduction, selective
Film, yellow-brown	Replenisher
Film duplicator	Replenisher pump
Film feed slot	Replenisher solutions
Film hangers	Restrainer
	Reticulation of emulsion
	Rinsing

Roller film transporter	Stirring rod
Room lighting	Sulfuric acid
Safelight filter	Tank, insert
Safelighting	Tank, master
Sodium carbonate	Tank, processing
Sodium sulfite	Thermometer
Sodium thiosulfate	Timer
Static electricity	Valve, mixing
Stirring paddle	

◼ INTRODUCTION

To produce high-quality diagnostic dental radiographs, dental x-ray film must be properly exposed and processed. Film processing procedures directly affect the quality of a dental radiograph. The dental radiographer must have a working knowledge of film processing procedures, problems, and solutions.

The purpose of this chapter is to detail film processing procedures, to describe darkroom requirements, to discuss manual and automatic film processing, and to explain film duplication procedures. In addition, this chapter discusses common processing problems and offers solutions to those problems.

◼ FILM PROCESSING

Film processing refers to a series of steps that collectively produces a visible permanent image on a dental radiograph. The purpose of film processing is twofold:

- to convert the latent (invisible) image on the film into a visible image

- to preserve the visible image so that it is permanent and does not disappear from the dental radiograph

Film Processing Fundamentals

As detailed in Chapter 7, the silver halide crystals in the film emulsion absorb x-radiation during x-ray exposure and store the energy from the radiation. The stored energy within the silver halide crystals forms a pattern and creates an invisible image within the emulsion on the exposed film. This pattern of stored energy on the exposed film cannot be seen and is referred to as the **latent image.** The latent image remains invisible within the film emulsion until it undergoes chemical processing procedures.

FROM LATENT IMAGE TO VISIBLE IMAGE

How does the latent image become a visible image? Under special darkroom conditions, a chemical reaction takes place when a film with a latent image is immersed in a series of special chemical solutions. During processing, a chemical reaction occurs, and the halide portion of the *exposed, energized* silver halide crystal is removed; chemically, this is referred to as a **reduction.** Reduction of the exposed silver halide crystals results in precipitated black metallic silver.

During film processing, selective reduction of the exposed silver halide crystals occurs. **Selective reduction** refers to the reduction of the energized, exposed silver halide crystals into black metallic silver, while the *unenergized, unexposed* silver halide crystals are removed from the film. The latent image is made visible through processing procedures (Fig. 9–1) and can be described as follows:

1. The film is placed in a chemical known as the **developer solution** for a specific amount of time and at a specific temperature. The developer distinguishes between the exposed and unexposed silver halide crystals. The developer initiates a chemical reaction that reduces the exposed silver halide crystals into black metallic silver and creates dark or black areas on a dental radiograph. At the same time, the unexposed silver halide crystals remain virtually unaffected by the developer.

2. Following the development process, the film is rinsed in water to remove any remaining developer solution.

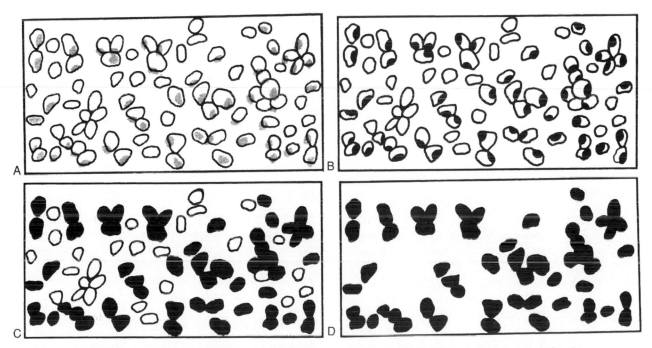

FIGURE 9–1. *A,* Schematic distribution of silver halide grains. The gray areas indicate a latent image produced by exposure. *B,* Partial development begins to produce metallic silver (black) in exposed grains. *C,* Development completed. *D,* Unexposed silver grains have been removed by fixation. (Reprinted courtesy of Eastman Kodak Company, Rochester, NY.)

3. Next, the film is placed in a special chemical known as the **fixer solution** for a specific amount of time. The fixer solution removes the unexposed silver halide crystals and creates white or clear areas on the dental radiograph. Meanwhile, the black metallic silver is not removed and remains on the film. Following the fixing process, the film is washed in water to remove any remaining traces of the chemical solutions and then dried.

THE VISIBLE IMAGE

The visible image that results on a dental radiograph is made up of black, white, and gray areas. The black areas seen on a dental radiograph are created by deposits of black metallic silver. The amount of deposited black metallic silver seen on a dental radiograph varies depending on the structures being radiographed. As discussed in Chapter 8, structures that permit the passage of the x-ray beam appear black, or radiolucent.

Radiolucent: A radiolucent structure is one that readily permits the passage of the x-ray beam and allows more x-rays to reach the film. If more x-rays reach the film, more silver halide crystals in the film emulsion are exposed and energized, thus resulting in increased deposits of black metallic silver. A radiograph with large deposits of black metallic silver appears black, or radiolucent.

The white areas on a dental radiograph result from the removal of the unexposed silver halide crystals. The amount of unexposed silver halide crystals removed depends on the structures being radiographed. As discussed in Chapter 8, structures that resist the passage of the x-ray beam appear white or radiopaque.

Radiopaque: A radiopaque structure is one that resists the passage of the x-ray beam and restricts or limits the amount of x-rays that reach the film. If no x-rays reach the film, no silver halide crystals in the film emulsion are exposed, and no deposits of black metallic silver are seen. A radiograph with areas of unexposed silver halide crystals that have been removed during processing and no black metallic silver deposits appears white, or radiopaque.

Film Processing Steps

There are five steps in film processing:

1. development
2. rinsing
3. fixation
4. washing
5. drying

DEVELOPMENT

The first step in film processing is **development.** A chemical solution known as the developer is used in the development process. The purpose of the developer is to chemically reduce the exposed, energized silver halide crystals into black metallic silver. The developer solution softens the film emulsion during this process.

RINSING

Following development, a water bath is used to wash or rinse the film. **Rinsing** is necessary to remove the developer from the film and stop the development process.

FIXATION

Following rinsing, **fixation** takes place. A chemical solution known as the fixer is used in the fixing process. The purpose of the fixer is to remove the unexposed, unenergized silver halide crystals from the film emulsion. The fixer hardens the film emulsion during this process.

WASHING

Following fixation, a water bath is used to wash the film. A washing step is necessary to thoroughly remove all excess chemicals from the emulsion.

DRYING

The final step in film processing is the drying of the films. Films may be air-dried at room temperature in a dust-free area or placed in a heated drying cabinet. Films must be completely dried before they can be handled for mounting and viewing.

Film Processing Solutions

Film processing solutions may be obtained in the following forms:

- powder
- ready-to-use liquid
- liquid concentrate

Both the powder and liquid concentrate forms must be mixed with distilled water. The liquid concentrate form is popular and is used in most dental offices; it is easy to mix and occupies little storage space (Fig. 9-2). It is important to follow the manufacturer's recommendations for the preparation of such solutions.

Fresh chemicals produce the best radiographs. To maintain freshness, film processing solutions must be replenished daily and changed every 3 to 4 weeks; more frequent changing of solutions may be necessary when large numbers of films are processed. Normal use is defined as 30 intraoral films per day.

As described under Film Processing Steps, two special chemical solutions are necessary for film processing:

- developer
- fixer

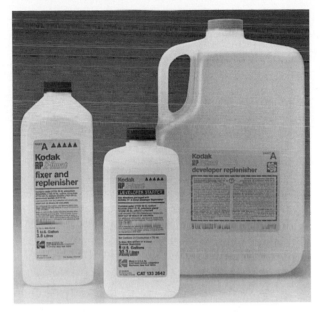

FIGURE 9-2. Liquid concentrates of developer and fixer. (Reprinted courtesy of Eastman Kodak Company, Rochester, NY.)

DEVELOPER SOLUTION

The developer solution contains four basic ingredients (Table 9-1).

Developing agent: The developing agent (also known as the reducing agent) contains two chemicals, hydroquinone (paradihydroxybenzene) and Elon (monomethy-para-aminophenol sulfate). The purpose of the developing agent is to reduce the exposed silver halide crystals chemically to black metallic silver. **Hydroquinone** generates the black tones and the sharp contrast of the radiographic image. Hydroquinone is temperature sensitive; it is inactive below 60°F and very active above 80°F. Because this chemical is sensitive to temperature, the temperature of the developing solution is critical. The optimal temperature for the developer solution is 68°F. **Elon,** also known as metol, acts quickly to produce a visible radiographic image. Elon generates the many shades of gray seen on a dental radiograph. This chemical is not temperature sensitive. If hydroquinone and Elon were used individually instead of in combination, Elon would produce a film that appeared gray with indistinct contrast, whereas hydroquinone would produce a film that

TABLE 9-1. Developer Composition

Ingredient	Chemical	Function
Developing agent	Hydroquinone	Converts exposed silver halide crystals to black metallic silver Slowly generates the black tones and contrast in the image
	Elon	Converts exposed silver halide crystals to black metallic silver Quickly generates the gray tones in the image
Preservative	Sodium sulfite	Prevents rapid oxidation of the developing agents
Accelerator	Sodium carbonate	Activates developer agents Provides necessary alkaline environment for developing agents Softens gelatin of the film emulsion
Restrainer	Potassium bromide	Prevents the developer from developing the unexposed silver halide crystals

appeared black and white. By using a combination of these chemicals, a film with black, white, *and* shades of gray is produced.

Preservative: The antioxidant **sodium sulfite** is the preservative used in the developer solution. The purpose of the preservative is to prevent the developer solution from oxidizing in the presence of air. The reducing agents hydroquinone and Elon are not stable in the presence of oxygen and readily absorb oxygen from the air. If these agents react with oxygen, the action of the developer solution is weakened. The preservative helps to prevent this weakening and to extend the useful life of hydroquinone and Elon.

Accelerator: The alkali **sodium carbonate** is used in the developer solution as an accelerator. The purpose of the accelerator (also called the activator) is to activate the developing agents. The developing agents are active only in an alkaline (high pH) environment. For example, hydroquinone and Elon do not develop when used alone; the presence of an alkaline accelerator is required. The accelerator not only provides the necessary alkaline environment for the developing agents but also softens the gelatin of the film emulsion so that the developing agents can reach the silver halide crystals more effectively.

Restrainer: The restrainer used in the developing solution is **potassium bromide.** The purpose of the restrainer is to control the developer and to prevent it from developing the exposed and unexposed silver halide crystals. Although the restrainer stops the development of both exposed and unexposed crystals, it is most effective in stopping development of the unexposed crystals. As a result, the restrainer prevents the radiographic image from appearing *fogged;* a fogged film appears dull gray, lacks contrast, and is nondiagnostic.

FIXER SOLUTION

The fixer solution contains four basic ingredients (Table 9–2).

Fixing agent: The fixing agent (also known as the clearing agent) is made up of **sodium thiosulfate** or **ammonium thiosulfate** and is commonly called **hypo.** The purpose of the fixing agent is to remove or clear all unexposed and undeveloped silver halide crystals from the film emulsion. This chemical "clears" the film so that the black image produced by the developer becomes readily distinguished.

Preservative: The same preservative used in the developer solution, sodium sulfite, is also used in the fixer solution. The purpose of the preservative is to prevent the chemical deterioration of the fixing agent.

Hardening agent: The hardening agent used in the fixer solution is **potassium alum.** The purpose of the **hardening agent,** as the name suggests, is to harden and shrink the gelatin in the film emulsion after it has been softened by the accelerator in the developer solution.

Acidifier: The acidifier used in the fixer solution is **acetic acid** or **sulfuric acid.** The purpose of the acidifier is to neutralize the alkaline developer. Any unneutralized alkali may cause the unexposed crystals to continue to develop in the fixer. The acidifier also produces the necessary acidic environment required by the fixing agent.

▇ THE DARKROOM

The primary function of a **darkroom** is to provide a completely darkened environment where x-ray film can be handled and processed to produce diagnostic radiographs. The darkroom must be properly designed and well equipped.

TABLE 9–2. Fixer Composition

Ingredient	Chemical	Function
Fixing agent	Sodium thiosulfate; ammonium thiosulfate	Removes all unexposed undeveloped silver halide crystals from the emulsion
Preservative	Sodium sulfite	Prevents deterioration of fixing agent
Hardening agent	Potassium alum	Shrinks and hardens the gelatin in the emulsion
Acidifier	Acetic acid; sulfuric acid	Neutralizes the alkaline developer and stops further development

Room Requirements

A well-planned darkroom makes processing easier. The ideal darkroom is the result of careful planning; it must be

- conveniently located
- of adequate size
- equipped with correct lighting
- arranged with ample work space with adequate storage
- temperature and humidity controlled

LOCATION AND SIZE

The location of the darkroom must be convenient; ideally, it should be located near the area where x-ray units are installed. The darkroom must be large enough to accommodate film processing equipment and to allow ample working space. A darkroom should measure at least 16 to 20 square feet and provide enough space for one person to work comfortably. The size of the darkroom is determined by a number of factors:

- the volume of radiographs processed
- the number of persons using the room
- the type of processing equipment used (processing tanks versus automatic processor)
- the space required for duplication of films and storage

LIGHTING

As the term darkroom suggests, this room must be completely dark and must exclude all visible white light. The term **light-tight** is often used to describe the darkroom. To be considered light-tight, no light leaks can be present. Any white light that "leaks" into the darkroom (e.g., from around a door or through a vent) is termed a **light leak.** In a darkroom, when all the lights are turned off and the door is closed, no white light should be seen. Any white light coming around the door, through a vent or keyhole, or through a wall or ceiling seam is a light leak and must be corrected with weather stripping or black tape. As previously discussed, x-ray film is extremely sensitive to visible white light. Any leaks of white light in the darkroom cause film fog. A fogged film appears dull gray, lacks contrast, and is nondiagnostic.

Two types of lighting are essential in a darkroom.

- room lighting
- safelighting

Room lighting: Incandescent **room lighting** is required for procedures not associated with the act of processing films. An overhead white light that provides adequate illumination for the size of the room is necessary to perform tasks such as cleaning, stocking materials, and mixing chemicals.

Safelighting: The special kind of lighting that is used to provide illumination in the darkroom is termed **safelighting.** It is a low-intensity light composed of long wavelengths in the red-orange portion of the visible light spectrum. Safelighting provides sufficient illumination in the darkroom to carry out processing activities safely without exposing or damaging the film. Safelighting does not rapidly affect unwrapped x-ray film and does not cause film fog.

A safelight typically consists of a lamp equipped with a low-wattage bulb (7½ or 15 watts) and a safelight filter. A **safelight filter** removes the short wavelengths in the blue-green portion of the visible light spectrum that are responsible for exposing and damaging x-ray film. At the same time, a safelight filter permits the passage of light in the red-orange range; consequently, the illumination in a darkroom is red. Most x-ray films have a reduced sensitivity to this red-orange range and are not affected by minimal exposure to the safelight.

Under safelight conditions, it is necessary to maintain an adequate safelight illumination distance and to keep film handling times to a minimum. Films that are unwrapped too close to the safelight or exposed to safelight illumination for more than 2 to 3 minutes appear fogged. A safelight must be placed a minimum of 4 feet (1.2 meters) away from the film and working area (Fig. 9–3), and unwrapped films must be processed immediately under safelight conditions.

A number of safelights with different types of filters are available for use in the darkroom; some safelights are used exclusively with intraoral films, some are used exclusively with extraoral films, and others are designed for use with both (Fig. 9–4). For example, a good universal safelight filter recommended for use in a darkroom in which both extraoral screen films and intraoral films are processed is the GBX-2 safelight filter by Kodak. Recommendations for specific safelights and filters depending on the type of film (intraoral or extraoral) are provided by the film manufacturer; such information is indicated on the outside of the film package.

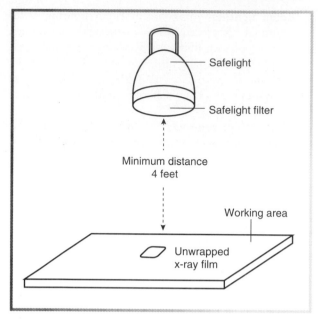

FIGURE 9–3. A minimum distance of 4 feet must exist between the safelight and working area.

MISCELLANEOUS

The **darkroom work space** must include an adequate counter area where films can be unwrapped prior to processing. A clean, organized work area is essential; the work area must be kept absolutely clean, dry, and free of processing chemicals, water, dust, and debris. If an unwrapped film comes into contact with any such substance prior to processing, an artifact results, and the quality of the dental radiograph is compromised.

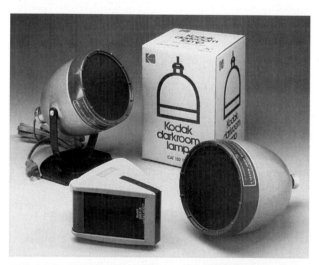

FIGURE 9–4. A variety of safelights are available for intraoral and extraoral films. (Reprinted courtesy of Eastman Kodak Company, Rochester, NY.)

The **darkroom storage space** must include ample room for chemical processing solutions, film cassettes, and other miscellaneous radiographic supplies. Storage of unopened boxes of film in the darkroom is *not* recommended; a reaction between the fumes from chemical processing solutions and the film emulsion may occur that will result in film fog. Boxes of opened extraoral film, however, must be stored in the darkroom. A light-tight storage drawer is necessary to protect opened boxes of unexposed extraoral film.

The temperature and **humidity level** of the darkroom must be controlled to prevent film damage. A room temperature of 70°F is recommended; if the room temperature exceeds 90°F, film fog results. A relative humidity level of between 50 and 70% should be maintained. When humidity levels are too high, the film emulsion does not dry, and when humidity levels are too low, static electricity becomes a problem and causes film artifacts.

The **darkroom plumbing** must include both hot and cold running water along with mixing valves to adjust the water temperature in the processing tanks. A utility sink with running water is also useful in the darkroom.

Other miscellaneous darkroom requirements include a wastebasket for the disposal of all film wrappings and an x-ray viewbox that is used to view radiographs.

Equipment Requirements

Dental x-ray film is processed in the darkroom using manual processing techniques or an automatic film processor. Special equipment is required for both manual film processing and automatic film processing.

PROCESSING TANK

Manual processing (also known as hand processing or tank processing) is a simple method that is used to develop, rinse, fix, and wash dental x-ray films. Manual processing equipment accessories, step-by-step manual processing procedures, and care and maintenance of equipment and supplies are discussed later in this chapter.

The essential piece of equipment required for manual processing is a **processing tank**. A processing tank is a container divided into compartments to hold the developer solution, water bath, and fixer solution. A processing tank has two insert tanks and one master tank (Fig. 9–5).

Insert tanks: Two removable 1-gallon insert tanks hold the developer and fixer solutions. Both are placed in the master tank. The developer solu-

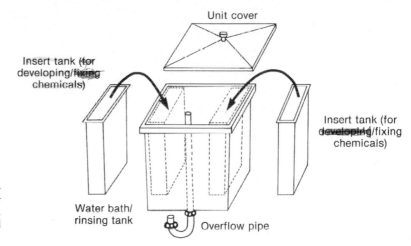

FIGURE 9–5. Processing tanks showing developing and fixing tank inserts in bath of running water with overflow drain. (From Goaz PW, White SC. Oral Radiology: Principles and Interpretation, 2nd ed. St. Louis, CV Mosby, 1987.)

tion is typically placed in the insert tank on the left and the fixer solution in the insert tank on the right. The water in the master tank separates the two insert tanks.

Master tank: The master tank suspends both insert tanks and is filled with circulating water. The water surrounds both insert tanks. An overflow pipe is used to control the water level in the master tank.

Ideally, the processing tank should be constructed of stainless steel, which does not react with processing solutions and is easy to clean. The processing tank should be equipped with a light-tight lid that is used to cover the solutions at all times. The cover protects the solutions from oxidation and evaporation, and during processing, it protects the developing films from exposure to light.

The temperatures of the developer and fixer solutions are controlled by the temperature of the circulating water in the master tank. A processing tank must be supplied with both hot and cold running water and a mixing valve. The water temperature is controlled through the use of a **mixing valve**, which functions like those found in bathroom showers. The mixing valve mixes the incoming hot and cold water to produce a water bath that maintains an optimum temperature of 68°F.

AUTOMATIC PROCESSOR

Automatic processing is another simple way of processing dental x-ray films. The essential piece of equipment required for automatic processing is the automatic film processing machine or **automatic processor.** The automatic processor automates all film processing steps. The component parts of the automatic processor, the mechanism of processing, step-by-step processing procedures, and care and maintenance of equipment and supplies are discussed later in this chapter.

A variety of automatic film processors are commercially available (Fig. 9–6). Some automatic processors are limited to certain sizes of x-ray film, whereas others are capable of processing a number of different sizes of x-ray film. Some automatic film processors are restricted to use under safelight conditions, whereas

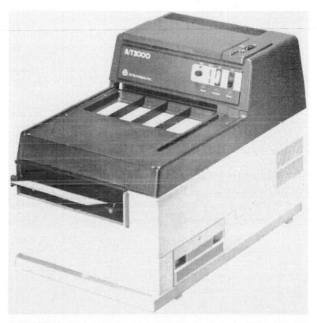

FIGURE 9–6. A typical automatic film processor used in the dental office. (Courtesy of Air Techniques, Hicksville, NY.)

others with **daylight loaders,** or light-shielded compartments, can be used in a room with white light (Fig. 9–7). Automatic processors also vary in regard to plumbing requirements and replenishment systems.

■ MANUAL FILM PROCESSING

Manual film processing is a simple method of developing, rinsing, fixing, and washing dental x-ray films. To process films manually, the dental radiographer must be knowledgeable about specific equipment requirements, step-by-step processing procedures, and care and maintenance of the equipment and supplies.

Equipment Accessories

In addition to a processing tank, a few accessory equipment items, including a thermometer, timer, and film hangers, are necessary for manual film processing.

THERMOMETER

A **thermometer** is necessary for manual processing and is used to determine the temperature of the developer solution. A floating thermometer or one that is clipped to the side of the developer tank may be used (Fig. 9–8).

A thermometer must be placed directly in the developer solution and *not* in the water bath. Why? As previously stated, the temperature of the water in the

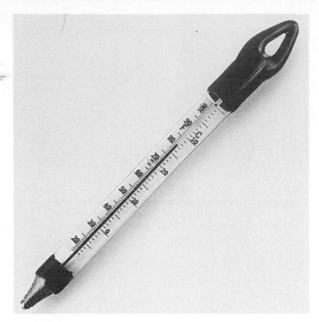

FIGURE 9–8. An example of a floating thermometer. (Courtesy of Rinn Corporation, Elgin, IL.)

master tank controls the temperature of the developer and fixer solutions in the insert tanks. The water in the master tank reaches the desired temperature almost as soon as it is turned on. The water, however, must circulate in the master tank for some time to equalize the temperatures of the processing solutions. Depending on the size of the insert tanks and the temperature of the solutions, the developer and fixer solutions may take up to 1 hour to reach the temperature of the water bath.

Using a thermometer, the developer temperature must be checked prior to processing. The optimum temperature for development is 68°F. Below 60°F, the chemicals work too slowly and result in underdevelopment. Over 80°F, the chemicals work too rapidly and produce film fog. The temperature of the developer determines development time. A time-temperature chart can be used to determine development time (Table 9–3).

TIMER

An accurate **timer** is also necessary for manual processing. X-ray film is processed in chemical solutions for specific time intervals indicated by the manufacturer of the processing solutions. A timer is used to indicate such time intervals (e.g., how long films have been placed in the developer solution, rinse water, fixer solution, and wash water). A timer is used to

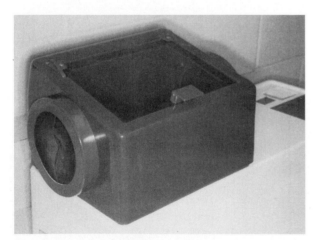

FIGURE 9–7. A small daylight loader. The filter in the top is generally safe for intraoral (direct exposure) film, but the daylight loader should not be used under bright overhead lights. (From Miles DA, Van Dis ML, Razmus TF: Basic Principles of Oral Maxillofacial Radiology. Philadelphia, WB Saunders, 1992.)

TABLE 9–3. Processing Temperatures and Times

Solution Temperature	Time in Developer (minutes)	Rinse Time (minutes)	Time in Fixer (minutes)	Wash Time (minutes)
65°F (18.5°C)	6.0	0.5	10–12	20
68°F (20.0°C)	5.0	0.5	10	20
70°F (21.0°C)	4.5	0.5	9–10	20
72°F (22.0°C)	4.0	0.5	8–9	20
75°F (24.0°C)	3.0	0.5	6–7	20
80°F (26.5°C)	2.5	0.5	5–6	20

signal the radiographer that the films must be removed from the current processing solution. Development time depends on the temperature of the developer solution and must be adjusted based on time-temperature guidelines (see Table 9–3).

FILM HANGERS

Film hangers, also known as film racks or processing hangers, are necessary for manual processing. A film hanger is a device equipped with clips used to hold films during processing (Fig. 9–9). Film hangers are made of stainless steel and include an identification tab or label. Film hangers are available in various sizes and can hold up to 20 intraoral films.

MISCELLANEOUS EQUIPMENT

A **stirring rod** or **stirring paddle** is a necessary piece of equipment for manual processing. A stirring rod is used to agitate the developer and fixer solutions prior to processing. The stirring action mixes the chemicals and equalizes the temperature of the solutions. The stirring rod or paddle may be plastic or glass. Another useful item for manual processing is a plastic apron; the apron is used to protect clothing during the processing of films and the mixing of chemicals.

Step-by-Step Procedures

Prior to manual film processing, the exposed dental x-ray film and necessary equipment must be present in the darkroom. Specific infection control procedures that pertain to manual film processing are detailed in Chapter 15. For step-by-step procedures, see "Procedure: Processing Film Manually."

Care and Maintenance

The processing solutions, equipment, and equipment accessories used in manual processing must be carefully maintained.

PROCESSING SOLUTIONS

The manufacturer's instructions for the storage, mixing, and use of processing solutions must be carefully followed. Processing solutions deteriorate with exposure to air, continued use, and chemical contamination. Exhausted processing solutions result in nondiagnostic radiographs and must be replaced. Processing solutions should be changed every 3 to 4 weeks; more frequent replacement of solutions may be necessary when large numbers of films are processed. Both the developer and fixer solutions should be changed at the same time. The processing solutions that require care and maintenance include the developer, fixer, and replenisher solutions.

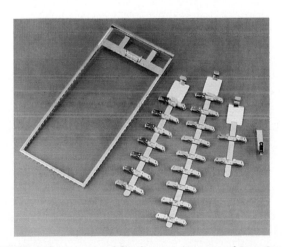

FIGURE 9–9. A variety of film hangers. (Courtesy of Rinn Corporation, Elgin, IL.)

PROCEDURE

Processing Film Manually

1. Determine which solution is the developer. Typically, the insert tank on the left is used for the developer, and the insert tank on the right is used for the fixer. The fixer solution is easily identified by its vinegarlike odor.

2. Check the levels of the developer and fixer solutions. If the developer level is low, add fresh developer. If the fixer level is low, add fresh fixer solution. *Never* add water to raise the level of the solutions; it dilutes the strength of the chemicals.

3. Stir the processing solutions using a stirring rod or paddle. To avoid chemical contamination, use different paddles to stir the developer and the fixer. Stirring the solutions mixes the chemicals and equalizes the temperature of the solutions.

4. Check the temperature of the developer solution. The optimum temperature for the developer is between 68°F and 70°F; however, temperatures between 65°F and 75°F may be used. If the temperature of the developer solution is outside of this range, the circulating water temperature must be adjusted accordingly. Sufficient time must then be allowed for the developer to reach the correct temperature.

5. Label the film hanger with the name of the patient and the date of exposure.

6. Close and lock the door of the darkroom, turn off the overhead white light, and turn on the safelights.

7. For intraoral films, carefully unwrap each exposed film over a clean working surface using proper infection control procedures (see Chapter 15). Dispose of all film packet wrappings. For extraoral films, carefully remove the film from the cassette. Handle all films by the edges only.

8. Clip each unwrapped film to the labeled film hanger (Fig. 9–10) (one film to a clip). Verify that each film is securely attached by running a finger along the film edge. Reattach any loose films.

9. Based on the temperature of the developer solution and the instructions of the manufacturer, set the timer. A time-temperature chart is used to determine such time intervals (see Table 9–3). If the optimal temperature of 68°F is used, the recommended development time is 4½ to 5 minutes.

10. Immerse the film hanger with films into the developer solution. Films must not contact other films or the side of the processing tank during development. Gently agitate the film hanger up and down several times to prevent air bubbles from clinging to the film. Hang the film rack on the edge of the insert tank and make certain that all films are immersed in the developer. Activate the timer and cover the processing tank.

11. When the timer goes off, uncover the processing tank; remove the film hanger with films from the developer solution and place it in the circulating water of the master tank. Agitate for 20 to 30 seconds. Remove and drain excess water for several seconds.

12. Based on the development time, determine the fixation time and set the timer. A time-temperature chart is used to determine such time intervals (see Table 9–3). Fixation time is approximately double the development time.

13. Immerse the film hanger with films in the fixer solution. Gently agitate it up and down several times. Hang the film rack on the edge of the insert tank and make certain that all films are immersed in the fixer. Activate the timer and cover the processing tank.

14. When the timer goes off, uncover the processing tank, remove the film hanger with films from the fixer, and allow the excess fixer to drain back into the fixer tank. Place the film hanger with films in the circulating water. Allow the films to wash for a minumum of 20 minutes.

15. Remove the film hanger with films from the wash water and gently shake off excess water. Cover the processing-tank. To air dry the films, suspend the film hanger with films from a rod or drying rack in a dust-free area over a drip pan. If a heated drying cabinet is used, the temperature should not exceed 120°F.

16. Remove the dry radiographs from the film hanger and place them in an envelope labeled with the patient's name and date of exposure. Outside the darkroom, use a view-box to examine the radiographs and place them in a labeled film mount.

17. After manual processing procedures have been completed, clean all processing equipment that was used and clean all work surfaces. A clean darkroom is essential for the production of diagnostic radiographs.

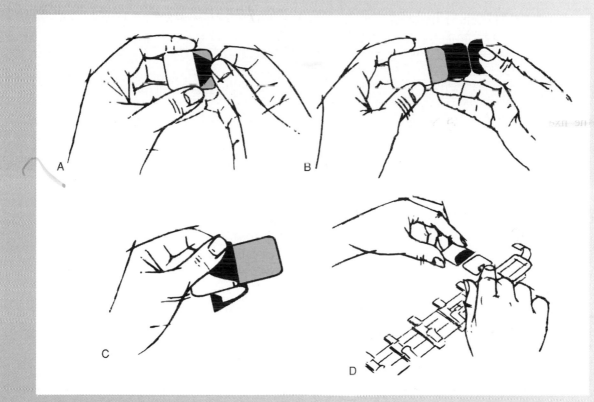

FIGURE 9–10. *A,* Pull up and out on the color-coded tab to tear open the top of the packet. *B,* Pull on the black paper tab until about half of the black paper is out of the packet. *C,* Fold the black paper away from the film, put the clip on the film, and carefully remove the film from the packet. *D,* Clip film on hanger—one film to a clip. (Reprinted courtesy of Eastman Kodak Company, Rochester, NY.)

Developer solution: The developer solution becomes depleted from evaporation and the removal of small amounts from the tank on the film hanger and films. With time and use, the developer solution decreases not only in volume but in strength as well. A weakened or exhausted developer solution does not fully develop the latent image and produces a nondiagnostic radiograph with reduced density and contrast.

Six ounces of developer solution should be added to the developer tank at the beginning of each day. When the tank is holding its maximum capacity (e.g., 1 gallon), 6 ounces must be removed before adding the replenisher.

Fixer solution: Fixer solution also decreases owing to evaporation and the removal of small amounts from the tank on the film hanger and films. In addition, the fixer solution is diluted with water each time films are transferred from the rinse water to the fixer; this gradual dilution weakens the solution.

With time and use, the fixer solution decreases not only in volume but in strength as well. A full-strength fixer ensures adequate "clearing" of the film and hardening of the film emulsion. An exhausted or depleted fixer does not stop the chemical reaction sufficiently to maintain film clarity; the films will turn a yellow-brown color, transmit less light, and lose their diagnostic quality.

Three ounces of fixer solution should be added to the fixer tank at the beginning of each day. When the tank is holding its maximum capacity (e.g., 1 gallon), 3 ounces must be removed before adding the replenisher.

Replenisher solutions: To maintain adequate freshness, strength, and solution levels, both the developer and fixer solutions must be replenished *daily.* A **replenisher** is a superconcentrated solution that is added to the processing solutions to compensate for the loss of volume and strength that results from oxidation. **Oxidation,**

or the process that occurs when developer and fixer solutions combine with oxygen and lose strength, takes place when the processing solutions are exposed to air. A breakdown of the chemicals in the processing solutions results, shortening the length of time the solutions can be used to produce diagnostic radiographs. Replenishment maintains adequate concentrations of chemicals, which ensures uniform results between solution changes.

PROCESSING TANK

The interaction between the mineral salts in water and the carbonate in the processing solutions produces deposits on the inside walls of the insert tanks. Such deposits contaminate the processing solutions. To produce diagnostic radiographs, the processing tank must be maintained in a clean state.

The master and insert tanks must be cleaned each time the solutions are changed. A commercial stainless steel tank cleaner or a solution of hydrochloric acid and water (1.5 ounces hydrochloric acid to 128 ounces of water) can be used to remove the mineral salts and carbonate deposits. Abrasive-type cleansers are not recommended for cleaning processing tanks; the cleansers may react unfavorably with the processing solutions.

For step-by-step cleaning procedures for the processing tank, see "Procedure: Cleaning the Processing Tank."

MISCELLANEOUS EQUIPMENT

Cleanliness of manual processing equipment is essential. Film hangers and stirring paddles must be cleaned after each use. Both must be thoroughly cleaned, rinsed, and dried. The plastic apron used to protect clothing should also be wiped clean after each use.

AUTOMATIC FILM PROCESSING

Automatic film processing is another simple method that is used to process dental x-ray films. The automatic processor automates all film processing steps. Automatic processing is often preferred over manual film processing for four reasons:

- less processing time is required
- time and temperatures are automatically controlled
- less equipment is used
- less space is required

PROCEDURE

Cleaning the Processing Tank

1. Pull the drain plugs in the insert tanks and master tank. Drain all liquid from each tank.

2. Pour cleaning solution into the master and insert tanks. If the insert tanks are heavily coated with deposits, allow the tanks to soak holding the cleaning solution for 30 minutes.

3. After soaking, use a brush to scrub all surfaces of the insert and master tanks as well as the tank cover. Rinse thoroughly with water, wipe clean, and dry.

4. Pour fresh developer solution into the left insert tank and fresh fixer solution into the right insert tank. Fill insert tanks until the solution level reaches the indicated fill-line, about 1 inch from the top of the tank. Fill the master tank with water.

5. Place the lid on the processing tank. The tank lid should be removed only when changing or adding solutions, when checking the developer temperature, or when processing films.

There are a number of advantages to automatic film processing. The major advantage is the time saved; an automatic processor requires only 4 to 6 minutes to develop, fix, wash, and dry a film, whereas manual film processing techniques require approximately 1 hour. Another advantage is the automatic control of time and temperature; the automatic processor maintains the correct temperature of solutions and controls the processing time, thus contributing to the uniformity of film processing.

Although automatic processing units have become very popular in recent years, many dental offices still maintain manual processing equipment for use when the automatic processor malfunctions. When the automatic processor and special processing solutions are properly maintained, this equipment consistently produces high-quality radiographs and provides less chance for operator error.

Component Parts of the Automatic Processor

The automatic processor uses a roller transport system to move the unwrapped dental x-ray film through the developer, fixer, water, and drying compartments. Each component of the automatic processor contributes to the mechanism of automatic film processing and has a specific function (Fig. 9–11).

The **processor housing** encases all of the component parts of the automatic processor.

The **film feed slot** is an opening on the outside of the processor housing that is used to insert unwrapped films into the automatic processor.

The **roller film transporter** is a system of rollers used to move the film rapidly through the developer, fixer, water, and drying compartments. The rollers are propelled by motor-driven gears or belts. The primary function of the rollers is to move the film through the automatic processor. In addition to moving the film, the rollers produce a wringing action that removes the excess solution from the emulsion as the film moves from compartment to compartment. The motion of the rollers also gently agitates the processing solutions, contributing to the uniformity of the processing.

The **developer compartment** holds the developer solution. The developer solution used in an automatic processor is a specially formulated, highly concentrated chemical solution designed to react at temperatures between 80°F and 95°F. As a result of the high temperatures, development occurs rapidly. The developer solution used in manual film processing is not the same as the developer used in automatic film processing and should *never* be used in an automatic processor.

The **fixer compartment** holds the fixer solution. The film is transported directly from the developer solution into the fixer *without* a rinsing step. The fixer solution used in an automatic processor is a specially formulated, highly concentrated chemical solution that contains additional hardening agents. In the fixer solution, the film is rapidly fixed or "cleared" and then hardened. The fixer solution used in manual film processing is not the same as the fixer used in automatic film processing and should *never* be used in an automatic processor.

The **water compartment** holds circulating water. Water is used to wash the films following fixation. After washing, the wet film is transported from the water compartment to a drying chamber.

The **drying chamber** holds heated air and is used to dry the wet film.

A **replenisher pump** and **replenisher solutions** are used to maintain proper solution concentration and levels automatically in some automatic processors, whereas other processors require the operator to add the necessary replenishing solutions.

The **film recovery slot** is an opening on the outside of the processor housing where the dry, processed radiograph emerges from the automatic processor.

Step-by-Step Procedures

Prior to processing, the exposed dental x-ray film and automatic processor (without daylight loader) must be present in the darkroom. Specific infection control procedures that pertain to automatic film processing are detailed in Chapter 15. For step-by-step procedures for automatic film processing, see "Procedure: Automatic Film Processing."

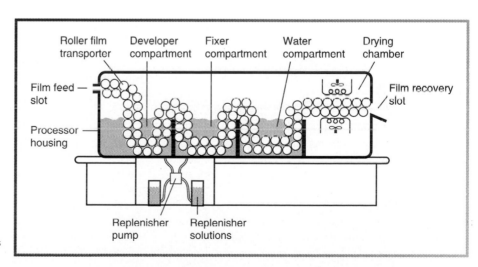

FIGURE 9–11. Component parts of the automatic processor.

PROCEDURE

Automatic Film Processing

1. Prepare darkroom. If a daylight loader is not part of the automatic processor, the films must be processed in the darkroom. Close and lock the door of the darkroom, turn off the overhead white light, and turn on the safelights.

2. Prepare films. For intraoral films, carefully unwrap each exposed film over a clean working surface using proper infection control procedures (see Chapter 15). Dispose of all film packet wrappings. For extraoral films, carefully remove the film from the cassette. Handle all films by the edges only.

3. Insert each unwrapped film into the film feed slot of the processor, one at a time. Allow at least 10 seconds between the insertion of each film. Alternate sides or slots whenever possible. Make certain that films are straight as they are inserted. (When films are turned sideways or inserted too quickly, they overlap during processing. Overlapped films result in nondiagnostic radiographs.) After films have been inserted into the automatic processor, allow 4 to 6 minutes for automated processing to occur.

4. Retrieve the processed radiographs from the film recovery slot on the outside of the automatic processor.

Care and Maintenance

The automatic processor and automatic processing solutions must be carefully maintained. The manufacturer's recommendations for care and maintenance must be followed meticulously.

AUTOMATIC PROCESSOR

The automatic processor requires routine preventive maintenance. Without proper cleaning and replenishment, the automatic processor will malfunction. A cleaning and replenishment schedule must be established and followed strictly to ensure optimum automatic processor performance.

Depending on the volume of films processed, the automatic processor requires daily or weekly cleaning. An extraoral-size **cleaning film** used to clean the rollers of the automatic processor must be run through

the processor at the beginning of each day. A cleaning film removes any residual gelatin or dirt from the rollers. On a weekly basis, the rollers must be removed from the automatic processor, cleaned in warm running water, and then soaked for 10 to 20 minutes. The manufacturer's recommendations for daily and monthly cleaning of the automatic processor must be carefully followed.

PROCESSING SOLUTIONS

Processing solution levels in the automatic processor must be checked at the beginning of each day and replenished as necessary. Failure to add replenisher results in exhausted solutions and nondiagnostic radiographs. Processing solutions in the automatic processor must be replaced every 2 to 6 weeks, depending on the number of films processed and the replenishment schedule. The manufacturer's recommendations for the changing of solutions must be carefully followed.

▰▰▰ FILM DUPLICATION

An identical copy of an intraoral or an extraoral radiograph is made through the process of film duplication. As discussed in Chapter 7, there are several uses for film duplication in dentistry. Duplicate radiographs may be used when referring patients to specialists, for insurance claims, and as teaching aids. The dental radiographer must be familiar with the equipment requirements for film duplication and with the step-by-step procedures for film duplication.

Equipment Requirements

The duplication of film requires the use of a **film duplicator** and **duplicating film.** A film duplicator is a light source that is commercially available from manufacturers, such as the Rinn Corporation (Fig. 9–12). A film duplicator provides a diffused light source that evenly exposes the special duplicating film. Duplicating film is discussed in Chapter 7.

Step-by-Step Procedures

Prior to film duplication, the films to be duplicated, the duplicating film, and the film duplicator must be present in the darkroom. Film duplication must take place in a light-tight darkroom. For step-by-step procedures for film duplication, see "Procedure: Film Duplication."

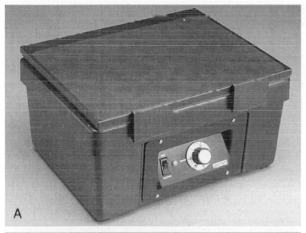

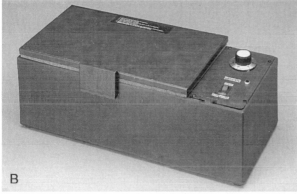

FIGURE 9–12. *A* and *B,* Examples of two film duplicators, available from the Rinn Corporation. (Courtesy of Rinn Corporation, Elgin, IL.)

PROCESSING PROBLEMS AND SOLUTIONS

Processing problems may result in nondiagnostic radiographs. As described in Chapter 8, a diagnostic radiograph is one that provides a great deal of information; the images have proper density and contrast, have sharp outlines, and are of the same shape and size as the object radiographed (Fig. 9–14).

Processing problems may occur for a number of reasons, including:

- time and temperature errors (Table 9–4)
- chemical contamination errors (Table 9–5)
- film handling errors (Table 9–6)
- lighting errors (Table 9–7)

Processing errors may cause a partial or total absence of images or obscure images that are present.

Films that appear light, dark, yellow-brown, or fogged are the result of processing errors. Films that appear scratched or contaminated with dirt, saliva, or fingerprints are the result of faulty film handling during processing. Reticulation and fingernail and static artifacts may also result from poor processing and film handling techniques.

Many processing errors can be attributed to one or more causes. The dental radiographer must be able to recognize the appearance of common processing errors, identify potential causes of such errors, and know what steps are necessary to correct such problems.

Time and Temperature

UNDERDEVELOPED FILM

Appearance. The film appears light (Fig. 9–15).

Problems. **Underdeveloped films** may result from:

- inadequate development time
- inaccurate timer
- low developer temperature
- inaccurate thermometer
- depleted or contaminated developer solution

Solution. To prevent underdeveloped films:

- check the temperature of the developer as well as the time the film must remain in the developer solution
- increase the time the film remains in the developer as needed
- replace faulty and inaccurate thermometers and timers
- if developer is depleted or contaminated, replace it with fresh developer solution

OVERDEVELOPED FILM

Appearance. The film appears dark (Fig. 9–16).

Problems. **Overdeveloped films** may result from:

- excess development time
- inaccurate timer
- high developer temperature
- inaccurate thermometer
- concentrated (overactive) developer solution

Solution. To prevent overdeveloped films:

- check the temperature of the developer and the time the film should remain in the developer solution
- decrease the time the film remains in the developer as needed

PROCEDURE

Film Duplication

1. Arrange radiographs. Place the dental radiographs to be duplicated on the light screen of the film duplicator. Use manufacturer-supplied film organizers to arrange the films and block out extraneous light (Fig. 9–13).

2. Place the duplicating film on top of the arranged radiographs. Place the emulsion side down. (The emulsion side will appear dull and gray or lavender in color.)

3. Secure duplicator lid. Close the lid of the film duplicator and fasten it securely to ensure adequate contact between the radiographs and the duplicating film. (To prevent blurring of the image, good contact must be maintained between the duplicating film and the films that are being duplicated. Without good contact, the duplicate film appears fuzzy and shows less detail than the original film.)

4. Select the exposure time, set the adjustable timer, and activate the light source to expose the duplicating film. (The exposure time is controlled by an adjustable timer on the film duplicator. The adjustable timer controls the amount of light emitted from the film duplicator; the light passes through the radiographs and exposes the duplicating film. The longer the duplicating film is exposed to light, the lighter it appears. This is the opposite of x-ray film; x-ray film appears darker with longer exposure to light. Exposure time depends on the type of duplicator used and the density of the radiographs that are being duplicated.)

5. Process the duplicating film using manual processing techniques or the automatic processor.

6. Label the processed duplicate radiographs with the patient's name and date of exposure. Also label the radiographs to indicate the patient's right and left sides.

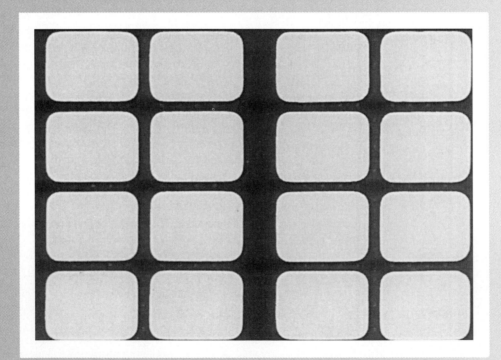

FIGURE 9–13. An x-ray "organizer" on which to place films for duplication. (From Miles DA, Van Dis ML, Jensen CW, Ferretti A: Radiographic Imaging for Dental Auxiliaries, 2nd ed. Philadelphia, WB Saunders, 1993.)

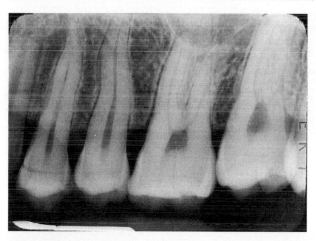

FIGURE 9-14. A diagnostic radiograph with images that exhibit proper density and contrast.

- replace faulty and inaccurate thermometers and timers
- if developer is overactive, replace it with fresh developer solution

RETICULATION OF EMULSION

Appearance. The film appears cracked (Fig. 9-17).

Problem. **Reticulation of emulsion** results when a film is subjected to a sudden temperature change between the developer solution and the water bath.

Solution. To prevent the reticulation of emulsion:

- check the temperature of the processing solutions and water bath

- avoid drastic temperature differences between the developer and the water bath

Chemical Contamination

DEVELOPER SPOTS

Appearance. Dark spots appear on the film (Fig. 9-18).

Problem. **Developer spots** are seen when the developer solution comes in contact with the film before processing.

Solution. To avoid developer spots:

- use a clean work area in the darkroom
- to ensure a clean working surface, place a paper towel on the work area before unwrapping films

FIXER SPOTS

Appearance. White spots appear on the film (Fig. 9-19).

Problem. **Fixer spots** are the result of fixer solution coming in contact with the film before processing.

Solution. To avoid fixer spots:

- use a clean work area in the darkroom
- to ensure a clean working surface, place a paper towel on the work area before unwrapping films

YELLOW-BROWN STAINS

Appearance. The film appears yellowish-brown (Fig. 9-20).

TABLE 9-4. Time and Temperature: Problems and Solutions

Example	Appearance	Problems	Solutions
Underdeveloped film	Light	Inadequate development time	Check development time
		Developer solution too cool	Check developer temperature
		Inaccurate timer or thermometer	Replace faulty timer or thermometer
		Depleted developer solution	Replenish developer with fresh solutions as needed
Overdeveloped film	Dark	Excessive developing time	Check development time
		Developer solution too hot	Check developer temperature
		Inaccurate timer or thermometer	Replace faulty timer or thermometer
		Concentrated developer solution	Replenish developer with fresh solutions as needed
Reticulation of emulsion	Cracked	Sudden temperature change between developer and water bath	Check temperature of processing solutions and water bath; avoid drastic temperature differences

TABLE 9–5. Chemical Contamination: Problems and Solutions

Example	Appearance	Problems	Solutions
Developer spots	Dark spots	Developer comes in contact with film before processing	Use a clean work area in the darkroom
Fixer spots	White spots	Fixer comes in contact with film before processing	Use a clean work area in the darkroom
Yellow-brown stains	Yellow-brown color	Exhausted developer or fixer Insufficient fixation time Insufficient rinsing	Replenish chemicals with fresh solutions as needed Use adequate fixation time Rinse for a minimum of 20 minutes

TABLE 9–6. Film Handling: Problems and Solutions

Example	Appearance	Problems	Solutions
Developer cut-off	Straight white border	Undeveloped portion of film due to low level of developer	Check developer level before processing; add solution if needed
Fixer cut-off	Straight black border	Unfixed portion of film due to low level of fixer	Check fixer level before processing; add solution if needed
Overlapped films	White or dark areas appear on film where overlapped	Two films contacting each other during processing	Separate films so that no contact takes place during processing
Air bubbles	White spots	Air trapped on the film surface after being placed in the processing solutions	Gently agitate film racks after placing in processing solutions
Fingernail artifact	Black crescent-shaped marks	Film emulsion damaged by the operator's fingernail during rough handling	Gently handle films by the edges only
Fingerprint artifact	Black fingerprint	Film touched by fingers that are contaminated with fluoride or developer	Wash and dry hands thoroughly before processing films
Static electricity	Thin, black, branching lines	Occurs when a film packet is opened quickly	Open film packets slowly
		Occurs when a film pack is opened before the radiographer touches a conductive object	Touch a conductive object before unwrapping films
Scratched film	White lines	Soft emulsion removed from the film by a sharp object	Use care when handling films and film racks

TABLE 9–7. Lighting: Problems and Solutions

Example	Appearance	Problems	Solutions
Light leak	Exposed area appears black	Accidental exposure of the film to white light	Examine film packets for defects before using Never unwrap films in the presence of white light
Fogged film	Gray; lack of detail and contrast	Improper safelighting Light leaks in darkroom Outdated films Improper film storage Contaminated solutions	Check the filter and bulb wattage of the safelight Check the darkroom for light leaks Check the expiration date on film packages Store films in a cool, dry, protected area Avoid contaminated solutions by covering tanks after each use
		Developer solution too hot	Check temperatures of developer

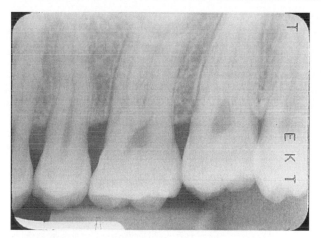

FIGURE 9–15. An underdeveloped film appears light.

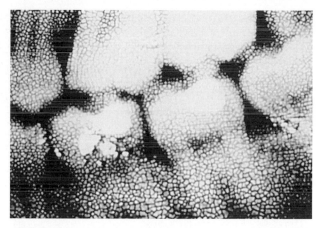

FIGURE 9–17. A film with a damaged emulsion appears cracked.

Problems. **Yellow-brown films** result from:

- use of exhausted developer or fixer
- insufficient fixation time
- insufficient rinsing

Solution. To prevent yellow-brown films:

- replace depleted developer and fixer solutions with fresh chemicals
- make certain that films have adequate fixation time and adequate rinse time
- rinse processed films for a minimum of 20 minutes in circulating cool water

Film Handling

DEVELOPER CUT-OFF

Appearance. A straight white border appears on the film (Fig. 9–21).

Problem. **Developer cut-off** results from a low level of developer solution and represents an undeveloped portion of the film. If the developer solution level is low, the films clipped at the very top of the film rack may not be completely immersed in the developer solution.

Solution. To avoid developer cut-off:

- check the developer level before processing films
- add proper replenisher solution if necessary
- make certain that all films on the film rack are completely immersed in the developer solution

FIXER CUT-OFF

Appearance. A straight black border appears on the film (Fig. 9–22).

Problem. **Fixer cut-off** results from a low level of fixer solution and represents an unfixed portion of the

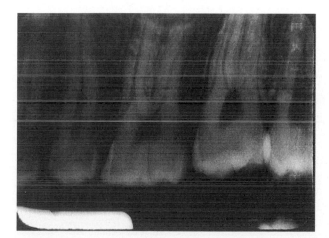

FIGURE 9–16. An overdeveloped film appears dark.

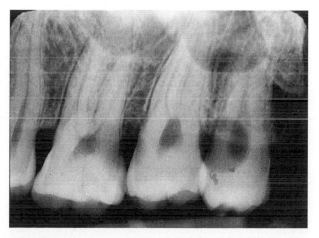

FIGURE 9–18. Developer spots appear dark or black.

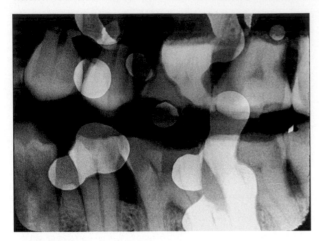

FIGURE 9–19. Fixer spots appear light or white.

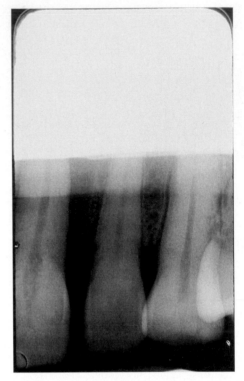

FIGURE 9–21. Developer cut-off appears as a straight white border on a film.

film. If the fixer solution is low, the films clipped at the very top of the film rack may not be completely immersed in the fixer solution.

Solution. To avoid fixer cut-off:

- check the fixer level before processing films
- add proper replenisher solution if necessary
- make certain that all films on the film rack are completely immersed in the fixer solution

OVERLAPPED FILMS

Appearance. White or dark areas appear on films where overlap has occurred (Figs. 9–23 and 9–24).

Problem. **Overlapped films** occur when two films come into contact with each other during manual or automatic processing techniques. Films that overlap in the developer have white areas that represent an unde-

veloped portion of the film. Films that overlap in the fixer have black areas that represent an unfixed portion of the film.

Solution. To avoid overlapped films, care should be taken to ensure that no film is permitted to come into contact with another film during processing.

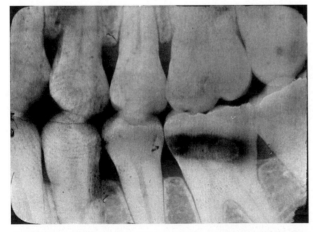

FIGURE 9–20. A number of processing errors may result in a yellow-brown film.

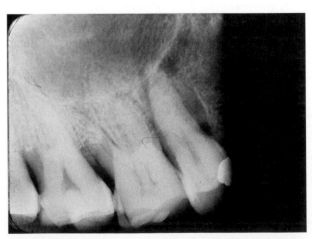

FIGURE 9–22. Fixer cut-off appears as a straight black border on a film.

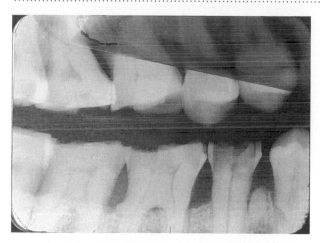

FIGURE 9–23. An overlapped film.

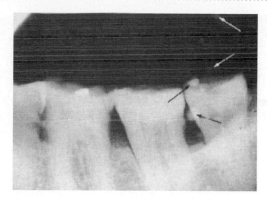

FIGURE 9–25. Air bubbles appear as tiny white spots (*arrows*). (From Langlais RP, Kasle MJ: Exercises in Radiographic Interpretation, 2nd ed. Philadelphia, WB Saunders, 1985.)

AIR BUBBLES

Appearance. White spots appear on the film (Fig. 9–25).

Problem. Air bubbles are seen when air is trapped on the film surface after the film is placed in the processing solution. Air bubbles prevent the chemicals from affecting the emulsion in that area.

Solution. To avoid air bubbles, gently agitate and stir film racks after placing them in the processing solution.

FINGERNAIL ARTIFACT

Appearance. Black crescent-shaped marks appear on the film (Fig. 9–26).

Problem. A **fingernail artifact** is seen when the film emulsion is damaged by the operator's fingernail during rough handling of the film.

Solution. To prevent a fingernail artifact, gently handle the film by the edges only.

FINGERPRINT ARTIFACT

Appearance. A black fingerprint appears on the film (Fig. 9–27).

Problem. A **fingerprint artifact** is seen when the film is touched by fingers contaminated with fluoride or developer.

Solution. To prevent fingerprint artifacts:

- wash and dry hands thoroughly before processing films
- work in a clean area to avoid contaminating the hands
- handle the films by the edges only

STATIC ELECTRICITY

Appearance. Thin, black branching lines appear on the film (Fig. 9–28).

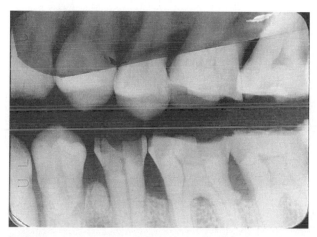

FIGURE 9–24. An overlapped film.

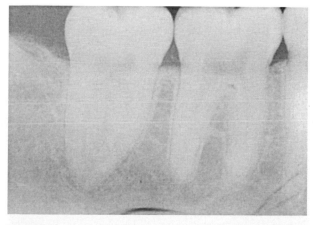

FIGURE 9–26. A fingernail artifact appears as a black crescent-shaped mark.

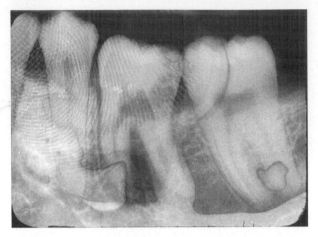

FIGURE 9–27. A black fingerprint artifact appears on the film.

Problems. **Static electricity** may result from:

- opening a film packet quickly
- opening a film packet before touching another object, such as the film processor or countertop in a carpeted office
- occurs most frequently during periods of low humidity

Solution. To prevent static electricity:

- always open film packets slowly
- in a carpeted office, touch a conductive object before unwrapping films

SCRATCHED FILM

Appearance. White lines appear on the film (Fig. 9–29).

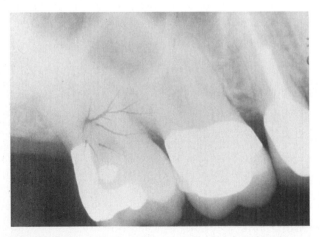

FIGURE 9–28. Static electricity appears as black branching lines.

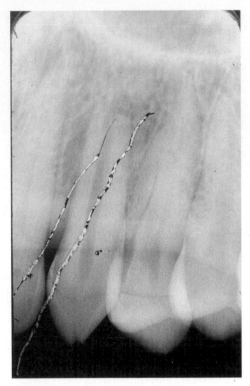

FIGURE 9–29. Scratches appear as thin white lines.

Problem. A **scratched film** results when the soft film emulsion is removed from the film base by a sharp object, such as a film clip or film hanger.

Solution. To prevent a scratched film:

- use care when placing a film rack in the processing solutions
- avoid contact with other film hangers

Lighting

LIGHT LEAK

Appearance. The exposed area appears black (Fig. 9–30).

Problems. A **light leak** results from:

- accidental exposure of the film to white light
- torn or defective film packets that expose a portion of the film to light

Solution. To prevent light leaks:

- examine film packets for minute tears or defects before use
- do not use film packets that are torn or defective
- never unwrap films in the presence of white light

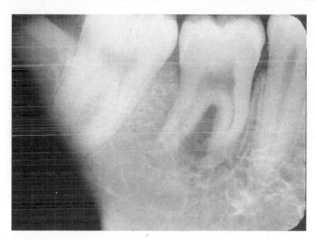

FIGURE 9–30. The portion of the film exposed to light appears black.

FOGGED FILM

Appearance. The film appears gray and lacks image detail and contrast (Fig. 9–31).

Problems. **Fogged films** result from:

- improper safelighting and light leaks in the darkroom
- improper film storage
- outdated films
- contaminated processing solutions
- high developer temperature

Solution. To prevent fogged films:

- check the filter and bulb wattage of the safelight
- minimize film exposure to the safelight and check the darkroom for light leaks

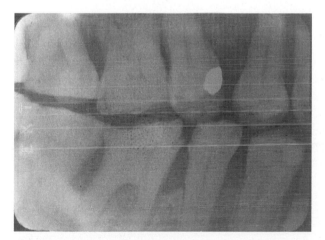

FIGURE 9–31. A fogged film appears gray and lacks detail and contrast.

- check the expiration date on film packages and store films in a cool, dry, and protected area
- avoid contamination of processing solutions by replacing tank covers after each use
- always check developer temperature before processing films

SUMMARY

- Film processing refers to a series of steps that collectively produce a visible permanent image on a dental radiograph.
- The pattern of stored energy on an exposed film is termed the latent image; this image remains invisible until it undergoes processing.
- The visible image that results on a dental radiograph is made up of black, white, and gray areas.
- There are five steps in film processing: development, rinsing, fixation, washing, and drying.
- A chemical solution known as the developer is used in the development process to chemically reduce the exposed, energized silver halide crystals to black metallic silver.
- The developer solution contains four basic ingredients: developing agent, preservative, accelerator, and restrainer.
- Following development, a water bath is used to wash or rinse the film.
- Following rinsing, fixation takes place.
- The fixer solution contains four basic ingredients: fixing agent, preservative, hardening agent, and acidifier.
- Following fixation, a water bath is used to wash the film and remove all excess chemicals from the emulsion.
- The final step in film processing is drying the film. Films must be completely dried before they can be handled for mounting and viewing.
- A darkroom is a completely darkened room where x-ray film can be handled and processed to produce diagnostic radiographs. The ideal darkroom should be conveniently located, of adequate size, equipped with correct lighting and ventilation, and arranged with ample work space and storage.
- The darkroom must be light-tight and must include proper safelighting. Safelighting provides illumination in the darkroom to carry out processing activities safely without exposing or damaging the film.
- Manual processing is a simple method used to develop, rinse, fix, and wash dental x-ray films. The essential piece of equipment required for manual film processing is a processing tank, which is a container divided into compartments for the developer solution, water bath, and fixer solution. Step-by-step manual processing procedures are detailed in this chapter.
- Automatic processing is another simple way to process dental x-ray film. The essential piece of equipment required for automatic processing is the automatic processor, which automates all film processing steps. Step-by-step automatic processing procedures are detailed in this chapter.
- An identical copy of an intraoral or extraoral radiograph is made through the process of film duplication. Duplication

of film requires the use of a film duplicator and duplicating film. Step-by-step procedures for film duplication are detailed in this chapter.

- A number of processing problems may result in nondiagnostic films. Processing problems may result from time and temperature errors (see Table 9–4), chemical contamination errors (see Table 9–5), film handling errors (see Table 9–6), and lighting errors (see Table 9–7).
- The dental radiographer must be able to recognize the appearance of common processing errors, identify the potential causes of such errors, and know what steps are necessary to correct such problems.

BIBLIOGRAPHY

Eastman Kodak Company: Film processing/mounting and viewing. *In* X-Rays in Dentistry. Rochester, Eastman Kodak Company, 1985, pp. 98–105.

Frommer HH: Film processing—the darkroom. *In* Radiology for Dental Auxiliaries, 6th edition. St. Louis, Mosby-Year Book, 1996, pp. 101–137.

Goaz PW, White SC: Processing x-ray film. *In* Oral Radiology: Principles of Interpretation, 3rd edition. St. Louis, Mosby-Year Book, 1994, pp. 106–125.

Haring JI, Lind LJ: Film exposure, processing and technique errors. *In* Radiographic Interpretation for the Dental Hygienist. Philadelphia, WB Saunders, 1993, pp. 159–166.

Kasle MJ, Langlais RP: The chemistry of image production and processing. *In* Basic Principles of Oral Radiography: Exercises in Dental Radiography, vol. 4. Philadelphia, WB Saunders, 1981, pp. 108–127.

Johnson ON, McNally MA, Essay CE: Dental x-ray film processing. *In* Essentials of Dental Radiography for Dental Assistants and Hygienists, 6th edition. Norwalk, Appleton and Lange, 1999, pp. 179–210.

Langland OE, Sippy FH: Processing and film mounting procedures. *In* Textbook of Dental Radiography, 2nd edition. Springfield, IL, Charles C Thomas, 1977, pp. 170–191.

Langland OE, Sippy FH, Langlais RP: Film processing and duplication. *In* Textbook of Dental Radiology, 2nd edition. Springfield, IL, Charles C Thomas, 1984, pp. 281–300.

Manson-Hing LR: Films, processing, darkroom, and duplicating. *In* Fundamentals of Dental Radiography, 3rd edition. Philadelphia, Lea & Febiger, 1990, pp. 20–35.

Matteson SR, Whaley C, Secrist VC: The film and the darkroom. *In* Dental Radiology, 4th edition. Chapel Hill, University of North Carolina Press, 1988, pp. 58–67.

Miles DA, Van Dis ML, Jensen CW, Ferretti A: Film processing and quality assurance. *In* Radiographic Imaging for Dental Auxiliaries, 3rd edition. Philadelphia, WB Saunders, 1999, pp. 49–71.

Miles DA, Van Dis ML, Razmus TF: Radiographic processing and processing quality assurance. *In* Basic Principles of Oral and Maxillofacial Radiology. Philadelphia, WB Saunders, 1992, pp. 156–177.

Quiz Questions ··

MULTIPLE CHOICE

_____ 1. The first step in film processing is:

    a. development
    b. rinsing
    c. fixation
    d. washing
    e. drying

_____ 2. In film processing, the rinsing step is necessary because:

    a. rinsing removes the silver halide crystals from the emulsion
    b. rinsing slows down the fixation process
    c. rinsing removes the developer from the film and stops the development process
    d. rinsing thoroughly removes all excess chemicals from the emulsion
    e. rinsing reduces the energized silver halide crystals to black metallic silver

_____ 3. The film emulsion is hardened during:

    a. development
    b. rinsing
    c. fixation
    d. washing
    e. drying

_____ 4. The hydroquinone in the developer brings out the _____ tones, whereas the Elon in the developer brings out the _____ tones on a dental radiograph.

    a. black/white
    b. white/black
    c. gray/gray
    d. white/gray
    e. black/gray

_____ 5. The optimal temperature for the developer solution is:

    a. 55°F
    b. 68°F
    c. 78°F
    d. 80°F
    e. 90°F

_____ 6. The size of a darkroom is determined by all of the following factors *except*:

    a. the volume of radiographs processed
    b. the type of processing equipment used
    c. the humidity level of the room
    d. the space required for duplication of films
    e. the number of persons using the room

_____ 7. Any leaks of white light into the darkroom will cause:

    a. film fog
    b. film reticulation
    c. overdeveloped films
    d. underexposed films
    e. any of the above

FILL IN THE BLANK

29. List the two equipment requirements for film duplication.

_____

30. Discuss how exposure time affects the density of duplicating film.

_____

MATCHING

For questions 31 to 36, describe the appearance of the processing error using one of the following words:

         a. light
         b. white
         c. black
         d. dark
         e. gray

_____ **31.** fogged film

_____ **32.** overdeveloped film

_____ **33.** underdeveloped film

_____ **34.** light leak

_____ **35.** developer cut-off

_____ **36.** fixer cut-off

IDENTIFICATION

For questions 37 to 45, describe or identify the processing error that causes the following:

37. black spots

_____

38. white spots

_____

39. yellow-brown stains

_____

40. cracked appearance

_____

41. straight white border

_____

42. straight black border

_____

43. black, crescent-shaped marks

_____

44. thin, black branching lines

_____

45. white lines

_____

TRUE OR FALSE

For questions 46 to 50, identify each statement as true or false.

_____ **46.** Film fog results from improper safelighting.

_____ **47.** Yellow-brown stains result from insufficient development time.

_____ **48.** Developer cut-off appears as a straight black border across the film.

_____ **49.** To avoid static electricity, touch a conductive object before unwrapping a film.

_____ **50.** Torn or defective film packets may allow a portion of the film to be exposed to light.

_____

Answers are supplied at the end of this book.

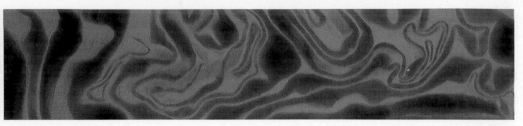

Quality Assurance in the Dental Office

OBJECTIVES

After completion of this chapter, the student will be able to:

- *Define the key words.*
- *List quality control tests and quality administration procedures that should be included in the quality assurance plan.*
- *Discuss the purpose and frequency of testing dental x-ray machines.*
- *Describe the tests used to check for fresh film and adequate film-screen contact. Discuss the frequency of testing and the interpretation of test results.*
- *Describe the test used to check for darkroom light leaks and proper safelighting. Discuss the frequency of testing and the interpretation of test results.*
- *Describe the test used to check the automatic processor. Discuss the frequency of testing and the interpretation of test results.*
- *List three tests used to check the strength of the developer solution.*
- *Describe the preparation of the reference radiograph and the standard stepwedge radiograph. Discuss the use of these radiographs to compare film densities and to monitor the strength of developer solution.*
- *Describe the test used to check the strength of the fixer. Discuss the frequency of testing and the interpretation of test results.*
- *Discuss the basic elements of a quality administration plan.*
- *Detail the importance of operator competence in dental radiographic procedures.*

KEY WORDS

Normalizing device	Radiograph, reference
Quality administration	Stepwedge
Quality assurance	Viewbox
Quality control tests	

INTRODUCTION

Quality assurance refers to special procedures that are used to *assure* the production of high-quality diagnostic radiographs. A quality assurance plan includes both quality control tests and quality administration procedures (Table 10–1). Although the dentist is ultimately responsible for the overall quality assurance plan, the dental radiographer can play an important role in the implementation and administration of such a plan. The dental radiographer must be knowledgeable about the quality assurance program used in the dental office.

The purpose of this chapter is to introduce the dental radiographer to quality control tests that are used to monitor dental x-ray equipment, supplies, and film processing. Quality administration procedures and operator competence for the dental office are also discussed.

QUALITY CONTROL TESTS

Quality control tests are specific tests that are used to maintain and monitor dental x-ray equipment, supplies, and film processing. To avoid excess exposure of

patients and personnel to x-radiation, the dental radiographer must have a clear understanding of the quality control procedures used to test specific equipment, supplies, and film processing in the dental office.

Equipment and Supplies

Quality control tests are necessary to monitor dental x-ray machines, dental x-ray film, screens and cassettes, and viewing equipment. To consistently produce diagnostic quality radiographs, dental x-ray equipment and supplies must be functioning properly and kept in good repair.

DENTAL X-RAY MACHINES

All dental x-ray machines must be inspected and monitored periodically. Some state and local regulatory agencies provide dental x-ray equipment inspection services as part of their registration and licensing procedures. Dental x-ray machines must also be calibrated, or adjusted for accuracy, at regular intervals. Calibration of dental x-ray equipment must be performed by a qualified technician to ensure consistent x-ray machine performance and the production of diagnostic radiographs.

The American Academy of Dental Radiology recommends a number of annual tests for dental x-ray machines. These tests are designed to identify minor malfunctions, including machine output variations, inadequate collimation, tubehead drift, timing errors, and inaccurate kilovoltage and milliamperage readings (see "Quality Control Tests for Dental X-ray Machines").

Annual tests for dental x-ray machines can be performed by the dentist, dental hygienist, dental assistant, or manufacturer's service representative. Most of the tests require some basic testing materials, film, and

TABLE 10–1. Quality Assurance Plan	
Quality Control Tests	**Quality Administration Procedures**
Dental x-ray machines	Description of plan
Dental x-ray film	Assignment of duties
Screens and cassettes	Monitoring schedule
Darkroom lighting	Maintenance schedule
Processing equipment	Record-keeping logs
Processing solutions	Evaluation and revision plan
	In-service training

QUALITY CONTROL TESTS FOR DENTAL X-RAY MACHINES

- X-ray output test
- Focal spot size test
- Collimation-beam alignment test
- Half-value layer (HVL) test
- Tubehead stability test
- Timer test
- Milliamperage test
- Kilovoltage test

test logs to record the results. Easy to follow, step-by-step procedures for performing each of these tests are described in a free pamphlet entitled *Quality Control Tests for Dental Radiography,* available from the Eastman Kodak Company, Rochester, New York (Kodak Publication No. ME-504a).

DENTAL X-RAY FILM

As discussed in Chapter 7, dental x-ray film must be properly stored, protected, and used before its expiration date. For quality control purposes, each box of film should be tested for freshness as it is opened.

The following fresh film test is recommended to check a newly opened box of film:

1. Prepare film. Unwrap one unexposed film from a newly opened box.
2. Process film. Use fresh chemicals to process the unexposed film.

The results of the fresh film test can be interpreted as follows:

- **Fresh film.** If the processed film appears clear with a slight blue tint, the film is fresh and has been properly stored and protected. Proceed with the use of this film.
- **Fogged film.** Film that has expired, has been improperly stored, or has been exposed to radiation appears fogged. If the film is fogged, it must not be used.

SCREENS AND CASSETTES

Extraoral intensifying screens used within a cassette holder should be periodically examined for dirt and scratches. Screens should be cleaned monthly with commercially available cleaners recommended by the screen manufacturer. After cleaning, an antistatic solution should be applied to the screen. Screens that appear visibly scratched should be replaced.

Cassette holders must be examined for worn closures, light leaks, and warping, which may result in fogged and blurred radiographs; these cassettes must be repaired or replaced. Cassettes must also be checked for adequate, screen-film contact.

The following film-screen contact test is recommended:

1. Insert one film between the screens in the cassette holder.
2. Place a wire mesh test object on top of the loaded cassette.

3. Position the position-indicating device (PID) using a 40-inch target-film distance while directing the central ray perpendicular to the cassette.
4. Expose the film using 10 mA, 70 kVp, and 15 impulses.
5. Process the exposed film.
6. View the film on a viewbox in a dimly lit room at a distance of 6 feet.

The results of the film-screen contact test can be interpreted as follows:

- **Adequate contact.** If the wire mesh image seen on the film exhibits a uniform density, good film-screen contact has taken place. Proceed with cassette and screen use.
- **Inadequate contact.** If the wire mesh image seen on the film exhibits varying densities, poor film-screen contact has taken place. Areas of poor film-screen contact appear darker than good contact areas (Fig. 10–1). Cassettes that provide inadequate film-screen contact and exhibit areas of poor contact in the central position must be repaired or replaced.

VIEWING EQUIPMENT

The **viewbox,** or illuminator, is a light source that is used to view dental radiographs (Fig. 10–2). A working viewbox is a necessary piece or equipment for the interpretation of dental radiographs. The viewbox contains fluorescent light bulbs that emit light through an opaque plastic or plexiglass front. The viewbox should emit a uniform and subdued light when it is function-

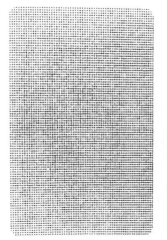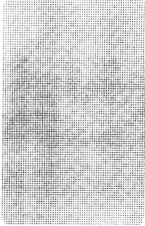

FIGURE 10–1. This illustration shows a cassette exhibiting good film-screen contact (*left*) and one exhibiting poor film-screen contact (*right*). (Reprinted courtesy of Eastman Kodak Company.)

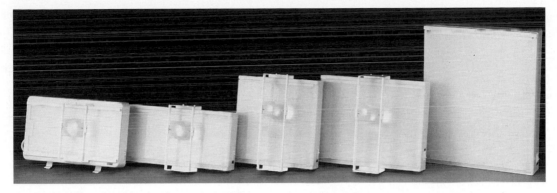

FIGURE 10–2. Examples of viewboxes in sizes to accommodate most dental viewing needs. (Courtesy of Rinn Corporation, Elgin, IL.)

ing properly. A photographic light meter can be used to determine proper viewing brightness.

The viewbox should be periodically examined for dirt and discoloration of the plexiglass surface. The surface of the viewbox should be wiped clean daily. Permanently discolored plexiglass surfaces must be replaced. Any blackened fluorescent light bulbs must also be replaced.

Film Processing

Film processing is one of the most critical areas in quality control and requires daily monitoring. Processing problems have the potential to result in a large number of nondiagnostic radiographs. Quality control tests must be performed routinely to determine whether or not the conditions for film processing are acceptable.

DARKROOM LIGHTING

The darkroom must be checked for light-tightness and proper safelighting every 6 months. The following light leak test is recommended for the darkroom:

1. Prepare darkroom. Close the darkroom door and turn off all lights, including the safelights.
2. Examine darkroom. Once your eyes are accustomed to the darkness, observe the areas around the door, the seams of the walls and ceiling, the vent areas, and the keyhole for light leaks.

The results of the light leak test can be interpreted as follows:

- **No light leaks.** If the darkroom is light-tight, no visible light is seen. Proceed with film processing.

- **Light leaks.** If present, light leaks are seen around the door, through the seams of the walls or ceiling, or through a vent or keyhole. Light leaks must be corrected with weather stripping or black tape before proceeding with film processing.

Only *after* the light-tightness of the darkroom has been established can the safelighting be checked. The following safelighting test, often referred to as the *coin test*, is recommended:

1. Prepare darkroom. Turn off all the lights in the darkroom, including the safelight.
2. Prepare film. Unwrap one unexposed film. Place on a flat surface at least 4 feet from the safelight. Place a coin on top of the film.
3. Turn on the safelight. Allow the film and coin to be exposed to the safelight for 3 to 4 minutes.
4. Remove the coin and process the film.

The results of the safelighting test can be interpreted as follows:

- **Proper safelighting.** If no visible image is seen on the processed radiograph, the safelighting is correct. Proceed with film processing.
- **Improper safelighting.** If the image of the coin and a fogged background appear on the processed radiograph, the safelight is *not* safe to use with that type of film (Fig. 10–3). As discussed in Chapter 9, to avoid safelighting problems, the dental radiographer must use the film manufacturer's recommended safelight filters and bulb wattages. In addition, the film must be unwrapped at least 4 feet away from the safelight.

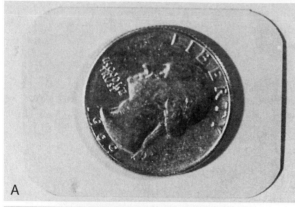

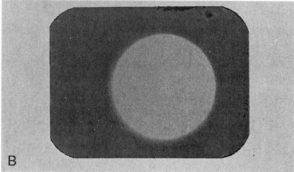

FIGURE 10–3. *A,* Coin test for safelighting. Coin placed on unexposed film under safelight. *B,* Developed film showing outline of coin indicating that safelight intensity is too great and is not safe. (From Frommer HH: Radiology for Dental Auxiliaries, 5th ed. St. Louis, Mosby-Year Book, 1992.)

Safelighting problems must be corrected before proceeding with film processing.

PROCESSING EQUIPMENT

Processing equipment must be meticulously maintained and monitored on a daily basis. As discussed in Chapter 9, the thermometer and timer must be checked for accuracy with manual processing techniques. The temperature and levels of the water bath, developer, and fixer solutions must also be monitored when manual processing techniques are used. The processing time and temperature recommendations of the film manufacturer must be strictly followed.

If automatic processing equipment is used, the water circulation system must be checked, and the solution levels, replenishment system, and temperatures must all be monitored. The manufacturer's procedure and maintenance directions must be carefully followed. Each day, two test films should be processed in the automatic processor. The following automatic processor test films are recommended:

1. Prepare films. Unwrap two unexposed films; expose one to light.
2. Process both films in the automatic processor.

The results of the automatic processor test films can be interpreted as follows:

- **Functioning processor.** If the unexposed film appears clear and dry and if the film exposed to light appears black and dry, the automatic processor is functioning properly. Proceed with processing.
- **Nonfunctioning processor.** If the unexposed film does not appear clear and dry and if the exposed film does not appear completely black and dry, then the processing solutions and dryer temperature must be checked. Corrections must be made before proceeding with processing.

PROCESSING SOLUTIONS

The most critical component of film processing quality control is the monitoring of the processing solutions. As discussed in Chapter 9, the processing solutions must be replenished daily and changed every 3 to 4 weeks as recommended by the manufacturer. As an alternative to using the calendar to determine the freshness of solutions, quality control tests can be used to monitor the strength of the developer and fixer solutions. Processing solutions must be evaluated each day *before* any patient films are processed.

Developer Strength. When the developer solution loses strength, the time-temperature recommendations of the manufacturer are no longer accurate. An easy way to check the strength of the developer solution is to compare film densities to a standard. One of the following tests can be used:

- reference radiograph
- stepwedge radiographs
- normalizing device (Table 10–2)

REFERENCE RADIOGRAPH. A **reference radiograph** is one that is processed under ideal conditions and then used to compare the film densities of radiographs that are processed daily. The following steps can be taken to create a reference radiograph:

1. Prepare film. Use fresh film to make a reference radiograph.
2. Expose the film using correct exposure factors.
3. Process the film using fresh chemicals at the recommended time and temperature.

TABLE 10-2. Quality Control Tests for Film Processing

Day	Solution Strength	Quality Control Tests	Test Results
1	Use fresh, full-strength processing solutions	Reference radiograph: Using correct exposure factors, expose and process one film. This film becomes the reference radiograph.	Reference radiograph: The reference radiograph demonstrates optimum film contrast and density.
		Stepwedge radiograph: Expose 20 stepwedge films; process *one* film. This film becomes the standard radiograph.	Stepwedge radiograph: The standard radiograph demonstrates optimum film contrast and density.
2, 3, etc.	Fresh processing solutions weaken with time and use; exhausted solutions result	Reference radiograph: Each day, expose and process one film to compare with the reference radiograph.	Compare films: Compare the daily film to the reference radiograph: If densities match, continue processing. If densities do not match, replace processing solutions.
		Stepwedge radiograph: Each day, process one of the previously exposed stepwedge films.	Compare films: Compare the daily film to the standard radiograph: If densities match, continue processing. If the densities differ by more than two steps on the stepwedge, replace processing solutions.

4. View the reference radiograph and the daily radiographs side by side on a viewbox. Compare the densities on the reference radiograph with the densities on the daily radiographs.

Comparison of daily radiographs with the reference radiograph can be interpreted as follows:

- **Matched densities.** If the densities seen on the reference radiograph match the densities seen on the daily radiographs, the developer solution strength is adequate. Proceed with processing.
- **Unmatched densities.** If the densities seen on the daily radiographs appear *lighter* than those seen on the reference radiograph, the developer solution is either weak or cold. If the densities seen on the daily radiographs appear *darker* than those seen on the reference radiograph, the developer solution is either too concentrated or too warm. Weakened or concentrated developer solution must be replaced. If the developer solution is too cool or too warm, the temperature must be adjusted.

STEPWEDGE RADIOGRAPHS. As described in Chapter 8, a **stepwedge** is a device constructed of layered aluminum steps. When a stepwedge is placed on top of a film and then exposed to x-rays, the different steps absorb varying amounts of x-rays. When processed, different film densities are seen on the dental radiograph as a result of the stepwedge (see Chapter 8, Fig. 8-6). The following steps can be taken to create stepwedge radiographs:

1. Prepare film. Use a total of 20 fresh films to create a supply of films for daily testing. Place an aluminum stepwedge on top of one film.
2. Expose the film. Repeat with the remaining films using the same stepwedge and exposure factors.
3. Using fresh chemicals, process only *one* of the exposed films. This processed radiograph will exhibit different densities as a result of the stepwedge and is known as the *standard* stepwedge radiograph.
4. Store the remaining 19 exposed films in a cool, dry area protected from x-radiation.
5. Each day, after the chemicals have been replenished, process one of the exposed stepwedge films.
6. View the standard radiograph and the daily radiograph side by side on a viewbox. Compare the densities seen on the daily radiograph with the densities seen on the standard radiograph.

Comparison of the daily stepwedge radiograph with the standard stepwedge radiograph can be interpreted as follows:

- **Matched densities.** Use the middle density seen on the standard stepwedge radiograph for comparison. If the density seen on the standard radiograph matches the density seen on the daily radiograph, the developer solution strength is adequate (Fig. 10–4). Proceed with processing.
- **Unmatched densities.** If the density on the daily radiograph differs from that on the standard radiograph by more than two steps on the stepwedge, the developer solution is depleted (Fig. 10–5). The developer solution must be changed before proceeding with processing.

NORMALIZING DEVICE. A dental radiographic normalizing and monitoring device can be used to monitor developer strength and film density (Fig. 10–6). The **normalizing device** is commercially available. For more information about the purchase and use of this device, contact Dental Radiographic Devices, P.O. Box 9294, Silver Spring, MD 20906.

Fixer Strength. As discussed in Chapter 9, the fixer solution removes the unexposed silver halide crystals on the film that result in "clear" areas on the processed dental radiograph. When the fixer solution loses strength, the film takes a longer time to clear, or become transparent in the unexposed areas. When the fixer is at full strength, a film should clear within 2 minutes, without agitation. To monitor fixer strength, the following clearing test can be used:

1. Prepare film. Unwrap one film and immediately place it in the fixer solution.

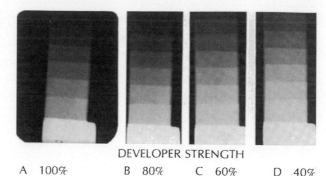

DEVELOPER STRENGTH

A   100%   B   80%   C   60%   D   40%

FIGURE 10–5. Four radiographs of stepwedges that were exposed at the same time and processed at different times. *A,* Radiograph processed when the processing chemicals were changed and complete development of image was obtained. *B,* Radiograph processed 2 weeks later when developer solution was weaker by 20%. A 20% increase in developing time is needed to obtain full development of latent image. *C,* Radiograph processed 4 weeks later when the developer was 60% of original strength. Full development requires a 40% increase in developing time. *D,* Radiograph processed in developer of 40% strength showing obvious underdevelopment of latent image. (From Manson-Hing LR: Fundamentals of Dental Radiography, 3rd ed. Philadelphia, Lea & Febiger, 1990.)

2. Check the film for clearing. Measure the amount of time the film takes to clear.

The results of the clearing test can be interpreted as follows:

- **Fast clearing.** If the film, clears in 2 minutes, the fixer is of adequate strength. Proceed with processing.
- **Slow clearing.** If the film is not completely clear after 2 minutes, reimmerse it in the fixer solution. If the film does not completely clear in 3 to 4 minutes, the fixer solution is depleted. The fixer solution must be replaced before proceeding with processing.

QUALITY ADMINISTRATION PROCEDURES

Quality administration refers to the management of the quality assurance plan in the dental office. Although many of the technical aspects of the quality assurance plan (e.g., quality control tests) may be delegated to the dental radiographer, the dentist is ultimately responsible for overall quality assurance. The basic elements of a quality administration program include the following:

- description of the plan
- assignment of duties

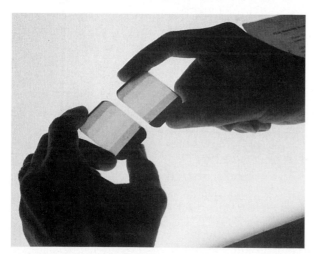

FIGURE 10–4. The daily check film should appear identical to the control film. (From Miles DA, Van Dis ML, Razmus TS: Basic Principles of Oral and Maxillofacial Radiology. Philadelphia, WB Saunders, 1991.)

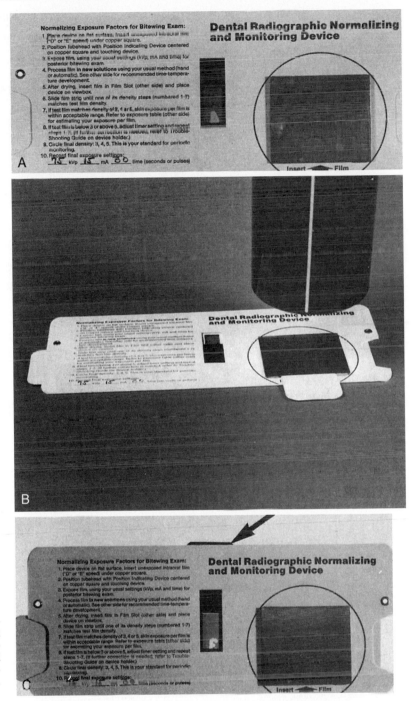

FIGURE 10-6. *A,* Dental radiographic normalizing and monitoring device. *B,* Test film inserted beneath copper plate and exposure made. *C,* Processed test film (*arrow*) inserted in device and compared with numbered densities. (From Frommer HH. Radiology for Dental Auxiliaries, 5th ed. St. Louis, Mosby-Year Book, 1992.)

- a monitoring schedule
- a maintenance schedule
- a record-keeping log
- a plan for evaluation and revision
- in-service training

A detailed, written description of the quality assurance plan used in the dental office should be on file and made available to all participating staff members. The standards of quality must be outlined by the dentist. Each staff member involved in the quality assurance plan must understand the standards of quality as well as the purpose and importance of maintaining quality control of radiographic procedures. A detailed, written assignment of quality assurance duties should also be on file and made available to all participating staff members. Each staff member assigned to perform a duty must understand the purpose and importance of that specific duty. Although the dentist may serve as the administrator of the quality assurance program, an assigned staff member may oversee the daily quality control testing and results.

A written monitoring schedule detailing all quality control tests and the frequency of testing for all dental x-ray equipment, supplies, and film processing should be posted in the office. A written maintenance schedule for the routine service and inspection of dental x-ray machines and processing equipment should also be posted in the office.

A record-keeping log of all quality control tests, including the specific test performed, the date performed, and the test results, should be carefully maintained and kept on file in the dental office. In addition, a processing solutions log that lists the dates of solution replacement, replenishment, and processor or tank cleaning should also be maintained. Examples of record-keeping logs can be found in the pamphlet *Quality Control Tests for Dental Radiography,* available from the Eastman Kodak Company.

A written plan for the periodic evaluation and revision of the existing quality assurance program should also be part of the quality administration plan. Last, periodic in-service training of staff members to upgrade and improve x-ray exposure techniques and film processing procedures is recommended.

OPERATOR COMPETENCE

The dentist is ultimately responsible for the diagnostic quality of *all* dental radiographs exposed in his or her office, regardless of who actually exposes and processes the film. As a result, the dentist depends on competent dental radiographers. Each dental radiographer must be competent in both exposure and processing techniques.

If the operator (dental radiographer) produces a nondiagnostic film, the film must be retaken. All retakes expose the patient to additional x-radiation; consequently, the number of retakes must be kept to an absolute minimum. Repeated operator errors and errors that require retakes should all be recorded. The use of a log to record retakes aids in identifying recurring problems that require attention. Continuing education courses or individualized instruction can be

used to upgrade and improve the competence of the dental radiographer.

SUMMARY

- A quality assurance plan ensures the production of high-quality radiographs and includes both quality control tests and quality administration procedures.
- Quality control tests are tests that are used to monitor dental x-ray equipment, supplies, and film processing. The following quality control tests are recommended:
  - **X-ray machines.** Dental x-ray machines should be tested for minor malfunctions, output variations, collimation problems, tubehead drift, timing errors, and inaccurate kilovoltage and milliamperage readings (see Table 10–2). These tests should be performed once a year.
  - **X-ray film.** The fresh film test can be used to determine whether dental x-ray film is fresh and has been properly stored and protected. This test should be performed each time a new box of film is opened.
  - **Screens and cassettes.** Cassettes should be examined periodically for adequate closure, light leaks, and warping. The film-screen contact test can be used to determine the adequacy of screen-film contact. This test should be performed periodically. More frequent testing is required if the screens and cassettes are used often.
  - **Darkroom lighting.** The light leak test can be used to evaluate the darkroom for light leaks, and the safelighting test can be used to check for proper safelighting conditions. These tests should be performed every 6 months.
  - **Processing equipment.** Manual and automatic processing equipment must be carefully maintained and monitored daily for potential problems. With manual processing techniques, the thermometer and timer must be accurate; the temperature and levels of the water bath, developer, and fixer solutions must also be checked. Automatic processor test films can be used to check the functioning of the automatic processor. These tests and checks must be performed daily.
  - **Processing solutions.** The developer strength can be monitored by a reference radiograph, stepwedge radiographs, or a normalizing device. The fixer solution can be checked by performing a clearing test. These tests must be performed daily.
- Quality administration procedures include a description of the quality assurance plan, the assignment of duties, a monitoring schedule, a maintenance schedule, record-keeping logs, a plan for evaluation and revision, and in-service training.
- The dentist is ultimately responsible for the overall quality assurance plan. In addition, the dentist is responsible for the diagnostic quality of all radiographs, regardless of who exposes and processes the film.
- To ensure the production of diagnostic radiographs, the dentist depends on the skill of competent dental radiographers. The dental radiographer must be competent in both exposure and processing techniques.

BIBLIOGRAPHY

Frommer HH: Radiation protection. *In* Radiology for Dental Auxiliaries, 6th edition. St. Louis, Mosby-Year Book, 1996, pp. 67–87.

Frommer HH: Film processing: the darkroom. *In* Radiology for Dental Auxiliaries, 6th edition. St. Louis, Mosby-Year Book, 1996, pp. 101–137.

Goaz PW, White SC: Health physics. *In* Oral Radiology: Principles and Interpretation, 3rd edition. St. Louis, Mosby-Year Book, 1994, p. 65.

Johnson ON, McNally MA, Essay CE: Radiation protection. *In* Essentials of Dental Radiography for Dental Assistants and Hygienists, 6th edition. Norwalk, CT, Appleton and Lange, 1999, pp. 105–130.

Johnson ON, McNally MA, Essay CE: Quality assurance in dental radiography. *In* Essentials of Dental Radiography for Dental Assistants and Hygienists, 6th edition. Norwalk, CT, Appleton and Lange, 1999, pp. 211–225.

Johnson ON, McNally MA, Essay CE: Identifying and correcting faulty radiographs. *In* Essentials of Dental Radiography for Dental Assistants and Hygienists, 6th edition. Norwalk, CT, Appleton and Lange, 1999, pp. 307–317.

Langland OE, Sippy FH, Langlais RP: Quality assurance. *In* Textbook of Dental Radiography, 2nd edition. Springfield, IL, Charles C Thomas, 1984, pp. 352–366.

Lusk LT: Peak performance. RDH The National Magazine for Dental Hygiene Professionals 14(3):32, 37–38, 1994.

Manson-Hing LR: Quality control in the dental office. *In* Fundamentals of Dental Radiography, 3rd edition. Philadelphia, Lea & Febiger, 1990, pp. 243–257.

Matteson SR, Whaley C, Secrist VC: The film and the darkroom. *In* Dental Radiology, 4th edition. Chapel Hill, University of North Carolina Press, 1988, pp. 62–64.

Miles DA, Van Dis ML, Jensen CW, Ferretti A: Film processing and quality assurance. *In* Radiographic Imaging for Dental Auxiliaries, 3rd edition. Philadelphia, WB Saunders, 1999, pp. 49–71.

Miles DA, Van Dis ML, Razmus TF: Radiographic processing and processing quality assurance. *In* Basic Principles of Oral and Maxillofacial Radiology. Philadelphia, WB Saunders, 1992, pp. 168–174.

Quiz Questions ....

MULTIPLE CHOICE

_____ 1. Calibration of dental x-ray equipment can be performed by the dentist, dental hygienist, or dental assistant.

    a. true
    b. false

_____ 2. Annual tests for dental x-ray machines can be performed by the dentist, dental hygienist, or dental assistant.

    a. true
    b. false

_____ 3. For quality control purposes, each new box of unopened film should be tested for film freshness and fog before it is used.

    a. true
    b. false

_____ 4. After processing, fresh film that has been properly stored and protected will appear:

    a. fogged
    b. clear with a slight blue tint
    c. clouded with a blue tint
    d. dark blue
    e. totally black

_____ 5. After performing the film-screen contact test, a wire mesh image of uniform density appears. These results indicate:

    a. adequate film-screen contact
    b. inadequate film-screen contact

_____ 6. When functioning properly, a viewbox should emit a uniform and brilliant light.

    a. true
    b. false

_____ 7. One of the most critical areas of quality control that requires _daily_ monitoring is:

    a. examination of the fluorescent bulbs inside the viewbox
    b. cleaning the extraoral intensifying screens
    c. examination of the darkroom for light-tightness
    d. processing of films
    e. all of the above

_____ 8. The coin test is used to check:

    a. proper safelighting
    b. strength of the processing solution
    c. film density
    d. film-screen contact
    e. beam collimation

9. The following must be closely monitored with manual processing techniques:

   a. temperature of the water bath
   b. levels of the processing solutions
   c. accuracy of the timer
   d. accuracy of the thermometer
   e. all of the above

10. On the average, processing solutions should be changed:

    a. once each day
    b. once each week
    c. every 3 to 4 weeks
    d. every 8 to 10 weeks
    e. every 3 to 4 months

11. On the average, processing solutions should be replenished:

    a. once each day
    b. once each week
    c. every 3 to 4 weeks
    d. every 8 to 10 weeks
    e. every 3 to 4 months

12. Fresh films and fresh chemicals must be used when preparing reference radiographs.

    a. true
    b. false

13. A reference radiograph is used to check:

    a. proper safelighting
    b. light-tightness of the darkroom
    c. strength of the fixer solution
    d. strength of the developer solution
    e. none of the above

14. The densities seen on the daily radiograph appear lighter than the densities seen on the reference radiograph; this result indicates that:

    a. the developer solution is too weak
    b. the developer solution is too concentrated
    c. the developer solution is too cold
    d. a or c
    e. b or c

15. The clearing test is used to monitor:

    a. developer strength
    b. fixer strength
    c. accuracy of the timer
    d. film density
    e. none of the above

16. Regardless of who actually exposes and processes radiographs, the dentist is ultimately responsible for the diagnostic quality of all dental radiographs.

    a. true
    b. false

Answers are supplied at the end of this book.

PART

three

Dental Radiographer Basics

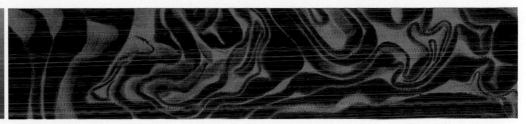

Dental Radiographs and the Dental Radiographer

OBJECTIVES

After completion of this chapter, the student will be able to:

- *Define the key words.*
- *Discuss the importance of dental radiographs.*
- *List the uses of dental radiographs.*
- *Discuss the benefits of dental radiographs.*
- *List examples of common dental conditions that may be evident on a dental radiograph.*
- *Discuss the knowledge and skill requirements of the dental radiographer.*
- *List the responsibilities that may be assigned to the dental radiographer.*
- *Discuss the professional goals of the dental radiographer.*

INTRODUCTION

The dental radiographer must understand the importance of dental radiographs and the reasons why dental radiographs are a necessary component of comprehensive patient care. As discussed throughout this text, the dental radiographer must have both sufficient knowledge and technical skills to perform dental radiographic procedures. In addition to background knowledge and technical skills, an understanding of the responsibilities and professional goals of the dental radiographer is necessary.

The purpose of this chapter is to review the importance and benefits of dental radiographs and the knowledge and skill requirements of the dental radiographer. The role of the dental radiographer is defined, and his or her duties and responsibilities are described. In addition, the professional goals of the dental radiographer are outlined.

DENTAL RADIOGRAPHS

A **dental radiograph** is a photographic image produced on film by the passage of x-rays through teeth and supporting structures. The dental radiographer must have a thorough understanding of the value and importance of dental radiographs. In addition, the dental radiographer must be familiar with the uses of dental radiographs, the benefits of dental radiographs, and the information that can be found on dental radiographs.

The Importance of Dental Radiographs

Dental radiographs are a necessary component of comprehensive patient care. In dentistry, a radiographic examination is essential for diagnostic purposes. Radiographs enable the dental professional to identify many conditions that may otherwise go undetected; dental radiographs allow the practitioner to see many conditions that are not apparent clinically. An oral examination without dental radiographs limits the practitioner

to a knowledge of what is seen clinically—the teeth and soft tissues. With the use of dental radiographs, the dental professional gains a great deal of information about the teeth and supporting bone.

Uses of Dental Radiographs

The uses of dental radiographs are many and varied. *Detection* is one of the most important uses of dental radiographs. Through the use of dental radiographs, the dental radiographer can detect diseases, lesions, and conditions of the teeth and bones that cannot be identified clinically. Many diseases and conditions produce no clinical signs or symptoms and are typically discovered *only* through the use of dental radiographs.

Dental radiographs are used not only for detection but also for confirming suspected diseases and assisting in the localization of lesions and foreign objects. Radiographs provide essential information during routine dental treatment; for example, the dentist depends on radiographs during root canal procedures. Dental radiographs can be used to examine the status of the teeth and bone during growth and development. Dental radiographs are indispensable for showing changes secondary to trauma, caries, and periodontal disease.

Dental radiographs are an essential component of the patient record. A radiograph contains an incredible amount of information, far more than a written record. An initial radiographic examination provides baseline information about the patient. Each radiograph serves to document the condition of a patient at a specific point in time. Any subsequent radiographs can be used for comparative purposes; follow-up radiographs can be compared with initial radiographs and examined for changes resulting from treatment, trauma, or disease.

Benefits of Dental Radiographs

Dental radiographs are taken to benefit the patient. The primary benefit is the detection of disease. When radiographs are properly prescribed, exposed, and processed, the benefit of disease detection far outweighs the risk of small doses of x-radiation. A discussion of the risk-versus-benefit concept is found in Chapter 4; guidelines for the proper prescription of dental radiographs are found in Chapter 5.

Through the proper use of dental radiographs, the dental professional can detect disease and ultimately benefit the patient by minimizing and preventing problems, such as tooth-related pain or the need for surgical procedures. By emphasizing the preventive aspect of dental radiography, the dental professional can save the patient time and money while maintaining the patient's oral health.

Information Found on Dental Radiographs

Numerous conditions of the teeth and jaws produce no clinical signs or symptoms and can *only* be detected on dental radiographs. Some of the more common diseases, lesions, and conditions found on dental radiographs include the following:

- missing teeth
- extra teeth
- impacted teeth
- dental caries
- periodontal disease
- tooth abnormalities
- retained roots
- cysts and tumors

Example radiographs can be used to educate the dental patient about some of these common conditions that are only detected through the use of dental radiographs.

THE DENTAL RADIOGRAPHER

The **dental radiographer** is any person who positions, exposes, and processes dental x-ray film. In the typical dental practice, the dental radiographer is a dental auxiliary, either a dental hygienist or a dental assistant. The dental radiographer must have both sufficient knowledge and technical skills to perform dental radiographic procedures. In addition, the dental radiographer must have an understanding of his or her responsibilities and professional goals.

Knowledge and Skill Requirements

To be a competent dental radiographer, a background knowledge of dental radiography is essential. The purpose of the first 10 chapters of this text has been to provide the dental radiographer with adequate background information to perform dental radiographic procedures. The dental radiographer must have a basic understanding of radiation history (Chapter 1) and a working knowledge of radiation physics (Chapter 2), radiation characteristics (Chapter 3), radiation biology (Chapter 4), and radiation protection (Chapter 5). In addition, the dental radiographer must be familiar with dental x-ray equipment (Chapter 6), dental x-ray film

(Chapter 7), dental x-ray image characteristics (Chapter 8), dental x-ray film processing (Chapter 9), and quality assurance in the dental office (Chapter 10).

In addition to background information, a knowledge of patient management basics (Chapters 12 to 15) must be mastered by the dental radiographer. Most important, the dental radiographer must be proficient in technique concepts and the technical skills used in dental radiography (Chapters 16 to 25).

Duties and Responsibilities

The dental auxiliary is a member of the dental team and has an important role in the practice. Each auxiliary employed in the dental office is assigned specific duties and responsibilities. The assigned duties and responsibilities vary, depending on the size and nature of the dental practice and the individual qualifications of the auxiliary. Assigned responsibilities in regard to dental radiography may include the following:

- the positioning and exposure of dental x-ray films
- the processing of dental x-ray films
- the mounting and identification of dental radiographs
- the education of patients about dental radiography
- the maintenance of darkroom facilities and processing equipment
- the implementation and monitoring of quality control procedures
- the ordering of dental x-ray film and related supplies

Professional Goals

The dental radiographer must have pride in his or her work and must always strive for professional improvement. The dental radiographer must have defined professional goals and be committed to achieving such goals. Priority goals for the dental radiographer include the following:

Patient protection: Patient protection must be a top priority and a primary concern of the dental radiographer. Whenever the dental radiographer performs radiographic procedures on patients, the lowest possible level of x-radiation must be used. Retakes resulting in unnecessary patient exposure to x-radiation must be avoided at all times. Patient protection techniques used prior to exposure include the proper prescribing of dental radiographs and the use of proper equipment. During exposure, a thyroid collar, lead apron, fast film, and film-holding devices can be used to protect the patient from excess exposure to radiation. In addition, proper selection of exposure factors and good technique can also be used to protect the patient. After exposure to x-rays, meticulous film handling and processing techniques are critical for the production of diagnostic radiographs. Specific patient protection techniques are discussed in Chapter 5.

Operator protection: Operator protection must also be a primary concern for the dental radiographer. To avoid occupational exposure to x-radiation, the dental radiographer must always avoid the primary beam and maintain an adequate distance, proper position, and proper shielding from x-rays during exposure. Radiation monitoring can also be used to protect the dental radiographer. Specific operator protection recommendations are discussed in Chapter 5.

Patient education: Patient education must also be a priority for the dental radiographer. The dental radiographer must play an active role in the education of patients concerning radiation exposure, patient protection, and the value and uses of dental radiographs (see Chapter 13).

Operator competence: Operator competence must always be a concern of the dental radiographer. The dental radiographer must strive to maintain or improve professional competence by attending continuing education courses and lectures, studying professional books and journals, and reviewing and updating radiographic techniques.

Operator efficiency: The dental radiographer must be committed to performing his or her assigned duties in a time-efficient manner. The dental radiographer must always work carefully but quickly when positioning and exposing dental x-ray films. Patients always appreciate the auxiliary who does not waste time and who works in a competent and efficient manner.

Production of quality radiographs: The dental radiographer must be committed to producing high-quality diagnostic radiographs. The dental radiographer must constantly strive to achieve perfection with each and every dental radiograph. To produce the perfect dental radiograph, the dental radiographer must carefully position and expose the film, correctly process it, and properly mount and identify the finished dental radiograph. The dental radiographer can take great professional pride in producing perfect dental radiographs.

When the dental radiographer attains professional goals such as those outlined, the patient receives the highest quality of care that is possible. Quality care benefits not only the patient but also the profession of dentistry.

■ SUMMARY

- The dental radiographer must understand the importance of dental radiographs and why dental radiographs are a necessary component of comprehensive patient care.
- Dental radiographs are essential for diagnostic purposes and enable the dental professional to identify many conditions that may otherwise go undetected.
- There are a number of uses of dental radiographs; however, the primary use is *detection* of diseases, lesions, and conditions of the teeth and bones.
- Dental radiographs are taken to benefit the patient. The primary benefit is disease detection; the benefit of disease detection far outweighs the risk of small doses of radiation.
- Much information can be obtained from a radiographic examination. Numerous conditions of the teeth and jaws produce no clinical signs or symptoms and can only be detected on dental radiographs.
- The dental radiographer is any person who positions, exposes, and processes dental x-ray film. The dental radiographer must have both sufficient knowledge and technical skills to perform dental radiographic procedures.
- Responsibilities of the dental radiographer may include the following: positioning, exposure, and processing of dental x-ray films; mounting and identification of dental radiographs; education of patients about dental radiography; maintenance of darkroom facilities and processing equipment; implementation and monitoring of quality control procedures; and the ordering of dental x-ray equipment and supplies.
- The dental radiographer must have defined professional goals and be committed to attaining such goals. Priority goals for the dental radiographer include patient protection, operator protection, patient education, operator competence, operator efficiency, and the production of high-quality radiographs.

BIBLIOGRAPHY

Frommer HH: Patient management and special problems. *In* Radiology for Dental Auxiliaries, 6th edition. St. Louis, Mosby-Year Book, 1996, pp. 245–2670.

Haring JI, Lind LJ: The importance of dental radiographs and interpretation. *In* Radiographic Interpretation for the Dental Hygienist. Philadelphia, WB Saunders, 1993, pp. 1–11.

Johnson ON, McNally MA, Essay CE: Patient relations and education. *In* Essentials of Dental Radiography for Dental Assistants and Hygienists, 6th edition. Norwalk, CT, Appleton and Lange, 1999, pp. 493–505.

Manson-Hing LR: Patient relations. *In* Fundamentals of Dental Radiography, 3rd edition. Philadelphia, Lea & Febiger, 1990, pp. 221–223.

Quiz Questions ●●

TRUE OR FALSE

_____ 1. Localization of foreign objects is the most important use of dental radiographs.

_____ 2. The benefit of disease detection does not outweigh the risk of small doses of x radiation.

_____ 3. Through the use of dental radiographs, the dental professional can detect diseases, lesions, and conditions of the jaws that cannot be identified clinically.

_____ 4. A radiograph contains less information than a written record.

_____ 5. Missing, extra, and impacted teeth can be identified on a dental radiograph.

_____ 6. The dental radiographer is any person who positions, exposes, and processes dental x-ray film.

_____ 7. The dental radiographer is assigned only to position and expose dental x-ray films.

_____ 8. The dental radiographer may be assigned to monitor quality control procedures.

_____ 9. Patient and operator protection must be primary concerns of the dental radiographer.

_____ 10. Operator competence is maintained by performing dental radiography duties.

Answers are supplied at the end of this book.

CHAPTER
12

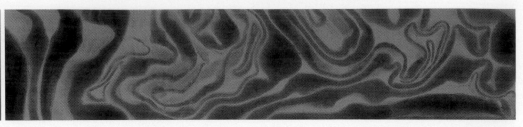

Patient Relations and the Dental Radiographer

OBJECTIVES

After completion of this chapter, the student will be able to:

- *Define the key words.*
- *Discuss verbal, nonverbal, and listening skills and explain how each can be used to enhance communication.*
- *Discuss how facilitative skills can be used to enhance patient trust.*
- *Define a relationship of trust between the dental professional and the patient.*
- *Discuss the importance of first impressions, chairside manner, and attitude and explain how each can enhance patient relations.*

Chairside manner   Interpersonal skills
Communication   Patient relations
Facilitation skills

INTRODUCTION

Patient relations are important for all dental professionals. The dental radiographer needs good interpersonal skills to communicate with patients and establish trusting relationships. Communicating with dental patients may be the most demanding professional challenge that a dental radiographer encounters. The purpose of this chapter is to discuss specific interpersonal skills that enhance communication between the dental radiographer and the patient and to review the importance of patient relations.

INTERPERSONAL SKILLS

Skills that promote good relationships between individuals are termed **interpersonal skills**. (The term interpersonal means between persons.) The dental radiographer must have effective interpersonal skills to establish trusting relationships with dental patients and promote patient confidence. Technical skills alone are not sufficient for providing optimal patient care. Interpersonal skills must be used in conjunction with technical skills to enhance the quality of patient care.

Communication Skills

Communication is a very important interpersonal skill. **Communication** can be defined as "the process by which information is exchanged between two or more persons." Effective communication is the basis for developing a successful radiographer-patient relationship.

VERBAL COMMUNICATION SKILLS

Verbal communication involves the use of language. The dental radiographer's choice of words is very important when talking with the dental patient. Certain words detract from the professional image of the dental radiographer. For example, the term *pull* sounds less professional than *extract,* and the word *fix* sounds less professional than *repair* or *restore.* Some words used in the dental setting (e.g., cut, drill, scrape, zap) are associated with negative images and must be avoided. In addition, excessive use of technical words may cause confusion and result in miscommunication. The dental radiographer should always choose words that can be easily understood by the patient.

Careless use of language can also contribute to miscommunication between the dental radiographer and the patient. The use of unnecessary words (e.g., you know, it's like, I mean) may make it difficult for the patient to understand exactly what the radiographer is saying. Excessive use of slang can also increase the chance of misunderstanding.

The delivery of speech is also important in verbal communication. The dental radiographer should always speak in a pleasant and relaxed manner. In the dental setting, the use of a soft tone of voice is preferred; a soft tone is soothing and effective for conveying warmth and concern. The use of a loud tone of voice is not appropriate in the dental setting and is often associated with fear, anger, or excitement. The dental radiographer should also avoid speaking in a rushed or tense manner.

NONVERBAL COMMUNICATION SKILLS

Nonverbal communication involves the use of body language. Nonverbal messages conveyed by the posture, body movement, and facial expressions of the dental radiographer are all very important when working with patients in the dental setting.

Nonverbal messages can be substituted for verbal messages. For example, a nod of the head indicates agreement, whereas a shake of the head signals disagreement. Nonverbal behavior can also be used to enhance communication. For example, if the statement "It's nice to see you" is accompanied by a smile, there is consistency between the verbal and nonverbal messages; the verbal message is enhanced by the nonverbal message. When nonverbal messages are consistent with verbal messages, the patient is more likely to relax and trust the dental professional. On the other hand, when nonverbal messages are not consistent with verbal messages, the patient is more likely to respond with apprehension and mistrust.

Posture and body movement are important nonverbal cues that convey the attitude of the dental radiographer. An attentive posture, leaning slightly toward the patient, and relaxed, still hands are nonverbal cues associated with interest and warmth. Conversely, a slumped posture, leaning away from the patient, with the arms folded across the chest and the fingers tapping are all nonverbal cues that signal indifference and coldness. Patients are more likely to understand and remember information presented by an interested health professional than by a professional whose nonverbal cues signal indifference.

Eye contact is another nonverbal means of communication that is very important in the dental setting. When listening to a patient, the dental radiographer should always maintain direct eye contact with the patient; the eyes should not wander. Direct eye contact is associated with interest and attention and plays a powerful role in the initiation and development of interpersonal relationships. A lack of eye contact is often interpreted as indifference or lack of concern.

LISTENING SKILLS

Listening involves more than just hearing; listening refers to the receiving and understanding of messages. When listening to a patient, the dental radiographer must receive and understand the information being presented. Careful attention to listening results in better communication and less chance for misunderstandings. The radiographer with good listening skills understands what the patient has said and in turn is able to communicate that understanding to the patient.

The good listener communicates attention and interest. When listening to a patient, the dental radiographer can use nonverbal cues such as a nod of the head or facial expressions to convey appropriate emotional responses. To communicate interest, the dental radiographer can paraphrase what the patient has just stated to confirm what has been heard.

To enhance communication, sometimes the dental radiographer may want to summarize the feelings of the patient rather than paraphrase the information that has been presented. When a patient is fearful and upset, and the dental radiographer can summarize and emphasize the feelings of the patient, interest and concern for the patient are conveyed.

When listening to a patient, the dental radiographer should give the patient undivided attention. The dental radiographer should never interrupt or correct the patient, finish the patient's sentences, look at a clock or watch, or distract the patient by fidgeting or playing with objects.

Facilitation Skills

Facilitation skills are interpersonal skills that are used to ease communication and develop a trusting relationship between the dental professional and the patient. (The term facilitation means the act of making easier.) In a trusting relationship, the patient feels cared for and understood by the dental professional. In the dental setting, trust involves the belief that the dental professional will interact with a patient in a beneficial way rather than a harmful way. A trusting relationship facilitates the delivery of patient care by reducing worry and psychological stress. When a patient trusts the dental professional, the patient is more likely to provide information, cooperate during procedures, comply with prescribed treatment, and return for further treatment.

Facilitative skills that enhance patient trust include encouraging questions, answering questions, responding with action, and warmth. The dental radiographer must encourage each patient to ask questions. Many patients may be hesitant to ask questions because they are intimidated by the dental professional or apprehensive about the dental visit. Inviting a patient to ask questions enhances communication. In addition, the dental radiographer must be prepared to answer patient questions directly. Whenever a patient asks a question, the dental radiographer should respond with accurate information in a direct manner and use language that can be easily understood by the patient.

The dental radiographer must also be prepared to respond with action or carry out patient requests. For example, if a patient requests a glass of water, the dental radiographer can respond by carrying out the request. The patient feels cared for when the dental radiographer responds to such requests. In addition, the dental radiographer must respond to patients with warmth. Warmth can be communicated through the voice and facial expression of the dental radiographer. The dental radiographer who responds to patients with warmth is friendly and smiling and shows interest in the patient. Warmth communicates the impression that the professional cares for the patient as a person.

■ PATIENT RELATIONS

In dentistry, the term **patient relations** refers to the relationship between the patient and the dental professional. Patient relations are important to all dental professionals—the dentist, the dental hygienist, and the dental assistant.

First Impressions and Patient Relations

The relationship between the patient and the dental professional begins with first impressions. The patient's first impression of the dental team most often involves the dental auxiliary; both the appearance of the auxiliary and how the auxiliary greets the patient are very important.

The professional appearance of the dental auxiliary is important. The dental auxiliary should always wear a clean uniform and appear well groomed. Strict attention must be paid to matters of personal hygiene such as handwashing and maintaining fresh breath. In addition, the dental auxiliary should never eat, drink, or chew gum while working with patients.

In many offices, the dental auxiliary is the first dental professional to meet and greet the patient. The dental auxiliary should always greet the patient in the reception room before escorting the patient to the treatment area. Patients should always be greeted by name. The dental auxiliary should address the patient using the patient's proper title (Miss, Ms., Mrs., Mr., Dr., Rev., etc.) and last name. If pronunciation of the name is uncertain, the dental auxiliary should verify the correct pronunciation with the patient. The dental auxiliary should always introduce himself or herself to the patient, using both a name and title. An example of a typical first greeting follows:

EXAMPLE

Hello, Mrs. Davis. My name is Kate Miller and I'm the dental assistant who will be working with you today. It's a pleasure to meet you. If you'll follow me to the patient treatment area, we can get started with today's appointment.

Chairside Manner and Patient Relations

The relationship between the patient and the dental professional develops as the professional works with the patient. **Chairside manner** refers to "the way a dental professional conducts oneself at the patient's chairside." The dental auxiliary must develop a relaxing chairside manner that makes the patient feel comfortable and at ease.

The dental auxiliary must also convey a confident chairside manner; the patient must be confident about the auxiliary's ability to perform radiographic proce-

dures. The dental radiographer must avoid comments such as "Oops!" and other statements that indicate a lack of control. The patient must feel that the operator is in control of all procedures being performed. One way to convey operator confidence is to explain to the patient exactly which procedures are about to be performed and then answer any questions the patient may have about the procedures.

In most dental offices, the dental auxiliary is responsible for performing radiographic procedures. However, some patients may be apprehensive about allowing a dental auxiliary to perform such procedures because they are accustomed to a dentist performing all procedures, including radiographic techniques. As a result, these patients may object to a dental auxiliary performing any services for them. In such cases, the dental auxiliary must try to establish a relationship with the patient by introducing the concept of the dental team. The dental auxiliary can educate and orient the patient to the dental team members and their respective roles and responsibilities. The dentist may then reinforce such information and reassure the patient before the dental auxiliary performs the radiographic procedures.

Attitude and Patient Relations

The attitude of the dental auxiliary will affect patient relations. Attitude can be defined as "a position of the body, or manner of carrying oneself, indicative of a mood." The attitude of all dental auxiliaries must be professional and should include the attributes of courtesy, patience, and honesty. The dental auxiliary must be courteous and polite toward all patients at all times. Patience, which includes both tolerance and understanding, is also necessary, especially when an uncooperative or difficult patient is encountered. Honesty is also an important part of a professional attitude. In dental radiography, some procedures are uncomfortable. In such instances, the dental auxiliary must be honest and inform the patient of the potential discomfort of the procedures.

◼ SUMMARY

- The relationship between the patient and the dental radiographer is an important one. Communication is a very important interpersonal skill and is the basis for developing a successful radiographer-patient relationship.
- Verbal communication involves the use of language. The

dental radiographer's choice of words is very important; words that detract from the professional image of dentistry and words that are associated with negative images must be avoided.

- Nonverbal communication involves the use of body language and includes messages conveyed by posture, body movement, and facial expressions. A patient will respond positively toward the dental professional whose nonverbal cues signal interest and warmth; a patient is less likely to respond to a dental professional whose nonverbal cues signal indifference and coldness.
- Communication also involves listening skills. The dental radiographer with good listening skills understands what the patient has said and, in turn, is able to communicate that understanding to the patient. The good listener communicates both attention and interest.
- Facilitation skills are interpersonal skills that make communication easier and develop a trusting relationship between the patient and the dental professional. Facilitative skills include encouraging patient questions, answering patient questions, responding to patient requests, and communicating with warmth.
- Patient relations refers to the relationship between the patient and the dental professional. The dental auxiliary must develop a relaxing and confident chairside manner that makes the patient feel comfortable.

BIBLIOGRAPHY

Frommer HH: Patient management and special problems. *In* Radiology for Dental Auxiliaries, 6th edition. St. Louis, Mosby-Year Book, 1996, pp. 245–267.

Gerrard BA, Boniface WJ, Love BH: Why health professionals need interpersonal skills. *In* Interpersonal Skills for Health Professionals. Reston, VA, Reston Publishing, 1980, pp. 2–3.

Gerrard BA, Boniface WJ, Love BH: Developing facilitation skills. *In* Interpersonal Skills for Health Professionals. Reston, VA, Reston Publishing, 1980, pp. 110–114.

Ingersoll BD: Verbal communication: Speaking and listening skills. *In* Patient Management Skills for Dental Assistants and Hygienists. Norwalk, CT, Appleton-Century-Crofts, 1986, pp. 10–23.

Ingersoll BD: Nonverbal communication. *In* Patient Management Skills for Dental Assistants and Hygienists. Norwalk, CT, Appleton-Century-Crofts, 1986, pp. 25–36.

Manson-Hing LR: Patient relations. *In* Fundamentals of Dental Radiography, 3rd edition. Philadelphia, Lea & Febiger, 1990, pp. 222–223.

O'Brien RC: Eighty-five percent of your success—your personality. *In* Dental Radiography: An Introduction for Dental Hygienists and Assistants, 4th edition. Philadelphia, WB Saunders, 1982, pp. 283–285.

Quiz Questions

TRUE OR FALSE

_____ 1. Skills that promote a good relationship between individuals are termed facilitation skills.

_____ 2. Technical skills alone are sufficient for providing optimal patient care.

_____ 3. The excessive use of technical words may confuse the patient and result in miscommunication.

_____ 4. The delivery of speech is important in verbal communication; the dental radiographer should speak in a pleasant, relaxed manner.

_____ 5. Nonverbal behavior cannot be used to enhance communication.

_____ 6. If verbal messages are consistent with nonverbal messages, the patient is likely to respond with apprehension and mistrust.

_____ 7. Patients are more likely to understand a dental professional whose nonverbal cues signal indifference.

_____ 8. Eye contact plays a powerful role in the development of interpersonal relationships.

_____ 9. Listening involves only hearing.

_____ 10. When listening to a patient, the dental radiographer can use facial expressions to convey appropriate emotional responses.

_____ 11. Interpersonal skills are skills that are used to make communication easier and develop a trusting relationship between the patient and the dental professional.

_____ 12. When a patient trusts the dental professional, the patient is more likely to comply with the prescribed treatment and return for further treatment.

_____ 13. The appearance of the dental auxiliary is important.

_____ 14. In many offices, the dental auxiliary is the first person to meet and greet the patient.

_____ 15. A patient should always be greeted by his or her first name.

_____ 16. It is appropriate for the dental auxiliary to chew gum while working with patients.

_____ 17. The dental auxiliary must develop a fast-paced, confident chairside manner.

_____ 18. In most dental offices, the dental auxiliary is responsible for performing radiographic procedures.

_____ 19. The attitude of the dental radiographer affects patient relations.

_____ 20. The dental radiographer does not need to be courteous if a patient is uncooperative or difficult.

Answers are supplied at the end of this book.

Patient Education and the Dental Radiographer

OBJECTIVES

After completion of this chapter, the student will be able to:

- *Summarize the importance of educating patients about dental radiographs.*
- *List three methods that can be used by the dental radiographer to educate patients about dental radiographs.*
- *Answer common patient questions about the need for dental radiographs, x-ray exposure, the safety of dental x-rays, and other miscellaneous concerns.*

INTRODUCTION

The dental radiographer must be able to educate patients about the importance of dental radiographs. The dental radiographer must also be prepared to answer common questions asked by patients about the need for dental radiographs, x-ray exposure, the safety of dental x-rays, and other miscellaneous concerns. The purpose of this chapter is to discuss the importance of patient education, to describe different methods of patient education, and to review common patient questions and answers about dental radiography.

IMPORTANCE OF PATIENT EDUCATION

Educating dental patients about the importance of dental radiographs is critical, yet patient education is often overlooked by dental professionals. Many patients do not understand the value of dental radiographs. Often the patient is simply told that "dental x-rays are required by the dentist," and very little information or additional explanation is provided. As a result, many patients fear the use of x-radiation. Others believe that dental radiographs are a way for the dentist to make extra money. To address such fears and misconceptions, the dental radiographer must be prepared to educate the patient about the value of dental radiographs.

Many patients have heard or have read about the damaging effects of x-radiation. Newspaper articles, magazine articles, and television magazine shows often highlight the damaging effects of radiation and cast doubt on the necessity and benefit of radiographic examinations. Such reports are often misleading and are not well researched. As a result, these reports cause the patient to fear the use of x-radiation and to avoid all radiation exposure.

Because of such information, the dental radiographer must take the time to educate the patient. In some instances, the patient must be completely reeducated. The dental radiographer must be prepared to explain exactly why dental radiographs are important (Chapter 11), how dental radiographs are used (Chapter 11), and how they benefit the patient (Chapters 4 and 11). In addition, the dental professional must be able to discuss common conditions and lesions that can be detected only through the use of dental radiographs (Chapter 11).

Comprehensive dental health education is one of the greatest services that a dental professional can provide for the patient. Education enhances understanding. A patient who is knowledgeable about the importance of dental radiographs is more likely to realize the benefit of dental radiographs, to accept prescribed treatment, and to follow prevention plans. Patient education is also likely to result in decreased fears of x-ray exposure, increased cooperation, and increased motivation for regular dental visits.

METHODS OF PATIENT EDUCATION

Patient education about dental radiographs can be accomplished in a number of ways. The dental radiographer can use an oral presentation, printed literature, or a combination of both to educate the dental patient.

An oral presentation, in conjunction with sample x-ray films, can be used to communicate the importance of dental radiographs. For example, the dental radiographer can show the patient a prepared series of radiographs illustrating typical normal and abnormal conditions. Through the use of such radiographs, the dental radiographer includes a visual component in the educational process; visual aids enhance patient comprehension. A prepared oral presentation with visual aids allows the patient to develop greater confidence in the expertise of the dental radiographer. A prepared presentation also communicates to the patient that the dental radiographer is organized and competent.

Printed information about dental radiographs can also be used to educate the dental patient. Brochures can be placed in the reception area of the dental office or distributed to patients before the radiographic examination. One example of the available printed literature is entitled *Dental X-rays: Your Dentist's Advice*. This pamphlet, which can be obtained from the American Dental Association, discusses dental x-rays and how dental radiographs benefit the patient. Other brochures about dental radiographs and x-ray exposure can be obtained from the American Dental Association and the Bureau of Radiologic Health. Printed literature about dental radiographs can also be custom designed by the dental professional and then produced for use in the dental office.

A combination of an oral presentation and printed literature is probably the most effective method of educating the dental patient about dental radiographs; the use of both can stimulate a question-and-answer discussion about dental radiographs.

COMMON QUESTIONS AND ANSWERS

The dental radiographer must be prepared to answer common questions by patients about the need for dental radiographs, x-ray exposure, the safety of dental x-rays, and other miscellaneous concerns. Many patients ask questions of the dental auxiliary rather than the dentist about x-radiation. Many patient questions can be answered by the dental radiographer. However, there are some questions that must be answered only by the dentist; such questions must be established by the dentist and understood by all members of the dental team. For example, questions about diagnosis must be answered only by the dentist.

Necessity Questions

Patients often ask questions about the need for dental x-rays, the frequency of dental x-rays for adults and children, the refusal of dental x-rays, and the use of dental x-rays from a previous dentist. Examples of questions and answers follow.

Question: **Are dental x-rays really necessary?**
Answer: Yes. There are many diseases and conditions, like tooth decay, gum disease, cysts, and tumors, that cannot be detected simply by looking into your mouth. Many diseases and conditions produce no signs or symptoms. Without dental x-rays, these conditions may go unnoticed for a long period of time. As these conditions progress, extensive damage and pain may occur, which in turn may result in more extensive and costly treatment. Some oral diseases can even affect your general health or become life threatening.

Dental radiographs are always taken to benefit you, the patient; the primary benefit is disease detection. Through the use of dental radiographs, conditions and diseases that cannot be detected in any other way can be identified early. Early identification and treatment minimize and prevent problems, such as pain and the need for surgical procedures.

Question: **How often should I have dental x-rays?**
Answer: The first step to limiting the amount of radiation that you receive is the proper prescribing, or

ordering, of dental radiographs. Decisions about the number, type, and frequency of dental x-rays are determined by the dentist based on your individual needs. Guidelines published by the American Dental Association are used by the dentist to aid in prescribing the number, type, and frequency of dental radiographs.

Because every patient's dental condition is different, the frequency of radiographic examinations is different as well; the frequency of your dental x-ray examinations is based on your individual needs. There is no set time interval between x-ray examinations. For example, a patient with tooth decay or gum disease needs more frequent radiographic examinations than a patient without such diseases.

Question: **How often should children have dental x-rays?**
Answer: The time interval between radiographic examinations should be based on the individual needs of the child. Because every child's dental condition is different, the frequency of radiographic examinations is different as well. There is no set time interval between x-ray examinations. For example, a child with tooth decay needs more frequent radiographic examinations than a child without tooth decay.

Question: **Can I refuse x-rays and be treated without them?**
Answer: No. When you refuse dental x-rays, the dentist cannot treat you. The standard of care requires that the dentist refuse treatment when a patient refuses x-rays that are necessary. Treatment without necessary radiographs is considered negligent. No document can be signed to release the dentist from liability. For example, if you were to sign a paper stating that you refused dental x-rays but released the dentist from any and all liability, you would be consenting to negligent care. Legally, you cannot consent to negligent care.

Question. **Instead of taking x-rays, can you use the x-rays from my previous dentist?**
Answer: Yes. Previous dental radiographs can be used, providing they are recent and of acceptable diagnostic quality. Additional dental radiographs may be necessary, however, based on your individual needs. If your previous dental radiographs are not of diagnostic quality, they will need to be retaken, even if they are recent.

Exposure Questions

Patients often ask questions about x-ray measurement, amounts of x-ray exposure, the use of the lead apron during exposure, the exposure of dental x-rays during pregnancy, and why the dental radiographer leaves the room during exposure. Examples of questions and answers follow.

Question: How are x-rays measured?

Answer: Special units are used to measure x-ray exposure and absorption. The radiation that reaches the surface of the skin is measured in roentgen units. The roentgen is a way of measuring radiation exposure. The unit for dose, or the amount of energy absorbed by a tissue, is termed **radiation absorbed dose.** Because of the small quantities of radiation used during radiographic procedures, very small multiples of these radiation units are used. The prefix milli, meaning 1/1000, is used to express the small quantities of exposure in milliroentgens and the dose in millirads.

Question: How much radiation will I receive from dental x-rays?

Answer: Because no amount of radiation is considered safe, we follow strict guidelines to limit the amount of x-radiation you receive. For example, prior to exposure the dentist will custom order your x-rays based on your individual needs. During exposure, a thyroid collar and lead apron, fast film, and a film-holding device will be used to protect you from excess radiation. Good technique and careful processing of the x-ray film will also be employed to limit your exposure to x-radiation.

The actual amount of x-radiation received will vary depending on the film speed, the technique used, and exposure factors. For example, when a single intraoral D-speed film is exposed, the x-rays expose a small area of skin; the exposure to the skin of the face is approximately 250 milliroentgens. With faster E-speed film, a single intraoral film results in a surface skin exposure of 125 milliroentgens. For dental x-rays to produce permanent skin damage, such as skin cancer, exposures in the range of thousands of roentgens are needed. Such exposures are inconceivable in dental radiography and are not possible with dental x-ray equipment.

Question: Why do you use a lead apron?

Answer: A lead apron and thyroid collar are used to protect your reproductive, blood-forming, and thyroid tissues from scatter radiation; the lead acts as a shield and actually prevents the radiation from reaching these radiosensitive organs. The lead apron protects you from unnecessary radiation exposure.

Question: Should dental x-rays be taken during pregnancy?

Answer: When a lead apron is used during dental radiographic procedures, the amount of radiation received in the gonadal region is nearly zero. There is no detectable exposure to the embryo or fetus with the use of the lead apron. The American Dental Association, in conjunction with the Food and Drug Administration, has stated in the *Guidelines for Prescribing Dental Radiographs* that the recommended guidelines "do not need to be altered because of pregnancy." Although scientific evidence indicates that dental x-ray procedures can be performed during pregnancy, many dentists elect to postpone such x-ray procedures owing to the concern of the patient.

Question: Why do you leave the room when x-rays are used?

Answer: When you are exposed to x-rays, you receive the diagnostic benefit of the dental radiographs; I do not receive any benefit. An individual should only be exposed to x-radiation when the benefit of disease detection outweighs the risk of exposure. Since I do not benefit from your x-ray exposure, I must use proper protection measures. One of the most effective ways for me to limit my x-ray exposure is to maintain adequate distance and shielding, which is why I step out of the room during your x-ray exposure.

Safety Questions

Patients often ask questions about the safety of dental x-rays and wonder whether dental x-rays cause cancer. Examples of questions and answers follow.

Question: Are dental x-rays safe?

Answer: All x-rays are harmful to living tissue. The amount of x-radiation used in dental radiography is small; however, biologic damage does occur. No amount of radiation is considered safe. As a result, dental x-rays must be prescribed only when the benefit of disease detection outweighs this risk of harm.

Question: **Will dental x-rays cause cancer?**

Answer: There is not a single recorded case of a patient's developing cancer from diagnostic x-rays. The radiation exposure that occurs during a dental x-ray examination is very small, and the chance that it will contribute to or cause cancer is extremely low. For example, the potential risk of dental radiography inducing a fatal cancer has been estimated to be 3 in 1,000,000. The risk of a person's developing cancer spontaneously is much higher, or 3300 in 1,000,000. When these two numbers are compared, it is evident that when cancer occurs, it is far more likely to be unrelated to radiation exposure.

Miscellaneous Questions

Other miscellaneous patient questions and answers about dental radiographs follow.

Question: **Can a panoramic x-ray be taken instead of a complete series?**

Answer: No. A panoramic radiograph cannot be substituted for a complete series of dental radiographs. A complete series of dental radiographs is required when information about the details of the teeth and surrounding bone are needed. A panoramic radiograph does not clearly reveal changes in teeth, like tooth decay, or the details of the supporting bone. The panoramic radiograph, however, is useful for showing the general condition of a patient's teeth and bone.

Question: **Who owns my dental radiographs?**

Answer: All of your dental records, including the dental radiographs, are the property of the dentist. As a patient, however, you have the privilege of reasonable access to your dental records. For example, this means that you can request a copy of your dental radiographs or request that a copy be sent to the dentist of your choice. Original dental radiographs, however, are typically retained by the dentist as part of the patient record.

◼ SUMMARY

- The dental radiographer must be able to educate patients about dental radiographs. A patient who is knowledgeable about the importance of dental radiographs is more likely to have decreased fears about x-ray exposure, to realize the benefits of dental radiographs, to accept prescribed treatment, and to follow prevention plans.
- The dental radiographer can use an oral presentation, printed literature, or a combination of both to educate the dental patient. A combination of an oral presentation and printed literature is probably the most effective method of educating the patient about radiographs.
- The dental radiographer must be prepared to answer common patient questions about the need for dental radiographs, x-ray exposure, the safety of dental x-rays, and other miscellaneous concerns.
- Some patient questions must be answered only by the dentist; such questions must be established by the dentist and understood by all members of the dental team. For example, all questions about diagnosis must be answered only by the dentist.

BIBLIOGRAPHY

Frommer HH: Radiation protection. *In* Radiology for Dental Auxiliaries, 6th edition. St. Louis, Mosby-Year Book, 1996, pp. 67–87.

Haring JI, Lind LJ: The importance of dental radiographs and interpretation. *In* Radiographic Interpretation for the Dental Hygienist. Philadelphia, WB Saunders, 1993, pp. 7–8.

Johnson ON, McNally MA, Essay CE: Patient relations and education. *In* Essentials of Dental Radiography for Dental Assistants and Hygienists, 6th edition. Norwalk, CT, Appleton and Lange, 1999, pp. 493–505.

Manson-Hing LR: Patient relations. *In* Fundamentals of Dental Radiography, 3rd edition. Philadelphia, Lea & Febiger, 1990, pp. 223–229.

Thunthy KH: X-rays: Detailed answers to frequently asked questions. Compendium of Continuing Education in Dentistry 14(3):394–398, 1993.

Quiz Questions

ESSAY

1. Summarize the importance of educating dental patients about dental radiographs.

2. List three methods the dental radiographer can use to educate patients about dental radiographs.

SHORT ANSWER

3. Are dental x-rays really necessary?

   yes because lesions, diseases cannot be detected by looking at the mouth

4. How often should adults have dental x-rays?

   every persons condition is different x-ray examination is based on individual needs.

5. How often should children have dental x-rays?

   each child is different so the need for x-ray is different too

6. Can a patient refuse dental x-rays and be treated without them?

   no because treatment without radiographs is considered negligent.

7. Can radiographs from a previous dentist be used instead of taking dental x-rays?

   yes but additional radiographs may be necessary based on individual needs.

8. How are x-rays measured?

   roentgen is a way of measuring radiation exposure

9. How much radiation is received from dental x-rays?

   -collor, lead apron, fast film and film holding device will be used to protect from excess radiation.

10. Why is a lead apron used during x-ray exposure?

    _____

11. Should dental x-rays be taken during pregnancy?

    yes but many dentist elect to postpone x-rays procedures

12. Why does the dental radiographer leave the room during x-ray exposure of the patient?

_____

13. Are dental x-rays safe?

_____

14. Will dental x-rays cause cancer?

_____

15. Can a panoramic x-ray be taken instead of a complete series?

_____

16. Who owns the dental radiographs, the dentist or the patient?

_____

_____

Answers are supplied at the end of this book.

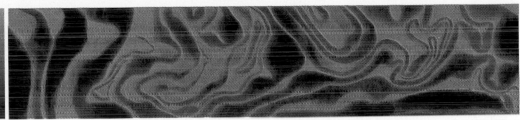

Legal Issues and the Dental Radiographer

OBJECTIVES

After completion of this chapter, the student will be able to:

- *Define the key words.*
- *List the federal and state regulations affecting the use of dental x-ray equipment.*
- *Describe the general application of federal and state regulations as they affect the dental auxiliary.*
- *Describe the licensure requirements for exposing dental radiographs.*
- *Define the legal concept of informed consent.*
- *Describe how to obtain informed consent from a patient.*
- *Discuss the legal significance of the dental record.*
- *Describe the legal implications of patient refusal to have dental radiographs exposed.*
- *Discuss how confidentiality laws affect the information in the dental record.*
- *Describe the patient's rights with regard to the dental record.*

INTRODUCTION

The dental auxiliary must be aware of the legal implications involved in taking dental radiographs. Laws exist that govern the use of ionizing radiation in dentistry, and the dental auxiliary must be informed of and comply with these regulations. Furthermore, because exposing dental radiographs has implications for patient care, including the diagnosis of dental disease and treatment planning, the possibility of negligent care exists when dental radiographs are not properly exposed or used.

The purpose of this chapter is to discuss general legal concepts, including various regulations as they apply to the dental radiographer who exposes dental radiographs for patient care. Additionally, the issues of confidentiality and documentation are addressed.

LEGAL ISSUES AND DENTAL RADIOGRAPHY

Federal and State Regulations

There are both federal and state regulations that control the use of dental x-ray equipment. The federal government has established requirements that include safety precautions affecting the use of dental x-ray machines made and sold in the United States. For example, the Consumer-Patient Radiation Health and Safety Act is a federal law that outlines requirements for the safe use of dental x-ray equipment. This law also establishes guidelines for the proper maintenance of x-ray equipment and requires persons who take dental radiographs to be properly trained and certified.

In addition to federal laws, there are state, county, and city laws that may affect the use of dental x-ray equipment. Most states have laws that require inspection of dental x-ray equipment on a regular basis, for instance, every 5 years. Some state laws also require that the dental radiographer be trained and certified or licensed to take dental radiographs.

Licensure Requirements

State law regulates the exposure of dental radiographs. In most cases, the licensed dentist and dental hygienist are not required to obtain additional certification to expose dental radiographs legally. The certification required for dental assistants to expose dental radiographs varies from state to state. Consequently, it is the responsibility of the dental auxiliary to become informed about the specific requirements relating to dental radiography in his or her particular state. These requirements may include the following:

- obtaining additional certification in dental radiography
- exposing dental radiographs only under the direct supervision of the dentist
- following restrictions concerning the types of dental radiographs that may be legally exposed

LEGAL ISSUES AND THE DENTAL PATIENT

Risk Management

Risk management is very important in dental radiography. **Risk management** refers to the policies and procedures that should be followed by the dental radiographer to reduce the chances that a patient will file legal action against the dental radiographer or the supervising dentist.

INFORMED CONSENT

Persons seeking health care services, including dental care, have the right to **self-determination**; they have the legal right to make choices about the care they receive, including the opportunity to consent to or to refuse treatment. Therefore, prior to receiving treatment, the dental patient should be informed of the various aspects of the proposed treatment, including such diagnostic procedures as the exposure of dental radiographs.

It is the responsibility of the dentist to discuss both diagnostic and treatment procedures with the patient. All patients must be informed of the need for dental radiographs. Information provided to the patient should include the following:

- the purpose and potential benefits of the radiographs
- the person responsible for exposing the radiographs
- the number and type of radiographs
- the possible harm that may result if the radiographs are not exposed
- the risks associated with x-ray exposure
- the alternative diagnostic aids that may serve the same purpose as the radiographs

This process of informing the patient about the particulars of exposing dental radiographs is termed **disclosure.** The disclosure process must be conducted by a competent dental professional. In many states, the prescribing of dental radiographs is the responsibility of the dentist, and the auxiliary is the person who exposes the radiographs under the dentist's supervision. In such cases, the dentist should be involved in the disclosure process and should be available to answer any patient questions.

It is important to standardize the disclosure process so that patients receive enough information to make informed choices. Patients must also be given the opportunity to ask questions and have their questions answered prior to x-ray exposure. Informed consent must be obtained from all patients. If the patient is a minor (generally under 18 years of age) or declared to be legally incompetent, informed consent must be obtained from a legal guardian. It is important that the person disclosing not misrepresent any of the information disclosed or threaten the patient into giving consent. The person disclosing information should use language that the patient can readily understand.

After the disclosure process has been completed, the patient may give or withhold consent for the exposure of dental radiographs. **Informed consent** is defined as consent given by a patient following complete disclosure. The governing standards for informed consent may vary from state to state; however, certain recognized elements of informed consent are summarized as follows: the purpose of the procedure and who will perform it, the potential benefits of receiving the procedure, the possible risks involved in having the procedure performed as well as the risks of not having it performed, and the opportunity for the patient to ask questions and obtain complete information.

A written consent form including these four elements may be used in obtaining consent for dental radiographic procedures.

If informed consent is not obtained from a patient prior to the exposure of dental radiographs, a patient may legally claim malpractice or negligence. A patient's consent to dental procedures is generally presumed valid if it is obtained in a manner consistent with state law, if it follows disclosure, and if it is obtained freely from the appropriate individual. Lack of informed consent may be shown by the following:

- complete lack of consent from the patient
- consent obtained from an individual who has no legal right to give it (e.g., a minor or incompetent adult)
- consent obtained from an individual who is under the influence of drugs or alcohol
- consent obtained by misrepresentation or fraudulent means
- consent obtained from an individual under duress
- consent obtained after incomplete disclosure

LIABILITY

When procedures are performed by a dental auxiliary, legal accountability is presumed to lie with both the supervising dentist and the dental auxiliary. According to state law, dentists are legally accountable or **liable** to supervise the performance of dental auxiliaries. Even though dental auxiliaries work under the supervision of a licensed dentist, they are also legally liable for their own actions. The trend in dental negligence or malpractice actions has historically been to sue the supervising dentist alone; however, cases exist in which the dentist and the dental auxiliary have both been sued for the actions of the dental auxiliary.

Malpractice Issues

Dental **malpractice** results when the dental practitioner is negligent in the delivery of dental care. **Negligence** in dental treatment occurs when the diagnosis made or the dental treatment delivered falls below the standard of care. The **standard of care** can be defined as the quality of care that is provided by dental practitioners in a similar locality under the same or similar conditions.

Negligent care may result from the action or lack of action of either the dentist or the dental auxiliary. Because dental radiographs are an essential part of diagnosis and treatment planning, negligence may result from the actions or inactions of the dental radiographer. For example, if informed consent is not obtained from the patient prior to the exposure of dental radiographs, negligence may be claimed unless the consent is implied. Negligence may also be claimed if radiographs are exposed improperly and the patient is injured in some way as a direct result. The following are examples of negligence if the patient is injured as a result: the incorrect number of radiographs is exposed or the radiographs are nondiagnostic.

State laws govern the time period during which a patient may bring a malpractice action against the dentist or the auxiliary. This time period is known as the **statute of limitations.** In many states, this time period begins when the patient discovers or should have discovered that an injury has occurred as a result of dental negligence. In such cases, the statute of limitations may not begin until years after the dental negligence occurred. Frequently, it is not until a patient seeks care from another dentist that he or she becomes aware that previous dental treatment may have been negligent. For example, if appropriate dental radiographs are not exposed, dental disease may be undiagnosed and untreated. Years later a patient may be informed that he or she has an irreversible condition (e.g., periodontal disease) that with early detection might have been prevented or more successfully treated. Even though such a dental disease is not life-threatening, the lack of diagnosis and treatment may result in significant harm to a patient. Examples of harm may include the loss of self-esteem, emotional distress, loss of income, and expenses incurred in seeking additional dental treatment.

Patient Records

A dental record must be established for every patient, and dental radiographs are an integral part of such a record. The dental record must accurately reflect all aspects of patient care. Complete dental records are important to ensure continuity of patient care and to provide legal documentation of a patient's condition.

DOCUMENTATION

It is very important that the dental record include documentation of the exposure of dental radiographs. The dental record must include documentation of the following:

- informed consent
- the number and type of radiographs exposed
- the rationale for exposing such radiographs
- the diagnostic information obtained from the interpretation of the radiographs

The prescribing and evaluation of radiographs are typically the responsibility of the dentist; therefore, entries in the dental record should be made by the dentist or under the dentist's supervision. Entries made in the dental record should never be erased or blocked out; if an error is made, the change should be added to the record.

CONFIDENTIALITY

All the information contained in the dental record, including dental radiographs, is **confidential,** or private, to the extent that state law does not otherwise require disclosure. State confidentiality laws protect this information and generally prohibit the transfer of this information to nonprivileged persons. A nonprivileged person refers to an individual who is not directly involved in the treatment of the patient. It is not appropriate for any dental professional to discuss a patient's care with another patient or to discuss a patient's care with office staff members who are not involved in the treatment of the patient. Likewise, sharing dental radiographs with others not involved in the patient's care may lead to a violation or breach of confidentiality laws.

OWNERSHIP AND RETENTION OF DENTAL RADIOGRAPHS

Legally, dental radiographs are the property of the dentist. The dentist owns the dental radiographs even though the radiographs were paid for by the patient or the patient's insurance company. The basis for this ownership of dental radiographs is that radiographs are indispensable to the dentist as part of the patient's record.

Patients do, however, have a right to reasonable access to their records. This includes the right to have their complete dental records, including a copy of the radiographs, forwarded to another dentist. When a patient transfers to another dentist, he or she can request in writing that his or her dental records be forwarded to that dentist. The original radiographs should not be forwarded; duplicates should be made and forwarded instead. The patient's written request should be placed in the dental record as evidence of the patient's directive. It is generally not advisable to release a copy of the dental record, including dental radiographs, directly to the patient. Instead, this information should be forwarded directly to the dentist assuming the responsibility for the patient's care.

Dental records and dental radiographs should be retained indefinitely. Because of the nature of varying state statute-of-limitation laws, it is often not possible to predict with certainty when to destroy or discard a patient record. It is necessary to store patient records carefully to maintain the integrity of these materials. All dental professionals must be aware of the importance and significance of maintaining patient records in good condition.

Patients Who Refuse Dental Radiographs

Patients may refuse dental radiographs. When this occurs, the situation must be carefully considered by the dentist. The dentist must then decide whether an accurate diagnosis can be made and whether treatment can be provided. In most cases, patient refusal of dental radiographs compromises the patient's diagnosis and treatment. In such cases, the dentist cannot treat the patient. As discussed in Chapter 13, every effort should be made to educate the patient about the importance and uses of dental radiographs. No document can be signed to release the dentist from liability. For example, if the patient signs a release and waiver that states that he or she is taking responsibility for any injury that may result and then an injury does result from negligence (e.g., failure to expose dental radiographs), the patient's consent may be invalidated. Legally, the patient cannot consent to negligent care; consent to negligent care is invalid.

▉ SUMMARY

- It is important for dental auxiliaries to understand their legal obligations in regard to the exposure of dental radiographs.

- The dentist is responsible for prescribing and interpreting dental radiographs, whereas the dental auxiliary is most often responsible for the exposure and processing of such radiographs.
- The dental auxiliary may also be responsible for disclosing the requisite information and obtaining informed consent from the patient prior to exposing radiographs.
- In many states, dental auxiliaries are employees who work under the supervision of a licensed dentist. In such cases, the dentist is liable for the actions of these dental personnel. In addition, dental auxiliaries are responsible for their own actions in providing patient care.
- The dental record must include documentation of informed consent and the exposure of radiographs (e.g., the number and type of films, the rationale for exposure, and the interpretation).
- Legally, dental radiographs are the property of the dentist. The patient, however, does have reasonable access to the dental radiographs.
- In most cases, the dentist cannot treat a patient who refuses dental radiographs; refusal compromises diagnosis and treatment. No document can be signed that releases the dentist from liability.

BIBLIOGRAPHY

Bundy AL: Radiology and the Law. Rockville, MD, Aspen Publishers, 1988.

Frommer HH: Legal considerations. *In* Radiology for Dental Auxiliaries, 6th edition. St. Louis, Mosby-Year Book, 1996, pp. 363–366.

Langland OE, Sippy FH, Langlais RP: Legal aspects and future of dental radiography. *In* Textbook of Dental Radiology, 2nd edition. Springfield, IL, Charles C Thomas, 1984, pp. 636–638.

Miles DA, Van Dis ML, Jensen CW, Ferretti A: Radiation biology and protection. *In* Radiographic Imaging for Dental Auxiliaries, 2nd edition. Philadelphia, WB Saunders, 1993, pp. 282–283.

Survey of legal provisions for delegating expanded functions to dental assistants and dental hygienists. Chicago, American Dental Association, 1995.

Quiz Questions ···

_____ 1. Informed consent is based on the concept that a patient receives:

   a. some disclosure
   b. no disclosure
   c. complete disclosure
   d. enough disclosure

_____ 2. The process of informing the patient about the particulars of exposing dental radiographs is termed:

   a. consent
   b. liability
   c. disclosure
   d. discussion

_____ 3. A dental assistant may have to take an additional certification/licensure examination to expose dental radiographs.

   a. true
   b. false

_____ 4. The right to self-determination means that the patient has the right to consent to or refuse treatment.

   a. true
   b. false

_____ 5. Which of the following may be liable for the actions of a dental auxiliary?

   a. the dentist
   b. the dental auxiliary
   c. both of the above
   d. none of the above

_____ 6. The improper exposure of dental radiographs may result in:

   a. phobia
   b. malpractice
   c. standard of care
   d. malfeasance

_____ 7. It is best to retain dental records for 6 years.

   a. true
   b. false

_____ 8. The following must be disclosed to the patient prior to obtaining informed consent:

   a. the purpose of the procedure and who will perform it
   b. the potential benefits of receiving the procedure
   c. the possible risks involved in having the procedure performed, including the risk of not having the procedure performed
   d. all of the above

9. Incomplete disclosure to the patient prior to obtaining his or her informed consent may:

   a. validate the consent
   b. serve as partial consent
   c. invalidate the consent
   d. none of the above

10. The dental record is a legal document.

   a. true
   b. false

Answers are supplied at the end of this book.

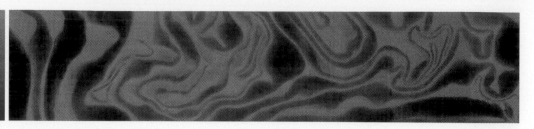

Infection Control and the Dental Radiographer

OBJECTIVES

After completion of this chapter, the student will be able to:

- *Define the key words.*
- *Describe the rationale for infection control.*
- *Describe three possible routes of disease transmission.*
- *Describe the conditions that must be present for disease transmission to occur.*
- *Discuss protective attire and barrier techniques, handwashing and care of hands, sterilization or disinfection of instruments, and the cleaning and disinfection of the dental unit and environmental surfaces.*
- *Detail infection control procedures necessary prior to x-ray exposure.*
- *Detail infection control procedures necessary during x-ray exposure.*
- *Detail infection control procedures necessary following x-ray exposure.*
- *Detail infection control procedures necessary for processing.*
- *Discuss film handling in the darkroom with and without barrier envelopes.*
- *Discuss film handling without barrier envelopes using the daylight loader of an automatic processor.*

INTRODUCTION

Infectious diseases present a significant hazard in the dental environment, and dental professionals are at an increased risk for acquiring such diseases. As a result, infection control is a major concern in dentistry. Infection control protocols are used in dentistry to minimize the potential for disease transmission. To protect both themselves and their patients, dental professionals must understand and use infection control protocols.

The infection control practices used in dentistry include radiographic procedures. The purpose of this chapter is to present the rationale for infection control and infection control terminology, to review the guidelines from the Centers for Disease Control and Prevention (CDC) entitled *Recommended Infection-Control Practices for Dentistry*, and to describe in detail the step-by-step infection control procedures used in dental radiography.

read

INFECTION CONTROL BASICS

To understand infection control practices, the dental professional must first understand the purpose of infection control and the terminology that is frequently used in infection control protocols.

Rationale for Infection Control

The primary purpose of infection control procedures is to prevent the transmission of infectious diseases. Infectious diseases may be transmitted from a patient to the dental professional, from the dental professional to

a patient, and from one patient to another patient. The use of recommended infection control guidelines can greatly reduce the transmission of infectious diseases.

Before the dental professional can use infection control practices to prevent disease transmission, an understanding of disease transmission in the dental environment is required. Disease transmission involves pathogens; a **pathogen** is a microorganism capable of causing disease. Dental professionals and dental patients may be exposed to a variety of pathogens that are present in the oral or respiratory secretions. These pathogens may include:

- cold and flu viruses and bacteria
- cytomegalovirus (CMV)
- hepatitis B virus (HBV)
- hepatitis C virus (HCV)
- herpes simplex virus (HSV-1, HSV-2)
- human immunodeficiency virus (HIV)
- *Mycobacterium tuberculosis*

In the dental environment, the general routes of disease transmission can be described as follows.

- direct contact with pathogens present in saliva, blood, respiratory secretions, or lesions
- indirect contact with contaminated objects or instruments
- direct contact with airborne contaminants present in spatter or aerosols of oral and respiratory fluids

For an infection to occur by one of these routes of transmission, three conditions must be present:

- a susceptible host
- a pathogen with sufficient infectivity and numbers to cause infection
- a portal of entry through which the pathogen may enter the host

Effective infection control practices are intended to alter one of these three conditions, thereby preventing disease transmission.

Infection Control Terminology

An understanding of the terminology related to infection control is important for the dental professional. The following terms are frequently used in discussions of infection control, in the infection control literature, and in infection control protocols.

Antiseptic: A substance that inhibits the growth of bacteria. This term is often used to describe handwashing or wound-cleansing procedures.

Asepsis: The absence of pathogens, or disease-causing microorganisms. This term is often used to describe procedures that prevent infection (e.g., aseptic technique).

Bloodborne pathogens: Pathogens present in blood that cause disease in humans.

Disinfect: The use of a chemical or physical procedure to inhibit or destroy pathogens. Highly resistant bacterial and mycotic (fungal) spores are *not* killed during disinfection procedures.

Disinfection: The act of disinfecting.

Exposure incident: A specific incident that involves contact with blood or other potentially infectious materials and that results from procedures performed by the dental professional.

Infectious waste: Waste that consists of blood, blood products, contaminated sharps, or other microbiologic products.

Occupational exposure: Contact with blood or other infectious materials that involves the skin, eye, or mucous membranes and that results from procedures performed by the dental professional.

Parenteral exposure: Exposure to blood or other infectious materials that results from piercing or puncturing the skin barrier (e.g., a needle-stick injury results in parenteral exposure).

Sharp: Any object that can penetrate skin, including, but not limited to, needles and scalpels.

Sterilize: The use of a physical or chemical procedure to destroy all pathogens, including the highly resistant bacterial and mycotic spores.

Sterilization: The act of sterilizing.

Universal precautions: A method of infection control in which all human blood and certain body fluids are treated as if known to be infectious for HIV, HBV, and other bloodborne pathogens.

RECOMMENDED INFECTION CONTROL PRACTICES FOR DENTISTRY

The CDC has published infection control guidelines entitled *Recommended Infection-Control Practices for Dentistry* (1993) (see box).

The recommended infection control practices are applicable to *all* settings in which dental treatment is provided. These recommendations must be observed in conjunction with the practices and procedures for worker protection required by the Occupational Safety

---

RECOMMENDED INFECTION-CONTROL PRACTICES FOR DENTISTRY

- vaccination of dental professionals
- use of protective attire and barrier techniques
- handwashing and care of hands
- proper use and care of sharp instruments and needles
- sterilization or disinfection of instruments
- cleaning and disinfection of the dental unit and environmental surfaces
- disinfection of the dental laboratory
- use and care of handpieces, antiretraction valves, and other intraoral dental devices attached to air and water lines of dental units
- single use of disposable instruments
- proper handling of biopsy specimens
- proper use of extracted teeth in dental educational settings
- proper disposal of waste materials
- implementation of recommendations

---

and Health Administration (OSHA) final rule on *Occupational Exposure to Bloodborne Pathogens*. The recommended infection control practices that directly relate to dental radiography procedures include:

- protective attire and barrier techniques
- handwashing and care of hands
- sterilization or disinfection of instruments
- cleaning and disinfection of dental unit and environmental surfaces

Protective Attire and Barrier Techniques

PROTECTIVE CLOTHING

All dental professionals must wear protective clothing (e.g., gown, lab coat, uniform) to prevent skin and mucous membrane exposure when contact with blood or other body fluids is anticipated. Protective clothing must be changed daily, or more frequently if it is visibly soiled. Protective garments should be removed before leaving the dental office and laundered according to the manufacturer's instructions.

GLOVES

All dental professionals must wear medical latex or vinyl gloves to prevent skin contact with blood, saliva, or mucous membranes. The dental professional must wear new gloves for each patient. Gloves must also be worn when touching contaminated items or surfaces.

Nonsterile gloves are recommended for examinations and nonsurgical procedures; sterile gloves are recommended for all surgical procedures.

In preparation for treating each patient, hands must be washed before gloves are worn. After treatment of each patient or exiting of the patient treatment area, gloves must be removed and discarded and the hands must be washed immediately. Dental professionals must always wash their hands and reglove between patients. During treatment, gloves must be removed and changed whenever they are torn, cut, or punctured. Gloves should never be washed before use or disinfected for reuse. Washing or disinfection causes defects and diminishes the barrier protection provided by the gloves.

MASKS AND PROTECTIVE EYEWEAR

Whenever spatter and aerosolized sprays of blood and saliva are likely, all dental professionals must use surgical masks and protective eyewear, or chin-length plastic face shields, to protect the eyes and face. When a mask is used, the mask must be changed between patients or during treatment if it becomes wet or moist. Following treatment, face shields and protective eyewear must be washed with appropriate cleaning agents; when such equipment is visibly soiled, it should be disinfected between patients.

Handwashing and Care of Hands

HANDWASHING

All dental professionals must thoroughly wash their hands before and after treating each patient (i.e., before gloving and after removing gloves), and after touching objects or surfaces contaminated by blood or saliva. For routine dental procedures, handwashing with plain soap is adequate. For surgical procedures, an antimicrobial handscrub preparation should be used.

CARE OF HANDS

All dental professionals must take precautions to avoid hand injuries during dental procedures. Dental professionals with exudative or weeping lesions on their hands must refrain from all direct patient contact and from handling patient care equipment until the condition resolves.

Sterilization or Disinfection of Instruments

All instruments in the dental practice can be classified as one of the following, depending on their risk of transmitting infection and the need to sterilize them between uses.

Critical instruments: Instruments that are used to penetrate soft tissue or bone are considered critical and must be sterilized after each use. Examples include forceps, scalpels, bone chisels, scalers, and surgical burs. In dental radiography, no critical instruments are used.

Semicritical instruments: Instruments that contact but do not penetrate soft tissue or bone are classified as semicritical. These devices must also be sterilized after each use. If the instrument can be damaged by heat and sterilization is not feasible, high-level disinfection is required. Examples include x-ray film-holding devices, mirrors, amalgam condensers, and burs.

Noncritical instruments: Instruments or devices that do not come in contact with the mucous membranes are considered noncritical. Because there is little risk of transmitting infection from noncritical devices, intermediate or low-level infection techniques are required for their care between uses in different patients. Examples include the position-indicating device (PID) of the dental x-ray tubehead, the exposure button, the x-ray control panel, and the lead apron.

Acceptable methods of sterilization include steam under pressure (autoclave), dry heat, and chemical vapor. The instructions of the manufacturers of the instruments and sterilizer must be followed. Proper functioning of sterilization cycles must be verified by periodic use of a biologic indicator, such as the spore test.

The U.S. Environmental Protection Agency (EPA) has classified certain chemicals as sterilants-disinfectants. These EPA-registered chemicals are classified as **high-level disinfectants** and can be used to disinfect heat-sensitive semicritical dental instruments.

Cleaning and Disinfection of Dental Unit and Environmental Surfaces

After each patient has been treated, dental unit surfaces and countertops that may have been contaminated with blood or saliva must be thoroughly cleaned with disposable toweling, using an appropriate cleaning agent and water as necessary. All surfaces must then be disinfected with a suitable chemical germicide. EPA-registered chemical germicides labeled as both hospital disinfectants and tuberculocidals are classified as **intermediate-level disinfectants** and are recommended for all surfaces that have been contaminated. Intermediate-level disinfectants include phenolics, iodophors, and chlorine-containing compounds. EPA-registered chemical germicides that are labeled only as hospital disinfectants are classified as **low-level disinfectants** and are recommended for general housekeeping purposes such as cleaning floors and walls.

INFECTION CONTROL IN DENTAL RADIOGRAPHY

In dentistry, all patients must be treated using universal precautions. The same infection control procedures must be used for each patient. There are no exceptions, and no "extra" precautions should be used on any patients. There are specific infection control procedures that pertain to dental radiography, and these procedures must also be used for each patient.

The areas designated for the exposure and processing of dental radiographs are not routinely associated with the spatter of blood or saliva; however, transmission of infectious diseases is still possible if the equipment, supplies, film packets, or cassettes used in the making of dental radiographs are contaminated. Therefore, specific infection control procedures that pertain to dental radiography must be used before, during, and following film exposure as well as during film processing (Tables 15–1 and 15–2).

Infection Control Procedures Used Prior to Exposure

Before dental x-ray films are exposed, the treatment area must be prepared using aseptic technique. Necessary supplies and equipment must also be prepared. Following such preparations, the dental radiographer can seat the patient. At that time, the dental radiographer can also complete the final infection control

---

TABLE 15–1. Checklist for Infection Control in Dental Radiography

Before Exposure	During Exposure	Following Exposure

Treatment Area
The following must be covered or disinfected:
  X-ray machine
  Dental chair
  Work area
  Lead apron
 	
Supplies and Equipment
The following must be prepared prior to seating the patient:
  Film
  Film-holding devices
  Cotton rolls
  Paper towel
  Disposable container
 	
Patient Preparation
The following must be performed prior to placing gloves:
  Adjust chair
  Adjust headrest
  Place lead apron
  Remove objects
 	
Radiographer Preparation
The following must be completed prior to exposure:
  Wash hands
  Put on gloves
  Prepare film-holding devices
	Film Handling
	Film-handling procedures must include the following:
	  After exposure, dry film with paper towel
	  Place dried film in disposable container
	
	Film-Holding Devices
	Film-holding devices must be handled as follows:
	  Transfer film-holding device from work area to mouth and back to work area
	  Never place film-holding devices on uncovered countertop
		Prior to Glove Removal
		  Dispose of all contaminated items
		  Place film-holding devices in area designated for contaminated instruments
		
		After Glove Removal
		  Wash hands
		  Remove lead apron

TABLE 15–2. Checklist for Film Handling During Processing

With Barrier Envelopes	Without Barrier Envelopes
Place disposable towel on work surface in darkroom	Place disposable towel on work surface in darkroom
Place container with contaminated films next to towel	Place container with contaminated films next to towel
Put on gloves	Put on gloves
Take one contaminated film out of container	Turn out darkroom lights and secure door
Tear open barrier envelope	Take one contaminated film out of container
Allow film to drop on paper towel	Open film packet tab and slide out lead foil backing and black paper
Do not touch film with gloved hands	Rotate foil away from black paper and discard
Dispose of barrier envelope	Without touching film, open the black paper wrapping
After all barrier envelopes have been opened, dispose of container	Allow film to drop on paper towel
Remove gloves and wash hands	Do not touch film with gloved hands
Turn out darkroom lights and secure door	Discard black paper wrapping
Unwrap and process films	After all barrier envelopes have been opened, dispose of container
Label a film mount, paper cup, or envelope with the patient's name and use to collect processed films	Remove gloves and wash hands
	Process films
	Label a film mount, paper cup, or envelope with the patient's name and use to collect processed films

procedures that are necessary prior to x-ray exposure.

PREPARATION OF TREATMENT AREA

The dental professional must prepare the surfaces that are likely to be touched during the x-ray exposure. All surfaces that are likely to be touched during treatment should be covered with impervious, disposable materials such as plastic wrap, plastic-backed paper, or aluminum foil. Covering the exposed surfaces with such disposable materials provides adequate protection while eliminating the need for surface cleaning and disinfection between patients. If disposable materials are not used, all contaminated areas must be disinfected following the manufacturer's instructions after the radiographic procedures have been completed. The following are examples of surfaces that must be covered or disinfected:

X-ray machine. The tubehead, PID, control panel, and exposure button must all be covered or disinfected.

Dental chair. The headrest, headrest adjustment, and chair adjustment controls must all be covered or disinfected.

Work area. The area where x-ray supplies (e.g., film) are placed during exposure must be covered or disinfected.

Lead apron. If contaminated, the lead apron must be wiped with a disinfectant between patients.

PREPARATION OF SUPPLIES AND EQUIPMENT

The dental professional must also prepare all anticipated supplies and equipment, such as film, sterilized film-holding devices, and other miscellaneous items. The following are examples of common items that must be prepared and made available in the work area:

Film. Dental x-ray films should be dispensed from a central supply area in a disposable container (e.g., coin envelope or paper cup). Commercially available plastic **barrier envelopes** that fit over intraoral films can be used to protect the film packets from saliva and minimize contamination after exposure of the film. Intraoral films may be inserted and sealed in plastic barrier envelopes (e.g., ClinAsept Barrier Envelopes, manufactured by Kodak) prior to dispensing films from a central supply area (Fig. 15–1).

Film-holding devices. Film-holding devices should be packaged in sterilized bags and dispensed from a central supply area.

Miscellaneous items. Other miscellaneous items include cotton rolls that can be used to stabilize film placement and paper towels that can be used to remove saliva from exposed films. A disposable container (e.g., paper cup or paper bag) labeled with the patient's name is also necessary to collect the exposed films. All miscellaneous items should also be dispensed from a central supply area.

PREPARATION OF THE PATIENT

The dental professional can seat the patient following preparation of the treatment area, supplies, and equipment. After seating the patient, the dental radiographer must complete the following procedures *before* washing the hands and putting on gloves:

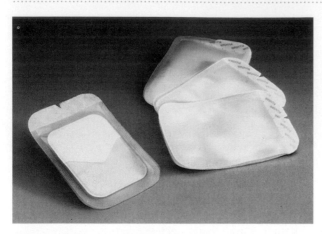

FIGURE 15–1. CLINASEPT Barrier Envelopes are easy to use. A film packet is inserted into the envelope and the exposure is made. Each envelope is then opened to release the film packet over a transfer container, such as a paper cup, taking care to blot any fluids from the envelope. The film is then processed as usual. Complete instructions are included with every carton. (Reprinted courtesy of Eastman Kodak Company, Rochester, NY.)

Chair adjustment. The chair must be positioned so that the patient is seated upright. The height of the chair should be adjusted to a comfortable working height for the dental radiographer.

Headrest adjustment. The headrest must be adjusted to support the patient's head. The patient's head should be positioned with the upper arch parallel with the floor.

Lead apron. The lead apron with the thyroid collar must be placed on the patient and secured prior to any x-ray exposure.

Miscellaneous objects. Miscellaneous objects belonging to the patient that may interfere with film exposure (e.g., eyeglasses, chewing gum, dentures) must be removed by the patient at this time.

PREPARATION OF THE DENTAL RADIOGRAPHER

Following patient preparation, a few final infection control procedures must take place. Prior to x-ray exposure of the patient, the dental radiographer must complete the following procedures:

Handwashing. Hands must be washed with soap or an antimicrobial solution in the presence of the patient.

Gloves. Immediately following handwashing, gloves must be placed.

Mask and eyewear. Because no aerosolized contaminants are created during radiographic exposures, the use of a surgical mask and protective eyewear is optional.

Film-holding devices. If film-holding devices are to be used during exposure, they must be removed from sterilized packages with gloved hands in the presence of the patient and then assembled.

Infection Control Procedures Used During Exposure

Once gloves have been put on and exposure of x-ray films begins, the dental radiographer should take special care to touch only covered surfaces. The best way the dental radiographer can minimize contamination is to touch as few surfaces as possible. During and immediately following film exposure, the dental radiographer must handle each film in a manner consistent with comprehensive infection control guidelines. Infection control procedures during exposure can be described as follows:

Drying of exposed films. After each film has been placed in the patient's mouth, exposed, and removed, it must be dried with a paper towel to remove excess saliva.

Collection of exposed films. Once dried, each film must be placed in a disposable container (paper bag or paper cup) labeled with the patient's name; this container is used to collect and transport the exposed films to the darkroom and must *not* be touched by gloved hands. To prevent film fog caused by scatter radiation, the container should not be placed in a room where additional films are being exposed. In addition, exposed films should never be placed in the dental radiographer's laboratory coat or uniform pocket.

Film-holding devices. During exposures, film-holding devices should be transferred from the covered work area to the patient's mouth and then back to the same area. Contaminated instruments should never be placed on an uncovered countertop.

Interruptions during exposure. If the dental radiographer is interrupted and must leave the room during exposure of films (e.g., in response to a telephone call), gloves must be removed and the hands must be washed before leaving the area. The hands must then be rewashed and new gloves put on before resuming with exposures.

Infection Control Procedures Used Following Exposure

Immediately following the completion of film exposures, all contaminated items must be discarded, and any uncovered areas must be disinfected. Contaminated items must be handled in a manner consistent with recommended infection control guidelines. Infection control procedures following exposure include the following:

Disposal of contaminated items. All contaminated items (cotton rolls, bite-wing tabs, cups, bags, and protective coverings) must be disposed of following local and state environmental regulations. Contaminated items must be discarded while the dental radiographer is still wearing gloves; this includes the disposable materials found on the protected surfaces. The dental radiographer must carefully unwrap all covered surfaces; the actual surfaces that are wrapped should not be touched by gloved hands. Ideally, the disposal of all contaminated items should take place in the presence of the patient.

Film-holding devices. While the dental radiographer is wearing gloves, the contaminated film-holding devices must be removed from the treatment area and placed in an area designated for contaminated instruments.

Handwashing. Following the removal and disposal of all contaminated items, the gloves must be removed and discarded and the hands must be washed.

Lead apron removal. After the hands have been washed, the lead apron can be removed from the patient, at which time the patient can be dismissed from the x-ray area.

Surface disinfection. Any uncovered areas that were contaminated during treatment must be cleaned and disinfected using an EPA-registered hospital-grade disinfectant and utility gloves.

Infection Control Procedures Used for Processing

Following the exposure of x-ray films, specific infection control guidelines must be followed during transport of the films to the darkroom, during film handling, and during film processing. Infection control procedures for processing include the following:

Film transport. As previously described, films contaminated with saliva must be placed in a labeled disposable container after exposure. The disposable container should never be touched by gloved hands. Only after the gloves have been removed, the hands have been washed, the patient has been dismissed, and the area has been cleaned, should the dental radiographer carry the disposable container holding the contaminated films to the darkroom.

Darkroom supplies. Paper towels and gloves are necessary for film handling prior to processing and must be available in the darkroom. Paper envelopes, paper cups, or film mounts, labeled with the patient's name, are used to hold films after processing and also should be available in the darkroom.

Film handling with barrier envelopes. Commercially available barrier envelopes help to minimize contamination in the darkroom. When exposed films are protected by barrier envelopes, the following film-handling procedure is recommended (Fig. 15–2):

1. Place disposable towel on work surface in darkroom.
2. Place container with contaminated films next to towel.
3. Put on gloves.
4. Take one contaminated film out of container.
5. Tear open barrier envelope.
6. Allow film to drop onto paper towel.
7. Do not touch film with gloved hands.
8. Dispose of barrier envelope.
9. After all barrier envelopes have been opened, dispose of container.
10. Remove gloves and wash hands.
11. Turn out darkroom lights and secure door.
12. Unwrap and process films.
13. Label a film mount, paper cup, or envelope with the patient's name and use to collect processed films.

Film handling without barrier envelopes. When exposed films are not protected by barrier envelopes, the following film-handling procedure is recommended (Fig. 15–3):

1. Place disposable towel on work surface in darkroom.
2. Place container with contaminated films next to towel.
3. Put on gloves.
4. Turn out darkroom lights and secure door.
5. Take one contaminated film out of container.
6. Open film packet tab and slide out lead foil backing and black paper. Discard film packet wrapping.
7. Rotate foil away from black paper and discard.

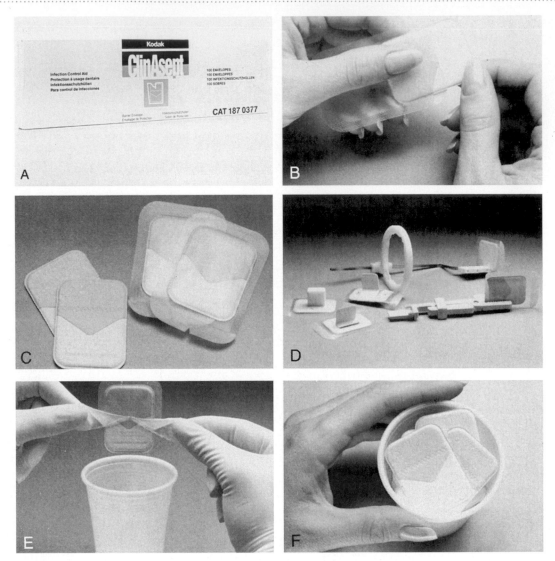

FIGURE 15–2. *A,* Commercial barrier envelope for dental film. Packaging of Kodak barrier envelope. *B,* Insertion of film into envelope. *C,* Protected and unprotected film. *D,* Bite-wing and periapical applications of protected film. *E,* Film packet removal from envelope without contamination. *F,* Uncontaminated film ready for processing. (Courtesy of Eastman Kodak Company, Rochester, NY.)

8. Without touching the film, open the black paper wrapping.
9. Allow film to drop onto paper towel.
10. Do not touch film with gloved hands.
11. Discard black paper wrapping.
12. After all film packets have been opened, dispose of container.
13. Remove gloves and wash hands.
14. Process films.
15. Label a film mount, paper cup, or envelope with the patient's name and use to collect processed films.

Disinfection of darkroom. Darkroom countertops and any areas touched by gloved hands must be disinfected with an EPA-registered hospital-grade disinfectant.

Daylight loader procedures. Infection control procedures for processing film without barrier envelopes in automatic film processors equipped with daylight loaders include the following:

1. Place paper cup and vinyl or nonpowdered gloves in daylight loader compartment.
2. Place container with contaminated films next to cup.

3. Close daylight loader lid and push hands through openings.
4. Put on gloves.
5. Take one contaminated film out of container.
6. Open film packets as described in *Film Handling Without Barrier Envelopes.*
7. Allow film to drop onto processor film feed slot area. (Do not touch film with gloved hands.)
8. Dispose of film packet wrappings in paper cup.
9. After all film packets have been opened, remove gloves and place in cup.
10. Feed all unwrapped films into processor.
11. Remove hands from daylight loader.
12. Wash hands.
13. Lift daylight loader lid to remove and discard cup with contaminated wrappings and container that held contaminated films.

14. Label a film mount, paper cup, or envelope with the patient's name and use to collect processed films.

SUMMARY

- To protect both themselves and patients, dental professionals must understand and use infection control protocols. The primary purpose of infection control procedures is to prevent the transmission of infectious diseases.
- Disease transmission involves pathogens, or microorganisms that are capable of causing disease. In dentistry, disease transmission may occur as a result of one of the following:
  - direct contact with pathogens in saliva, blood, respiratory secretions, or lesions

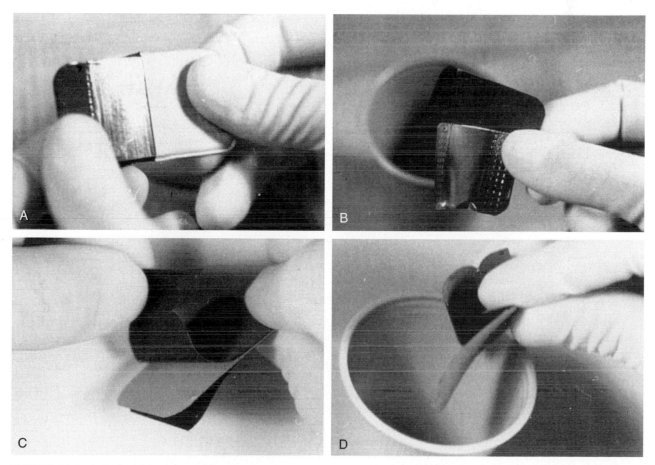

FIGURE 15–3. *A,* Method for removing films from packet without touching them with contaminated gloves. Open tab and slide lead foil and black interleaf paper from wrapping. Illustration of the steps used to open a size 2 film packet without contaminating film. *B,* Rotate foil away from black paper and discard. *C,* Open paper wrapping. *D,* Allow film to fall into a clean cup. (From Goaz PW, White SC: Oral Pathology: Principles and Interpretation, 3rd ed. St. Louis, Mosby-Year Book, 1994.)

- indirect contact with contaminated objects or instruments
- direct contact with airborne contaminants present in spatter or aerosols or oral and respiratory fluids
- For infection to occur via one of the described routes of transmission, three conditions must be present:
  - a susceptible host
  - a pathogen with sufficient infectivity and numbers to cause infection
  - a portal of entry through which the pathogen may enter the host
- The Centers for Disease Control and Prevention has published infection control guidelines entitled *Recommended Infection-Control Practices for Dentistry* (1993). This document outlines specific infection control measures that pertain to dentistry; these measures are described in this chapter.
- The recommended infection control practices are applicable to all settings in which dental treatment is provided. The same infection control procedures must be used for each patient. There are no exceptions, and no "extra" precautions should be used on any select patients.
- Specific infection control procedures are recommended before x-ray exposure, during exposure, following exposure, and during processing. This chapter describes each of these procedures.

BIBLIOGRAPHY

Centers for Disease Control and Prevention: Recommended Infection-Control Practices for Dentistry. MMWR 42 (No. RR-8):1–12, 1993.

Cottone JA, Terezhalmy GT, Molinari JA: Infection control in dental radiology. *In* Practical Infection Control in Dentistry. Philadelphia, Lea & Febiger, 1991, pp. 167–175.

Cottone JA, Terezhalmy GT, Molinari JA: Rationale for practical infection control in dentistry. *In* Practical Infection Control in Dentistry. Philadelphia, Lea & Febiger, 1991, pp. 71–79.

Cottone JA, Terezhalmy GT, Molinari JA: Appendix B. *In* Practical Infection Control in Dentistry. Philadelphia, Lea & Febiger, 1991, pp. 229–231.

Eastman Kodak Company: Infection control in dental radiography. *In* Infection Control in the Dental Office. Rochester, Eastman Kodak Company, 1989, pp. 1–11.

Frommer HH: Infection control. *In* Radiology for Dental Auxiliaries, 6th edition. St. Louis, Mosby-Year Book, 1996, pp. 89–99.

Goaz PW, White SC: Radiographic infection control. *In* Oral Radiology: Principles and Interpretation, 3rd edition. St. Louis, CV Mosby, 1994, pp. 219–226.

Katz JO, Cottone JA, Hardman PK, et al: Infection control protocol for dental radiology. Journal of the Academy of General Dentistry 38(4):261–264, 1990.

Manson-Hing LR: Infection control. *In* Fundamentals of Dental Radiography, 3rd edition. Philadelphia, Lea & Febiger, 1990, pp. 230–242.

Quiz Questions ··

MATCHING

For questions 1 to 10, match each term with its definition.

a. disinfect
b. sterilize
c. asepsis
d. infectious waste
e. pathogen
f. noncritical instrument
g. critical instrument
h. semicritical instrument
i. parenteral exposure
j. occupational exposure
k. antiseptic

_____ 1. Use of a chemical or physical procedure to destroy all pathogens, including spores.

_____ 2. Microorganism capable of causing disease.

_____ 3. Exposure to infectious material that occurs as a result of procedures performed by the dental professional.

_____ 4. Exposure to infectious materials that occurs as a result of piercing or puncturing the skin.

_____ 5. Use of a chemical or physical procedure to destroy all pathogens except spores.

_____ 6. Instrument used to penetrate soft tissue or bone.

_____ 7. Instrument that contacts but does not penetrate soft tissue or bone.

_____ 8. Instrument that does not contact mucous membranes.

_____ 9. Waste that consists of blood, blood products, contaminated sharps, and other microbiologic products.

_____ 10. Absence of pathogens.

FILL IN THE BLANK

11. What is the primary purpose of infection control?

_____

12. List the three possible routes of disease transmission.

_____

13. List the three conditions that must be present for disease transmission to occur.

_____

MULTIPLE CHOICE

_____ 14. Identify the FALSE statement concerning protective clothing. Protective clothing

    a. must be worn by all dental professionals
    b. must be worn to prevent contact with infectious materials
    c. must be changed weekly
    d. must be removed before leaving the dental office

_____ 15. Identify the FALSE statement concerning gloves.

    a. Gloves must be worn by all dental professionals
    b. Gloves must be washed before use
    c. Gloves must be worn for each patient
    d. Gloves must be sterile for surgical procedures

_____ 16. Identify the FALSE statement concerning masks and protective eyewear.

    a. Masks and protective eyewear are optional for dental radiographic procedures
    b. Masks must be changed between patients
    c. When visibly soiled, protective eyewear must be disinfected between patients
    d. Protective shield must be worn during radiographic procedures

_____ 17. Identify the TRUE statements concerning handwashing. Hands must be washed

(1) before and after gloving; (2) before and after each patient; (3) after touching contaminated surfaces; (4) with plain soap for routine dental procedures.

    a. 1, 2, 3, 4
    b. 1, 2, 3
    c. 1, 2, 4
    d. 2, 3, 4

_____ 18. Examples of critical instruments include:

(1) film-holding device; (2) scalpel; (3) scaler; (4) amalgam condenser

    a. 1, 2, 3, 4
    b. 1, 2, 3
    c. 2, 3, 4
    d. 2, 3

_____ 19. EPA-registered chemical germicides labeled as both hospital disinfectants and tuberculocidal are classified as:

    a. high-level disinfectants
    b. sterilant disinfectants
    c. low-level disinfectants
    d. intermediate-level disinfectants

_____ 20. EPA-registered chemical germicides labeled only as hospital disinfectants are classified as:

    a. high-level disinfectants
    b. sterilant disinfectants
    c. low-level disinfectants
    d. intermediate-level disinfectants

ESSAY

21. Describe the infection control procedures that are necessary *before* to x-ray exposure.

22. Describe the infection control procedures that are necessary *during* x-ray exposure.

23. Describe the infection control procedures that are necessary *following* x-ray exposure.

24. Describe the infection control procedures that are necessary for processing.

25. Discuss film handling in the darkroom with and without barrier envelopes.

Answers are supplied at the end of this book.

Technique Basics

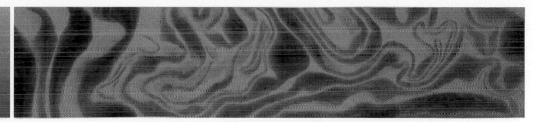

Introduction to Radiographic Examinations

OBJECTIVES

After completion of this chapter, the student will be able to:

- *Define the key words.*
- *List the three types of intraoral radiographic examinations.*
- *Describe the purpose and the type of film and technique used for each of the three types of intraoral radiographic examinations.*
- *List the films that comprise a CMRS.*
- *List the general diagnostic criteria for intraoral radiographs.*
- *List examples of extraoral radiographic examinations.*
- *Discuss the prescribing of dental radiographs.*
- *Describe when prescribing a CMRS for a new patient is warranted.*

KEY WORDS

CMRS (complete mouth radiographic series)	Film, occlusal
	Film, periapical
	Interproximal examination
Dentulous	
Edentulous	Intraoral radiographic examination
Extraoral radiographic examination	
	Occlusal examination
Film, bite-wing	Periapical examination
Film, extraoral	Radiograph, diagnostic
Film, intraoral	Tooth-bearing areas

INTRODUCTION

The dental radiographer must have a working knowledge of radiographic techniques. Prior to the discussion of technique basics, an understanding of the different types of radiographic examination is necessary. Dental radiographic examinations may involve either intraoral films (films placed *inside* the mouth) or extraoral films (films placed *outside* the mouth).

The purpose of this chapter is to introduce the dental radiographer to the different intraoral radiographic examinations used in dentistry, to define the complete mouth radiographic series, and to describe in detail the diagnostic criteria of intraoral radiographs. In addition, the extraoral radiographic examinations used in dentistry are introduced.

THE INTRAORAL RADIOGRAPHIC EXAMINATION

The **intraoral radiographic examination** is a radiographic inspection of teeth and intraoral adjacent structures. Such intraoral examinations are the foundation of dental radiography. The intraoral radiographic examination requires the use of intraoral film (see Chapter 7); **intraoral film** is film that is placed inside the mouth and is used to examine the teeth and supporting structures.

Types of Intraoral Radiographic Examinations

There are three common types of radiographic examination that use intraoral film:

- the periapical examination
- the interproximal examination
- the occlusal examination

Each of these examinations has a certain purpose and requires the use of a specific type of film and technique.

PERIAPICAL EXAMINATION

Purpose. The **periapical examination** is used to examine the entire tooth (crown and root) and supporting bone.

Film Type. The **periapical film** (see Chapter 7) is used in the periapical examination. The term periapical is derived from the Greek word *peri* (meaning around) and the Latin word *apex* (referring to the terminal end of a tooth root). As the term periapical suggests, this type of film shows the terminal end of the tooth root and surrounding bone as well as the crown.

Technique. There are two methods for obtaining periapical radiographs: the paralleling technique (see Chapter 17) and the bisecting technique (see Chapter 18).

INTERPROXIMAL EXAMINATION

Purpose. The **interproximal examination** is used to examine the crowns of both the maxillary (upper) and mandibular (lower) teeth on a single film. As the term proximal suggests, this examination is useful in examining adjacent tooth surfaces and crestal bone.

Film Type. The **bite-wing film** (see Chapter 7) is used in the interproximal examination. The bite-wing film has a "wing" or tab attached to the film; the patient "bites" on the "wing" to stabilize the film—hence the term bite-wing.

Technique. The bite-wing technique (see Chapter 19) is used in the interproximal examination.

OCCLUSAL EXAMINATION

Purpose. The **occlusal examination** is used to examine large areas of the maxilla (upper jaw) or the mandible (lower jaw) on one film.

Film Type. The **occlusal film** (see Chapter 7) is used in the occlusal examination. The film is so-named because the patient "occludes," or bites on, the entire film.

Technique. The occlusal technique (see Chapter 21) is used in the occlusal examination.

Complete Mouth Radiographic Series

The **complete mouth radiographic series,** abbreviated CMRS, is also known as a full-mouth series or complete series. The CMRS can be defined as a series of intraoral dental radiographs that shows *all* of the tooth-bearing areas of the upper and lower jaws. **Tooth-bearing areas** are the regions of the maxilla and mandible where the 32 teeth of the human dentition are normally located. Tooth-bearing areas include **dentulous** areas, or areas that exhibit teeth, as well as **edentulous** areas, or areas where teeth are no longer present.

The CMRS consists of periapical radiographs alone or a combination of periapical and bite-wing radiographs. Bite-wing films are used only in areas where teeth have interproximal contact with other teeth to examine the contact areas for caries (decay). To include every tooth and all tooth-bearing areas, a total of 14 to 19 films may be included in the CMRS.

The number of films is dictated by the radiographic technique used to expose the films and the number of teeth present. For example, in the patient without teeth, 14 periapical films are usually sufficient to cover the edentulous arches. In the dentulous patient, the number of periapical films varies depending on which technique, the paralleling or bisecting technique, is used. Film size is also dictated by the technique used.

Diagnostic Criteria for Intraoral Radiographs

A **diagnostic radiograph,** as described in Chapter 8, provides a great deal of information. Specific diagnostic criteria for each radiographic exposure are described in the technique chapters (paralleling, bisecting, bitewing, occlusal). Criteria for intraoral radiographs are outlined in "General Diagnostic Criteria for Intraoral Radiographs."

■ THE EXTRAORAL RADIOGRAPHIC EXAMINATION

The **extraoral radiographic examination** is a radiographic inspection of large areas of the skull or jaws. The extraoral radiographic examination requires the use of extraoral film (see Chapter 7); **extraoral film** is

---

GENERAL DIAGNOSTIC CRITERIA FOR INTRAORAL RADIOGRAPHS

....

- Dental radiographs must show images with optimum density, contrast, definition, and detail.
- Dental radiographs must show images with the least amount of distortion possible; radiographic images must be of the same shape and size as the object being radiographed.
- The CMRS must include radiographs that show all tooth-bearing areas, including dentulous and edentulous regions.
- Periapical radiographs must show the entire crowns and roots of the teeth being examined as well as 2 to 3 mm beyond the root apices.
- Bite-wing radiographs must show open contacts, or interproximal tooth surfaces that are not overlapped.

---

film that is placed outside the mouth. Examples of common extraoral radiographs include the panoramic radiograph as well as the lateral jaw, lateral cephalometric, posteroanterior, Waters, submentovertex, reverse Towne, transcranial, and tomographic projections. Each of these extraoral examinations has a specific purpose and requires the use of certain films and techniques; the purposes, films, and techniques used in extraoral radiography are described in Chapters 22 and 23.

■ PRESCRIBING OF DENTAL RADIOGRAPHS

As discussed in Chapter 5, the prescribing of dental radiographs is based on the individual needs of the patient. The professional judgment of the dentist is used to make decisions about the number, type, and frequency of dental radiographs. Every patient's dental condition is different, and therefore every patient must be evaluated for dental radiographs on an individual basis.

For example, not all patients need a CMRS. As detailed in the *Guidelines for Prescribing Dental Radiographs* (see Table 5–1), a CMRS is appropriate when a new adult patient presents with clinical evidence of generalized dental disease or a history of extensive dental treatment. Otherwise, a combination of bitewing films, selected periapical films, and/or a panoramic film should be prescribed based on the patient's individual needs.

SUMMARY

- Dental radiographic examinations may involve either intraoral films (films placed inside the mouth) or extraoral films (films placed outside the mouth).
- The intraoral radiographic examination is a radiographic inspection of teeth and intraoral structures. There are three common types of intraoral radiographic examinations: periapical, interproximal, and occlusal.
- The periapical examination is used to inspect the crowns and roots of teeth as well as the supporting bone. Periapical film is used in the periapical examination. Either the paralleling or the bisecting technique can be used to expose periapical films.
- The interproximal examination is used to examine the crowns of both the maxillary and mandibular teeth on a single film. The bite-wing film and bite-wing technique are used in the interproximal examination.
- The occlusal examination is used to examine large areas of the maxilla or mandible on one film. The occlusal film and occlusal technique are used in the occlusal examination.
- The complete mouth radiographic series (CMRS) is an intraoral series of dental radiographs that shows all of the tooth-bearing areas of the maxilla and mandible. The CMRS consists of a total of 14 to 19 films; such films include either periapical radiographs alone, or a combination of periapical and bite-wing radiographs. The number and size of film used in the CMRS are dictated by the radiographic technique used and the number of teeth present.
- An intraoral radiograph is considered diagnostic if it shows images with optimum density, contrast, definition and detail, and minimal distortion. In addition, a diagnostic periapical radiograph shows the entire crowns and roots of the teeth being examined, and a diagnostic bite-wing radiograph should show open contacts.
- The extraoral radiographic examination is a radiographic inspection of large areas of the skull or jaws.

BIBLIOGRAPHY

Goaz PW, White SC: Intraoral radiographic examinations. *In* Oral Radiology: Principles and Interpretation, 3rd edition. St. Louis, CV Mosby, 1994, p. 151.

Johnson ON, McNally MA, Essay CE: Intraoral radiographic procedures. *In* Essentials of Dental Radiography for Dental Assistants and Hygienists, 6th edition. Norwalk, CT, Appleton and Lange, 1999, pp. 319–337.

Langland OE, Sippy FH, Langlais RP: Intraoral radiographic techniques. *In* Textbook of Dental Radiography, 2nd edition. Springfield, IL, Charles C Thomas, 1984, pp. 206–209.

Miles DA, Van Dis ML, Jensen CW, Ferretti A: Intraoral radiographic technique. *In* Radiographic Imaging for Dental Auxiliaries, 3rd edition. Philadelphia, WB Saunders, 1999, pp. 1–47.

Quiz Questions ···

MATCHING

For questions 1 to 10, match each term with its definition.

        a. dentulous
        b. edentulous
        c. periapical film
        d. bite-wing film
        e. occlusal film
        f. intraoral film
        g. extraoral film
        h. maxilla
        i. mandible
        j. occlude
        k. occlusion

_____ 1. A film placed inside of the mouth.

_____ 2. The lower jaw.

_____ 3. Without teeth.

_____ 4. To close or to bite.

_____ 5. A film used to examine a large area of the maxilla or mandible in one film.

_____ 6. A film used to examine the crowns of the upper and lower teeth on a single film.

_____ 7. A film placed outside of the mouth.

_____ 8. With teeth.

_____ 9. The upper jaw.

_____ 10. A film used to examine the entire tooth and supporting bone.

SHORT ANSWER

11. List the three types of intraoral radiographic examinations.

12. Describe the purpose, type of film, and technique used for each of the three types of intraoral radiographic examinations.

13. List the general diagnostic criteria for intraoral radiographs.

14. List examples of extraoral radiographic examinations.

15. Discuss the prescribing of dental radiographs.

_____

Answers are supplied at the end of this book.

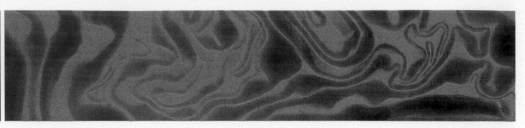

Paralleling Technique

OBJECTIVES

After completion of this chapter, the student will be able to:

- *Define the key words.*
- *State the basic principle of the paralleling technique and illustrate the placement of the film, film holder, position-indicating device (PID), and central ray.*
- *Discuss how object-film distance affects the radiographic image and how target-film distance is used to compensate for such changes.*
- *List the film holders that can be used with the paralleling technique.*
- *Describe why a film holder is necessary with the paralleling technique.*
- *Identify and label the parts of the Rinn XCP instruments.*
- *Describe the different sizes of film used with the paralleling technique and how each film is placed in the bite-block.*
- *State the five basic rules of the paralleling technique.*
- *Describe the patient and equipment preparations that are necessary prior to using the paralleling technique.*
- *Discuss the exposure sequence for 15 periapical film placements using the paralleling technique.*
- *Describe each of the 15 periapical film placements recommended for use with the XCP instruments.*

- *Summarize the guidelines for periapical film positioning.*
- *Explain the modifications in the paralleling technique that are used for a patient with a shallow palate, bony growths, or a sensitive premolar region.*
- *List the advantages and disadvantages of the paralleling technique.*

KEY WORDS

Angle, right	Long axis (tooth)
Central ray	Object-film distance
Exposure sequence	Palate
Film holder	Parallel
Film holder, EEZEE-	Paralleling technique
Grip	Perpendicular
Film holder, hemostat	Target-film distance
Film holder, Precision	Teeth, anterior
Film holder, Stabe	Teeth, posterior
Film placement	Tori, mandibular
Instruments, Rinn XCP	Torus, maxillary
Intersecting	Torus, tori

INTRODUCTION

In dentistry, the radiographer must master a variety of intraoral radiographic techniques. The paralleling technique is a very important technique that is used to expose periapical radiographs. Before the dental radiographer can use this important technique, an understanding of the basic concepts and required equipment is necessary. In addition, the dental radiographer must comprehend patient preparation, equipment preparation, exposure sequencing, and the film placement procedures used in the paralleling technique.

The purpose of this chapter is to present basic concepts and to describe patient preparation, equipment preparation, and film placement procedures used in the paralleling technique. In addition, this chapter also describes modifications of this technique that can be used in patients with certain anatomic conditions, outlines the advantages and disadvantages of the paralleling technique, and reviews helpful hints.

BASIC CONCEPTS

The **paralleling technique** (also known as the *extension cone paralleling [XCP] technique, right-angle technique,* and *long-cone technique*) is one method that can be used to expose periapical films. Before the dental radiographer can competently perform the paralleling technique, a thorough understanding of the terminology, principles, and basic rules governing this technique is necessary. In addition, a knowledge of the film holders and film used with the paralleling technique is also required.

Terminology

Prior to describing the paralleling technique, an understanding of a number of basic terms is necessary.

Parallel: Moving or lying in the same plane, always separated by the same distance and not intersecting (Fig. 17–1*A*).

Intersecting: To cut across or through (Fig. 17–1*B*).

Perpendicular: Intersecting at or forming a right angle (Fig. 17–1*C*).

Right angle: An angle of 90 degrees formed by two lines perpendicular to each other (Fig. 17–1*D*).

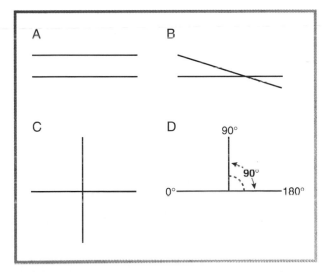

FIGURE 17–1. *A,* Parallel lines are always separated by the same distance and do not intersect. *B,* Intersecting lines cross one another. *C,* Perpendicular lines intersect one another to form right angles. *D,* A right angle measures 90 degrees and is formed by two perpendicular lines.

Long axis of the tooth: An imaginary line that divides the tooth longitudinally into two equal halves (Fig. 17–2).

Central ray: The central portion of the primary beam of x-radiation.

Principles

As the term paralleling suggests, this technique is based on the concept of parallelism. The basic principles of the paralleling technique can be described as follows (Fig. 17–3):

- The film is placed in the mouth *parallel* to the long axis of the tooth being radiographed.
- The central ray of the x-ray beam is directed *perpendicular* (at a right angle) to the film and long axis of the tooth.
- A film holder must be used to keep the film parallel with the long axis of the tooth. The patient *cannot* hold the film.

To achieve parallelism between the film and the tooth, the film must be placed *away* from the tooth and toward the middle of the oral cavity. Because of the anatomic configuration of the oral cavity (e.g., curvature of the palate), the **object-film distance** (distance between the film and the tooth) must be increased to keep the film parallel with the long axis of the tooth (Fig. 17–4). Because the film is placed away from the tooth, image magnification and loss of definition result. As discussed in Chapter 8, increased object-film distance results in increased image magnification.

To compensate for image magnification, the **target-film distance** (distance between the source of x-rays and the film) must also be increased to ensure that only the most parallel rays will be directed at the tooth

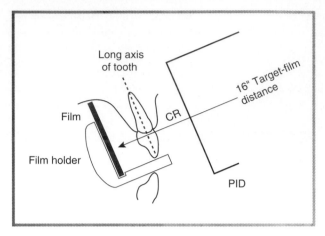

FIGURE 17–3. Positions of the film, teeth, and central ray of the x-ray beam in the paralleling technique. The film and long axis of the tooth are parallel. The central ray is perpendicular to the tooth and film. An increased target-film distance (16 inches) is required.

and film. As a result, a long (16-inch) target-film distance must be used with the paralleling technique. The paralleling technique is sometimes referred to as the *long-cone technique;* "long" refers to the length of the cone, or position-indicating device (PID), that is used. The use of a long target-film distance in the paralleling technique results in less image magnification and increased definition.

Film Holders

The paralleling technique requires the use of a film-holding instrument to position the film parallel to the long axis of the tooth. A **film holder,** as defined in Chapter 6, is a device that is used to position an intraoral film in the mouth and retain the film in position during exposure. Film holders eliminate the need for the patient to stabilize the film. Examples of commercially available intraoral film holders include the following:

- **Rinn XCP Instruments** (Rinn Corporation, Elgin, IL). The XCP (X = extension, C = cone, P = paralleling) instruments include plastic bite-blocks, plastic aiming rings, and metal indicator arms (Fig. 17–5A). To reduce the amount of radiation the patient receives, a snap-on ring collimator can be added to the plastic aiming ring.
- **Precision Film Holders** (Masel Company, Philadelphia, PA). The Precision instruments include metal collimating shields and film-holding devices that restrict the size of the x-ray beam to the size of the film (Fig. 17–5B).

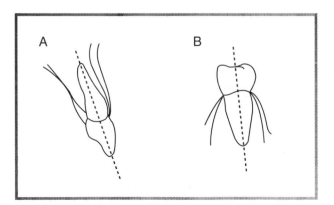

FIGURE 17–2. *A,* The long axis of the maxillary incisor divides the tooth into two equal halves. *B,* The long axis of a mandibular premolar divides the tooth into two equal halves.

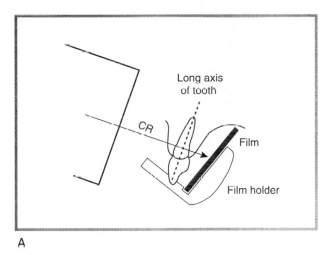

A

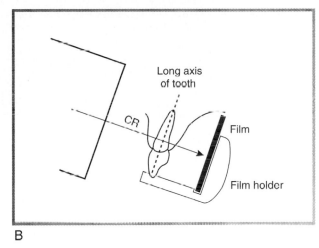

B

FIGURE 17–4. *A,* The film is placed close to the tooth and is not parallel to the long axis of the tooth. *B,* Increased object-film distance. The film is placed away from the tooth and is now parallel with the long axis of the tooth.

- **Stabe Bite-Block** (Rinn Corporation). The Stabe bite-block is a disposable film holder that is designed for one-time use only (Fig. 17–5C).
- **EEZEE-Grip Film Holder** (Rinn Corporation). Formerly known as the Snap-A-Ray, this film-holding device can be used to stabilize a film (Fig. 17–5D).
- **Hemostat with Bite-Block.** A hemostat (a small surgical clamp) inserted through a rubber bite block can also be used to stabilize a film (Fig. 17–5E).

Some film holders are disposable (e.g., Stabe bite-block) and are designed for one-time use only. Other film holders are reusable (e.g., XCP instruments, Precision film holders, EEZEE-Grip film holder, hemostat with bite-block) and must be sterilized following each use.

Of all the film holders listed, the Rinn XCP instruments with snap-on ring collimators and the Precision film holders are recommended for exposure of periapical films. These film holders are recommended because both include aiming rings that aid in the alignment of the PID with the film, and both significantly reduce the amount of patient exposure to x-rays. These instruments are simple to position and easy to sterilize. Although only the Rinn XCP instruments are illustrated in this text, the same principles apply to all of the film holders listed.

Film

The size of the intraoral film used with the paralleling technique depends on the teeth being radiographed.

- In the anterior regions, Size 1 film is used; this narrow film is needed to permit film placement high in the palate without bending or curving the film. Size 1 film is always positioned with the long portion of the film in a *vertical* (upright) direction.
- In the posterior regions, Size 2 film is used. Size 2 film is always placed with the long portion of the film in a *horizontal* (sideways) direction.

Rules

There are five basic rules to follow when using the paralleling technique.

- **Film placement.** The film must be positioned to cover the prescribed area of teeth to be examined. Specific film placements are detailed in the Procedures section of this chapter.
- **Film position.** The film must be positioned *parallel* to the long axis of the tooth. The film, in the film holder, must be placed away from the teeth and toward the middle of the oral cavity (see Fig. 17–3).
- **Vertical angulation.** The central ray of the x-ray beam must be directed *perpendicular* (at a right angle) to the film and the long axis of the tooth (see Fig. 17–3).
- **Horizontal angulation.** The central ray of the x-ray beam must be directed through the contact areas between the teeth (Fig. 17–6).
- **Film exposure.** The x-ray beam must be centered on the film to ensure that all areas of the film are exposed. Failure to center the x-ray beam results in a partial image on the film or a "cone-cut" (Fig. 17–7). Cone-cutting is discussed in Chapter 20.

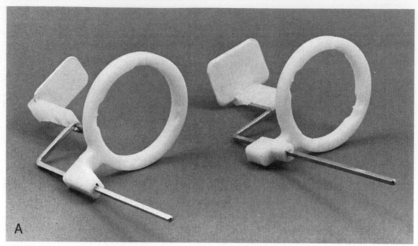

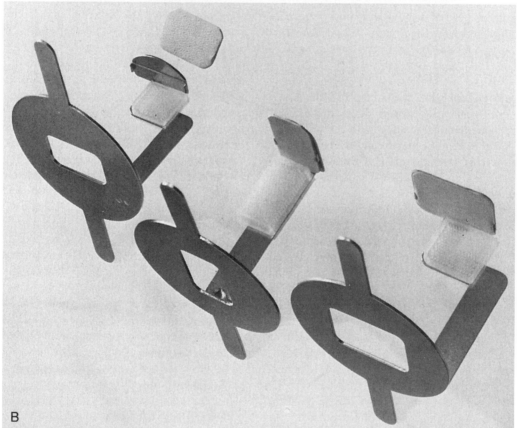

FIGURE 17–5. *A,* Film-holding instruments. XCP instruments: instrument for anterior views *(left):* instrument for posterior views *(right). B,* Precision x-ray film holders showing instruments for posterior projections *(left and right)* instrument for anterior projections *(middle).* In use, the PID is positioned against the face-shield.

STEP-BY-STEP PROCEDURES

Step-by-step procedures for the exposure of periapical films using the paralleling technique include the following: patient preparation, equipment preparation, and film placement methods. Prior to exposing any dental radiographs using the paralleling technique, infection control procedures (as detailed in Chapter 15) must be completed.

Patient Preparation

Following the completion of infection control procedures and the preparation of the treatment area and supplies, the patient should be seated. After seating-

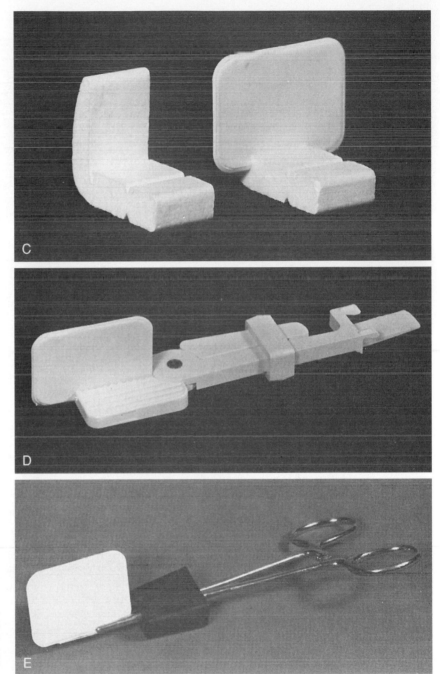

FIGURE 17–5. *Continued. C,* Stabe disposable film holders. *D,* Snap-A-Ray intraoral film holder. *E,* Hemostat and rubber bite block. (From Goaz PW, White SC: Oral Radiology: Principles and Interpretation, 3rd edition. St. Louis, Mosby-Year Book, 1994.)

the patient, and prior to the exposure of any films, the dental radiographer must prepare the patient for the exposure of x-rays (see "Procedure: Patient Preparation for Paralleling Technique").

Equipment Preparation

Following patient preparation, equipment must also be prepared prior to the exposure of any films (see "Procedure: Equipment Preparation").

Exposure Sequence for Film Placements

When using the paralleling technique, an **exposure sequence**, or definite order for periapical film placement and exposure, must be followed. The dental radiographer must have an established exposure routine to prevent errors and use time efficiently. Working without an exposure sequence may result in omitting an area or exposing an area twice.

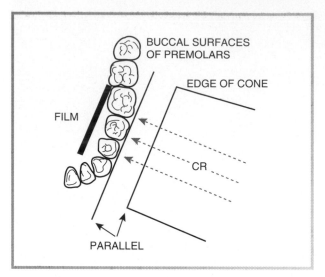

FIGURE 17–6. In this diagram, the x-rays pass through the contact areas of the premolars because the central ray is directed through the contacts and perpendicular to the film. If the central ray is not directed through the contacts, overlap of the premolar contacts occurs.

ANTERIOR EXPOSURE SEQUENCE

When exposing periapical films with the paralleling technique, *always* start with the **anterior teeth** (canines and incisors) because:

- The film (Size 1) used for the anterior exposures is small, less uncomfortable, and easier for the patient to tolerate.
- The more tolerable anterior film placements allow the patient to become accustomed to the film holder used in paralleling technique.
- The anterior film placements are less likely to cause the patient to gag; once the gag reflex is stimulated, the patient may gag on films that could normally be tolerated. Management of the patient with a hypersensitive gag reflex is discussed in Chapter 25.

With Size 1 film, a total of seven anterior film placements are used in the paralleling technique: four maxillary exposures and three mandibular exposures. If Size 2 film is used instead, there are six anterior film placements: three maxillary exposures and three mandibular exposures. The authors of this text recommend the use of Size 1 film; the recommended anterior periapical exposure sequence for the Rinn XCP instruments illustrated in this text is as follows (Table 17–1):

1. Assemble the anterior XCP instrument.
2. Begin with the maxillary right canine (tooth No. 6).

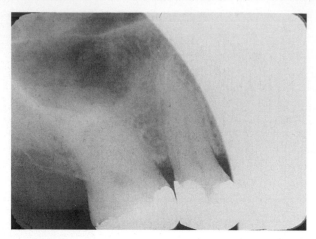

FIGURE 17–7. This radiograph demonstrates a cone-cut, that is, a clear, unexposed area on the film. The PID was positioned too far distally, so that the anterior portion of the film received no exposure.

3. Expose all of the maxillary anterior teeth from *right to left.*
4. End with the maxillary left canine (tooth No. 11).
5. Next, move to the mandibular arch.
6. Begin with the mandibular left canine (tooth No. 22).
7. Expose all of the mandibular anterior teeth from *left to right.*

PROCEDURE

Patient Preparation for Paralleling Technique

1. Briefly explain the radiographic procedures to the patient before the procedure begins.

2. Adjust the chair so that the patient is positioned upright in the chair. The level of the chair must be adjusted to a comfortable working height for the dental radiographer.

3. Adjust the headrest to support and position the patient's head. The patient's head must be positioned so that the upper arch is parallel to the floor, and the midsagittal (midline) plane is perpendicular to the floor.

4. Place and secure the lead apron with thyroid collar on the patient.

5. Remove all objects from the mouth (e.g., dentures, retainers, chewing gum) that may interfere with film exposure. Eyeglasses must be removed also.

TABLE 17-1. Exposure Sequence for Anterior Film Placements (with Rinn XCP Instruments)

Exposure Number	Arch	Side	Tooth	Tooth Number
1	Maxillary	Right	Canine	6
2	Maxillary	Right	Lateral incisor	7
	Maxillary	Right	Central incisor	8
3	Maxillary	Left	Central incisor	9
	Maxillary	Left	Lateral incisor	10
4	Maxillary	Left	Canine	11
5	Mandibular	Left	Canine	22
6	Mandibular	Left	Lateral incisor	23
	Mandibular	Left	Central incisor	24
	Mandibular	Right	Central incisor	25
	Mandibular	Right	Lateral incisor	26
7	Mandibular	Right	Canine	27

8. Finish with the mandibular right canine (tooth No. 27).

When the dental radiographer works from right to left in the maxillary arch and then from left to right in the mandibular arch, no wasted movement or shifting of the PID occurs (Fig. 17–10). In addition, when working from right to left and then from left to right, the teeth are exposed in increasing numerical order:

teeth 6 → 7 → 8 → 9 → 10 → 11, and then
teeth 22 → 23 → 24 → 25 → 26 → 27

This exposure sequence allows the dental radiographer to keep track of the last exposure easily if interrupted.

POSTERIOR EXPOSURE SEQUENCE

Following anterior film placement, the **posterior teeth** (premolars and molars) are exposed. In each quadrant, *always* expose the premolar film first and then the molar film because:

- Premolar film placement is easier for the patient to tolerate.
- Premolar exposure is less likely to evoke the gag reflex.

Eight posterior film placements are used in the paralleling technique: four maxillary exposures and four mandibular exposures. The recommended exposure sequence for the posterior film placements varies depending on the film holder used. The recommended posterior periapical exposure sequence for the Rinn XCP instruments illustrated in this text is as follows Table 17–2):

1. Begin with the maxillary right quadrant.

2. Assemble the posterior XCP instrument for this area.
3. Expose the premolar film (teeth No. 4 and 5) first and then expose the molar film (teeth No. 1, 2, and 3).
4. Without reassembling the XCP instrument, move to the mandibular left quadrant.
5. Expose the premolar film (teeth No. 20 and 21) first and then expose the molar film (teeth No. 17, 18, and 19).
6. Move to the maxillary left quadrant and reassemble the posterior XCP instrument for this area.
7. Expose the premolar film (teeth No. 12 and 13) first and then the molar film (teeth No. 14, 15, and 16).
8. Finish with the mandibular right quadrant.
9. Expose the premolar film (teeth No. 28 and 29) first and then end with the exposure of the molar film (teeth No. 30, 31, and 32).

Film Placement

When exposing a complete mouth radiographic series (CMRS) using the paralleling technique, each periapical exposure has a prescribed **film placement**. Film placement, or the specific area where the film must be positioned before exposure, is dictated by the teeth and surrounding structures that must be included on the resultant radiograph. Prescribed film placements for the anterior teeth are described in the "Prescribed Placements for Anterior Periapical Films" chart and illustrated in Figure 17–11; posterior placements are described in the "Prescribed Placements for Posterior Periapical Films" chart and illustrated in Figure 17–12.

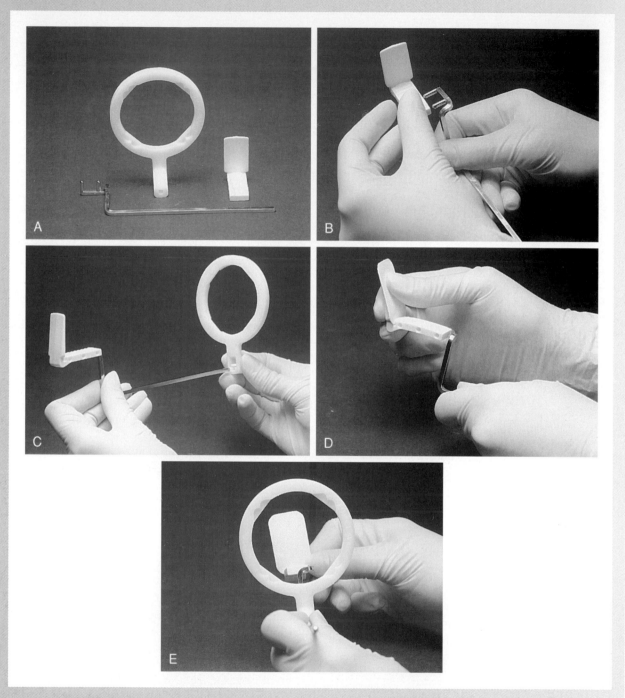

FIGURE 17–8. *A,* Parts of the anterior XCP instrument. *B,* Assembly of the anterior XCP instrument. Insert the two prongs of the anterior indicator arm into the openings in the anterior bite-block as shown. *C,* Insert the anterior indicator arm into the opening on the anterior aiming ring as shown. *D,* Flex the plastic backing of the bite-block to open the film slot for easy insertion of the anterior film packet. *E,* The anterior XCP instrument is correctly assembled when the film is seen centered in the middle of the aiming ring.

1. Set the exposure factors (kilovoltage, milliamperage, and time) on the x-ray unit according to the recommendations of the film manufacturer.

2. Open the sterilized package containing the film holder, and, if necessary, assemble the film holder. Some film holders require assembly (e.g., XCP and Precision instruments), and others do not (e.g., Stabe and EEZEE-Grip film holders). Assembly of the anterior XCP instrument is illustrated in Figure 17–8; posterior XCP instrument assembly is illustrated in Figure 17–9. For assembly instructions on other film holders, refer to information provided by the manufacturer.

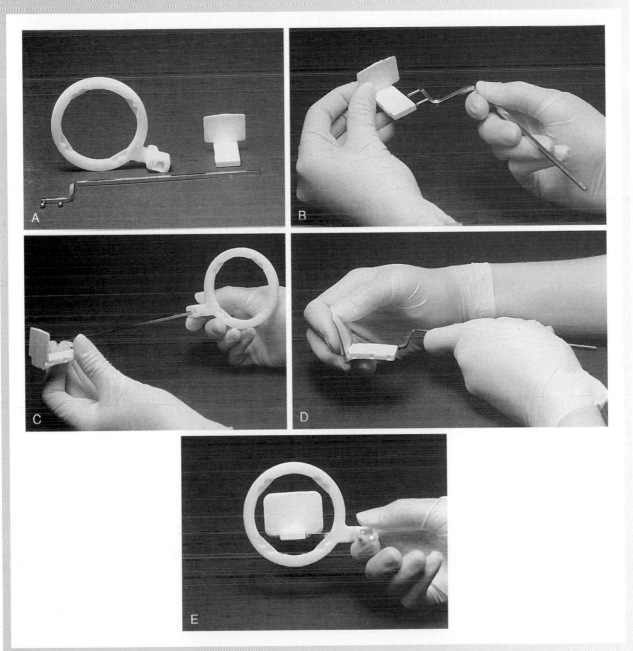

FIGURE 17–9. *A,* Parts of the posterior XCP instrument. *B,* Assembly of the posterior XCP instrument. Insert the two prongs of the posterior indicator arm into the openings in the posterior bite-block shown. *C,* Insert the posterior indicator arm into the opening on the posterior aiming ring as shown. *D,* Flex the plastic backing of the bite-block to open the film slot for easy insertion of the posterior film packet. *E,* The posterior XCP instrument is correctly assembled when the film is seen centered in the middle of the aiming ring.

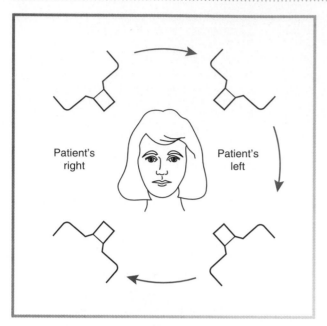

FIGURE 17–10. When exposing maxillary anterior films, work from the right to the left. Then expose the mandibular anterior films from left to right. No unnecessary movements of the PID result.

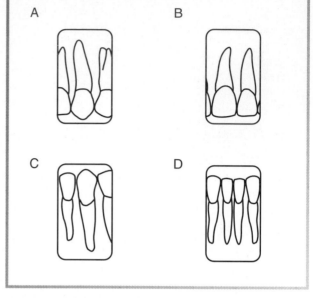

FIGURE 17–11. Prescribed placements for anterior periapical films. *A,* The maxillary canine exposure. *B,* The maxillary lateral and central incisor exposure. *C,* The mandibular canine exposure. *D,* The mandibular lateral and central incisor exposure.

The specific film placements described in this chapter are for a 15-film periapical series using Size 1 films for the anterior exposures and Size 2 films for the posterior exposures. Variations in film placement or the number of total films may be recommended by other reference sources or individual practitioners. Guidelines for periapical film positioning used with the paralleling technique are summarized in the "Guidelines for Film Placement" chart.

ANTERIOR FILM PLACEMENT

The anterior XCP instrument is used for all anterior film placements. After the anterior XCP instrument has

been assembled, a Size 1 film packet is inserted vertically into the bite-block and secured in the slot. Anterior film placements include the following: two maxillary canine exposures, two maxillary incisor exposures, two mandibular canine exposures, and one mandibular incisor exposure (see the respective Procedures).

POSTERIOR FILM PLACEMENT

The posterior XCP instrument is used for all posterior film placements. After the posterior XCP instrument has been assembled, a Size 2 film packet is inserted horizontally into the bite-block and secured in the slot.

TABLE 17–2. Exposure Sequence for Posterior Film Placements (with Rinn XCP Instruments)

Exposure Number	Arch	Side	Teeth	Teeth Numbers
1	Maxillary	Right	Premolars	4, 5
2	Maxillary	Right	Molars	1, 2, 3
3	Mandibular	Left	Premolars	20, 21
4	Mandibular	Left	Molars	17, 18, 19
5	Maxillary	Left	Premolars	12, 13
6	Maxillary	Left	Molars	14, 15, 16
7	Mandibular	Right	Premolars	28, 29
8	Mandibular	Right	Molars	30, 31, 32

PRESCRIBED PLACEMENTS FOR ANTERIOR PERIAPICAL FILMS

Maxillary Canine Exposure

The entire crown and root of the canine, including the apex and surrounding structures, must be seen on this radiograph. In addition, the interproximal alveolar bone and mesial contact of the canine must also be visible. The lingual cusp of the first premolar usually obscures the distal contact of the canine.

Maxillary Incisor Exposure

The entire crowns and roots of one lateral and one central incisor, including the apices of the teeth and surrounding structures, must be seen on this radiograph. In addition, the interproximal alveolar bone between the central and lateral, the mesial and distal contact areas, and the surrounding regions of bone must also be visible. The mesial contact of the adjacent central incisor and mesial contact of the adjacent canine should also be seen on this exposure.

Mandibular Canine Exposure

The entire crown and root of the canine, including the apex and surrounding structures, must be seen on this radiograph. In addition, the interproximal alveolar bone and mesial and distal contacts must also be visible.

Mandibular Incisor Exposure

The entire crowns and roots of the four mandibular incisors, including the apices of the teeth and surrounding structures, must be seen on this radiograph. In addition, the contacts between the central incisors, and between the central and lateral incisors, must also be visible. In most cases, it is not necessary to see the distal contacts of the lateral incisors.

PRESCRIBED PLACEMENTS FOR POSTERIOR PERIAPICAL FILMS

Maxillary Premolar Exposure

All crowns and roots of the first and second premolars and first molar, including the apices, alveolar crests, contact areas, and surrounding bone, must be seen on this radiograph. In addition, the distal contact of the maxillary canine must be visible in this projection.

Maxillary Molar Exposure

All crowns and roots of the first, second, and third molars, including the apices, alveolar crests, contact areas, surrounding bone, and tuberosity region, must be seen on this radiograph.

Mandibular Premolar Exposure

All crowns and roots of the first and second premolars and first molar, including the apices, alveolar crests, contact areas, and surrounding bone, must be seen on this radiograph. In addition, the distal contact of the mandibular canine should also be visible.

Mandibular Molar Exposure

All crowns and roots of the first, second, and third molars, including the apices, alveolar crests, contact areas, and surrounding bone, must be seen on this radiograph.

Posterior film placements include the following: two maxillary premolar exposures, two maxillary molar exposures, two mandibular premolar exposures, and two mandibular molar exposures (see the respective Procedures).

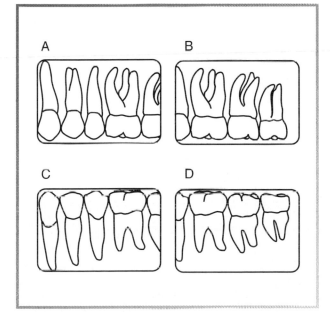

FIGURE 17-12. Prescribed placements for posterior periapical films. *A,* The maxillary premolar exposure. *B,* The maxillary molar exposure. *C,* The mandibular premolar exposure. *D,* The mandibular molar exposure.

GUIDELINES FOR FILM PLACEMENT

- The white side of the film always faces the teeth.
- The anterior films are always placed vertically.
- The posterior films are always placed horizontally.
- The identification dot on the film is always placed in the slot of the film holder, toward the occlusal end of the film. (Place the "dot in the slot.")
- When placing the film in the mouth, always lead with the apical end of the film and rotate the film holder.
- When positioning the film holder, always place the film away from the teeth and toward the middle of the oral cavity.
- When positioning the film holder, always center the film over the area to be examined (as defined in the prescribed film placements).
- When positioning the film holder, ask the patient to "slowly close" on the bite-block; always make certain that the bite-block is stabilized by the teeth and not the lips.

Text continued on page 244

PROCEDURE

Maxillary Canine Exposure (Fig. 17–13)

1. Center the film holder and film packet on the canine.

2. Position the film as far away from the teeth as possible.

3. Instruct the patient to "slowly close" on the bite-block and slide the aiming ring down the indicator arm to the skin surface. Align the PID with the aiming ring and expose the film.

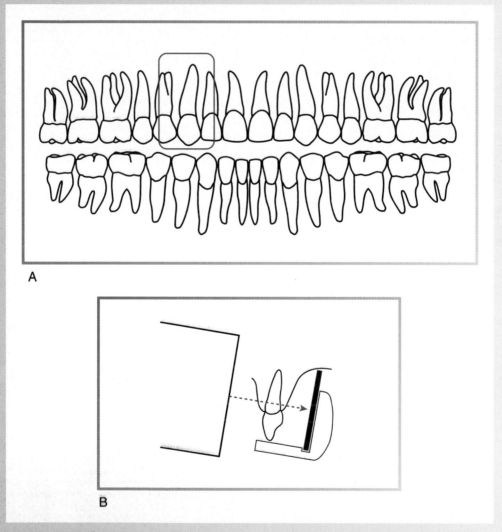

A

B

FIGURE 17–13. The maxillary canine exposure. *A,* Film placement. *B,* Relationship of film, teeth, XCP instrument, and PID.

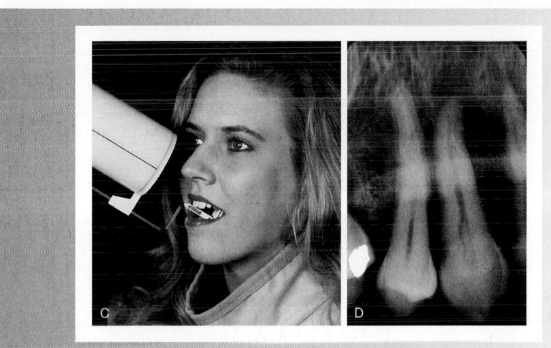

FIGURE 17–13. *Continued. C,* Exposure of film. *D,* Resultant radiograph.

PROCEDURE

Maxillary Incisor Exposure (Fig. 17–14)

1. Center the film holder and film packet on the contact between the central incisor and the lateral incisor.

2. Position the film as far away from the teeth as possible.

3. Instruct the patient to "slowly close" on the bite-block and slide the aiming ring down the indicator arm to the skin surface. Align the PID with the aiming ring and expose the film.

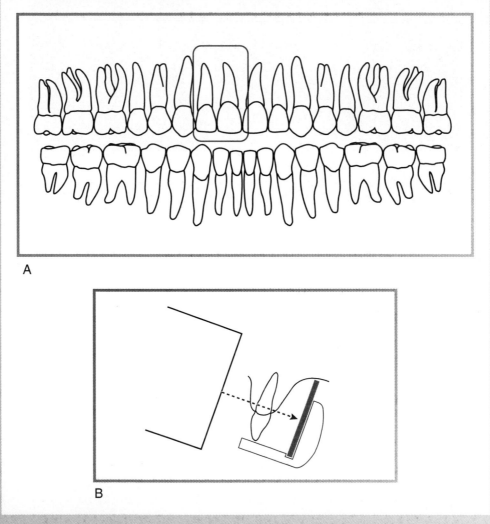

A

B

FIGURE 17–14. The maxillary incisor exposure. _A,_ Film placement. _B,_ Relationship of film, teeth, XCP instrument, and PID.

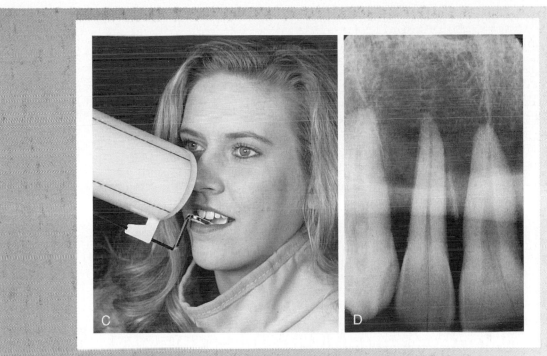

FIGURE 17–14. *Continued. C,* Exposure of film. *D,* Resultant radiograph.

PROCEDURE

Mandibular Canine Exposure (Fig. 17–15)

1. Center the film holder and film packet on the canine.

2. Position the film as far away from the teeth as possible.

3. Instruct the patient to "slowly close" on the bite-block and slide the aiming ring down the indicator arm to the skin surface. Align the PID with the aiming ring and expose the film.

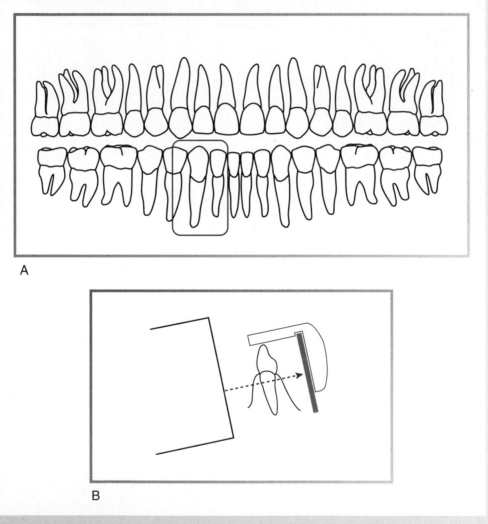

A

B

FIGURE 17–15. The mandibular canine exposure. *A,* Film placement. *B,* Relationship of film, teeth, XCP instrument, and PID.

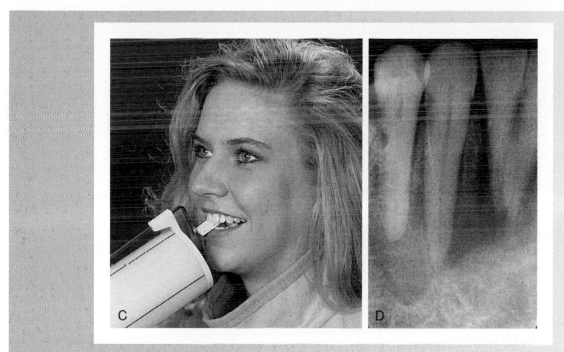

FIGURE 17-15. *Continued. C,* Exposure of film. *D,* Resultant radiograph.

PROCEDURE

Mandibular Incisor Exposure (Fig. 17–16)

1. Center the film holder and film packet on the contact between the two central incisors.

2. Position the film as far away from the teeth as possible.

3. Instruct the patient to "slowly close" on the bite-block and slide the aiming ring down the indicator arm to the skin surface. Align the PID with the aiming ring and expose the film.

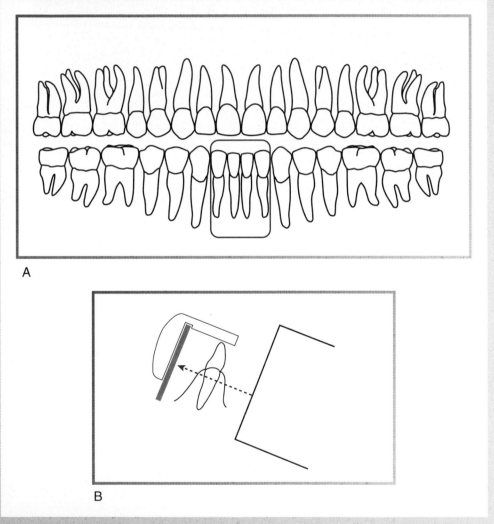

FIGURE 17–16. The mandibular incisor exposure. *A,* Film placement. *B,* Relationship of film, teeth, XCP instrument, and PID.

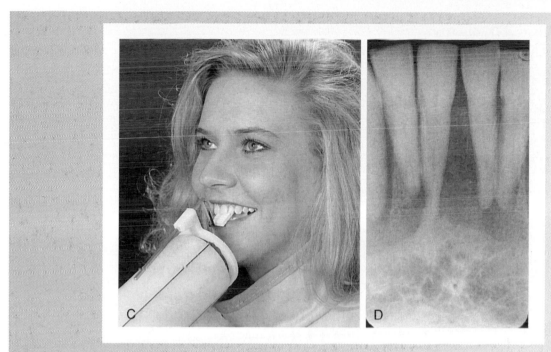

FIGURE 17–16. *Continued. C,* Exposure of film. *D,* Resultant radiograph.

PROCEDURE

Maxillary Premolar Exposure (Fig. 17–17)

1. Center the film holder and film packet on the second premolar; the front edge of the film should cover the canine.

2. Position the film as far away from the teeth as possible.

3. Instruct the patient to "slowly close" on the bite-block, and slide the aiming ring down the indicator arm to the skin surface. Align the PID with the aiming ring and expose the film.

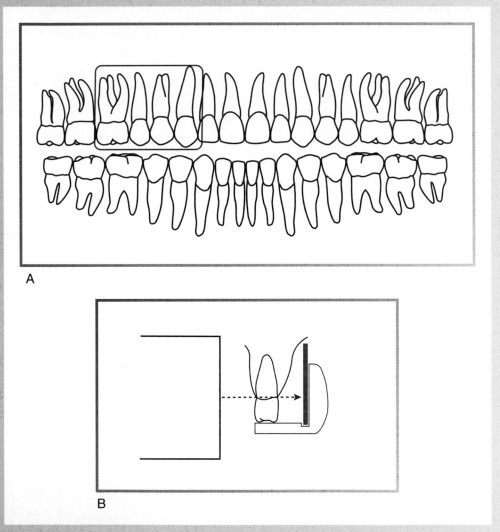

FIGURE 17–17. The maxillary premolar exposure. *A,* Film placement. *B,* Relationship of film, teeth, XCP instrument, and PID.

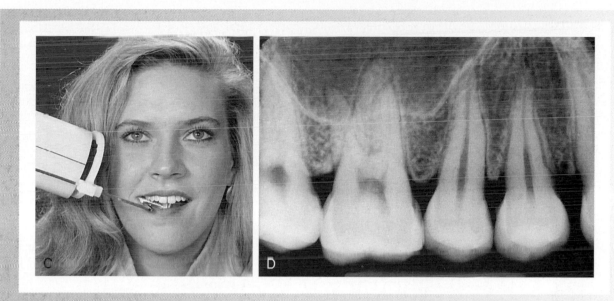

FIGURE 17–17. *Continued. C,* Exposure of film. *D,* Resultant radiograph.

PROCEDURE

Maxillary Molar Exposure (Fig. 17–18)

1. Center the film holder and film packet on the second molar; the front edge of the film should be aligned with the midline of the second premolar.

2. Position the film as far away from the teeth as possible.

3. Instruct the patient to "slowly close" on the bite-block and slide the aiming ring down the indicator arm to the skin surface. Align the PID with the aiming ring and expose the film.

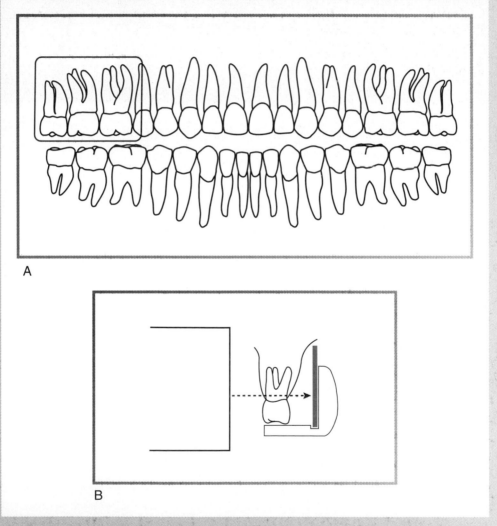

FIGURE 17–18. The maxillary molar exposure. *A,* Film placement. *B,* Relationship of film, teeth, XCP instrument, and PID.

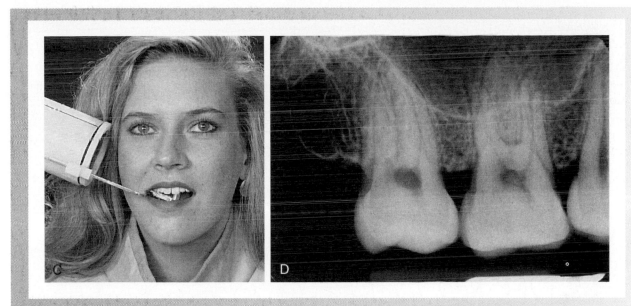

FIGURE 17–18. *Continued. C,* Exposure of film. *D,* Resultant radiograph.

PROCEDURE

Mandibular Premolar Exposure (Fig. 17–19)

1. Center the film holder and film packet on the second premolar; the front edge of the film should cover the canine.

2. Position the film as far away from the teeth as possible.

3. Instruct the patient to "slowly close" on the bite-block and slide the aiming ring down the indicator arm to the skin surface. Align the PID with the aiming ring and expose the film.

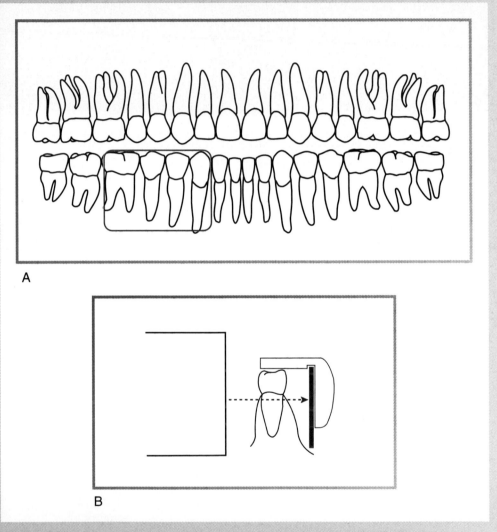

FIGURE 17–19. The mandibular premolar exposure. *A*, Film placement. *B*, Relationship of film, teeth, XCP instrument, and PID.

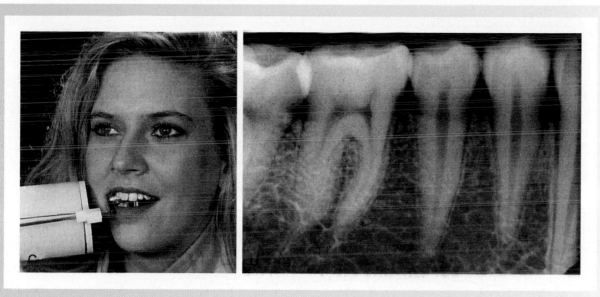

FIGURE 17–19. *Continued. C,* Exposure of film. *D,* Resultant radiograph.

PROCEDURE

Mandibular Molar Exposure (Fig. 17–20)

1. Center the film holder and film packet on the second molar; the front edge of the film should be aligned with the midline of the second premolar.

2. Position the film as far away from the teeth as possible.

3. Instruct the patient to "slowly close" on the bite-block and slide the aiming ring down the indicator arm to the skin surface. Align the PID with the aiming ring and expose the film.

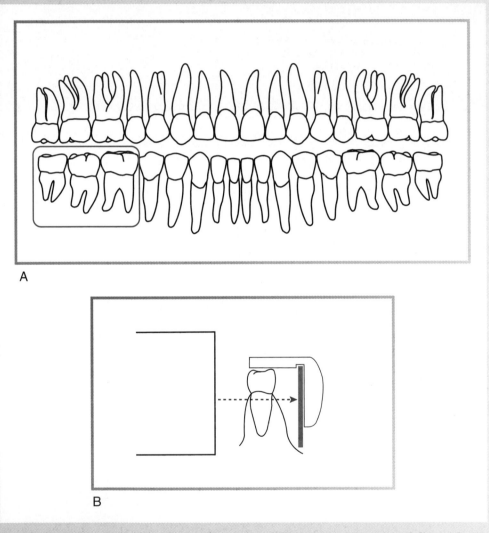

FIGURE 17–20. The mandibular molar exposure. *A,* Film placement. *B,* Relationship of film, teeth, XCP instrument, and PID.

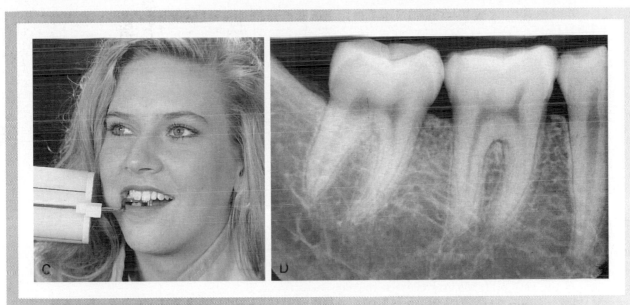

FIGURE 17–20. *Continued. C,* Exposure of film. *D,* Resultant radiograph.

▉ MODIFICATIONS IN TECHNIQUE

Modifications in the paralleling technique may be used to accommodate variations in anatomic conditions. Such modifications may be necessary when a patient has a shallow palate, bony growths, or a sensitive mandibular premolar region.

Shallow Palate

Parallelism between the film and the long axis of the tooth is difficult to accomplish in a patient with a shallow **palate** (roof of the mouth), also known as a low palatal vault. In a patient with a shallow palate, tilting of the bite-block occurs, which results in a lack of parallelism between the film and the long axis of the tooth. If the lack of parallelism between the film and the long axis of the tooth does not exceed 20 degrees, the resultant radiograph is generally acceptable (Fig. 17–21). When the lack of parallelism is greater than 20 degrees, a modification in technique is necessary.

- **Cotton rolls.** To position the film parallel to the long axis of the tooth, two cotton rolls can be used, one placed on each side of the bite-block (Fig. 17–22). As a result, however, periapical coverage is reduced.
- **Vertical angulation.** To compensate for the lack of parallelism, the vertical angulation can be increased by 5 to 15 degrees more than the XCP

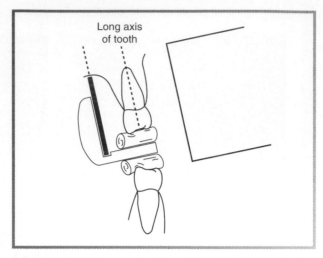

FIGURE 17–22. Two cotton rolls can be used to position the film parallel to the long axis of the tooth.

instrument indicates. As a result, however, image distortion occurs.

Bony Growths

A **torus** (plural, **tori**) is a bony growth seen in the oral cavity. A **maxillary torus** (torus palatinus) is a nodular mass of bone seen along the midline of the hard palate (Fig. 17–23). **Mandibular tori** (torus mandibularis) are bony growths along the lingual aspect (tongue side) of the mandible (Fig. 17–24). When using the paralleling technique, maxillary and mandibular tori can cause problems with film placement, and modifications in technique are necessary.

- **Maxillary torus.** The film must be placed on the far side of the torus (not *on* the torus) and then exposed (Fig. 17–25).
- **Mandibular tori.** The film must be placed between the tori and the tongue (not *on* the tori) and then exposed (Fig. 17–26).

Mandibular Premolar Region

The anterior floor of the mouth area can be a very sensitive region. When periapical film placements cause discomfort in the mandibular premolar region, a modification in technique is neccessary.

- **Film placement.** The film must be placed under the tongue to avoid impinging on muscle attachments and the sensitive lingual gingiva. When inserting the film holder into the mouth, the film is tipped away from the tongue and toward the

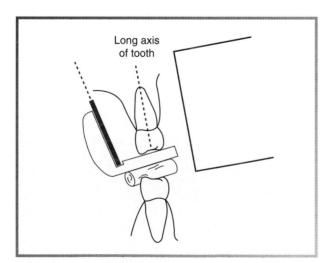

FIGURE 17–21. Tilting of the bite-block results in a lack of parallelism between the film and the long axis of the tooth. When the lack of parallelism is less than 20 degrees (as shown in this diagram) the radiograph is generally acceptable.

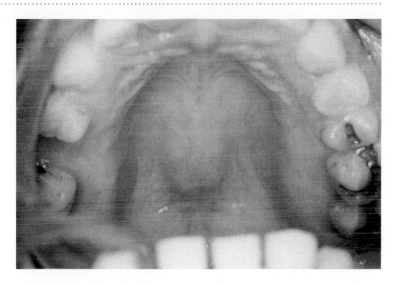

FIGURE 17–23. A maxillary torus.

teeth being examined while the bite-block is placed firmly on the mandibular premolars. When the patient closes on the bite-block, the film is moved into the proper position (Fig. 17–27).

- **Film.** The lower edge of the film can be gently curved, or softened, to prevent discomfort. Bending or creasing the film, however, must be avoided.

ADVANTAGES AND DISADVANTAGES

As with all intraoral techniques, the paralleling technique has both advantages and disadvantages. The ad-

vantages of the paralleling technique, however, outweigh the disadvantages.

Advantages

The primary advantage of the paralleling technique is that it produces a radiographic image without dimensional distortion. In addition, it is uncomplicated and can be easily repeated when serial radiographs are indicated. The advantages of the paralleling technique, can be summarized as follows:

- **Accuracy.** The paralleling technique produces an image that has dimensional accuracy; the image is very representative of the actual tooth. The radiographic image is free of distortion and exhibits maximum detail and definition.

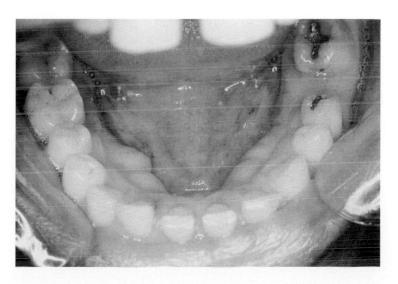

FIGURE 17–24. Mandibular tori.

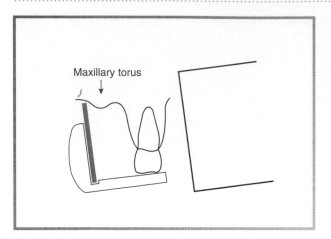

FIGURE 17–25. If a maxillary torus is present, the film must be placed on the far side of the torus and then exposed.

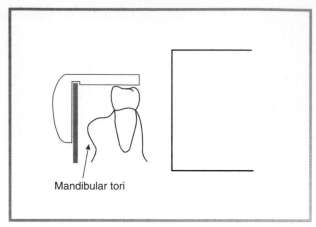

FIGURE 17–26. If mandibular tori are present, the film must be placed on the far side of the tori and then exposed.

- **Simplicity.** The paralleling technique is simple and is easy to learn and use. The use of a film holder with a beam alignment device eliminates the need for the dental radiographer to determine horizontal and vertical angulations and also eliminates the chances of dimensional distortion.
- **Duplication.** The paralleling technique is easy to standardize and can be accurately duplicated, or repeated, when serial radiographs are indicated. As a result, comparisons of serial radiographs exposed using the paralleling technique have great validity.

Disadvantages

The primary disadvantage of the paralleling technique is film placement. In addition, patient dis-

comfort may also be a problem. The disadvantages of the paralleling technique can be summarized as follows:

- **Film placement.** Because a film-holding device must be used with the paralleling technique, film placement may be difficult for the dental radiographer. Difficulties may be encountered with the child patient or with adult patients with a small mouth or a shallow palate. Such film placements become less problematic as the dental radiographer becomes more proficient at using the paralleling technique.
- **Discomfort.** The film-holding device used to position the film in the paralleling technique may impinge on the oral tissues and cause discomfort for the patient.

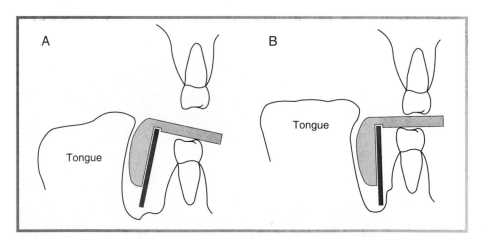

FIGURE 17–27. Positioning of the XCP instrument in the sensitive mandibular premolar area. *A,* The film is tipped away from the tongue while the bite-block is placed firmly on the mandibular premolars. *B,* When the patient closes on the bite-block, the film is moved into proper position.

HELPFUL HINTS • • • • • • • • • • • • • • • • • •
in Using the Paralleling Technique

- ➤ **DO** set all exposure factors (kilovoltage, milliamperage, time) before placing any films in the mouth.
- ➤ **DO** ask patients to remove all intraoral objects and eyeglasses prior to placing any films in the mouth.
- ➤ **DO** use a definite order (exposure sequence) when exposing films to avoid errors and make efficient use of time.
- ➤ **DO** place each film in the bite-block with the "dot in the slot." The identification dot must be located at the occlusal or incisal end of the film; this facilitates film mounting and ensures that the dot will not interfere with a diagnosis in the periapical area.
- ➤ **DO** explain the radiographic procedures that will be performed; instruct patients on how to close and remain still during the exposure.
- ➤ **DO** communicate with patients; patients are more likely to be tolerant of discomfort when they understand why a film must be placed in a specific area.
- ➤ **DO** use the word *please;* instruct patients to "open please."
- ➤ **DO** use praise; tell cooperative patients how much they are helping you.
- ➤ **DO** instruct patients to *"slowly close";* when patients close slowly, their musculature relaxes and less discomfort results.
- ➤ **DO** align the PID so that the opening of the PID is flush with the aiming ring of the XCP instrument.
- ➤ **DON'T** bend or crimp a film packet; excessive film bending causes distortion of the image.
- ➤ **DON'T** use words like *hurt.* Instead, inform patients that the procedure will be "momentarily uncomfortable."
- ➤ **DON'T** make comments like "Oops!" or other statements that indicate a lack of control in a situation. Patients will lose confidence in your abilities.
- ➤ **DON'T** pick up a film packet if it drops. Leave it on the floor; it is contaminated. Instead, remove it during cleaning of the treatment area.
- ➤ **DON'T** allow patients to dictate how you should perform your duties. Some patients must be handled firmly. The dental radiographer must always remain in control of the procedures.
- ➤ **DON'T** begin with posterior exposures; posterior film placements may cause patients to gag. Instead, always start with anterior exposures.
- ➤ **DON'T** position films on top of a torus (tori); the apical regions of the teeth will not be seen on the resultant radiograph. Instead, always position the films behind the torus (tori).

▰ SUMMARY

- The paralleling technique is one technique that is used to expose periapical films. The film is placed in the mouth parallel to the long axis of the tooth, and the central ray is

directed perpendicular to the film and the long axis of the tooth. To achieve parallelism between the film and the tooth, the film must be placed away from the tooth and toward the middle of the oral cavity.

- In the paralleling technique, a film holder must be used to position the film parallel to the long axis of the tooth. The patient cannot hold the film. A variety of film holders are commercially available.
- The size of the intraoral film used with the paralleling technique will depend on the teeth being radiographed. With the anterior teeth, Size 1 film is used; with the posterior teeth, Size 2 film is used.
- There are five basic rules to follow in the paralleling technique: (1) the film must cover the prescribed area of interest, (2) the film must be positioned parallel to the long axis of the tooth, (3) the central ray must be directed perpendicular to the film and long axis of the tooth, (4) the central ray must be directed through the contact areas between the teeth, and (5) the x-ray beam must be centered over the film to ensure that all areas of the film are exposed.
- Prior to film exposure using the paralleling technique, the dental radiographer must complete infection control procedures, preparation of the treatment area and supplies, seating of the patient, explanation of radiographic procedures to be performed, chair and headrest adjustments, placement of the lead apron, removal of intraoral objects and eyeglasses, setting of the exposure factors, and assembly of film-holding devices.
- An exposure sequence for periapical film placements must be followed using the paralleling technique. Always begin with the anterior exposures; anterior exposures are easier for the patient to tolerate, more comfortable, and less likely to cause gagging. Following the anterior exposures, the posterior teeth are exposed. In each quadrant, always expose the premolar film first, then the molar film.
- When exposing a CMRS using the paralleling technique, each periapical exposure has a prescribed film placement. Prescribed film placements are detailed in charts and illustrated in Figures 17–11 and 17–12.
- Modifications in the paralleling technique may be necessary when a patient has a low or shallow palate, bony growths, or a sensitive mandibular premolar region; these modifications are described in this chapter.
- The advantages of the paralleling technique are as follows: the paralleling technique produces images with dimensional accuracy, is simple and easy to learn and use, is easy to standardize, and can be accurately repeated.
- The disadvantages of the paralleling technique are as follows: film placements may be difficult for the dental radiographer, and the film-holding device may cause the patient discomfort.

BIBLIOGRAPHY

Eastman Kodak Company: Intraoral—the paralleling technic (long cone). *In* X-Rays in Dentistry. Rochester, Eastman Kodak Company, 1985, pp. 52–69.

Frommer HH: Intraoral radiographic technique: The paralleling method. *In* Radiology for Dental Auxiliaries, 6th edition. St. Louis, Mosby-Year Book, 1996, pp. 139–180.

Goaz PW, White SC: Intraoral radiographic examinations. *In* Oral Radiology: Principles and Interpretation, 3rd edition. St. Louis, CV Mosby, 1994, pp. 151–179.

Johnson ON, McNally MA, Essay CE: Intraoral radiographic procedures. *In* Essentials of Dental Radiography for Dental Assistants and Hygienists, 6th edition. Norwalk, Appleton and Lange, 1999, pp. 319–337.

Johnson ON, McNally MA, Essay CE: The periapical examination. *In* Essentials of Dental Radiography for Dental Assistants and Hygienists, 6th edition. Norwalk, Appleton and Lange, 1999, pp. 339–375.

Langland OE, Sippy FH, Langlais RP: Intraoral radiographic techniques. *In* Textbook of Dental Radiography, 2nd edition. Springfield, IL, Charles C Thomas, 1984, pp. 206–255.

Manson-Hing LR: The paralleling technic. *In* Fundamentals of Dental Radiography, 3rd edition. Philadelphia, Lea & Febiger, 1990, pp. 53–62.

Manson-Hing LR: Comparing technics and evaluating technical errors. *In* Fundamentals of Dental Radiography, 3rd edition. Philadelphia, Lea & Febiger, 1990, pp. 53–62.

Matteson SR, Whaley C, Secrist VC: Intraoral radiographic techniques. *In* Dental Radiology, 4th edition. Chapel Hill, University of North Carolina Press, 1988, pp. 77–105.

Miles DA, Van Dis ML, Jensen CW, Ferretti A: Intraoral radiographic technique. *In* Radiographic Imaging for Dental Auxiliaries, 3rd edition. Philadelphia, WB Saunders, 1993, pp: 1–47.

Miles DA, Van Dis ML, Razmus TF: Intraoral radiographic techniques. *In* Basic Principles of Oral and Maxillofacial Radiology. Philadelphia, WB Saunders, 1992, pp. 73–85.

Quiz Questions

MATCHING

For questions 1 to 8, refer to Figure 17–28. Match the letters of the appropriate items with the descriptions below.

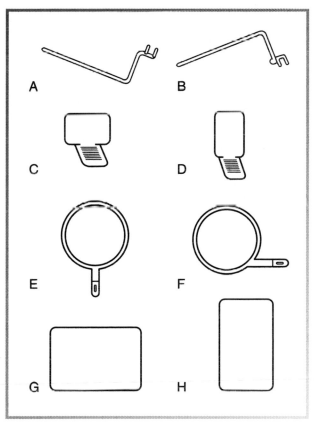

FIGURE 17–28

_H_	**1.** Film, No. 1
_G_	**2.** Film, No. 2
_F_	**3.** XCP aiming ring, posterior
_E_	**4.** XCP aiming ring, anterior
_A_	**5.** XCP indicator arm, posterior
_B_	**6.** XCP indicator arm, anterior
_C_	**7.** XCP bite-block, posterior
_D_	**8.** XCP bite-block, anterior

FILL IN THE BLANK

9. What happens to the radiographic image when the object-film distance is increased?

_____

10. What piece of equipment is required to hold the film parallel to the long axis of the tooth in the paralleling technique?

_____

11. What do the letters X, C, and P stand for?

_____

12. What size film is used with the anterior XCP instrument?

_____

13. What size film is used with the posterior XCP instrument?

_____

14. Which film holders are recommended for use with the paralleling technique because they reduce patient exposure?

_____

15. How is the patient's head positioned prior to exposing films?

_____

MULTIPLE CHOICE

_____ 16. Why is an increased target-film distance required in the paralleling technique?

    a. to avoid image magnification
    b. to avoid distortion
    c. to reduce scatter radiation
    d. to improve film placement

_____ 17. Which of the following describes the relationship of the central ray to the film in the paralleling technique?

    a. 20 degrees to the long axis of the tooth
    b. 90 degrees to the film and long axis of the tooth
    c. 75 degrees to the long axis of the tooth
    d. 15 degrees to the film and long axis of the tooth

_____ 18. Which of the following definitions is incorrect?

    a. parallel: always separated by the same distance
    b. intersecting: to cut through
    c. right angle: formed by two parallel lines
    d. central ray: central portion of the x-ray beam

_____ 19. Which of the following describes the relationship of the film and the long axis of the tooth in the paralleling technique?

    a. the film and tooth are parallel to each other
    b. the film and tooth are at right angles to each other
    c. the film and tooth are perpendicular to each other
    d. the film and tooth are intersecting each other

_____ 20. Which of the following describes the distance between the film and tooth in the paralleling technique?

    a. the film is placed as close as possible to the tooth
    b. the film is placed away from the tooth and toward the middle of the oral cavity
    c. a or b
    d. none of the above

_____ 21. Which of the following is correct concerning film placement?
(1) anterior films are placed horizontally, (2) anterior films are placed vertically, (3) posterior films are placed horizontally, (4) posterior films are placed vertically

    a. 1, 2, 3
    b. 2, 3, 4
    c. 2, 3
    d. 1, 4

_____ 22. Which of the following is incorrect concerning the exposure sequence for periapical films?

    a. anterior films are always exposed before posterior films
    b. either anterior or posterior films may be exposed first
    c. in posterior quadrants, the premolar film is always exposed before the molar film
    d. when exposing anterior films, work from the patient's right to left in the upper arch, and then from left to right in the lower arch

_____ 23. Which of the following is correct concerning the lack of parallelism between the film and the long axis of the tooth?

    a. if greater than 30 degrees, the film is generally acceptable
    b. if less than 20 degrees, the film is generally acceptable
    c. if less than 50 degrees, the film is generally acceptable
    d. if greater than 50 degrees, the film is generally acceptable

_____ 24. Which of the following are advantages of the paralleling technique?
(1) increased accuracy, (2) simplicity of use, (3) ease of duplication, (4) ease of film placement

    a. 1, 2, 3, 4
    b. 1, 2, 3
    c. 2, 3, 4
    d. 1, 3, 4

_____ 25. The advantages of the paralleling technique outweigh the disadvantages.

    a. true
    b. false

ESSAY

26. State the basic principle of the paralleling technique.

27. Describe why a film holder must be used in the paralleling technique.

28. State the five rules of the paralleling technique.

29. Discuss the patient and equipment preparations that are necessary prior to using the paralleling technique.

30. Discuss the exposure sequence for 15 periapical film placements using the paralleling technique.

31. Describe each of the 15 periapical film placements that are recommended for use with the XCP instruments.

32. Summarize the guidelines for periapical film positioning.

33. Explain the modifications in the paralleling technique that are used for a shallow palate, bony growths, or a sensitive premolar region.

Answers are supplied at the end of this book.

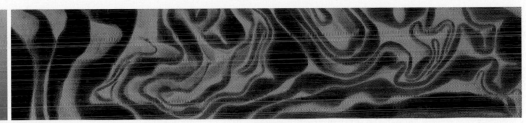

Bisecting Technique

OBJECTIVES

After completion of this chapter, the student will be able to:

- *Define the key words.*
- *State the rule of isometry.*
- *State the basic principles of the bisecting technique and illustrate the location of the film, tooth, imaginary bisector, central ray, and position-indicating device (PID).*
- *List the film holders that can be used with the bisecting technique.*
- *Describe the finger-holding method of film stabilization.*
- *List the disadvantages of the finger-holding method.*
- *Describe the film size used with the bisecting technique.*
- *Describe correct and incorrect horizontal angulation.*
- *Describe correct and incorrect vertical angulation.*
- *State each of the recommended vertical angulation ranges used for periapical exposures in the bisecting technique.*
- *State the basic rules of the bisecting technique.*
- *Describe the patient and equipment preparations necessary prior to using the bisecting technique.*
- *Discuss the exposure sequence used for the 14 periapical film placements used in the bisecting technique.*

- *Describe each of the 14 periapical film placements recommended for use with the bisecting technique.*
- *List the advantages and disadvantages of the bisecting technique.*

KEY WORDS

Angle	Foreshortening
Angulation	Hypotenuse
Angulation, horizontal	Isometry
Angulation, vertical	Isometry, rule of
Bisect	Long axis of the tooth
Bisecting technique	Teeth, anterior
Bisector, imaginary	Teeth, posterior
Central ray	Triangle
Elongation	Triangle, equilateral
Exposure sequence	Triangle, right
Film holder	Triangles, congruent
Film placement	
Finger-holding method	

INTRODUCTION

The dental radiographer must master a variety of intraoral radiographic techniques. As discussed in Chapter 17, the paralleling technique is one method for exposing periapical films. Another method is the bisecting technique. Before the dental radiographer can use this technique, an understanding of the basic concepts, including terminology and principles, is necessary. In addition, the dental radiographer must comprehend patient preparation, equipment preparation, exposure sequencing, and film placement procedures used in the bisecting technique.

The purpose of this chapter is to present basic concepts and to describe patient preparation, equipment preparation, and film placement procedures used in the bisecting technique. This chapter also describes the advantages and disadvantages of the bisecting technique and reviews helpful hints.

BASIC CONCEPTS

The **bisecting technique** (also known as the *bisecting-angle technique, bisection-of-the-angle technique,* and

short-cone technique) is another method that can be used to expose periapical films.

Terminology

Prior to describing the bisecting technique, an understanding of a number of basic terms is necessary.

Angle: In geometry, a figure formed by two lines diverging from a common point (Fig. 18–1A).

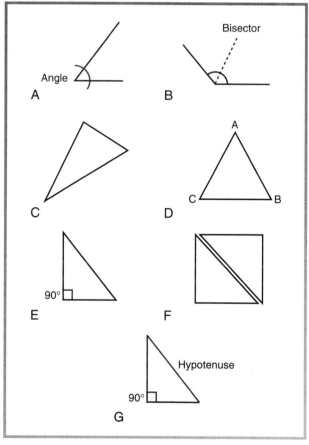

FIGURE 18–1. *A,* An angle is formed by two lines that diverge from a common point. *B,* A bisector divides an angle into equal angles. *C,* A triangle. *D,* An equilateral triangle has three equal sides (AB = BC = CA). *E,* A right triangle has one 90-degree angle. *F,* Congruent triangles are identical. *G,* The hypotenuse is the side of a right triangle opposite the right angle.

Bisect: To divide into two equal parts (bisector, *n.*) (Fig. 18–1*B*).

Triangle: In geometry, a figure formed by connecting three points not in a straight line by three straight-line segments (Fig. 18–1*C*). As the term triangle suggests, this figure has three angles.

Triangle, equilateral: In geometry, a triangle with three equal sides (Fig. 18–1*D*).

Triangle, right: In geometry, a triangle with one 90-degree angle (right angle) (Fig. 18–1*E*).

Triangles, congruent: Triangles that are identical and correspond exactly when superimposed (Fig. 18–1*F*).

Hypotenuse: In geometry, the side of a right triangle opposite the right angle (Fig. 18–1*G*).

Isometry: Equality of measurement.

Long axis of the tooth: An imaginary line that divides the tooth longitudinally into two equal halves (Fig. 18–2).

Central ray: The central portion of the primary beam of x-radiation.

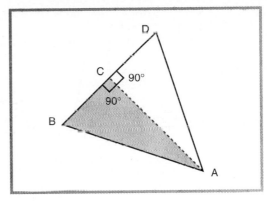

FIGURE 18–3. Angle A is bisected by line AC. Line AC is perpendicular to line BD. Angle BAC is equal to angle DAC. Angle ACB is equal to angle ACD.

The rule of isometry. The two triangles have two angles that are equal and a common side; therefore, triangle BAC (shaded) is equal to triangle DAC.

Principles

The bisecting technique is based on a simple geometric principle known as the rule of isometry. The **rule of isometry** states that two triangles are equal if they have two equal angles and share a common side (Fig. 18–3). In dental radiography, this geometric principle is applied to the bisecting technique to form two imaginary equal triangles (Fig. 18–4). The bisecting technique can be described as follows:

- The film must be placed along the lingual surface of the tooth.

- At the point where the film contacts the tooth, the plane of the film and the long axis of the tooth form an angle.

- The dental radiographer must visualize a plane that divides in half, or bisects, the angle formed by the film and the long axis of the tooth. This plane is termed the **imaginary bisector.** The imaginary bisector creates two equal angles and provides a common side for the two imaginary equal triangles.

- The dental radiographer must then direct the central ray of the x-ray beam perpendicular to the imaginary bisector. When the central ray is directed 90 degrees to the imaginary bisector, two imaginary equal triangles are formed.

- The two imaginary triangles that result are **right triangles** and are **congruent.** The **hypotenuse** of one imaginary triangle is represented by the long axis of the tooth; the other hypotenuse is represented by the plane of the film.

When this rule of isometry is followed strictly, the radiographic image of the tooth is accurate; when the angle formed by the plane of the film and the long axis of the tooth is bisected and the x-ray beam is directed at a right angle to the imaginary bisector, the actual tooth and the image of the tooth on the film are the same length (Fig. 18–5).

Film Stabilization

In the bisecting technique, film-holding instruments or the patient's finger may be used to position and stabilize the film.

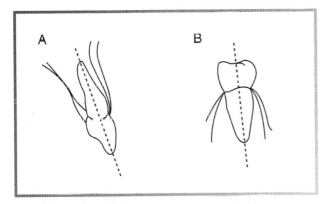

FIGURE 18–2. *A,* The long axis of the maxillary incisor divides the tooth into two equal halves. *B,* The long axis of a mandibular premolar divides the tooth into two equal halves.

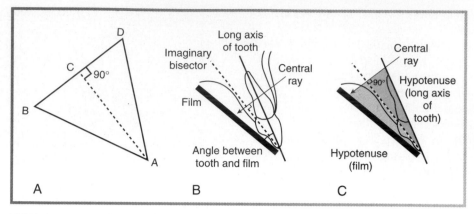

FIGURE 18–4. *A,* The film (line BA) is placed along the lingual surface of the tooth. At the point where the film contacts the tooth, the plane of the film and the long axis of the tooth (DA) form an angle (BAD). The imaginary bisector divides this angle into two equal angles (BAC and DAC). The central ray (BD) is directed perpendicular to the imaginary bisector and completes the third sides (BC and CD) of the two triangles. *B,* Bisecting technique showing the central ray directed at a right angle to the imaginary bisector. *C,* The two imaginary triangles that result are right triangles and congruent. The hypotenuse of each triangle is represented by the long axis of the tooth and the plane of the film.

FILM HOLDERS

A **film holder,** as defined in Chapter 6, is a device used to position an intraoral film in the mouth and retain the film in position during exposure. *With the bisecting technique, film holders are recommended because they eliminate the need for the patient to stabilize the film.* Examples of commercially available intraoral film holders that can be used with the bisecting technique include the following:

- **Rinn BAI Instruments** (Rinn Corporation, Elgin, IL). The BAI (B = bisecting, A = angle, I =

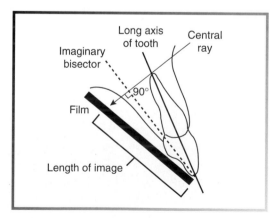

FIGURE 18–5. The image on the film is equal to the length of the tooth when the central ray is directed at 90 degrees to the imaginary bisector. A tooth and its radiographic image will be equal in length when two equal triangles are formed that share a common side (imaginary bisector).

instrument) film holders include plastic bite-blocks, plastic aiming rings, and metal indicator arms (Fig. 18–6). To reduce the amount of radiation received by the patient, snap-on ring collimators can be added to the plastic aiming rings. The BAI instruments have been designed to aid in the determination of horizontal and vertical angulations, minimize distortion from film bending, and prevent cone-cutting.

- **Stabe Bite-Block** (Rinn Corporation). The Stabe bite-block is a film holder that can be used with the paralleling technique or the bisecting technique (see Fig. 17–5C). For use with the bisecting technique, the scored front section is removed and the film is placed as close to the teeth as possible.
- **EEZEE-Grip Film Holder** (Rinn Corporation). Formerly known as the Snap-A-Ray, this film-holding device is used to stabilize a film in either the paralleling technique or the bisecting technique (see Fig. 17–5D).

The Stabe bite-block is disposable and is designed for one-time use only. The BAI instruments and the EEZEE-Grip film holder are reusable and must be sterilized following each use.

The BAI instruments with collimators are the film holders recommended for the bisecting technique; these holders are recommended because they include aiming rings that aid in the alignment of the PID and collimators that significantly reduce the amount of pa-

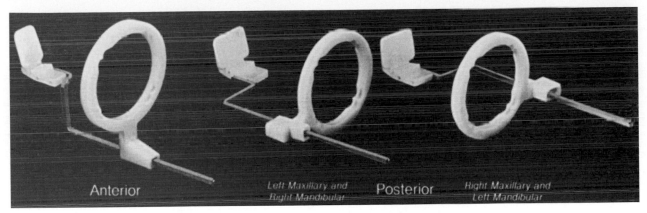

FIGURE 18–6. Rinn BAI instruments used with the bisecting technique.

tient exposure. The BAI instruments are simple to assemble and position. For information about the use of the BAI instruments or other film holders available for the bisecting technique, the dental radiographer should refer to the instructions provided by the manufacturer.

FINGER-HOLDING METHOD

The use of a film holder is not required in the bisecting technique; however, it is strongly recommended. The **finger-holding method** (also known as the *digital method*) is the alternative to using a film holder in the bisecting technique. In the finger-holding method, the patient's finger or thumb is used to stabilize the periapical film. *The finger or thumb is always placed behind the film and teeth.* With this method, the patient's thumb is used to position the maxillary films, and the patient's index finger is used to stabilize the mandibular films. The patient's left hand is used for exposures on the right side of the mouth, and the right hand is used for exposures on the left side.

Although the finger-holding method has remained popular with practitioners for years, it remains the least desirable method for exposing films using the bisecting technique. The disadvantages of the finger-holding method can be summarized as follows:

- The patient's hand is in the path of the primary beam, resulting in unnecessary radiation exposure.
- The patient may use excessive force to stabilize the film, causing the film to bend and resulting in image distortion.
- The patient may allow the film to slip from its position, resulting in inadequate exposure of the prescribed area.

- Without the use of a film holder with aiming ring, the dental radiographer may align the PID incorrectly, causing a partial image or cone-cut (cone-cutting is discussed in Chapter 20).

Because a film holder may not always be available or because the dental radiographer is unfamiliar with the available film holder, the use of the finger-holding method is demonstrated in this text.

Film

Traditionally, Size 2 intraoral film is used with the bisecting technique. In the anterior regions, Size 2 film is always placed with the long portion of the film in a *vertical* (upright) direction. In the posterior regions, Size 2 film is always placed with the long portion of the film in a *horizontal* (sideways) direction.

PID Angulations

In the bisecting technique, the angulation of the PID is critical. **Angulation** is a term used to describe the alignment of the central ray of the x-ray beam in the horizontal and vertical planes. Angulation can be varied by moving the PID in either a horizontal or vertical direction. The use of the BAI instruments with aiming rings dictates the proper PID angulation. However, when the finger-holding method is employed, the dental radiographer must determine both the horizontal and vertical angulations.

HORIZONTAL ANGULATION

Horizontal angulation refers to the positioning of the tubehead and direction of the central ray in a horizon-

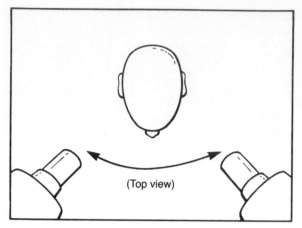

FIGURE 18–7. Horizontal angulation of the cone refers to cone placement in a side-to-side (ear-to-ear) direction. (From Haring JI, Lind LJ: Radiographic Interpretation for the Dental Hygienist. Philadelphia, WB Saunders, 1993.)

tal or side-to-side plane (Fig. 18–7). The horizontal angulation does not differ according to the radiographic technique used; the paralleling, bisecting, and bite-wing techniques all use the same principles of horizontal angulation.

Correct Horizontal Angulation. With correct horizontal angulation, the central ray is directed perpendicular to the curvature of the arch and *through* the contact areas of the teeth (Fig. 18–8). As a result, the contact areas on the radiograph appear to be "opened."

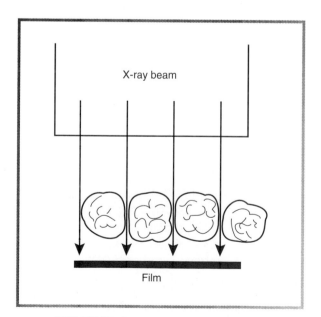

FIGURE 18–8. Correct horizontal angulation.

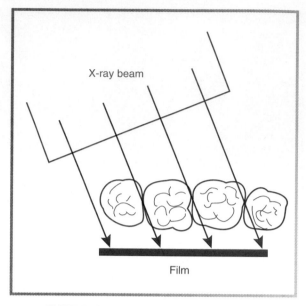

FIGURE 18–9. Incorrect horizontal angulation.

Incorrect Horizontal Angulation. Incorrect horizontal angulation results in overlapped (unopened) contact areas (Fig. 18–9). A film with overlapped interproximal contact areas cannot be used to examine the interproximal areas of the teeth (Fig. 18–10).

VERTICAL ANGULATION

Vertical angulation refers to the positioning of the PID in a vertical or up and down plane (Fig. 18–11). Vertical angulation is measured in degrees and is registered on the outside of the tubehead. The vertical angulation differs according to the radiographic technique used: (1) with the paralleling technique, the ver-

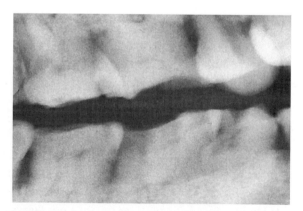

FIGURE 18–10. Overlapped contacts. (From Haring JI, Lind LJ: Radiographic Interpretation for the Dental Hygienist. Philadelphia, WB Saunders, 1993.)

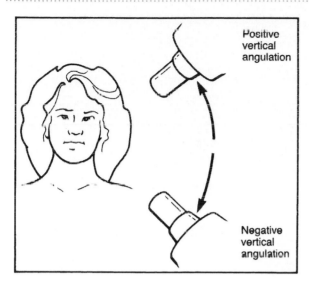

FIGURE 18–11. Vertical angulation of the cone refers to cone placement in an up-and-down (head-to-toe) direction. (From Haring JI, Lind LJ: Radiographic Interpretation for the Dental Hygienist. Philadelphia, WB Saunders, 1993.)

tical angulation of the central ray is directed *perpendicular to the film and the long axis of the tooth;* (2) with the bisecting technique, the vertical angulation is determined by the imaginary bisector; the central ray is directed *perpendicular to the imaginary bisector;* and (3) with the bite-wing technique, the vertical angulation is predetermined; the central ray is directed at *+10 degrees to the occlusal plane* (see Chapter 19).

Correct Vertical Angulation. Correct vertical angulation results in a radiographic image that is the same length as the tooth. Some recommended vertical angulation ranges for the bisecting technique are listed in Table 18–1.

TABLE 18–1. Recommended Vertical Angulation Ranges (Bisecting Technique)*

	Maxillary Vertical Angulation (degrees)	Mandibular Vertical Angulation (degrees)
Canines	+45 to +55	−20 to −30
Incisors	+40 to +50	−15 to −25
Premolars	+30 to +40	−10 to −15
Molars	+20 to +30	−5 to 0

*Using the finger-holding method.

Incorrect Vertical Angulation. Incorrect vertical angulation results in a radiographic image that is not the same length as the tooth; instead, the image appears longer or shorter. Elongated or foreshortened images are not diagnostic.

FORESHORTENED IMAGES. Foreshortened images refer to images of the teeth that appear shortened. **Foreshortening** of images results from excessive vertical angulation. When the vertical angulation is too steep, the image of the tooth on the film appears shorter than the actual tooth (Fig. 18–12). Foreshortening also occurs if the central ray is directed perpendicular to the plane of the film rather than perpendicular to the imaginary bisector.

ELONGATED IMAGES. Elongated images refer to images of the teeth that appear too long. **Elongation** of images results from insufficient vertical angulation. When the vertical angulation is too flat, the image of the tooth on the film appears longer than the actual tooth (Fig. 18–13). Elongation also occurs if the central ray is directed perpendicular to the long axis of the tooth rather than perpendicular to the imaginary bisector.

Rules

Five basic rules should be followed in the bisecting technique.

- **Film placement.** The film must be positioned to cover the prescribed area of teeth to be examined. Specific film placements are described in the Procedures section of this chapter.
- **Film position.** The film must be placed against the lingual surface of the tooth. The occlusal end of the film (indicated by the raised identification dot) must extend approximately 1/8 inch beyond the incisal or occlusal surfaces (Fig. 18–14). The apical end of the film must rest against the palatal or alveolar tissues. If the finger-holding method is used to stabilize the film, the patient should be instructed to press the film gently against the cervical portion (where the crown meets the root) of the tooth (Fig. 18–15).
- **Vertical angulation.** The central ray of the x-ray beam must be directed *perpendicular* (at a right angle) to the imaginary bisector that divides the angle formed by the film and the long axis of the tooth.
- **Horizontal angulation.** The central ray of the

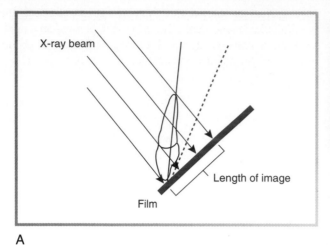

A

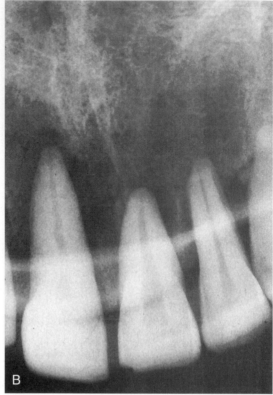

B

FIGURE 18–12. *A,* If the vertical angulation is too steep, the image on the film is shorter than the actual tooth. *B,* Foreshortened images. (From Haring JI, Lind LJ: Radiographic Interpretation for the Dental Hygienist. Philadelphia, WB Saunders, 1993.)

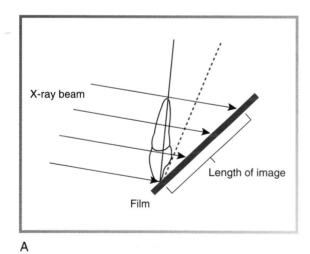

A

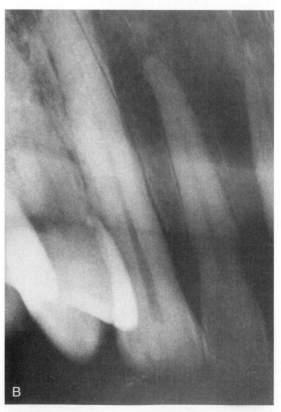

B

FIGURE 18–13. *A,* If the vertical angulation is too flat, the image on the film is longer than the actual tooth. *B,* Elongated images. (From Haring JI, Lind LJ: Radiographic Interpretation for the Dental Hygienist. Philadelphia, WB Saunders, 1993.)

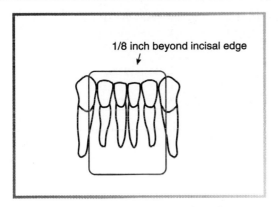

FIGURE 18-14. Approximately 1/8 inch of the film must appear beyond the incisal edges of the teeth.

x-ray beam must be directed through the contact areas between the teeth.

- **Film exposure.** Center the x-ray beam on the film to ensure that all areas of the film are exposed. Failure to center the x-ray beam results in a partial image on the film or a cone-cut.

STEP-BY-STEP PROCEDURES

Step-by-step procedures for the exposure of periapical films using the bisecting technique include the follow-

ing: patient preparation, equipment preparation, and film placement methods. Prior to exposing any dental radiographs using the bisecting technique, infection control procedures (as detailed in Chapter 15) must be completed.

Patient Preparation

Following the completion of infection control procedures and the preparation of the treatment area and supplies, the patient should be seated. After seating the patient, and prior to the exposure of any films, the dental radiographer must prepare the patient for film exposure (see "Procedure: Patient Preparation for Bisecting Technique").

Equipment Preparation

Following patient preparation, the dental radiographer must complete equipment preparations before exposing any films (see "Procedure: Equipment Preparation").

Exposure Sequence for Film Placements

When using the bisecting technique, an **exposure sequence,** or definite order for periapical film placements and exposures, must be followed. The dental

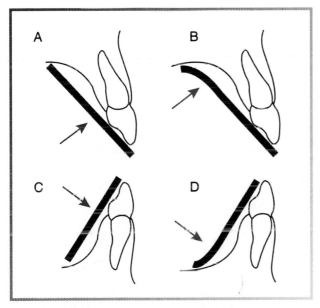

FIGURE 18-15. Correct and incorrect finger placement (arrows indicate finger pressure holding film in place). *A,* Correct finger placement at crown-gingival junction. *B,* Incorrect finger placement on palatal tissues. *C,* Correct finger placement at crown-gingival junction. *D,* Incorrect finger placement on alveolar tissues.

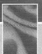

PROCEDURE

Patient Preparation for Bisecting Technique

1. Briefly explain the radiographic procedure to the patient before the procedure begins.

2. Position the patient upright in the chair. The level of the chair must be adjusted to a comfortable working height for the dental radiographer.

3. Adjust the headrest to support the patient's head. The patient's head must be positioned so that the arch that is being radiographed is parallel to the floor and the midsagittal plane is perpendicular to the floor.

4. Place and secure the lead apron with thyroid collar over the patient.

5. Remove all objects from the patient's mouth (e.g., dentures, retainers, chewing gum) that may interfere with film exposure. Eyeglasses must also be removed.

PROCEDURE

Equipment Preparation

1. Set the exposure factors (kilovoltage, milliamperage, and time) on the x-ray unit according to the recommendations of the film manufacturer. Either a short (8-inch) or long (16-inch) cone may be used with the bisecting technique; typically the short cone is preferred.

2. If film holders are used with the bisecting technique, open the sterilized package containing the film holder, and, if necessary, assemble the film holder.

radiographer must have an established exposure routine to prevent errors and use time efficiently. Working without an exposure sequence may result in omitting an area or exposing an area twice.

ANTERIOR EXPOSURE SEQUENCE

When exposing periapical films with the bisecting technique, *always* start with the **anterior teeth** (canines and incisors). The rationale for beginning with anterior film placements is as follows: anterior film placements are less likely to cause the patient to gag. Once the gag reflex has been stimulated, the patient may gag on films that could normally be tolerated. Management of the patient with a hypersensitive gag reflex is discussed in Chapter 25.

With Size 2 film, a total of six anterior film placements are used in the bisecting technique: three maxillary exposures and three mandibular exposures. The recommended anterior periapical exposure sequence for the bisecting technique using the finger-holding method is as follows (Table 18–2):

1. Begin with the maxillary right canine (tooth No. 6).
2. Expose all of the maxillary anterior teeth from *right to left.*
3. End with the maxillary left canine (tooth No. 11).
4. Next, move to the mandibular arch.
5. Begin with the mandibular left canine (tooth No. 22).
6. Expose all of the mandibular anterior teeth from *left to right.*
7. Finish with the mandibular right canine (tooth No. 27).

As previously discussed in Chapter 17, when the dental radiographer works from right to left in the maxillary arch and then from left to right in the mandibular arch, no wasted movement or shifting of the PID occurs (see Fig. 17–10). In addition, when working from right to left and then from left to right, the teeth are exposed in increasing numerical order. This exposure sequence allows the dental radiographer easily to keep track of the last exposure if interrupted.

POSTERIOR EXPOSURE SEQUENCE

Following anterior film placements, the **posterior teeth** (premolars and molars) are exposed. In each quadrant, *always* expose the premolar film first and then the molar film. The rationale for exposing the premolar film first is as follows:

- Premolar film placement is easier for the patient to tolerate.

TABLE 18–2. Exposure Sequence for Anterior Film Placement (Bisecting Technique)*

Exposure Number	Arch	Side	Tooth	Tooth Number
1	maxillary	right	canine	6
2	maxillary	right	lateral incisor	7
	maxillary	right	central incisor	8
	maxillary	left	central incisor	9
	maxillary	left	lateral incisor	10
3	maxillary	left	canine	11
4	mandibular	left	canine	22
5	mandibular	left	lateral incisor	23
	mandibular	left	central incisor	24
	mandibular	right	central incisor	25
	mandibular	right	lateral incisor	26
6	mandibular	right	canine	27

*Using the finger-holding method.

TABLE 18-3. Exposure Sequence for Posterior Film Placement (Bisecting Technique)*

Exposure Number	Arch	Side	Teeth	Teeth Numbers
1	maxillary	right	premolars	4, 5
2	maxillary	right	molars	1, 2, 3
3	mandibular	right	premolars	28, 29
4	mandibular	right	molars	30, 31, 32
5	maxillary	left	premolars	12, 13
6	maxillary	left	molars	14, 15, 16
7	mandibular	left	premolars	20, 21
8	mandibular	left	molars	17, 18, 19

*Using the finger-holding method.

- Premolar exposure is less likely to evoke the gag reflex.

Eight posterior film placements are used in the bisecting technique: four maxillary exposures and four mandibular exposures. The recommended posterior periapical exposure sequence for the bisecting technique using the finger-holding method is as follows (Table 18-3):

1. Begin with the maxillary right quadrant.
2. Expose the premolar film (teeth No. 4 and 5) first and then the molar film (teeth No. 1, 2, and 3).
3. Move to the mandibular right quadrant.
4. Expose the premolar film (teeth No. 28 and 29) first and then the molar film (teeth No. 30, 31, and 32).
5. Move to the maxillary left quadrant.
6. Expose the premolar film (teeth No. 12 and 13) first and then the molar film (teeth No. 14, 15, and 16).
7. Finish with the mandibular left quadrant.
8. Expose the premolar film (teeth No. 20 and 21) first and then end with exposure of the molar film (teeth No. 17, 18, and 19).

Film Placement

When exposing a complete mouth radiographic series (CMRS) using the bisecting technique, each periapical exposure has a prescribed **film placement**. Film placement, or the specific area where the film must be positioned prior to exposure, is dictated by the teeth and surrounding structures that must be included on the resultant radiograph. Prescribed film placements for the anterior teeth are detailed in the "Prescribed Placements for Anterior Periapical Films" chart and illustrated in Figure 18-16; posterior placements are detailed in the "Prescribed Placements for Posterior Periapical Films" chart and illustrated in Figure 18-17.

The specific film placements described in this chapter are for a 14-film periapical series using Size 2 films for all anterior and posterior exposures. Variations in film placement or the number of total films used may be recommended by other reference sources or individual practitioners (see the "Guidelines for Film Placements" chart).

PRESCRIBED PLACEMENTS FOR ANTERIOR PERIAPICAL FILMS

Maxillary Canine Exposure
The entire crown and root of the canine, including the apex and surrounding structures, must be seen on this radiograph. The interproximal alveolar bone and mesial contact of the canine must also be visible. The lingual cusp of the first premolar usually obscures the distal contact of the canine.

Maxillary Incisor Exposure
The entire crowns and roots of all four maxillary incisors, including the apices of the teeth and surrounding structures, must be seen on this radiograph. The interproximal alveolar bone between the central incisors and the central and lateral incisors must also be visible.

Mandibular Canine Exposure
The entire crown and root of the canine, including the apex and surrounding structures, must be seen on this radiograph. The interproximal alveolar bone and mesial and distal contacts must also be visible.

Mandibular Incisor Exposure
The entire crowns and roots of the four mandibular incisors, including the apices of the teeth and surrounding structures, must be seen on this radiograph. The contacts between the central incisors and between the central and lateral incisors must also be visible. In most cases, it is not necessary to see the distal contacts of the lateral incisors.

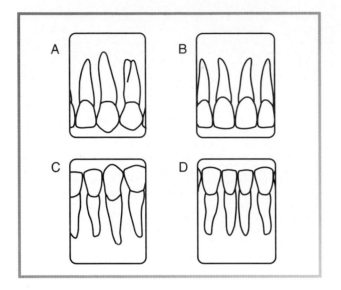

FIGURE 18–16. Prescribed placements for anterior periapical films. *A,* The maxillary canine exposure. *B,* The maxillary incisor exposure. *C,* The mandibular canine exposure. *D,* The mandibular incisor exposure.

FIGURE 18–17. Prescribed placements for posterior periapical films. *A,* The maxillary premolar exposure. *B,* The maxillary molar exposure. *C,* The mandibular premolar exposure. *D,* The mandibular molar exposure.

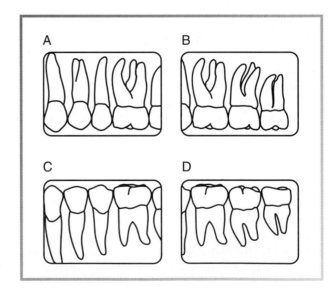

PRESCRIBED PLACEMENTS FOR POSTERIOR PERIAPICAL FILMS

Maxillary Premolar Exposure

All crowns and roots of the first and second premolars and first molar, including the apices, alveolar crests, contact areas, and surrounding bone, must be seen on this radiograph. In addition, the distal contact of the maxillary canine must be visible in this projection.

Maxillary Molar Exposure

All crowns and roots of the first, second, and third molars, including the apices, alveolar crests, contact areas, surrounding bone, and tuberosity region, must be seen on this radiograph.

Mandibular Premolar Exposure

All crowns and roots of the first and second premolars and first molar, including the apices, alveolar crests, contact areas, and surrounding bone, must be seen on this radiograph. In addition, the distal contact of the mandibular canine should be visible.

Mandibular Molar Exposure

All crowns and roots of the first, second, and third molars, including the apices, alveolar crests, contact areas, and surrounding bone, must be seen on this radiograph.

GUIDELINES FOR FILM PLACEMENT

- The white side of the film always faces the teeth.
- Anterior films are always placed vertically.
- Posterior films are always placed horizontally.
- The incisal or occlusal edge of the film must extend approximately 1/8 inch beyond the teeth.
- When positioning the film, always center the film over the area to be examined (as defined in the prescribed film placements).
- When positioning the patient's finger to stabilize the film, instruct the patient to "gently" push the film against the lingual surface of the tooth.

ANTERIOR FILM PLACEMENT

Anterior film placements include two maxillary canine exposures, one maxillary incisor exposure, two mandibular canine exposures, and one mandibular incisor exposure (see the respective Procedures). Size 2 film is used for all anterior film placements and is positioned vertically.

POSTERIOR FILM PLACEMENT

Posterior film placements include two maxillary premolar exposures, two maxillary molar exposures, two mandibular premolar exposures, and two mandibular molar exposures (see the respective Procedures). Size 2 film is used for all posterior placements and is positioned horizontally.

PROCEDURE

Maxillary Canine Exposure (Fig. 18–18)

1. Center the film packet on the canine.

2. Position the lower edge of the film parallel to the occlusal plane so that 1/8 inch extends below the incisal edge of the canine.

3. Instruct the patient to hold the film, using the thumb on the hand opposite the side on which the film is placed. Instruct the patient to exert light but firm pressure behind the film in the area where the teeth meet the gingival tissues.

4. Establish the correct vertical angulation by bisecting the angle and directing the central ray perpendicular to the imaginary bisector.

5. Establish the correct horizontal angulation by directing the central ray between the contacts of the canine and first premolar.

6. Position the PID using the correct vertical and horizontal angulations. Center the PID over the film to avoid cone-cutting.

7. Expose the film.

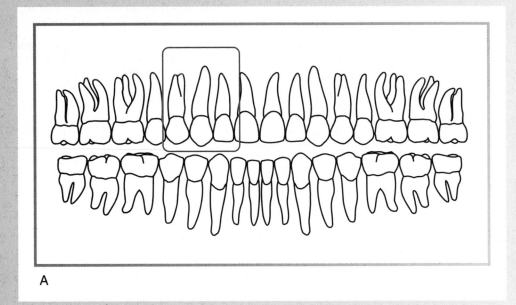

A

FIGURE 18–18. The maxillary canine exposure. *A,* Film placement.

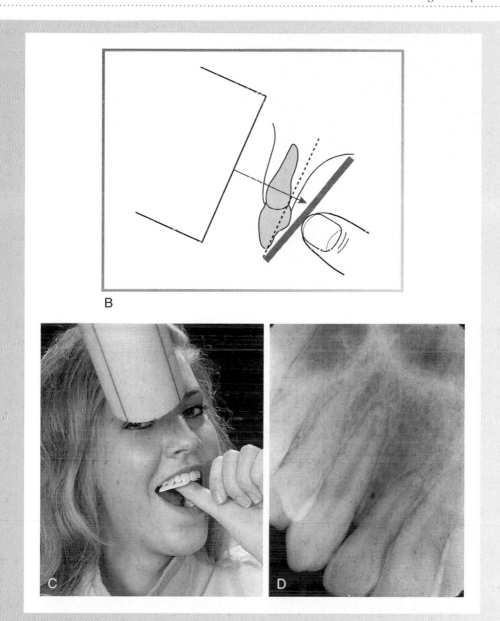

FIGURE 18–18. *Continued. B,* Relationship of film, teeth, imaginary bisector, and central ray. *C,* Exposure of film. *D,* Resultant radiograph.

PROCEDURE

Maxillary Incisor Exposure (Fig. 18–19)

1. Center the film packet on the contact between the two central incisors.

2. Position the lower edge of the film parallel to the occlusal plane so that 1/8 inch extends below the incisal edges of the teeth.

3. Instruct the patient to hold the film, using the thumb of either hand. Instruct the patient to exert light but firm pressure behind the film in the area where the teeth meet the gingival tissues.

4. Establish the correct vertical angulation by bisecting the angle and directing the central ray perpendicular to the imaginary bisector.

5. Establish the correct horizontal angulation by directing the central ray between the contacts of the central incisors.

6. Position the PID using the correct vertical and horizontal angulations. Center the PID over the film to avoid cone-cutting.

7. Expose the film.

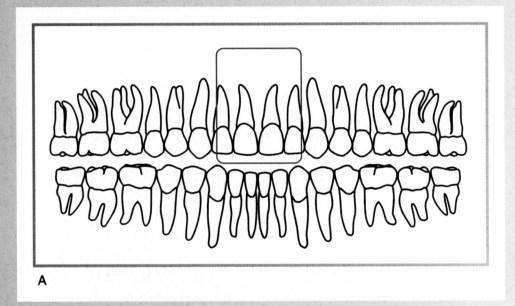

A

FIGURE 18–19. The maxillary incisor exposure. *A*, Film placement.

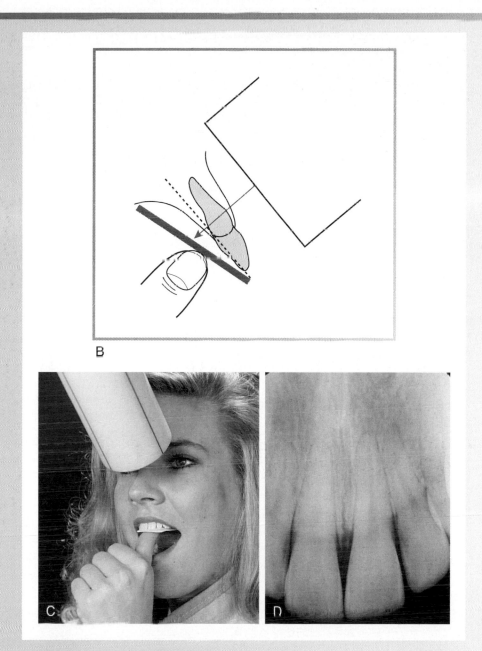

FIGURE 18–19. *Continued. B,* Relationship of film, teeth, imaginary bisector, and central ray. *C,* Exposure of film. *D,* Resultant radiograph.

PROCEDURE

Mandibular Canine Exposure (Fig. 18–20)

1. Center the film packet on the canine.

2. Position the upper edge of the film parallel to the occlusal plane so that 1/8 inch extends above the incisal edge of the canine.

3. Instruct the patient to hold the film, using the index finger on the hand opposite the side on which the film is placed. Instruct the patient to exert light but firm pressure behind the film in the area where the teeth meet the gingival tissues.

4. Establish the correct vertical angulation by bisecting the angle and directing the central ray perpendicular to the imaginary bisector.

5. Establish the correct horizontal angulation by directing the central ray between the contacts of the canine and first premolar.

6. Position the PID using the correct vertical and horizontal angulations. Center the PID over the film to avoid cone-cutting.

7. Expose the film.

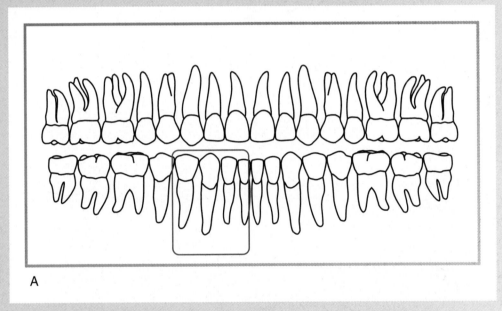

A

FIGURE 18–20. The mandibular canine exposure. *A,* Film placement.

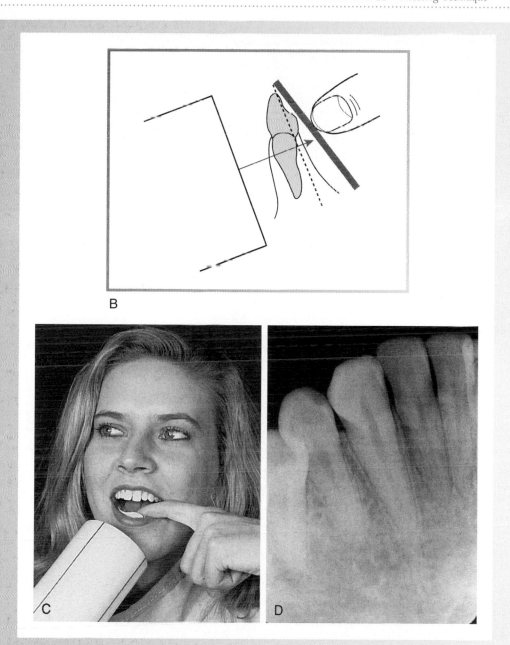

FIGURE 18–20. *Continued. B,* Relationship of film, teeth, imaginary bisector, and central ray. *C,* Exposure of film. *D,* Resultant radiograph.

PROCEDURE

Mandibular Incisor Exposure (Fig. 18–21)

1. Center the film packet on the contact between the two central incisors.

2. Position the upper edge of the film parallel to the occlusal plane so that 1/8 inch extends above the incisal edges of the teeth.

3. Instruct the patient to hold the film, using the index finger of either hand. Instruct the patient to exert light but firm pressure behind the film in the area where the teeth meet the gingival tissues.

4. Establish the correct vertical angulation by bisecting the angle and directing the central ray perpendicular to the imaginary bisector.

5. Establish the correct horizontal angulation by directing the central ray between the contacts of the central incisors.

6. Position the PID using the correct vertical and horizontal angulations. Center the PID over the film to avoid cone-cutting.

7. Expose the film.

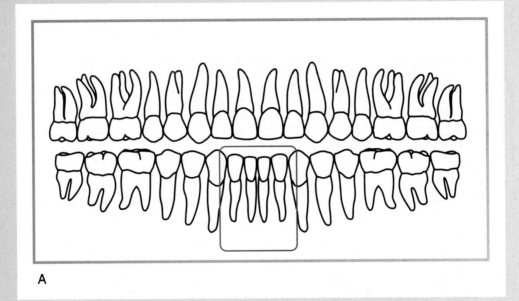

A

FIGURE 18–21. The mandibular incisor exposure. A, Film placement.

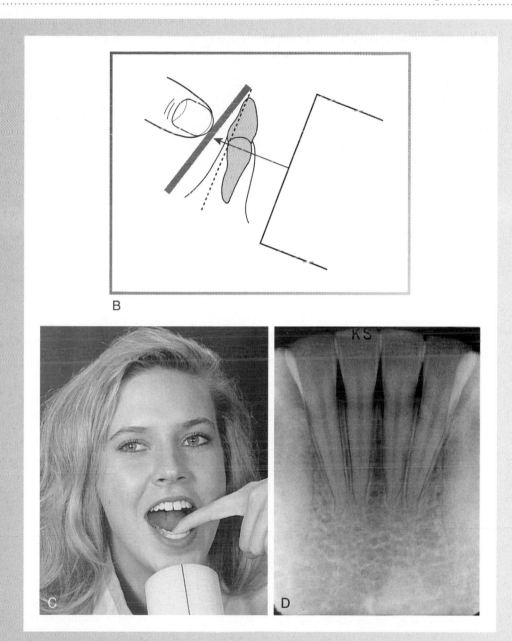

FIGURE 18-21. Continued. B, Relationship of film, teeth, imaginary bisector, and central ray. C, Exposure of film. D, Resultant radiograph.

PROCEDURE

Maxillary Premolar Exposure (Fig. 18–22)

1. Center the film packet on the second premolar, the front edge of the film should be aligned with the midline of the canine.

2. Position the lower edge of the film parallel to the occlusal plane so that 1/8 inch extends below the occlusal edges of the teeth.

3. Instruct the patient to hold the film, using the thumb on the hand opposite the side on which the film is placed. Instruct the patient to exert light but firm pressure behind the film in the area where the teeth meet the gingival tissues.

4. Establish the correct vertical angulation by bisecting the angle and directing the central ray perpendicular to the imaginary bisector.

5. Establish the correct horizontal angulation by directing the central ray between the contacts of the premolars.

6. Position the PID using the correct vertical and horizontal angulations. Center the PID over the film to avoid cone-cutting.

7. Expose the film.

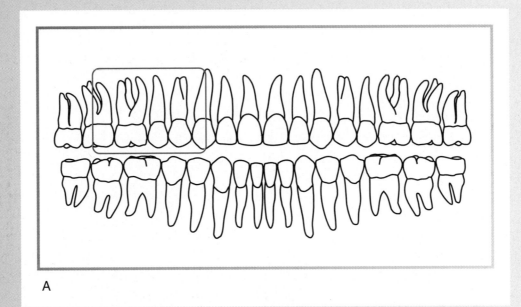

A

FIGURE 18–22. The maxillary premolar exposure. *A*, Film placement.

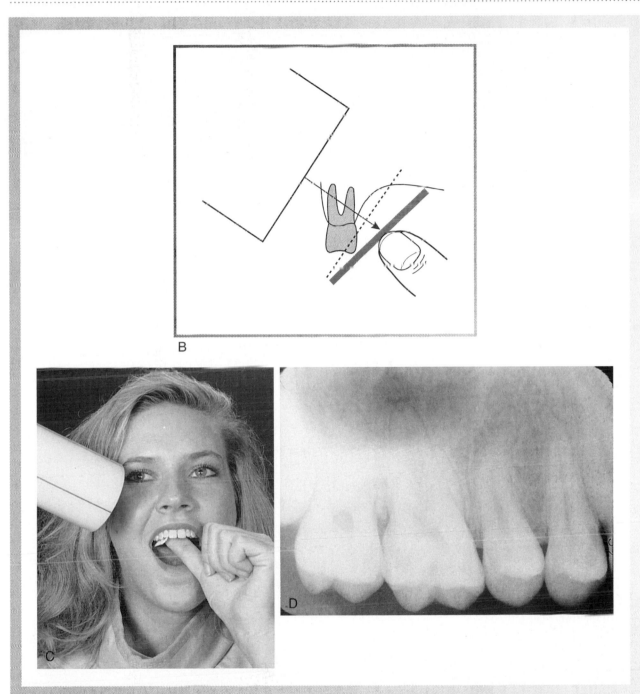

FIGURE 18-22. *Continued. B,* Relationship of film, teeth, imaginary bisector, and central ray. *C,* Exposure of film. *D,* Resultant radiograph.

PROCEDURE

Maxillary Molar Exposure (Fig. 18–23)

1. Center the film holder and film packet on the second molar; the front edge of the film should be aligned with the midline of the second premolar.

2. Position the lower edge of the film parallel to the occlusal plane so that 1/8 inch extends below the occlusal edges of the teeth.

3. Instruct the patient to hold the film, using the thumb on the hand opposite the side on which the film is placed. Instruct the patient to exert light but firm pressure behind the film in the area where the teeth meet the gingival tissues.

4. Establish the correct vertical angulation by bisecting the angle and directing the central ray perpendicular to the imaginary bisector.

5. Establish the correct horizontal angulation by directing the central ray between the contacts of the molars.

6. Position the PID using the correct vertical and horizontal angulations. Center the PID over the film to avoid cone-cutting.

7. Expose the film.

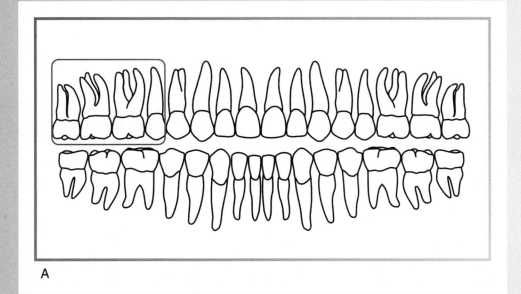

A

FIGURE 18–23. The maxillary molar exposure. *A,* Film placement.

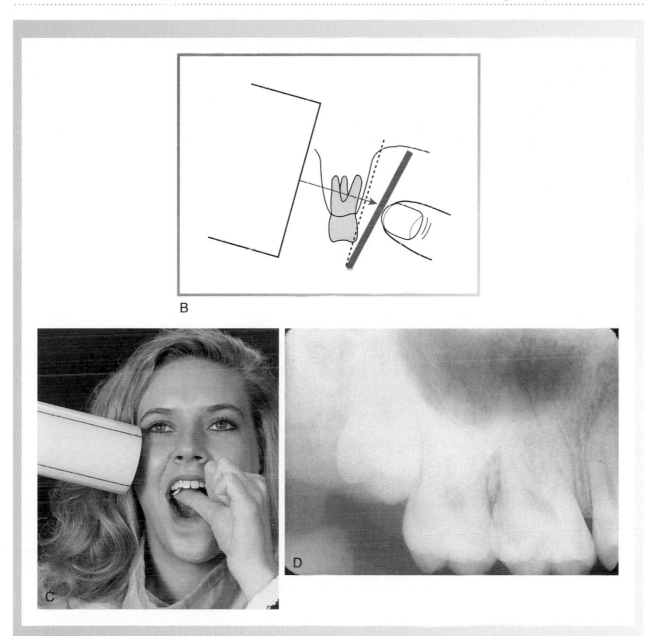

FIGURE 18-23. *Continued. B,* Relationship of film, teeth, imaginary bisector, and central ray. *C,* Exposure of film. *D,* Resultant radiograph.

PROCEDURE

Mandibular Premolar Exposure (Fig. 18–24)

1. Center the film holder and film packet on the second premolar; the front edge of the film should be aligned with the mesial of the canine.

2. Position the upper edge of the film parallel to the occlusal plane so that 1/8 inch extends above the occlusal edges of the teeth.

3. Instruct the patient to hold the film, using the index finger on the hand opposite the side on which the film is placed. Instruct the patient to exert light but firm pressure behind the film in the area where the teeth meet the gingival tissues.

4. Establish the correct vertical angulation by bisecting the angle and directing the central ray perpendicular to the imaginary bisector.

5. Establish the correct horizontal angulation by directing the central ray between the contacts of the premolars.

6. Position the PID using the correct vertical and horizontal angulations. Center the PID over the film to avoid cone-cutting.

7. Expose the film.

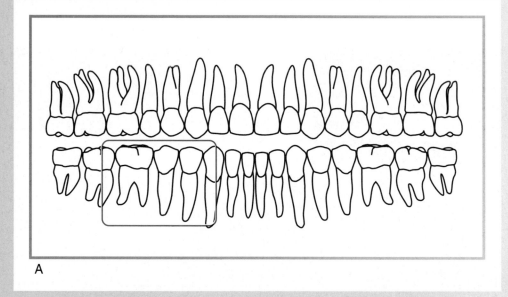

A

FIGURE 18–24. The mandibular premolar exposure. *A,* Film placement.

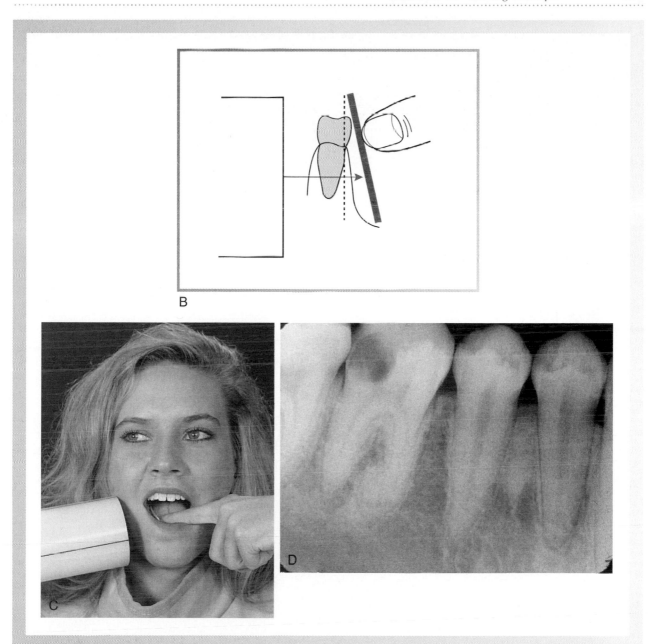

FIGURE 18–24. *Continued. B,* Relationship of film, teeth, imaginary bisector, and central ray. *C,* Exposure of film. *D,* Resultant radiograph.

PROCEDURE

Mandibular Molar Exposure (Fig. 18–25)

1. Center the film holder and film packet on the second molar; the front edge of the film should be aligned with the midline of the second premolar.

2. Position the upper edge of the film parallel to the occlusal plane so that 1/8 inch extends above the occlusal edges of the teeth.

3. Instruct the patient to hold the film, using the index finger on the hand opposite the side on which the film is placed. Instruct the patient to exert light but firm pressure behind the film in the area where the teeth meet the gingival tissues.

4. Establish the correct vertical angulation by bisecting the angle and directing the central ray perpendicular to the imaginary bisector.

5. Establish the correct horizontal angulation by directing the central ray between the contacts of the molars.

6. Position the PID using the correct vertical and horizontal angulations. Center the PID over the film to avoid cone-cutting.

7. Expose the film.

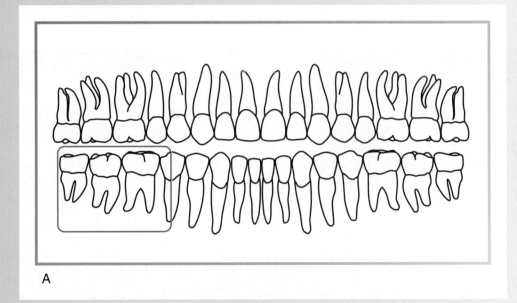

A

FIGURE 18–25. The mandibular molar exposure. *A,* Film placement.

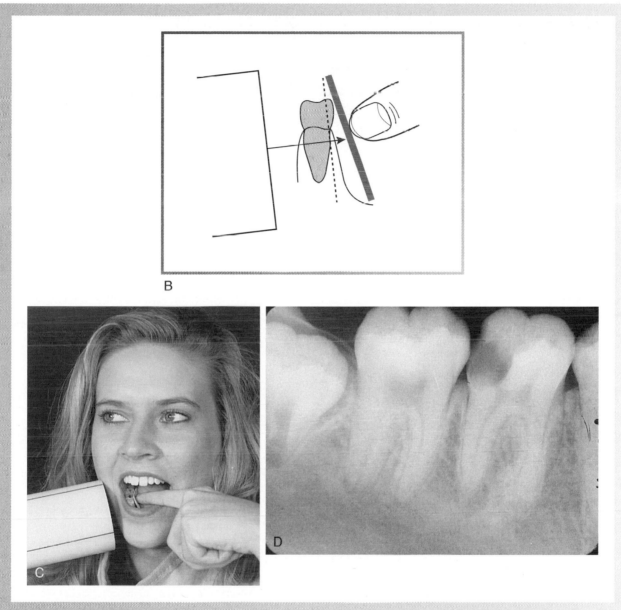

FIGURE 18-25. *Continued. B,* Relationship of film, teeth, imaginary bisector, and central ray. *C,* Exposure of film. *D,* Resultant radiograph.

ADVANTAGES AND DISADVANTAGES

As with all intraoral techniques, the bisecting technique has both advantages and disadvantages. The disadvantages of the bisecting technique, however, outweigh the advantages. Therefore, *the paralleling technique is preferred over the bisecting technique* for exposure of periapical films and should be used whenever possible.

Advantages

The primary advantage of the bisecting technique is that it can be used without a film holder when the anatomy of the patient (shallow palate, bony growths, sensitive mandibular premolar area) precludes the use of a film-holding device. Another advantage is decreased exposure time. When a short (8-inch) PID is used with the bisecting technique, a shorter exposure time is recommended.

Disadvantages

The primary disadvantage of the bisecting technique is dimensional distortion. The disadvantages of the bisecting technique can be summarized as follows:

- **Image distortion.** Distortion occurs when a short PID is used; with a short PID there is an increased divergence of x-rays, resulting in image magnification. Distortion also occurs when a tooth (three-dimensional structure) is projected onto a film (two-dimensional structure); structures that are farther away from the film appear more elongated than those closer to the film.
- **Angulation problems.** Without the use of a film holder and aiming ring, it is difficult for the dental radiographer to visualize the imaginary bisector and then determine the vertical angulation. Any error in vertical angulation will result in image distortion (elongation or foreshortening).
- **Unnecessary exposure.** If a film holder is not used, and the patient stabilizes the film with a finger, the patient's hand is unnecessarily exposed to the primary beam of x-radiation.

HELPFUL HINTS
in Using the Bisecting Technique

- ➤ **DO** set all exposure factors (kilovoltage, milliamperage, time) before placing any films in the mouth.
- ➤ **DO** ask patients to remove all intraoral objects and eyeglasses prior to placing any films in the mouth.
- ➤ **DO** use a definite order (exposure sequence) when exposing films to avoid errors and make efficient use of time.
- ➤ **DO** place each film in the patient's mouth with the identification dot oriented toward the occlusal edge of the film; this facilitates film mounting and ensures that the dot will not interfere with a diagnosis in the periapical area.
- ➤ **DO** explain the radiographic procedures that will be performed.
- ➤ **DO** instruct patients on exactly how to hold the film and remain still during the exposure.
- ➤ **DO** make certain the finger or thumb stabilizing the film is always positioned *behind* the film and teeth.
- ➤ **DO** memorize the recommended vertical angulation ranges for each periapical exposure and use these ranges as a guide when determining PID placement.
- ➤ **DO** direct the central ray perpendicular to the imaginary bisector.
- ➤ **DO** align the opening of the PID parallel to the imaginary bisector.
- ➤ **DO** use the word *please;* instruct patients to "open please."
- ➤ **DO** use praise; tell cooperative patients how much they are helping you.
- ➤ **DON'T** bend or crimp a film packet; film bending causes distortion of the image.
- ➤ **DON'T** use words such as *hurt.* Instead, inform patients that the procedure will be "momentarily uncomfortable."
- ➤ **DON'T** make comments like "Oops." Patients will lose confidence in your abilities.
- ➤ **DON'T** pick up a film packet if it drops. Leave it on the floor; it is contaminated. Instead, remove it during cleaning of the treatment area.
- ➤ **DON'T** allow patients to dictate how you should perform your duties. The dental radiographer must always remain in control of the procedures.
- ➤ **DON'T** begin with posterior exposures; posterior film placements may cause patients to gag. Instead, always start with anterior exposures.

SUMMARY

- The bisecting technique is a technique used to expose periapical films. As the term bisecting suggests, this technique is based on the concept of bisecting the angle that is formed by the film and the long axis of a tooth.
- The bisecting technique can be described as follows: (1) the film is placed along the lingual surface of the tooth;

(2) at the point where the film contacts the tooth, the plane of the film and the long axis of the tooth form an angle; (3) an imaginary bisector divides the angle in half, or bisects it; and (4) the central ray of the x-ray beam is directed perpendicular to the imaginary bisector.

- In the bisecting technique, film-holding instruments or the patient's finger may be used to stabilize the film. A variety of film holders are commercially available.
- The finger-holding method is not recommended for the following reasons: the patient's hand receives unnecessary radiation exposure; the patient may cause the film to bend, which results in image distortion; the patient may allow the film to slip, resulting in inadequate exposure of the prescribed area; without the use of a film holder and aiming ring, the dental radiographer may align the PID incorrectly, causing a partial image (cone-cut).
- Size 2 intraoral film is used with the bisecting technique. For anterior exposures, the film is always positioned vertically; for posterior exposures, the film is always positioned horizontally.
- Horizontal angulation refers to the positioning of the PID in a side-to-side plane. With correct horizontal angulation, the central ray is directed through the contact areas of the teeth; as a result, the contact areas on the radiograph appear "opened." Incorrect horizontal angulation results in overlapped (unopened) contacts.
- Vertical angulation refers to the positioning of the PID in an up-and-down plane. With the bisecting technique, the vertical angulation is determined by the imaginary bisector; the central ray is directed perpendicular to the imaginary bisector. Correct vertical angulation results in a radiographic image that is the same length as the tooth.
- Incorrect vertical angulation results in a radiographic image that is not the same length as the tooth. Foreshortening of the images occurs with excessive vertical angulation, whereas elongation of the images results with insufficient vertical angulation.
- Five basic rules must be followed in the bisecting technique: (1) the film must cover the prescribed area of interest; (2) the film must be positioned with 1/8 inch extending beyond the incisal or occlusal surfaces; (3) the central ray must be directed perpendicular to the imaginary bisector that divides the angle formed by the tooth and the film; (4) the central ray must be directed through the contact areas between the teeth; and (5) the x-ray beam must be centered over the film to ensure that all areas of the film are exposed.
- Prior to film exposure using the bisecting technique, the dental radiographer must complete infection control procedures, prepare the treatment area and supplies, seat the patient, explain the radiographic procedures to be performed, make chair and headrest adjustments, place the lead apron, remove intraoral objects and eyeglasses, set the exposure factors, and, if film holders are used, assemble the filmholding devices.

- An exposure sequence for periapical film placements must be followed when using the bisecting technique. The radiographer should always begin with the anterior exposures; anterior exposures are less likely to cause gagging. Following the anterior exposures, the posterior teeth are exposed. In each quadrant, the premolar film is always exposed first, and then the molar film.
- When exposing a complete mouth radiographic series using the bisecting technique, each of the 14 periapical exposures has a prescribed film placement. Prescribed film placements are described in charts and illustrated in Figures 18–16 and 18–17.
- The advantages of the bisecting technique are as follows: this technique can be used without a film holder and has a shorter exposure time.
- The disadvantages of the bisecting technique include the following: image distortion, angulation problems, and excess radiation exposure to the patient's hand.
- The paralleling technique is preferred to the bisecting technique and should be used whenever possible.

BIBLIOGRAPHY

Frommer HH: Accessory radiographic techniques. *In* Radiology for Dental Auxiliaries, 6th edition. St. Louis, Mosby-Year Book, 1996, pp. 181–204.

Goaz PW, White SC: Intraoral radiographic examinations. *In* Oral Radiology: Principles and Interpretation, 3rd edition. St. Louis, CV Mosby, 1994, pp. 180–199.

Johnson ON, McNally MA, Essay CE: Intraoral radiographic procedures. *In* Essentials of Dental Radiography for Dental Assistants and Hygienists, 6th edition. Norwalk, CT, Appleton and Lange, 1999, pp. 319–337.

Johnson ON, McNally MA, Essay CE: The periapical examination. *In* Essentials of Dental Radiography for Dental Assistants and Hygienists, 6th edition. Norwalk, CT, Appleton and Lange, 1999, pp. 339–375.

Langland OE, Sippy FH, Langlais RP: Intraoral radiographic techniques. *In* Textbook of Dental Radiography, 2nd edition. Springfield, IL, Charles C Thomas, 1984, pp. 255–265.

Manson-Hing LR: The bisecting-the-angle technic. *In* Fundamentals of Dental Radiography, 3rd edition. Philadelphia, Lea & Febiger, 1990, pp. 63–71.

Manson-Hing LR: Comparing technics and evaluating technical errors. *In* Fundamentals of Dental Radiography, 3rd edition. Philadelphia, Lea & Febiger, 1990, pp. 76–81.

Miles DA, Van Dis ML, Razmus TF: Intraoral radiographic techniques. *In* Basic Principles of Oral and Maxillofacial Radiology. Philadelphia, WB Saunders, 1992, pp. 86–99.

O'Brien RC: Exposing periapical films of the mandibular arch. *In* Dental Radiography: An Introduction for Dental Hygienists and Assistants, 4th edition. Philadelphia, WB Saunders, 1982, pp. 100–107.

O'Brien RC: Exposing periapical films of the maxillary arch. *In* Dental Radiography: An Introduction for Dental Hygienists and Assistants, 4th edition. Philadelphia, WB Saunders, 1982, pp. 83–97.

O'Brien RC: The bisection of the angle technique. *In* Dental Radiography: An Introduction for Dental Hygienists and Assistants, 4th edition. Philadelphia, WB Saunders, 1982, pp. 73–82.

Quiz Questions

MATCHING

For questions 1 to 4, refer to Figure 18–26. Match the letter of the item shown with the description below.

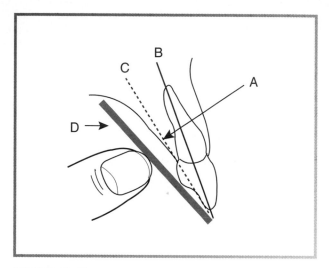

FIGURE 18–26

_____ **1.** Plane of the film

_____ **2.** Long axis of the tooth

_____ **3.** Imaginary bisector

_____ **4.** Central ray

IDENTIFICATION

For questions 5 to 10, refer to Figures 18–27, 18–28, and 18–29. Write in the letter of the item defined in each question.

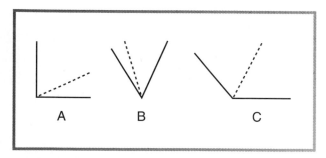

FIGURE 18–27

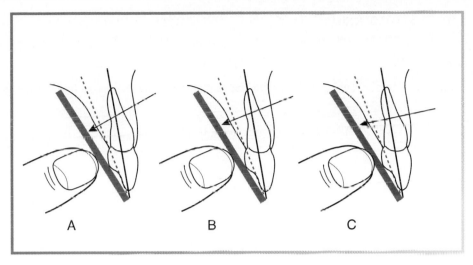

FIGURE 18-28

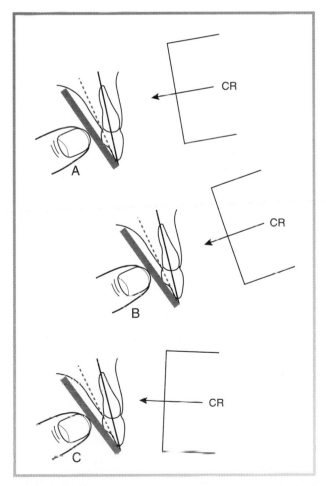

FIGURE 18-29

———— **5.** In Figure 18–27, identify the angle that is bisected.

———— **6.** In Figure 18–28, identify the central ray that is perpendicular to the imaginary bisector.

———— **7.** In Figure 18–29, identify the PID that is aligned correctly.

———— **8.** In Figure 18–29, identify the vertical angulation that results in foreshortening.

———— **9.** In Figure 18–29, identify the vertical angulation that results in elongation.

———— **10.** In Figure 18–29, identify the correct vertical angulation.

FILL IN THE BLANK

11. What happens to the radiographic image when a short (8-inch) PID is used?

_____

12. Which size film is used with the bisecting technique?

_____

13. Which film holder is recommended for use with the bisecting technique because it aids in alignment of the PID and reduces patient exposure?

_____

14. How is the patient's head positioned prior to exposing maxillary periapical films with the bisecting technique?

_____

15. How is the patient's head positioned prior to exposing mandibular periapical films with the bisecting technique?

_____

MULTIPLE CHOICE

———— **16.** Which of the following describes the proper direction of the central ray in the bisecting technique?

    a. 90 degrees to the long axis of the tooth
    b. 90 degrees to the film and long axis of the tooth
    c. 90 degrees to the film
    d. 90 degrees to the imaginary bisector

———— **17.** Which of the following describes the distance between the film and the tooth in the bisecting technique?

    a. the film is placed as close as possible to the tooth
    b. the film is placed away from the tooth and toward the middle of the oral cavity
    c. the film is placed parallel to the tooth
    d. none of the above

———— **18.** Which of the following are advantages of the bisecting technique? (1) increased accuracy, (2) simplicity of use, (3) shorter exposure time

    a. 1, 2, 3
    b. 1, 2
    c. 2, 3
    d. 3 only

_____ 19. The disadvantages of the bisecting technique outweigh the advantages.

  a. true
  b. false

ESSAY

20. State the rule of isometry.

21. In Figure 18–30, discuss the significance of the shaded areas.

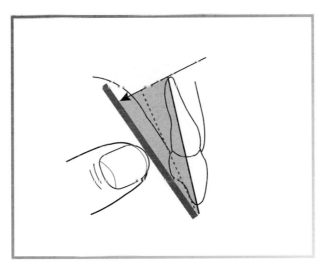

FIGURE 18–30

22. State the five rules of the bisecting technique.

23. Discuss the patient and equipment preparations necessary prior to using the bisecting technique.

24. Discuss the exposure sequence for the 14 periapical film placements using the bisecting technique.

25. Describe each of the 14 periapical film placements recommended for use with the bisecting technique.

26. Describe the finger-holding method of film stabilization.

27. List the disadvantages of the film-holding method.

28. Describe correct and incorrect horizontal angulation.

29. State the recommended vertical angulations for each maxillary periapical exposure using the bisecting technique.

30. State the recommended vertical angulations for each mandibular periapical exposure using the bisecting technique.

_____

Answers are supplied at the end of this book.

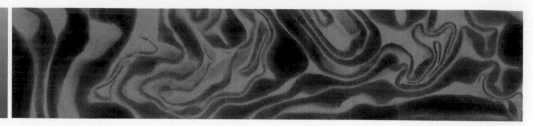

Bite-Wing Technique

OBJECTIVES

After completion of this chapter, the student will be able to:

- *Define the key words.*
- *Describe the purpose and use of the bite-wing film.*
- *Describe the appearance of opened and overlapped contact areas on a dental radiograph.*
- *State the basic principles of the bite-wing technique.*
- *List the two ways a film can be stabilized in the bite-wing technique and identify which one is recommended for bite-wing exposures.*
- *List the four film sizes that can be used in the bite-wing technique and identify which film size is recommended for exposures in the adult patient.*
- *Describe correct and incorrect horizontal angulation.*
- *Describe the difference between positive and negative vertical angulation.*
- *State the recommended vertical angulation for all bite-wing exposures.*
- *State the basic rules for the bite-wing technique.*
- *Describe the patient and equipment preparations that are necessary before using the bite-wing technique.*
- *Discuss the exposure sequence for a complete mouth radiographic series (CMRS) that includes both periapical and bite-wing exposures.*

- *Describe the premolar and molar bite-wing film placements.*
- *Describe the purpose and use of vertical bite-wings. List the number of exposures and the size of film used in the vertical bite-wing technique.*

KEY WORDS

Angulation	Contact areas
Angulation, horizontal	Contacts, open
Angulation, negative vertical	Contacts, overlapped
	Edentulous
Angulation, positive vertical	Exposure sequence
	Film, bite-wing
Angulation, vertical	Film holder
Bite-wing, vertical	Film placement
Bite-wing tab	Interproximal
Bite-wing technique	Interproximal examination
Bone, alveolar	
Bone, crestal	Tori, mandibular
Caries	Torus, tori

INTRODUCTION

In dentistry, the radiographer must master a variety of intraoral radiographic techniques. The bite-wing technique is used to examine the interproximal surfaces of teeth. A bite-wing radiograph includes the crowns of the maxillary and mandibular teeth, the interproximal areas, and the areas of crestal bone on the same film. Bite-wing radiographs are used to detect interproximal caries (tooth decay) and are particularly useful in detecting early carious lesions that are not clinically evident. Bite-wing radiographs are also useful in examining the crestal bone levels between teeth.

Before the dental radiographer can use this important technique, an understanding of the basic concepts, including the terminology and principles relating to it, is necessary. In addition, the dental radiographer must comprehend patient preparation, equipment preparation, exposure sequencing, and the film placement procedures used in the bite-wing technique.

The purpose of this chapter is to present basic concepts and to describe patient preparation, equipment preparation, and film placement procedures used in the bite-wing technique. This chapter also outlines the advantages and disadvantages of the bite-wing technique and reviews helpful hints.

BASIC CONCEPTS

The **bite-wing technique** (also known as the *interproximal technique*) is a method used to examine the interproximal surfaces of teeth. Before the dental radiographer can competently use this technique, a thorough understanding of the terminology, principles, and basic rules of the bite-wing technique is necessary. In addition, a knowledge of the film holders, sizes of film, and position-indicating device (PID) angulations used with the bite-wing technique is also required.

Terminology

Interproximal: Between two adjacent surfaces.

Interproximal examination: Intraoral radiographic examination used to inspect the crowns of both the maxillary and mandibular teeth on a single film.

Bite-wing film: Type of film used in the interproximal examination. As the term bite-wing suggests, this film has a "wing" or tab. The patient *bites* on the *wing* to stabilize the film—hence the term bite-wing.

Alveolar bone: Bone that supports and encases the roots of the teeth (Fig. 19–1).

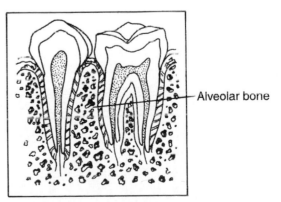

FIGURE 19–1. Alveolar bone. (From Haring JI, Lind LJ: Radiographic Interpretation for the Dental Hygienist. Philadelphia, WB Saunders, 1993.)

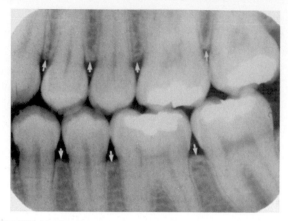

FIGURE 19–2. Crestal bone is the most coronal portion of alveolar bone found in between the teeth. (From Haring JI, Lind LJ: Radiographic Interpretation for the Dental Hygienist. Philadelphia, WB Saunders, 1993.)

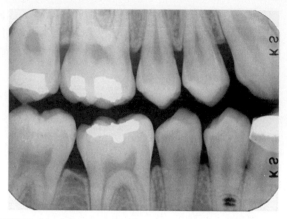

FIGURE 19–4. The open contacts in the premolar region appear as thin radiolucent lines. Note that the occlusal plane is postioned horizontally along the midline of the long axis of the film. (From Haring JI, Lind LJ: Radiographic Interpretation for the Dental Hygienist. Philadelphia, WB Saunders, 1993.)

Crestal bone: Coronal portion of alveolar bone found between the teeth (also known as the *alveolar crest*) (Fig. 19–2).

Contact areas: Area of a tooth that touches an adjacent tooth; the area where adjacent tooth surfaces contact each other (Fig. 19–3).

Contacts, open: On a dental radiograph, open contacts appear as thin radiolucent lines between adjacent tooth surfaces (Fig. 19–4).

Contacts, overlapped: On a dental radiograph, the area where the contact area of one tooth is superimposed over the contact area of an adjacent tooth is referred to as overlapped contacts (Fig. 19–5).

Principles

The basic principles of the bite-wing technique can be described as follows (Fig. 19–6):

- The film is placed in the mouth *parallel* to the crowns of both the upper and lower teeth.
- The film is stabilized when the patient bites on the bite-wing tab or bite-wing film holder.
- The central ray of the x-ray beam is directed through the contacts of the teeth, using a +10-degree vertical angulation.

Film Holder and Bite-Wing Tab

In the bite-wing technique, either a film holder or bite-wing tab is used to stabilize the film.

BITE-WING FILM HOLDER

A **film holder,** as defined in Chapter 6, is a device used to position an intraoral film in the mouth and

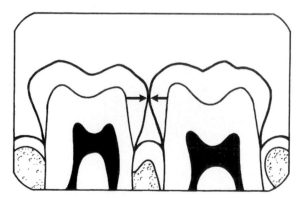

FIGURE 19–3. Contact areas are areas where adjacent tooth surfaces contact each other. (From Haring JI, Lind LJ: Radiographic Interpretation for the Dental Hygienist. Philadelphia, WB Saunders, 1993.)

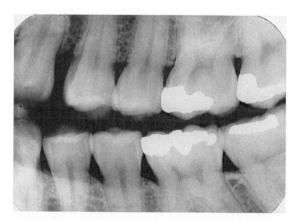

FIGURE 19–5. A nondiagnostic bite-wing with overlapped interproximal contacts. (From Haring JI, Lind LJ: Radiographic Interpretation for the Dental Hygienist. Philadelphia, WB Saunders, 1993.)

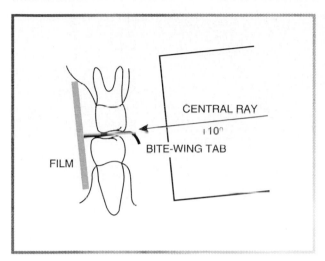

FIGURE 19-6. Positions of the film, bite-wing tab, and central ray in the bite-wing technique. The film is parallel to the crowns in the upper and lower teeth. The central ray is directed downward (+10 degrees vertical angulation.)

retain the film in position during the exposure. Film holders eliminate the need for the patient to stabilize the film. An example of a commercially available intraoral bite-wing film holder is the XCP bite-wing instrument.

- **Rinn XCP Bite-Wing Instruments** (Rinn Corporation, Elgin, IL). The XCP bite-wing instruments include plastic bite-blocks, plastic aiming rings, and metal indicator arms (Fig. 19–7). To reduce the amount of radiation the patient receives, a snap-on ring collimator can be added to the plastic aiming

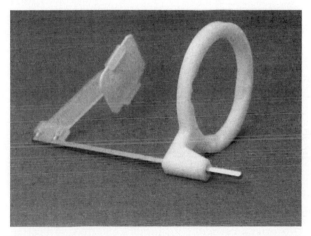

FIGURE 19-7. Film-holding device for bite-wing radiographs. Note external localizing ring used for postion-aiming tube of the x-ray machine to ensure that the entire film is in the x-ray beam. (From Goaz PW, White SC: Oral Radiology: Principles and Interpretation, 3rd edition. St. Louis, Mosby-Year Book, 1994.)

ring. These film holders are reusable and must be sterilized following each use.

- The Rinn XCP bite-wing instruments with collimators are recommended for bite-wing exposures; these holders include aiming rings that aid in the alignment of the PID and collimators that significantly reduce the amount of radiation exposure. These instruments are simple to position and easy to sterilize. For information about the use of the Rinn XCP bite-wing instruments, the dental radiographer should refer to the instructions provided by the manufacturer.

BITE-WING TAB

As an alternative to a film-holding device, a film can be fitted with a **bite-wing tab** (also called a *bite loop* or *bitetab*). The bite-wing tab is a heavy paperboard tab or loop fitted around a periapical film and used to stabilize the film during the exposure (Fig. 19–8A). A bite-wing film is a periapical film that has been fitted with a bite-wing tab; the periapical film is oriented in the bite loop so that the tab portion extends from the white side (tube side) of the film. Bite-wing films may be purchased with the tabs attached to the film, or they may be constructed from a periapical film and bite-wing tab. Bite loops are available in various sizes; adhesive bitetabs are also available (Fig. 19–8B).

Film

As described in Chapter 7, four sizes of bite-wing film (0, 1, 2, and 3) are available. Table 7–2 summarizes the measurements and uses of these films.

Size 0: Size 0 film is used to examine the posterior teeth of children with primary dentitions. This film is always placed with the long portion of the film in a *horizontal* (sideways) direction.

Size 1: Size 1 film is used to examine the posterior teeth of children with mixed dentitions. In the posterior regions, Size 1 film is always placed with the long portion of the film in a *horizontal* direction. Size 1 film can also be used to examine the anterior teeth of adults (in vertical bite-wing exposures). In the anterior regions, Size 1 film is always placed with the long portion of the film in a *vertical* (up-and-down) direction.

Size 2: Size 2 film is used to examine the posterior teeth in adults and may be placed horizontally or vertically. For most bite-wing exposures, Size 2 film is placed with the long portion of the film in a *horizontal* direction. When vertical posterior bite-wing exposures are indicated, Size 2 film is

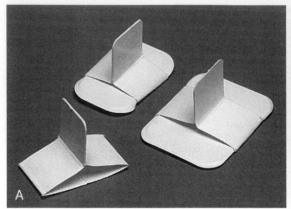

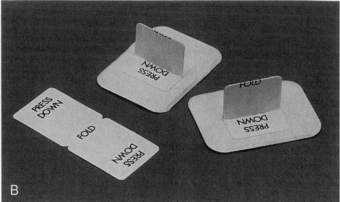

FIGURE 19–8. *A,* Bite-wing tabs. *B,* Adhesive bite-wing tabs.

placed with the long portion of the film in a *vertical* direction.

Size 3: Size 3 film is longer and narrower than the standard Size 2 film and is used *only* for bite-wings. One film is exposed on each side of the arch to examine all of the premolar and molar contact areas. Size 3 film is placed with the long portion of the film in a *horizontal* direction.

In the adult patient, Size 2 film is recommended for bite-wing exposures. Size 3 film is *not* recommended. With Size 3 film, overlapped contacts result because of the difference in the curvature of the arch between the premolar and molar areas. In addition, the crestal bone areas may not be adequately seen on the radiographs of patients with bone loss because of the narrow shape of the film.

PID Angulations

In the bite-wing technique, the angulation of the PID is critical. As defined in Chapter 18, **angulation** is a term used to describe the alignment of the central ray of the x-ray beam in the horizontal and vertical planes. Angulation can be varied by moving the PID in either a horizontal or vertical direction. Use of the XCP bite-wing instruments with aiming rings dictates the proper PID angulation. However, when a bite-wing tab is used, the dental radiographer must determine both the horizontal and vertical angulations.

HORIZONTAL ANGULATION

As described in Chapter 18, **horizontal angulation** refers to the positioning of the central ray in a horizontal or side-to-side plane (see Fig. 18–7). The bite-wing, paralleling, and bisecting techniques all use the same principles of horizontal angulation.

Correct Horizontal Angulation. With correct horizontal angulation, the central ray is directed perpendicular to the curvature of the arch and *through* the contact areas of the teeth (see Fig. 18–8). As a result, the contact areas on the exposed radiograph appear "opened" and can be examined for evidence of caries (see Fig. 19–4).

Incorrect Horizontal Angulation. Incorrect horizontal angulation results in overlapped (unopened) contact areas (see Fig. 18–9). A film with overlapped interproximal contact areas cannot be used to examine the interproximal areas of the teeth for evidence of caries (see Fig. 19–5).

VERTICAL ANGULATION

As described in Chapter 18, **vertical angulation** refers to the positioning of the PID in a vertical or up and down plane (Fig. 19–9). Vertical angulation may be positive or negative and is measured in degrees on the outside of the tubehead (Fig. 19–10). If the PID is positioned *above* the occlusal plane and the central ray is directed downward, the vertical angulation is termed **positive** (+). If the PID is positioned *below* the occlusal plane and the central ray is directed upward, the vertical angulation is termed **negative** (−).

Correct Vertical Angulation. A +10-degree vertical angulation is recommended for the bite-wing radiograph. The +10-degree vertical angulation is used to compensate for the slight bend of the upper portion of the film and the slight tilt of the maxillary teeth (Fig. 19–11).

Incorrect Vertical Angulation. Incorrect vertical angulation used in the exposure of a bite-wing film results in a distorted image. For example, if a negative vertical angulation is used, the occlusal surfaces of the maxillary teeth are evident, and the apical regions of

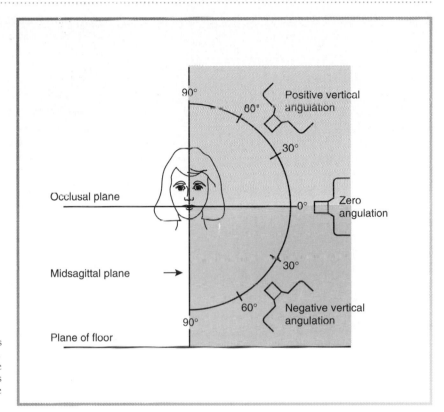

FIGURE 19–9. All vertical angulations above the occlusal plane are termed positive. Vertical angulations below the occlusal plane are termed negative. Zero angulation is achieved when the PID and central ray are parallel to the floor.

the mandibular teeth are seen (Fig. 19–12). A bite-wing radiograph exposed with an excessive negative vertical angulation is nondiagnostic.

Rules

Five basic rules must be followed in the bite-wing technique.

- **Film placement.** The film must be positioned to cover the prescribed area of teeth to be examined. Specific film placements are detailed in the following procedures.
- **Film positions.** The film must be positioned *parallel* to the crowns of both the upper and lower teeth. The film must be stabilized when the patient bites on the bite-wing tab or bite-wing holder.
- **Vertical angulation.** The central ray of the x-ray beam must be directed at +10 degrees (see Fig. 19–6).
- **Horizontal angulation.** The central ray of the x-ray beam must be directed through the contact areas between the teeth.
- **Film exposure.** The x-ray beam must be centered on the film to ensure that all areas of the film are exposed. Failure to center the x-ray beam results in a partial image on the film or a cone-cut.

STEP-BY-STEP PROCEDURES

Step-by-step procedures for the exposure of bite-wing films include patient preparation, equipment preparation, and film placement methods. Prior to exposing any dental radiographs using the bite-wing technique,

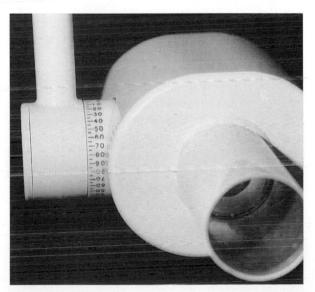

FIGURE 19–10. Vertical angulation is measured in degrees on the outside of the tubehead.

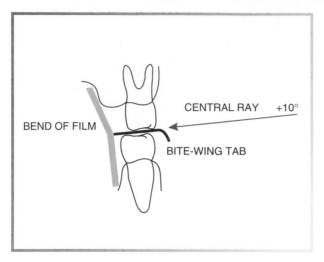

FIGURE 19–11. A +10 degree vertical angulation is used to compensate for the slight bend of the upper portion of the film and the tilt of the maxillary teeth.

infection control procedures (as described in Chapter 15) must be completed.

Patient Preparation

Following the completion of infection control procedures and the preparation of the treatment area and supplies, the patient should be seated. After seating the patient and before exposing any films, the dental radiographer must prepare the patient for film exposure (see "Procedure: Patient Preparation").

Equipment Preparation

Following patient preparation, equipment must also be prepared prior to the exposure of any films (see "Procedure: Equipment Preparation").

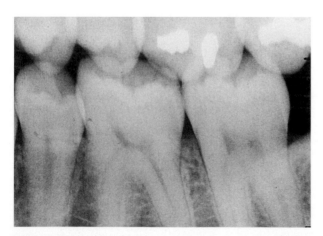

FIGURE 19–12. Negative vertical angulation.

PROCEDURE

Patient Preparation

1. Briefly explain the radiographic procedure to the patient before the procedure begins.

2. Position the patient upright in the chair. Adjust the level of the chair to a comfortable working height for the dental radiographer.

3. Adjust the headrest to support and position the patient's head. The patient's head must be positioned so that the upper arch is parallel to the floor and the midsagittal (midline) plane is perpendicular to the floor.

4. Place and secure the lead apron with thyroid collar on the patient.

5. Remove all objects from the mouth (e.g., dentures, retainers, chewing gum) that may interfere with film exposure. Eyeglasses must also be removed.

Exposure Sequence for Film Placements

When using the bite-wing technique, an **exposure sequence,** or definite order for film placement and exposure, must be followed. The dental radiographer must have an established exposure routine to prevent errors and make efficient use of time. Working without an exposure sequence may result in omitting an area or exposing an area twice.

As discussed in Chapter 16, a CMRS (complete mouth radiographic series) is an intraoral series of dental radiographs that shows all of the toothbearing areas of the upper and lower jaws. The CMRS may

PROCEDURE

Equipment Preparation

1. Set the exposure factors (kilovoltage, milliamperage, and time) on the x-ray unit according to the recommendations of the film manufacturer. Either a short (8-inch) or long (16-inch) cone may be used with the bite-wing technique.

2. If a film holder is used with the bite-wing technique, open the sterilized package containing the film holder, and assemble the film holder.

consist of periapical radiographs alone or a combination of periapical and bite-wing radiographs. Bite-wing films are used only in areas where teeth have interproximal contact with other teeth.

The number of bite-wing films necessary is based on the curvature of the arch and the number of teeth present in the posterior areas. The curvature of the arch often differs in the premolar and molar areas (Fig. 19–13). If the curvature of the arch differs, it is impossible to open all of the posterior contact areas on one bite-wing film. Consequently, two bite-wing films are typically exposed on each side of the arch. Because the curvature of the arch differs in most adult patients, a total of four bite-wing films is exposed: one right premolar, one right molar, one left premolar, and one left molar.

When posterior teeth are missing (e.g., in patients in whom the premolars have been extracted as part of orthodontic treatment), one bite-wing film on each side of the arch (instead of two) may be sufficient to cover the number of teeth present.

In the patient who requires both periapical and bite-wing radiographs, the following exposure sequence is recommended:

1. Expose all anterior periapical films first (see Chapters 17 and 18).
2. Follow with posterior periapical films (see Chapters 17 and 18).
3. Finish with the bite-wing exposures.

The exposure sequence ends with the bite-wing films because these films are relatively easy for the patient to tolerate. It is unwise to end the radiographic examination with difficult exposures (e.g., painful film placements or placements that elicit the gag reflex).

In the patient who requires bite-wing radiographs only, the following exposure sequence is recommended for *each* side of the mouth:

1. Expose the premolar bite-wing film first. (This film is easier for the patient to tolerate and is less likely to evoke the gag reflex.)
2. Expose the molar bite-wing film last.

Film Placement

When exposing bite-wing films, each exposure has a prescribed **film placement**. Film placement, or the specific area where the film must be positioned prior to exposure, is dictated by the teeth and surrounding structures that must be included on the resulting bite-wing radiograph. The specific film placements described in this chapter are for a four-film posterior

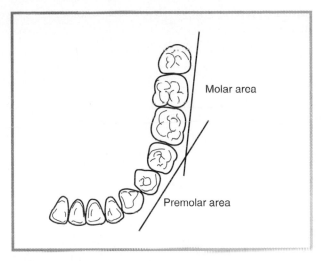

FIGURE 19–13. Notice the difference in the curvature of the arch in the premolar and molar areas.

bite-wing series using Size 2 film and bite-wing tabs. Variations in film placement, film size, or total number of films exposed may be recommended by other reference sources or individual practitioners (see Guidelines for Film Placement).

BITE-WING FILM PLACEMENTS

Film placements for the four posterior bite-wing exposures include the following: right and left premolar exposures and right and left molar exposures. It is important to note that in the step-by-step procedures that follow for both the premolar and molar bite-wing exposures, the film is placed *after* both the *vertical* and *horizontal* angulations have been set (see "Procedure: Premolar Bite-Wing Exposure" and "Procedure: Molar Bite-Wing Exposure").

GUIDELINES FOR FILM PLACEMENT

- The white side of the film always faces the teeth.
- In the posterior bite-wing series, the films are placed horizontally.
- The identification dot on the film has no significance in bite-wing film placement.
- When positioning the film, always center the film over the area to be examined (as defined in the prescribed film placements).
- When positioning the film, ask the patient to "slowly bite" on the bite-wing tab or bite-block of the film holder.

Premolar Bite-Wing Exposure (Fig. 19–14)

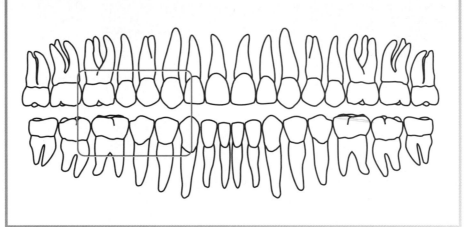

A

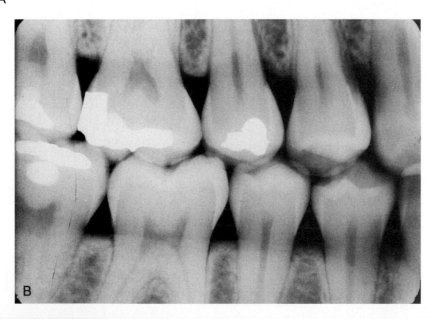

B

FIGURE 19–14. The premolar bite-wing. *A*, Film placement. *B*, Resultant radiograph.

1. Set vertical angulation at +10 degrees (Fig. 19-15)

2. To set the horizontal angulation, stand in front of the patient. Examine the posterior curvature of the arch. To better visualize the curvature of the arch, place your index finger along the premolar area. Align the open end of the PID parallel with your index finger and the curvature of the arch in the premolar area and direct the central ray through the contact areas (Fig. 19-16)

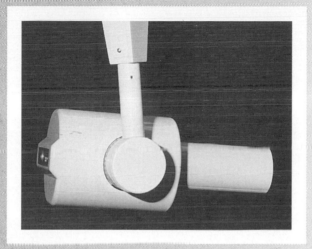

FIGURE 19-15. Vertical angulation is set at +10 degrees.

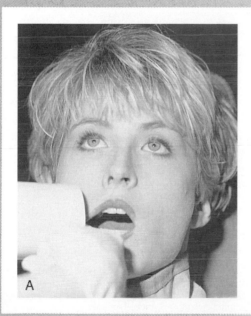

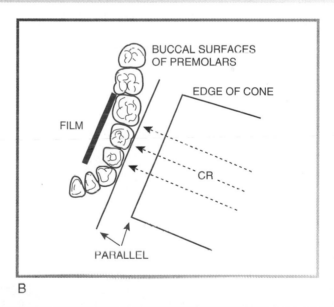

FIGURE 19-16. *A,* To better visualize the curvature of the arch, place your index finger along the premolar area. *B,* Correct horizontal angulation.

Procedure continued on following page

3. Make certain that the PID is positioned far enough forward to *cover both the maxillary and mandibular canines* and is positioned evenly over the mandibular and maxillary arches to avoid a cone-cut. The middle of the PID should be directed at the level of the occlusal plane (Fig. 19–17). After the vertical angulation, horizontal angulation, and PID position have been established the PID should not be adjusted, and the film should be placed without moving the PID.

4. Fold the bite-wing tab in half and crease it. Insert the film into the patient's mouth and place the lower half of the film between the tongue and the teeth. Place the biting surface of the tab on the occlusal surfaces of the teeth. Center the film on the second premolar; the front edge of the film should be aligned with the midline of the mandibular canine. Using your index finger, hold the bite-wing tab against the buccal surfaces of the premolars (Fig. 19–18). Hold in place during steps 5 and 6.

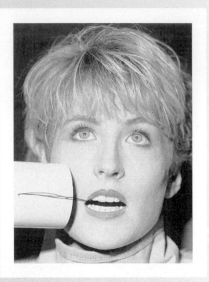

FIGURE 19–17. The middle of the position-indicating device should be directed at the level of the occlusal plane.

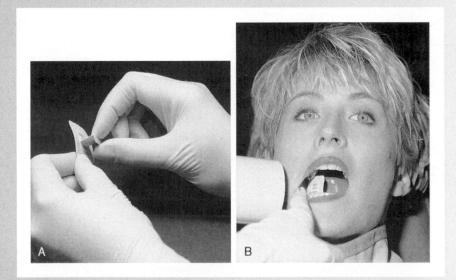

FIGURE 19–18. *A,* Crease the middle of the bite-wing before placing the film in the patient's mouth. *B,* Place the biting area of the tab on the occlusal surfaces of the teeth while holding the tab against the buccal surfaces of the premolars. The front edge of the film should be aligned with the middle of the mandibular canine.

5. Make certain that the patient's occlusal plane is parallel with the floor. If necessary, instruct the patient to lower the chin (Fig. 19–19).

6. To check for cone-cut, stand directly behind the tubehead and look along the side of the PID. No portion of the film should be visible; the film should be covered by the opening of the PID (Fig. 19–20). If the film is not visible, instruct the pa-

tient to "slowly close" while holding the bite-wing tab. If any portion of the film is visible, a cone-cut will result. In such instances, the PID must be adjusted to cover the film. After the PID has been positioned properly, instruct the patient to "slowly close" while holding the bite-wing tab.

7. Expose the film.

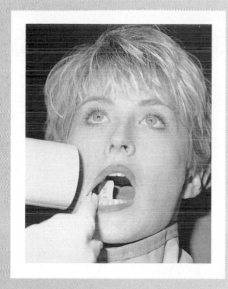

FIGURE 19–19. The patient's occlusal plane must be parallel with the floor.

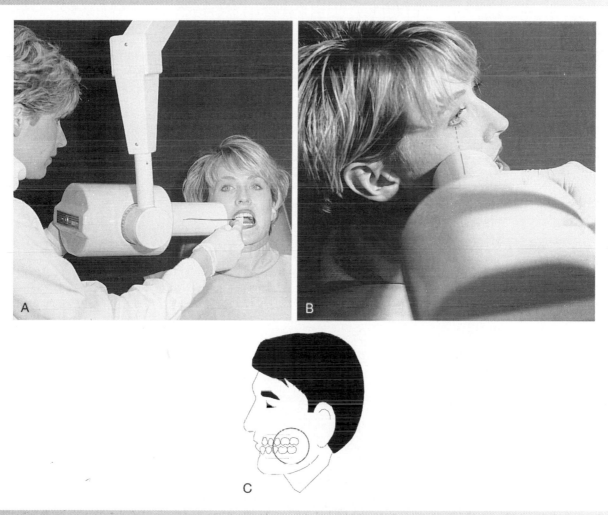

A

B

C

FIGURE 19–20. *A,* To check for cone-cuts, stand behind the tubehead and look along the side of the PID. *B,* No portion of the film should be visible. *C,* A cone-cut results when any portion of the film is visible.

PROCEDURE

Molar Bite-Wing Exposure (Fig. 19–21)

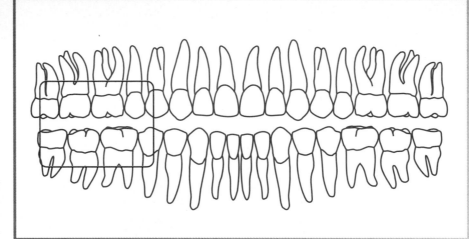

A

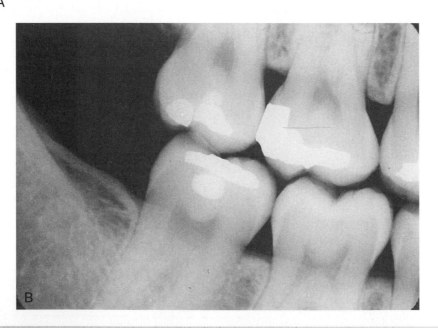

B

FIGURE 19–21. The molar bite-wing. A, Film placement. B, Resultant radiograph.

Procedure continued on following page

1. Set the vertical angulation at +10 degrees (see Fig. 19–15).

2. To set the horizontal angulation, stand in front of the patient. Examine the posterior curvature of the arch. To better visualize the curvature of the arch, place your index finger along the molar area. Align the open end of the PID parallel with your index finger and the curvature of the arch in the molar area and direct the central ray through the contact areas (Fig. 19–22).

3. Make certain that the PID is positioned far enough forward to *cover both the maxillary and mandibular second premolars* and is positioned evenly over both the mandibular and maxillary arches to avoid a cone-cut. The middle of the PID should be directed at the level of the occlusal plane (see Fig. 19–17). After the vertical angulation, horizontal angulation, and PID position have been established, the PID should not be adjusted, and the film should be placed without moving the PID.

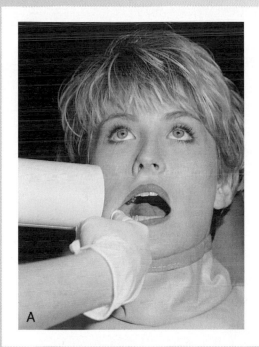

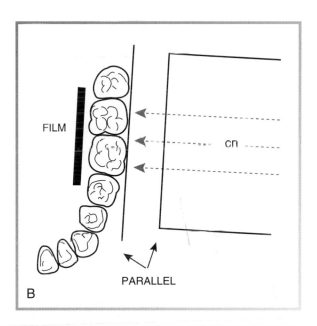

FIGURE 19–22. *A,* To better visualize the curvature of the arch, place your index finger along the molar area. *B,* Correct horizontal angulation.

4. Fold the bite-wing tab in half and crease it. Insert the film into the patient's mouth and place the lower half of the film between the tongue and teeth. Place the biting surface of the tab on the occlusal surfaces of the teeth. Center the film on the second molar; the front edge of the film should be aligned with the midline of the mandibular second premolar. Using your index finger, hold the bite-wing tab against the buccal surfaces of the molars (Fig. 19–23). Hold in place during steps 5 and 6.

5. Make certain that the patient's occlusal plane is parallel with the floor. If necessary, instruct the patient to lower the chin (see Fig. 19–19).

6. To check for cone-cut, stand directly behind the tubehead and look along the side of the PID. No portion of the film should be visible; the film should be covered by the opening of the PID (Fig. 19–24). If the film is not visible, instruct the patient to "slowly close" while still holding the bite-wing tab. If any portion of the film is visible, a cone-cut will result. In such instances, the PID must be adjusted to cover the film. After the PID has been positioned properly, instruct the patient to "slowly close" while still holding the bite-wing tab.

7. Expose the film.

Procedure continued on following page

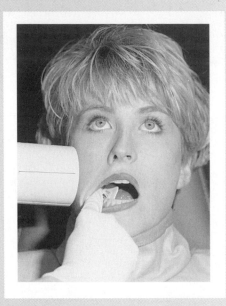

FIGURE 19–23. Place the biting area of the tab on the occlusal surfaces of the teeth while holding the tab against the buccal surfaces of the premolars. The front edge of the film should be aligned with the middle of the mandibular second molar.

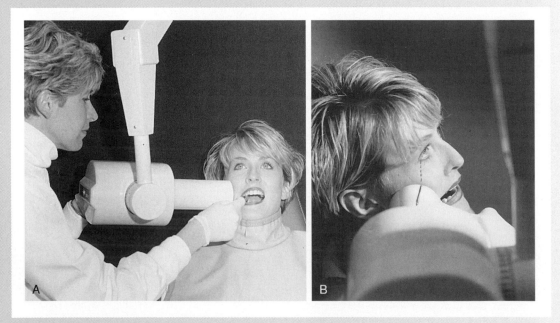

FIGURE 19–24. *A,* To check for cone-cuts, stand behind the tubehead and look along the side of the PID. *B,* No portion of the film should be visible.

VERTICAL BITE-WINGS

A **vertical bite-wing** can be used to examine the level of alveolar bone in the mouth. As the word vertical suggests, this bite-wing is placed with the long portion of the film in a *vertical* direction (Fig. 19–25). Vertical bite-wings are often used as post-treatment or follow-up films for patients with bone loss due to periodontal disease. The vertical bite-wing examination uses one-half the number of exposures included in a complete series of periapicals.

A total of seven films (three anterior and four posterior) are used to cover the canine, midline, premolar, and molar areas. Size 2 film may be used for all exposures, or a combination of Size 1 film (anterior teeth) and Size 2 film (posterior teeth) may be used. In the anterior regions, a longer bite-wing tab is often necessary. The patient should be instructed to bite on the tab in an end-to-end occlusal relationship (Fig. 19–26).

MODIFICATIONS IN TECHNIQUE

Modifications in the bite-wing technique may be used to accommodate variations in anatomic conditions.

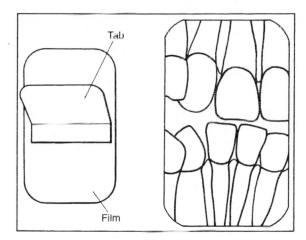

FIGURE 19–25. A vertical bite-wing can be used to evaluate the level of the supporting bone. (From Haring JI, Lind LJ: Radiographic Interpretation for the Dental Hygienist. Philadelphia, WB Saunders, 1993.)

Such modifications may be necessary in patients who have edentulous spaces or bony growths.

Edentulous Spaces

As described in Chapter 16, an **edentulous** space is an area where teeth are no longer present. An edentulous

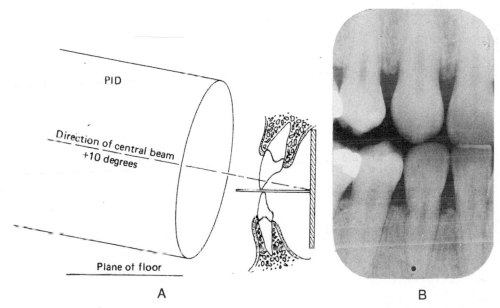

FIGURE 19–26. Anterior interproximal area. *A,* Center film packet vertically at midline and stabilize patient by gently closing on tab at incisal edges of teeth. Teeth meet tab in end-to-end position. Suggested vertical angulation is +10 degrees toward the center of the film; horizontally the x-ray beam is directed through the interproximal spaces. *B,* Bite-wing film of the right canine area. (From DeLyre WR, Johnson ON: Essentials of Dental Radiography for Dental Assistants and Hygienists, 4th edition. Norwalk, CT, Appleton and Lange, 1990.)

space may cause a problem with bite-wing film placement, and a modification in technique is necessary. A cotton roll must be placed in the area of the missing tooth (or teeth) to support the bite-wing tab or film holder. When the patient closes, the opposing teeth occlude on the cotton roll and support the bite-wing tab or film holder. Failure to support the bite-wing tab or film holder results in a tipped occlusal plane on the resulting radiograph.

Bony Growths

As described in Chapter 17, a **torus** (plural, tori) is a bony growth in the oral cavity. **Mandibular tori** are bony growths along the lingual aspect (tongue side) of the mandible. When using the bite-wing technique, mandibular tori may cause problems with film placement, and a modification in technique is necessary.

The film must be placed between the tori and the tongue (not *on* the tori) and then exposed. With large tori, the film is pushed away from the teeth. As a result, the patient bites on the very end of the bite-wing tab to stabilize the film, thus making it difficult for the dental radiographer to establish film placement. In such cases, a bite-wing film holder is recommended.

HELPFUL HINTS
For Using the Bite-Wing Technique

- ➤ **DO** set all exposure factors (kilovoltage, milliamperage, time) before placing any films in the mouth.
- ➤ **DO** ask patients to remove all intraoral objects and eyeglasses prior to placing any films in the mouth.
- ➤ **DO** use a definite order (exposure sequence) when exposing films to avoid errors and make efficient use of time.
- ➤ **DO** explain the radiographic procedures to be performed.
- ➤ **DO** instruct patients on how to close on the bite-wing tab and remain still during the exposure; make certain that the patient *remains* closed on the bite-wing tab during the exposure.
- ➤ **DO** set the vertical angulation at +10 degrees.
- ➤ **DO** direct the central ray through the contact areas of the teeth and align the opening of the PID parallel with the curvature of the arch.
- ➤ **DO** check for cone-cuts prior to exposing the film.
- ➤ **DO** use the word *please;* instruct patients to "open please."
- ➤ **DO** use praise; tell cooperative patients how much they are helping you.
- ➤ **DON'T** bend or crimp a film packet; excessive film bending causes distortion of the image.

- ➤ **DON'T** use words such as *hurt*. Instead, inform patients that the procedure will be "momentarily uncomfortable."
- ➤ **DON'T** make comments like "Oops." Patients will lose confidence in your abilities.
- ➤ **DON'T** pick up a film packet if it drops. Leave it on the floor; it is contaminated. Instead, remove it during cleaning of the treatment area.
- ➤ **DON'T** allow patients to dictate how you should perform your duties. The dental radiographer must always remain in control of the procedures.
- ➤ **DON'T** begin with the molar bite-wing exposure; molar film placements may cause patients to gag. Instead, always start with the premolar bite-wing.
- ➤ **DON'T** position a film on top of a torus (tori). Instead, always position the film between the torus and the tongue.

■ SUMMARY

- A bite-wing radiograph includes the crowns of the maxillary and mandibular teeth, the interproximal areas, and the areas of crestal bone on the same film. Bite-wing radiographs are useful for examining the interproximal surfaces of the teeth, detecting caries, and examining the crestal bone levels between the teeth.
- As the term bite-wing suggests, the film has a "wing" or tab. The patient *bites* on the *wing* to stabilize the film—hence the term bite-wing.
- The principles of the bite-wing technique can be summarized as follows:
  - the film is placed parallel to the crowns of both the upper and lower teeth
  - the film is stabilized when the patient bites on the bite-wing tab or bite-wing film holder
  - the central ray of the x-ray beam is directed through the contacts using a +10-degree vertical angulation
- In the bite-wing technique, a film holder or bite-wing tab may be used to stabilize the film. The Rinn XCP bite-wing film holder with collimator is recommended for bite-wing exposures. As an alternative to the holder, a film can be fitted with a bite-wing tab. Bite-wing tabs are available in various sizes; adhesive bitetabs are also available.
- Four sizes of film (0, 1, 2, and 3) can be used in the bite-wing technique; in the adult patient, Size 2 film is recommended.
- Horizontal angulation refers to the positioning of the PID in a side-to-side plane. With correct horizontal angulation, the central ray is directed through the contact areas of the teeth; as a result, the contact areas on the radiograph appear "opened." Incorrect horizontal angulation results in overlapped (unopened) contacts.
- Vertical angulation refers to the positioning of the PID in an up-and-down plane. A +10-degree vertical angulation is recommended for bite-wing radiographs to compensate for the slight bend of the upper portion of the film and the slight tilt of the maxillary teeth.
- Five basic rules must be followed in the bite-wing technique:

- the film must cover the prescribed area of interest
- the film must be positioned parallel to the crowns of the upper and lower teeth and stabilized by the bite-wing tab or film holder
- the vertical angulation must be directed at +10-degrees
- the central ray must be directed through the contact areas between the teeth
- the x-ray beam must be centered over the film to ensure that all areas of the film are exposed
- Prior to film exposure using the bite-wing technique, the dental radiographer must complete infection control procedures, prepare the treatment area and supplies, seat the patient, explain the radiographic procedures to be performed, make chair and headrest adjustments, place the lead apron, remove any intraoral objects and eyeglasses, set the exposure factors, and, if a film-holding device is used, assemble the film holder.
- An exposure sequence for film placements must be followed when using the bite-wing technique. When exposing bite-wing radiographs only, the radiographer always begins with the premolar bite-wing exposure; the premolar is easier for the patient to tolerate and is less likely to cause gagging. Following the premolar exposure, the molar teeth are exposed.
- When exposing films using the bite-wing technique, the premolar and molar exposures have prescribed film placements (see Figs. 19-16 and 19-23).
- A vertical bite-wing can be used to examine the level of alveolar bone. This bite-wing is placed with the long portion of the film in a vertical direction. Vertical bite-wings are often used as post-treatment films for patients with bone loss due to periodontal disease.
- Modifications in the bite-wing technique may be necessary when a patient has edentulous spaces or bony growths.

BIBLIOGRAPHY

Frommer HH: Intraoral radiographic technique: The paralleling method. *In* Radiology for Dental Auxiliaries, 6th edition. St. Louis, Mosby-Year Book, 1996, pp. 139–180

Goaz PW, White SC: Intraoral radiographic examinations. *In* Oral Radiology: Principles and Interpretation, 3rd edition. St. Louis, CV Mosby, 1994, pp. 200–205.

Johnson ON, McNally MA, Essay CE: The bitewing examination. *In* Essentials of Dental Radiography for Dental Assistants and Hygienists, 6th edition. Norwalk, CT, Appleton and Lange, 1999, pp. 377–390.

Manson-Hing LR: The bitewing radiograph. *In* Fundamentals of Dental Radiography, 3rd edition. Philadelphia, Lea & Febiger, 1990, pp. 72–75.

Matteson SR, Whaley C, Secrist VC: Intraoral radiographic techniques. *In* Dental Radiology, 4th edition. Chapel Hill, University of North Carolina Press, 1988, pp. 96–97.

Miles DA, Van Dis ML, Jensen CW, Ferretti A: Intraoral radiographic technique. *In* Radiographic Imaging for Dental Auxiliaries, 3rd edition. Philadelphia, WB Saunders, 1999, pp. 1–47.

Miles DA, Van Dis ML, Razmus TF: Intraoral radiographic techniques. *In* Basic Principles of Oral and Maxillofacial Radiology. Philadelphia, WB Saunders, 1992, pp. 104–108.

O'Brien RC: Bite-wing exposures. *In* Dental Radiography: An Introduction for Dental Hygienists and Assistants, 4th edition. Philadelphia, WB Saunders, 1982, pp. 110–118.

Quiz Questions ···

FILL IN THE BLANK

1. What does the term bite-wing refer to?

   _____

2. What size film is recommended for use with the bite-wing technique in the adult patient?

   _____

3. What size film is recommended for use with the bite-wing technique in the child patient with a primary dentition?

   _____

4. How is the patient's head positioned prior to exposing films in the bite-wing technique?

   _____

5. What are bite-wing films primarily used to detect?

   _____

6. What size film is used to include all the posterior teeth in one bite-wing exposure?

   _____

7. What type of angulation is determined by the up-and-down movement of the PID?

   _____

8. What type of angulation is determined by the side-to-side movement of the PID?

   _____

9. When the central ray is not directed through the contact areas, what is seen on the resulting radiograph?

   _____

10. When does a cone-cut result?

    _____

MULTIPLE CHOICE

 11. Which of the following describes the primary use of the bite-wing radiograph?

   a. examination of the apical areas of teeth
   b. examination of the apical and interproximal areas of teeth
   c. examination of the interproximal areas of teeth
   d. examination of the pulp chambers of teeth

_____C_____ **12.** Which of the following is the correct vertical angulation used with the bite-wing technique?

    a. −10 degrees
    b. −20 degrees
    c. +10 degrees
    d. +15 degrees

_____A_____ **13.** Which of the following describes the relationship of the film to the maxillary and mandibular teeth in the bite-wing technique?

    a. the film and teeth are parallel to each other
    b. the film and teeth are at right angles to each other
    c. the film and teeth are perpendicular to each other
    d. the film and teeth intersect each other

_____B_____ **14.** Which of the following is correct concerning film placement?
(1) anterior bite-wings may be placed horizontally, (2) anterior bite-wings may be placed vertically, (3) posterior bite-wings may be placed horizontally, (4) posterior bite-wings may be placed vertically

    a. 1, 2, 3
    b. 2, 3, 4
    c. 2, 3
    d. 1, 4

_____D_____ **15.** Which of the following is incorrect concerning the exposure sequence for a CMRS that includes periapicals and bite-wings?

    a. anterior periapicals are always exposed first
    b. posterior periapicals are exposed after anterior periapicals
    c. bite-wings are exposed last
    d. none of the above

ESSAY

16. State the basic principles of the bite-wing technique.

17. Describe the two ways to stabilize a film in the bite-wing technique.

18. State the basic rules of the bite-wing technique.

19. Discuss the patient and equipment preparations necessary prior to using the bite-wing technique.

20. Discuss the exposure sequence for a CMRS that includes both periapical films and bite-wing films.

21. Describe premolar and molar bite-wing film placements.

22. Explain the modifications in the bite-wing technique that are used for patients with edentulous spaces or bony growths.

23. Describe why a +10 degree vertical angulation is used with the bite-wing technique.

Answers are supplied at the end of this book.

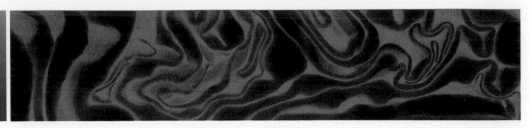

Exposure and Technique Errors

OBJECTIVES

After completion of this chapter, the student will be able to:

- *Define the key words.*
- *Identify and describe the appearance of the following film exposure errors: unexposed film, film exposed to light, underexposed film, and overexposed film.*
- *Describe horizontal and vertical angulation.*
- *Identify and describe the appearance of the following periapical technique errors: incorrect horizontal angulation, incorrect vertical angulation (foreshortened images and elongated images), and incorrect beam alignment (cone-cut images).*
- *Describe and identify proper film placement for bite-wing radiographs.*
- *Identify and describe the appearance of the following bite-wing technique errors: incorrect horizontal angulation, incorrect vertical angulation, and incorrect position-indicating device (PID) alignment (cone-cut images).*
- *Identify and describe the appearance of the following miscellaneous technique errors: film bending, film creasing, phalangioma, double exposure, movement, and reversed film.*

INTRODUCTION

The dental radiographer must remember that radiographs are taken to benefit the patient. However, only *diagnostic* radiographs benefit the patient. A diagnostic dental radiograph is one that has been properly placed, exposed, and processed; errors in any one of these three areas may result in nondiagnostic films. In many instances, nondiagnostic radiographs must be retaken. Retakes result in additional exposure of the patient to ionizing radiation, which does not benefit the patient.

The dental radiographer must have a working knowledge of film exposure, technique, and processing errors; processing errors have been previously discussed in Chapter 9. The purpose of this chapter is to describe film exposure problems and periapical, bitewing, and miscellaneous technique errors.

FILM EXPOSURE ERRORS

Film exposure errors result in nondiagnostic films. Exposure problems include films that are not exposed, accidentally exposed to light, overexposed, and underexposed. All of these errors produce films that are too light or too dark. The dental radiographer must be able to recognize film exposure errors, identify their causes, and know what steps are necessary to correct such problems.

Exposure Problems

UNEXPOSED FILM

Appearance. The film appears clear (Fig. 20–1).

Cause. The film was not exposed. Causes include failure to turn on the x-ray machine, electrical failure, or malfunction of the x-ray machine.

FIGURE 20–1. An unexposed film appears clear.

Correction. To ensure proper exposure of the film, make certain that the x-ray machine is turned on and listen for the audible exposure signal.

FILM EXPOSED TO LIGHT

Appearance. The film appears black (Fig. 20–2).

Cause. The film was accidentally exposed to white light.

Correction. To protect the film, do not unwrap it in a room with white light. Check the darkroom for

FIGURE 20–2. A film exposed to light appears black. (From Haring JI, Lind LJ: Radiographic Interpretation for the Dental Hygienist. Philadelphia, WB Saunders, 1993.)

possible light leaks. Turn off all lights in the darkroom (except for safelights) before unwrapping the film.

Time and Exposure Factor Problems

OVEREXPOSED FILM

Appearance. The film appears dark (Fig. 20–3).

Cause. The film was overexposed. An **overexposed film** results from excessive exposure time, kilovoltage, milliamperage, or a combination of these factors.

Correction. To prevent overexposure, check the exposure time, kilovoltage, and milliamperage settings on the x-ray machine before exposing the film. Reduce exposure time, kilovoltage, or milliamperage as needed.

UNDEREXPOSED FILM

Appearance. The film appears light (Fig. 20–4).

Cause. The film was underexposed. An **underexposed film** results from inadequate exposure time, kilovoltage, milliamperage, or a combination of these factors.

Correction. To prevent underexposure, check the exposure time, kilovoltage, and milliamperage settings on the x-ray machine before exposing the film. Increase exposure time, kilovoltage, or milliamperage as needed.

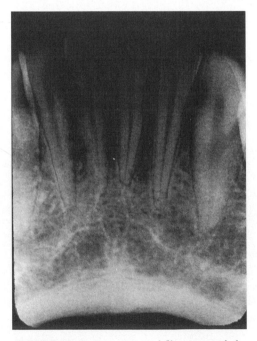

FIGURE 20–3. An overexposed film appears dark.

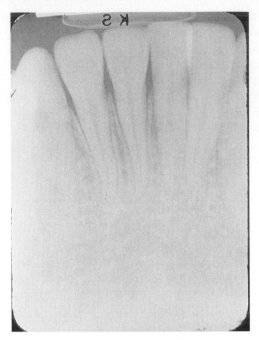

FIGURE 20–4. An underexposed film appears light.

▓ TECHNIQUE ERRORS (PERIAPICAL FILMS)

Just as film exposure errors may result in nondiagnostic radiographs, errors in technique may also result in nondiagnostic films. Periapical technique errors include film placement, angulation, and beam alignment problems. The dental radiographer must be able to recognize periapical technique errors, identify their causes, and know what steps are necessary to correct such problems.

Film Placement Problems

CORRECT FILM PLACEMENT

As described in Chapter 16, the periapical film shows the entire tooth, including the apex and surrounding structures (Fig. 20–5). For a periapical film to be considered diagnostic, film placement must be correct. Specific periapical film placements for incisors, canines, premolars, and molars are described in Chapters 17 and 18. Each periapical film must be positioned in a certain way to show specific teeth and related anatomic structures. In addition, the edge of the periapical film must be placed parallel to the incisal or occlusal surfaces of the teeth and extend 1/8 inch beyond the incisal or occlusal surfaces.

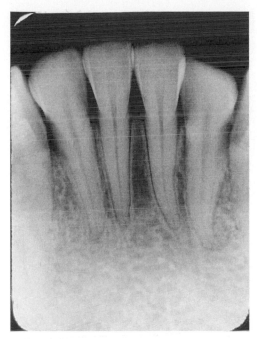

FIGURE 20–5. Correct periapical film placement demonstrates the entire tooth, including the apex and surrounding structures.

INCORRECT FILM PLACEMENT

A nondiagnostic periapical film may result from improper placement of a film over the area of intended interest, inadequate coverage of the apical regions, or a dropped film corner.

Absence of Apical Structures

APPEARANCE. No apices appear on the film (Fig. 20–6).

CAUSE. The film was not positioned in the patient's mouth to cover the apical regions of the teeth. As a result, no apical structures appear on the radiograph, and there is an excessive margin of film edge (which appears as a black band). This error occurs with both the paralleling and bisecting techniques.

CORRECTION. To make sure that apical structures appear on a periapical radiograph, make certain that no more than 1/8 inch of the film edge extends beyond the incisal-occlusal surfaces of the teeth. Such film placement ensures adequate coverage of the tooth apices.

Dropped Film Corner

APPEARANCE. The occlusal plane appears tipped or tilted (Fig. 20–7).

CAUSE. The edge of the film was not placed parallel to the incisal-occlusal surfaces of the teeth. As a result, the occlusal plane appears tipped on the radiograph. If the patient is not instructed to hold the film firmly against the tooth, a corner of the film may drop or slip. This error occurs when the finger-holding method is used with the bisecting technique.

CORRECTION. To prevent a dropped film corner, make certain that the edge of the film is placed parallel to the incisal-occlusal surfaces of the teeth. Instruct the patient to hold the film firmly in place.

Angulation Problems

Angulation is a term used to describe the alignment of the central ray of the x-ray beam in the horizontal and vertical planes. Angulation can be varied by moving the PID in either a horizontal or vertical direction.

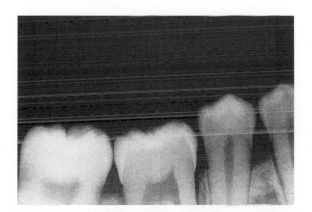

FIGURE 20–6. Improper film placement; no apices appear on this film. (From Haring JI, Lind LJ: Radiographic Interpretation for the Dental Hygienist. Philadelphia, WB Saunders, 1993.)

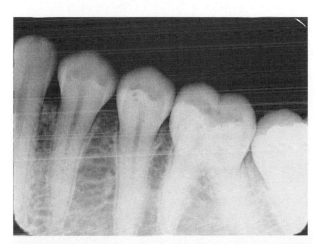

FIGURE 20–7. Improper film placement. a dropped film corner is seen when the edge of the film is not placed parallel to the incisal or occlusal surfaces of the teeth.

Horizontal angulation refers to the positioning of the PID in a horizontal or side-to-side plane. **Vertical angulation** refers to the positioning of the PID in a vertical or up-and-down plane. Correct horizontal and vertical angulation of periapical films is described in Chapter 18.

INCORRECT HORIZONTAL ANGULATION

Appearance. Overlapped contacts appear on the film (Fig. 20–8).

Cause. The central ray was not directed through the interproximal spaces. As a result, the proximal surfaces of adjacent teeth appear overlapped in the periapical film. Overlapped contacts prevent the examination of interproximal areas. This error occurs with both the paralleling and bisecting techniques.

Correction. To avoid overlapped contacts on a periapical film, direct the x-ray beam *through* the interproximal regions. The use of Rinn instruments minimizes errors in horizontal angulation.

INCORRECT VERTICAL ANGULATION

Incorrect vertical angulation results in a radiographic image that is not the same length as the tooth; instead the image appears either longer or shorter. Elongated or foreshortened images are nondiagnostic.

Foreshortened Images

APPEARANCE. Short teeth with blunted roots appear on the film (Fig. 20–9).

CAUSE. The vertical angulation was excessive (too steep). As a result, images that are shorter than the actual teeth, or **foreshortened images,** are seen on the

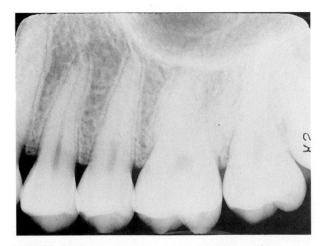

FIGURE 20–8. Incorrect horizontal angulation results in overlapped contact areas.

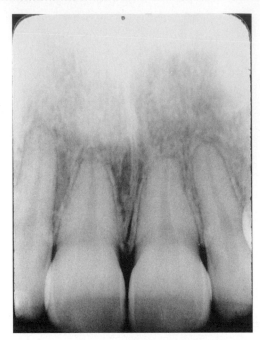

FIGURE 20–9. If the vertical angulation is too steep, the image of the tooth on the film is shorter than the actual tooth; the images are foreshortened.

radiograph. This error occurs with the bisecting technique.

CORRECTION. To avoid foreshortened images, do not use excessive vertical angulation with the bisecting technique. The use of Rinn instruments minimizes errors in vertical angulation.

Elongated Images

APPEARANCE. Long, distorted teeth appear on the film (Fig. 20–10).

CAUSE. The vertical angulation was insufficient (too flat). As a result, images that are longer than the actual teeth, or **elongated images,** are seen on the radiograph. This error occurs with the bisecting technique.

CORRECTION. To avoid elongated images, use adequate vertical angulation with the bisecting technique. The use of Rinn instruments minimizes errors in vertical angulation.

PID Alignment Problems

If the PID is misaligned and the x-ray beam is not centered over the film, a partial image is seen on the resultant radiograph. The PID, or cone, is said to "cut" the image—hence the term cone-cut. A **cone-cut** appears as a clear, unexposed area on a dental radio-

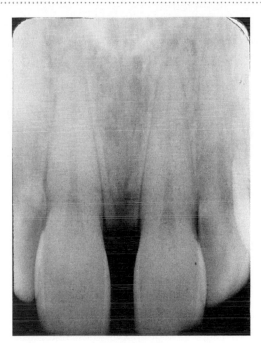

FIGURE 20–10. If the vertical angulation is too flat, the image of the tooth on the film is longer than the actual tooth; the images are elongated.

graph and may occur with either a rectangular or round PID.

CONE-CUT WITH FILM HOLDER

Appearance. A clear (unexposed) area appears on the film (Fig. 20–11).

Cause. The PID was not properly aligned with the periapical film holder and the x-ray beam did not expose the entire film. As a result, a clear, unexposed area resembling the outline of the PID is seen on the radiograph.

Correction. To avoid a cone-cut on a periapical film using a film holder, position the PID carefully. If a film holder with an aiming ring is used, make certain that the PID and aiming ring are aligned. If an aiming ring is not used, make certain that the x-ray beam is centered over the film.

CONE-CUT WITHOUT FILM HOLDER

Appearance. A clear (unexposed) area appears on the film (Fig. 20–12).

Cause. The PID was not directed at the center of the film, and the x-ray beam did not expose the entire film. As a result, a clear, unexposed area resembling the outline of the PID is seen on the radiograph.

Correction. To avoid a cone-cut on a periapical film without using a film holder, position the PID carefully. Make certain that the x-ray beam is centered over the film and that the entire film is covered by the diameter of the PID.

TECHNIQUE ERRORS (BITE-WING FILMS)

Just as errors in the periapical technique may result in nondiagnostic films, errors in the bite-wing technique may also result in films that are nondiagnostic. Bite-wing technique errors include film placement, angulation, and beam alignment problems. The dental radiog-

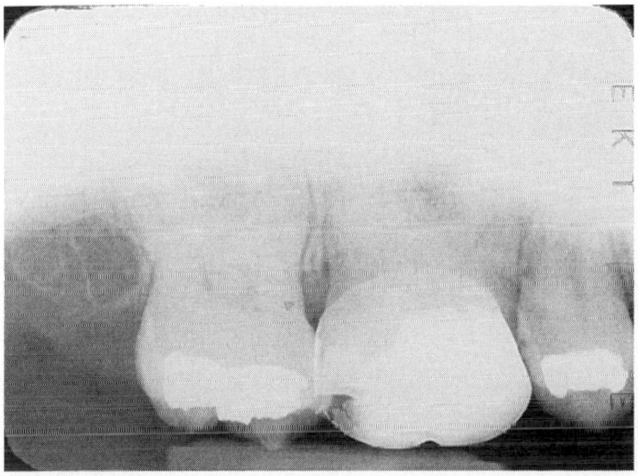

FIGURE 20–11. A cone-cut is seen when the PID is not properly aligned with the periapical film-holding device.

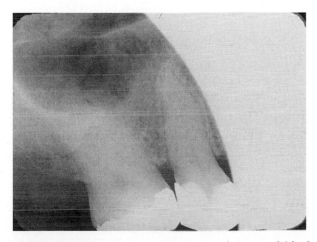

FIGURE 20–12. A cone-cut appears as a curved unexposed (clear) area on a radiograph.

rapher must be able to recognize bite-wing technique errors, identify their causes, and know what steps are necessary to correct such problems.

Film Placement Problems

CORRECT FILM PLACEMENT

As described in Chapter 19, the bite-wing film includes the crowns of both the maxillary and mandibular teeth, the interproximal contact areas, and crestal bone. For a bite-wing film to be considered diagnostic, film placement must be correct. Specific bite-wing film placements for premolars and molars are described in Chapter 19. In addition to placement over the prescribed areas, the radiograph must show an occlusal plane that is positioned horizontally, along the long axis of the film.

Premolar Bite-Wing

The premolar bite-wing must be positioned so that the resulting film shows both the maxillary and mandibular premolars and the distal contact areas of both canines (Fig. 20–13). To ensure that the distal surfaces of the canines are evident on the resulting radiograph, the film must be positioned so that the front edge of the film is aligned with the midline of the mandibular canine.

Molar Bite-Wing

The molar bite-wing must be positioned so that the resulting film shows both the maxillary and mandibular molars. The molar bite-wing must be centered over the mandibular second molar (Fig. 20–14). To ensure

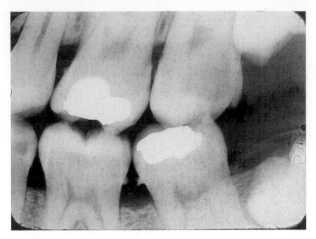

FIGURE 20–14. Correct film placement for the molar bite-wing.

correct film placement, the film must be positioned so that the front edge of the film is aligned with the midline of the mandibular second premolar.

INCORRECT FILM PLACEMENT

Incorrect bite-wing film placement may result in an absence of specific teeth or tooth surfaces on a film, a tipped occlusal plane, overlapped interproximal contacts, or a distorted image. Such errors may render a bite-wing film nondiagnostic.

Premolar Bite-Wing

APPEARANCE. Distal surfaces of the canines are not visible on the film (Fig. 20–15).

CAUSE. The bite-wing film was positioned too far posteriorly in the mouth; the front edge of the film

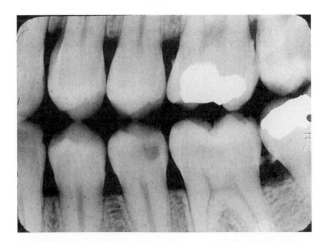

FIGURE 20–13. Correct film placement for the premolar bite-wing.

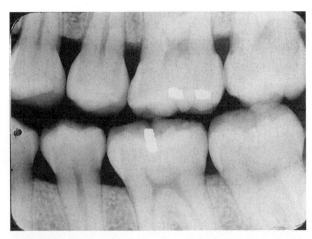

FIGURE 20–15. Incorrect film placement for the premolar bite-wing.

was not placed at the midline of the mandibular canine. As a result, the distal surfaces of the canines are not seen on the radiograph.

CORRECTION. To prevent this error, make certain that the anterior edge of the bite-wing film is positioned at the midline of the mandibular canine.

Molar Bite-Wing

APPEARANCE. Third molar regions are not visible on the film (Fig. 20–16).

CAUSE. The bite-wing film was positioned too far anteriorly in the mouth; the front edge of the film was not placed at the midline of the mandibular second premolar. As a result, the third molar areas are not seen on the radiograph.

CORRECTION. To prevent this error, make certain that the anterior edge of the bite-wing film is positioned at the midline of the mandibular second premolar. *Always* center the molar bite-wing on the mandibular second molar, even when no erupted third molars are present.

Angulation Problems

To produce diagnostic bite-wing radiographs, the dental radiographer must be prepared to choose the correct horizontal and vertical angulations. Correct horizontal and vertical angulation of bite-wing films is described in Chapter 19. Incorrect horizontal angulation results in overlapped interproximal contacts, and incorrect vertical angulation results in distorted images.

INCORRECT HORIZONTAL ANGULATION

Appearance. Overlapped contacts appear on the film (Fig. 20–17).

Cause. The central ray was not directed through the interproximal spaces. As a result, the proximal surfaces of adjacent teeth appear overlapped in the bite-wing film. **Overlapped contacts** prevent examination of interproximal areas.

Correction. To avoid overlapped contacts on a bite-wing film, direct the x-ray beam *through* the interproximal regions. When the contacts are opened, a thin radiolucent line is seen between the proximal surfaces of the teeth. The use of Rinn bite-wing instruments minimizes errors in horizontal angulation.

INCORRECT VERTICAL ANGULATION

Appearance. Images appear distorted on the film (Fig. 20–18).

Cause. The vertical angulation was incorrect. As a result, distorted images are seen on the radiograph. In this example, a negative vertical angulation was used. Note the occlusal surfaces of the maxillary teeth and the apical regions of the mandibular teeth.

Correction. To avoid incorrect vertical angulation, always use a +10-degree vertical angulation with the bite-wing technique. This vertical angulation compensates for the slight tilt of the maxillary teeth and the slight lingual bend of the upper half of the film caused by the hard palate.

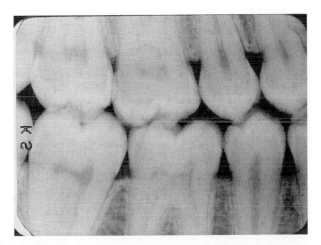

· **FIGURE 20–16.** Incorrect film placement for the molar bite-wing.

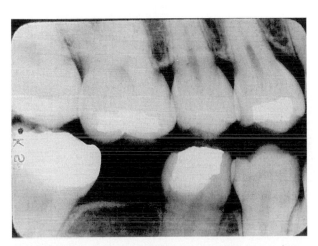

FIGURE 20–17. Overlapped interproximal contacts occur due to incorrect horizontal angulation.

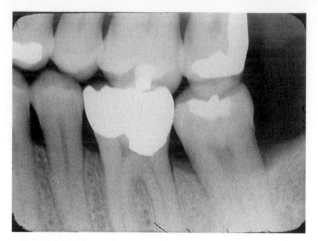

FIGURE 20–18. Incorrect vertical angulation causes the images to appear distorted.

PID Alignment Problems

As previously described in this chapter, if the PID is misaligned and the x-ray beam is not centered over the film, a partial image known as a cone-cut is seen on the resulting bite-wing radiograph.

CONE-CUT WITH FILM HOLDER

Appearance. A clear (unexposed) area appears on the film (Fig. 20–19).

Cause. The PID was not properly aligned with the bite-wing film holder, and the x-ray beam did not expose the entire film. As a result, a clear, unexposed area resembling the outline of the PID is seen on the radiograph.

Correction. To avoid a cone-cut on a bite-wing film using a film holder, position the PID carefully and make certain that the PID and aiming ring are aligned.

CONE-CUT WITHOUT FILM HOLDER

Appearance. A clear (unexposed) area appears on the film (Fig. 20–20).

Cause. The PID was not directed at the center of the film, and the x-ray beam did not expose the entire film. As a result, a clear, unexposed area resembling the outline of the PID is seen on the radiograph.

Correction. To avoid a cone-cut on a bite-wing film without using a film holder, position the PID carefully. Make certain that the x-ray beam is centered over the film and that the entire film is covered by the diameter of the PID.

▨ MISCELLANEOUS TECHNIQUE ERRORS

Miscellaneous technique errors may be seen on either periapical or bite-wing radiographs. Miscellaneous technique errors include film bending, film creasing, phalangioma, double exposure, patient movement, and the reversed film. The dental radiographer must be able to recognize these miscellaneous technique errors, identify their causes, and know what steps are necessary to correct such problems.

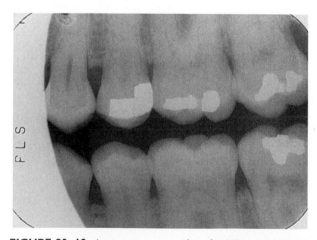

FIGURE 20–19. A cone-cut is seen when the PID is not properly aligned with the bite-wing film-holding device.

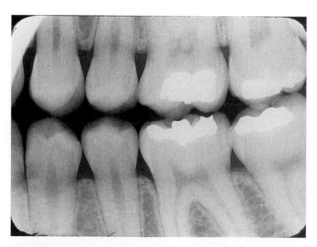

FIGURE 20–20. A cone-cut appears as a curved unexposed (clear) area on a radiograph.

Film Bending

Appearance. Images appear stretched and distorted (Fig. 20–21).

Cause. The film was bent excessively owing to the curvature of the hard palate or heavy finger pressure on the film. As a result, stretched and distorted images are seen on the radiograph.

Correction. To avoid film bending, always check film placement before exposure. If the patient's finger pressure is excessive, instruct the patient to stabilize the film gently. If the film is bent because of the curvature of the hard palate, cotton rolls can be used with the paralleling technique, or the bisecting technique can be used. Film-holding devices are helpful in preventing film bending.

Film Creasing

Appearance. A thin radiolucent line appears on the film (Fig. 20–22).

Cause. The film was creased and the film emulsion cracked. As a result, a thin radiolucent line is seen on the resultant radiograph.

Correction. To avoid film creasing, do not bend or crease the film excessively. Instead, gently soften the corners of the film before placing it in the patient's mouth.

Phalangioma

Appearance. The patient's finger appears on the film (Fig. 20–23).

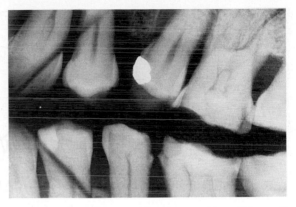

FIGURE 20–22. A film crease appears as a thin radiolucent line. (From Haring JI, Lind LJ: Radiographic Interpretation for the Dental Hygienist. Philadelphia, WB Saunders, 1993.)

Cause. The patient's finger was incorrectly positioned in front of the film instead of behind the film. As a result, the patient's finger appears on the radiograph. The term **phalangioma** was coined by Dr. David F. Mitchell of the Indiana University School of Dentistry; it refers to the distal phalanx of the finger seen in the radiograph. (A phalanx [plural, phalanges] is any bone of a finger or toe.) This error occurs when the finger-holding method is used with the bisecting technique.

Correction. To avoid a phalangioma, make certain that the patient's finger used to stabilize the film is placed *behind* the film and not in front of it.

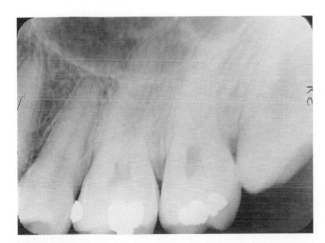

FIGURE 20–21. A bent film appears distorted.

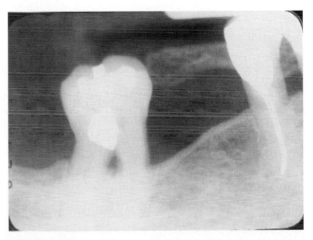

FIGURE 20–23. This film demonstrates a phalangioma; the bones of a patient's finger appear on the film.

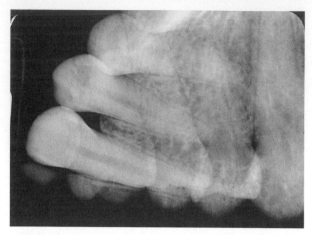

FIGURE 20–24. This film demonstrates a double exposure.

Double Exposure

Appearance. A double image appears on the film (Fig. 20–24).

Cause. The film was exposed in the patient's mouth twice. As a result, a double image appears on the radiograph. A double exposure is a serious technique error and results in two retakes, one of each area previously exposed.

Correction. To avoid a double exposure, always separate exposed and unexposed films. Once a film has been exposed, place it in a designated area (e.g., a disposable cup or bag) away from unexposed films. If exposed films are always separated from unexposed films, this error will not occur.

Movement

Appearance. Blurred images appear on the film (Fig. 20–25).

Cause. The patient moved during the exposure of the film. As a result, blurred images are seen on the radiograph.

Correction. To prevent movement errors, stabilize the patient's head before exposing the radiograph and instruct the patient to remain still. Never expose a film when a patient is moving. As necessary, reposition the patient, the film, or the PID, and then expose the film.

Reversed Film

Appearance. Light images with a herringbone pattern appear on the film (Fig. 20–26).

Cause. The film was placed in the mouth backward (reversed) and then exposed. The x-ray beam was attenuated by the lead foil backing in the film packet; consequently, a decreased amount of the x-ray beam exposed the film. As a result, light images with a **herringbone pattern** (also known as the tire-track pattern) are seen on the radiograph. The herringbone pattern on the radiograph is representative of the actual pattern embossed on the lead foil (see Chapter 7).

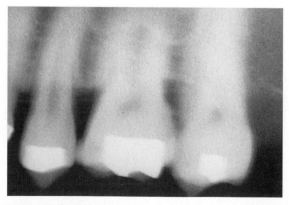

FIGURE 20–25. Movement results in a blurred image. (From Haring JI, Lind LJ: Radiographic Interpretation for the Dental Hygienist. Philadelphia, WB Saunders, 1993.)

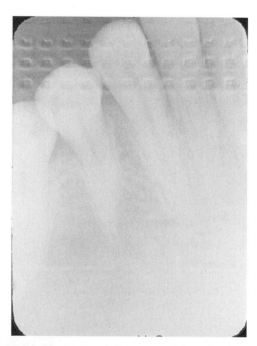

FIGURE 20–26. A reversed film appears light with a herringbone or tire-track pattern. The tire-track pattern is seen on the lead-foil backing within the film packet.

Correction. To avoid a reversed film, always place the white side of the film adjacent to the teeth. Always note the front and back sides of the film before placing a film in the patient's mouth.

SUMMARY

- The dental radiographer must have a working knowledge of the film exposure and technique errors that result in nondiagnostic films. (Processing errors are discussed in Chapter 9.)
- Film exposure problems include films that are not exposed, accidentally exposed to white light, overexposed, or underexposed. All these errors produce nondiagnostic radiographs that are too light or too dark.
- Periapical and bite-wing technique errors include film placement, angulation, and PID alignment problems.
- Miscellaneous technique errors include film bending, film creasing, phalangioma, double exposure, patient movement, and the reversed film.
- The dental radiographer must be able to recognize and identify the causes of exposure and technique errors. In addition, the dental radiographer must know what steps are necessary to correct such errors.

BIBLIOGRAPHY

Haring JI, Lind LJ: Film exposure, processing and technique errors. *In* Radiographic Interpretation for the Dental Hygienist. Philadelphia, WB Saunders, 1993, pp. 159–180.

Johnson ON, McNally MA, Essay CE: Identifying and correcting faulty radiographs. *In* Essentials of Dental Radiography for Dental Assistants and Hygienists, 6th edition. Norwalk, CT, Appleton and Lange, 1999, pp. 297–317.

Manson-Hing LR: Radiographic quality and artifacts. *In* Fundamentals of Dental Radiography, 3rd edition. Philadelphia, Lea & Febiger, 1990, pp. 40–47.

Miles DA, Van Dis ML, Jensen CW, Ferretti A: Technique/processing errors and troubleshooting. *In* Radiographic Imaging for Dental Auxiliaries, 3rd edition. Philadelphia, WB Saunders, 1999, pp. 101–128.

Miles DA, Van Dis ML, Razmus TF: Intraoral radiographic techniques. *In* Basic Principles of Oral and Maxillofacial Radiology. Philadelphia, WB Saunders, 1992, pp. 114–121.

O'Brien RC: The five most common errors in technique. *In* Dental Radiography: An Introduction for Dental Hygienists and Assistants, 4th edition. Philadelphia, WB Saunders, 1982, pp. 223–228.

O'Brien RC: Processing errors. *In* Dental Radiography: An Introduction for Dental Hygienists and Assistants, 4th edition. Philadelphia, WB Saunders, 1982, pp. 238–245.

Quiz Questions ··

IDENTIFICATION

For questions 1 to 10 refer to Figures 20–27 through 20–36. Identify the film exposure or technique error seen in each radiograph.

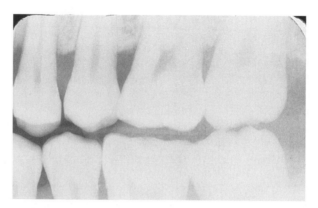

FIGURE 20–27

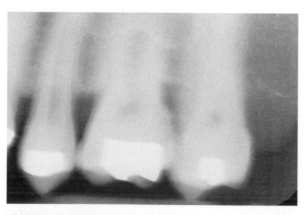

FIGURE 20–28

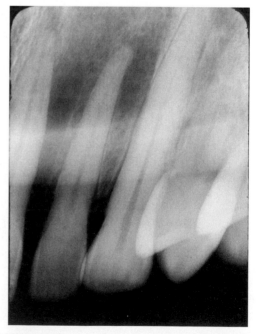

FIGURE 20–29

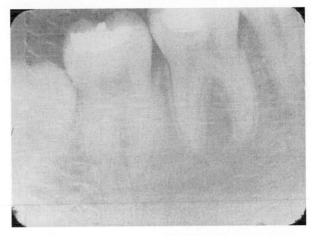

FIGURE 20–30

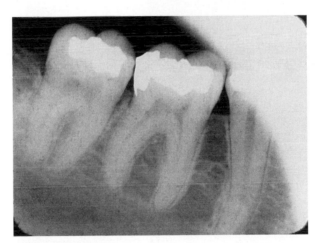

FIGURE 20–31

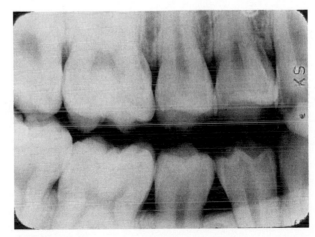

FIGURE 20–32

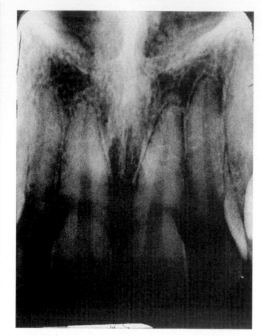

FIGURE 20–33

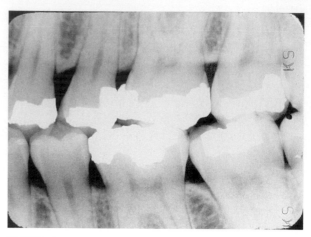

FIGURE 20–34

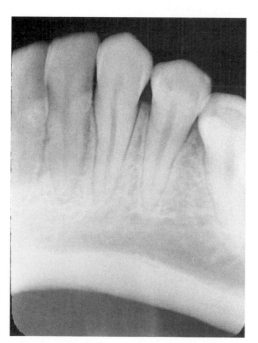

FIGURE 20–35

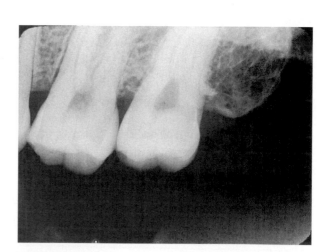

FIGURE 20–36

MATCHING

For questions 11 to 15, describe the appearance of each film error using one of these words:

> a. clear
> b. black
> c. light
> d. dark

_____ 11. overexposed film

_____ 12. underexposed film

_____ 13. film exposed to light

_____ 14. unexposed film

_____ 15. reversed film

MULTIPLE CHOICE

_____ 16. Too much vertical angulation results in images that are:

   a. elongated
   b foreshortened
   c. overlapped
   d. none of the above

_____ 17. Too little vertical angulation results in images that are:

   a. elongated
   b. foreshortened
   c. overlapped
   d. none of the above

_____ 18. Incorrect horizontal angulation results in images that are:

   a. elongated
   b. foreshortened
   c. overlapped
   d. none of the above

_____ 19. Which of the following errors can occur with the bite-wing technique?
         (1) elongation, (2) overlapped contacts, (3) cone-cut, (4) phalangioma

   a. 1, 2, 3, 4
   b. 1, 2, 3
   c. 2, 4
   d. 2, 3

_____ 20. Which of the following errors can occur with the bisecting technique?
         (1) elongation, (2) overlapped contacts, (3) cone-cut, (4) phalangioma

   a. 1, 2, 3, 4
   b. 1, 2, 3
   c. 2, 4
   d. 2, 3

_____

Answers are supplied at the end of this book.

CHAPTER 21

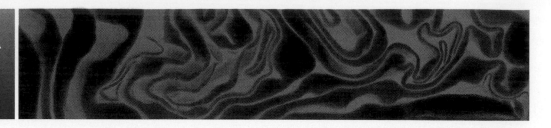

Occlusal and Localization Techniques

Objectives
Key Words
Introduction
Occlusal Technique
    Basic Concepts
    Step-by-Step Procedures
Helpful Hints

Localization Techniques
    Basic Concepts
    Step-by-Step Procedures
Summary
Bibliography
Quiz Questions

OBJECTIVES

After completion of this chapter, the student will be able to:

- *Define the key words.*
- *Describe the purpose of the occlusal examination.*
- *List the uses of the occlusal examination.*
- *Describe the patient and equipment preparations necessary prior to using the occlusal technique.*
- *State the recommended vertical angulations for the following maxillary occlusal projections: topographic, lateral (right or left), and pediatric.*
- *State the recommended vertical angulations for the following mandibular occlusal projections: topographic, cross-sectional, and pediatric.*
- *State the purpose of localization techniques.*
- *Describe the buccal object rule.*
- *Describe the right-angle technique.*
- *List the patient and equipment preparations that are necessary prior to using the buccal object rule or the right-angle technique.*
- *Describe the film placements for the buccal object rule and compare the resulting radiographs.*
- *Describe the film placements for the right-angle technique and compare the resulting radiographs.*

INTRODUCTION

In addition to mastering periapical and interproximal examination techniques, the dental radiographer must also master occlusal and localization techniques. Before the dental radiographer can use these important techniques, an understanding of the basic concepts, patient preparation, equipment preparation, and film placement procedures is necessary.

The purpose of this chapter is to present basic concepts and to describe patient preparation, equipment preparation, and film placement procedures for both the occlusal and localization techniques.

OCCLUSAL TECHNIQUE

The **occlusal technique** is used to examine large areas of the upper or lower jaw. Before the dental radiographer can use the occlusal technique, a thorough understanding of basic concepts is necessary. In addition, a knowledge of step-by-step procedures is required.

Basic Concepts

TERMINOLOGY

Before describing the principles of the occlusal technique, a number of basic terms must be defined.

Occlusal surfaces: The chewing surfaces of the posterior teeth.

Occlusal examination: A type of intraoral radiographic examination used to inspect large areas of the maxilla or mandible on one film.

Occlusal technique: The method used to expose a film in the occlusal examination.

Occlusal film: In the occlusal technique Size 4 intraoral film is used. The film is so named because the patient "occludes" or bites on the entire film. Size 4 film is the largest size of intraoral film, measuring 3 by $2\frac{1}{4}$ inches. In adults, Size 4 film is used in the occlusal examination. In children, however, Size 2 film is used.

PURPOSE AND USE

The occlusal technique is a supplementary radiographic technique that is usually used in conjunction with periapical or bite-wing radiographs. The occlusal technique is used when large areas of the maxilla or mandible must be visualized. The occlusal radiograph is preferred when the area of interest is larger than a periapical film or when the placement of periapical films is too difficult for the patient. Occlusal radiographs can be used for the following purposes:

- to locate retained roots of extracted teeth
- to locate supernumerary (extra), unerupted, or impacted teeth
- to locate foreign bodies in the maxilla or mandible
- to locate salivary stones in the duct of the submandibular gland
- to locate and evaluate the extent of lesions (e.g., cysts, tumors, malignancies) in the maxilla or mandible
- to evaluate the boundaries of the maxillary sinus
- to evaluate fractures of the maxilla or mandible
- to aid in the examination of patients who cannot open their mouths more than a few millimeters
- to examine the area of a cleft palate
- to measure changes in the size and shape of the maxilla or mandible

PRINCIPLES

The basic principles of the occlusal technique can be described as follows.

- The film is positioned with the white side facing the arch that is being exposed.
- The film is placed in the mouth between the occlusal surfaces of the maxillary and mandibular teeth.
- The film is stabilized when the patient gently bites on the surface of the film.

Step-by-Step Procedures

Step-by-step procedures for the exposure of occlusal films include the following: patient preparation, equipment preparation, and film placement methods. Before exposing any occlusal films, infection control procedures (as described in Chapter 15) must be completed.

PATIENT PREPARATION

Following the completion of infection control procedures and the preparation of the treatment area and supplies, the patient should be seated. After seating the patient, and before exposing any films, the dental radiographer must prepare the patient for film exposure (see "Procedure: Patient Preparation").

EQUIPMENT PREPARATION

Following patient preparation, equipment must also be prepared prior to the exposure of any films (see "Procedure: Equipment Preparation").

PROCEDURE

Patient Preparation

1. Briefly explain the radiographic procedure to the patient.

2. Position the patient upright in the chair. The level of the chair must be adjusted to a comfortable working height for the dental radiographer.

3. Adjust the headrest to support and position the patient's head. For *maxillary occlusal films,* the patient's head must be positioned so that the upper arch is parallel with the floor and the midsagittal (midline) plane is perpendicular to the floor. For some *mandibular occlusal films,* the patient's head must be reclined and positioned so that the occlusal plane is perpendicular to the floor. For others, it is positioned parallel with the floor.

4. Place the lead apron with thyroid collar on the patient and secure it.

5. Remove all objects from the mouth (e.g., dentures, retainers, chewing gum) that may interfere with film exposure. Eyeglasses must also be removed.

PROCEDURE

Equipment Preparation

Set the exposure factors (kilovoltage, milliamperage, and time) on the x-ray unit according to the recommendations of the film manufacturer. Either a short (8-inch) or long (16-inch) PID may be used with the occlusal technique.

MAXILLARY OCCLUSAL PROJECTIONS

There are three different maxillary occlusal projections: topographic, lateral (right or left), and pediatric.

TOPOGRAPHIC PROJECTION

The **maxillary topographic occlusal projection** is used to examine the palate and the anterior teeth of the maxilla (Fig. 21–1). (See "Procedure: Maxillary Topographic Occlusal Projection.")

LATERAL (RIGHT OR LEFT) PROJECTION

The **maxillary lateral occlusal projection** is used to examine the palatal roots of the molar teeth. It may also be used to locate foreign bodies or lesions in the posterior maxilla (Fig. 21–2). (See "Procedure: Maxillary Lateral Occlusal Projection.")

PEDIATRIC PROJECTION

The **maxillary pediatric occlusal projection** is used to examine the anterior teeth of the maxilla and is recommended for use in children 5 years old or younger (Fig. 21–3). (See "Procedure: Maxillary Pediatric Occlusal Projection.")

MANDIBULAR OCCLUSAL PROJECTIONS

There are three different mandibular occlusal projections: topographic, cross-sectional, and pediatric.

TOPOGRAPHIC PROJECTION

The **mandibular topographic occlusal projection** is used to examine the anterior teeth of the mandible (Fig. 21–4). (See "Procedure: Mandibular Topographic Occlusal Projection.")

CROSS-SECTIONAL PROJECTION

The **mandibular cross-sectional occlusal projection** is used to examine the buccal and lingual aspects of the mandible (Fig. 21–5). It is also used to locate foreign bodies or salivary stones in the region of the floor of the mouth. (See "Procedure: Mandibular Cross-Sectional Occlusal Projection.")

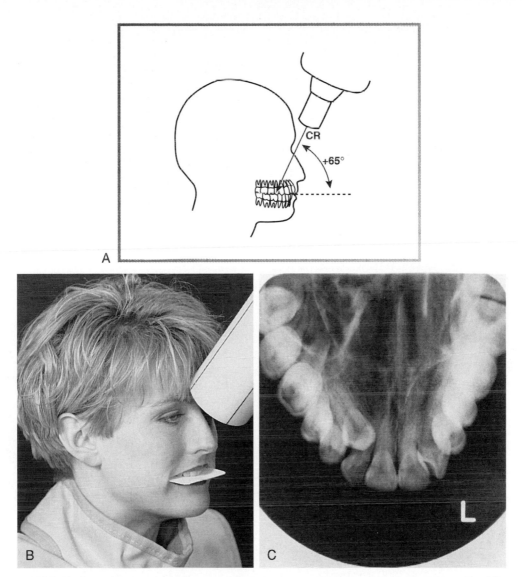

FIGURE 21–1. *A,* The central ray (CR) is directed at +65 degrees to the plane of the film. *B,* Relationship of film and PID. *C,* Maxillary occlusal topographic projection. (*A* and *C* reprinted courtesy of Eastman Kodak Company.)

PROCEDURE

Maxillary Topographic Occlusal Projection

1. Position the maxillary arch parallel with the floor.

2. Position a Size 4 film with the white side facing the maxilla and the long edge in a side-to-side direction. Insert the film into the patient's mouth, placing it as far posteriorly as the anatomy of the patient permits.

3. Instruct the patient to bite gently on the film and retain the position of the film in an end-to-end bite.

4. Position the PID so that the central ray is di-

rected through the midline of the arch toward the center of the film.

5. Position the PID so that the central ray is directed at +65 degrees toward the center of the film. The top edge of the PID is placed between the eyebrows on the bridge of the nose.

6. As recommended by the Eastman Kodak Company, use the following exposure factors for E-speed film: 65 kVp, 10 mA, 15 impulses, or 90 kVp, 10 mA, 5 impulses.

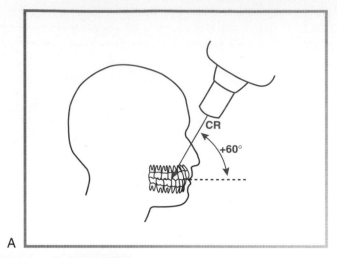

A

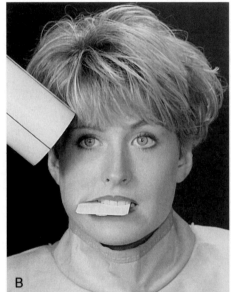

B

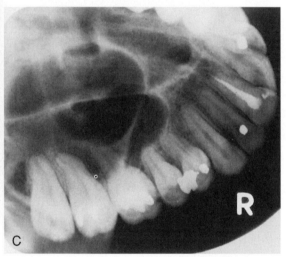

C

FIGURE 21–2. *A,* The central ray (CR) is directed at +60 degrees to the plane of the film. *B,* Relationship of film and PID. *C,* Maxillary occlusal lateral projection. (*A* and *C* reprinted courtesy of Eastman Kodak Company.)

PROCEDURE

Maxillary Lateral Occlusal Projection

1. Position the maxillary arch parallel with the floor.
2. Position a Size 4 film with the white side facing the maxilla and the long edge in a front-to-back direction. Insert the film into the patient's mouth and place it as far posteriorly as the anatomy of the patient permits. Shift the film to the side (right or left) of intended interest. The long edge of the film should extend approximately 1/2 inch beyond the buccal surfaces of the posterior teeth.
3. Instruct the patient to bite gently on the film, retaining the position of the film in an end-to-end bite.
4. Position the PID so that the central ray is directed through the contact areas of intended interest.
5. Position the PID so that the central ray is directed at +60 degrees toward the center of the film. The top edge of the PID is placed above the corner of the eyebrow.
6. As recommended by the Eastman Kodak Company, use the following exposure factors for E-speed film: 65 kVp, 10 mA, 15 impulses, or 90 kVp, 10 mA, 5 impulses.

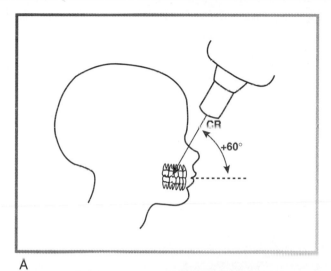

A

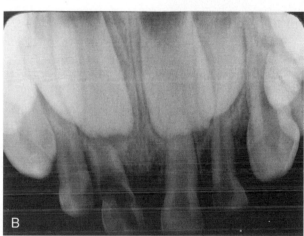

B

FIGURE 21–3. *A*, The central ray (CR) is directed at +60 degrees to the plane of the film. *B*, Maxillary occlusal pediatric projection.

PROCEDURE

Maxillary Pediatric Occlusal Projection

1. Position the maxillary arch parallel with the floor.

2. Position a Size 2 periapical film with the white side facing the maxilla and the long edge in a side-to-side direction. Insert the film into the child's mouth.

3. Instruct the child to bite gently on the film, retaining the position of the film in an end-to-end bite.

4. Position the PID so that the central ray is directed through the midline of the arch toward the center of the film.

5. Position the PID so that the central ray is directed at +60 degrees toward the center of the film. The top edge of the PID is placed between the eyebrows on the bridge of the nose.

6. As recommended by the Eastman Kodak Company, use the following exposure factors for E-speed film: 65 kVp, 10 mA, 10 impulses, or 90 kVp, 10 mA, 3 impulses.

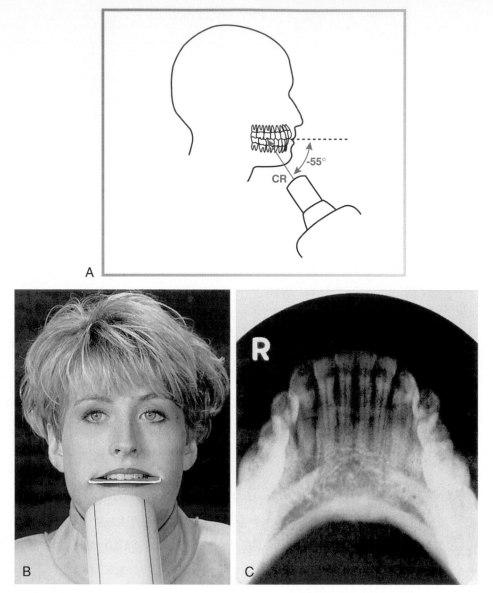

FIGURE 21–4. *A,* The central ray (CR) is directed at −55 degrees to the plane of the film. *B,* Relationship of film and PID. *C,* Mandibular occlusal topographic projection. (*A* and *C* reprinted courtesy of Eastman Kodak Company.)

PROCEDURE

Mandibular Topographic Occlusal Projection

1. Position the mandibular arch parallel with the floor.

2. Position a Size 4 film with the white side facing the mandible and the long edge in a side-to-side direction. Insert the film into the patient's mouth, placing it as far posteriorly as the anatomy of the patient permits.

3. Instruct the patient to bite gently on the film, retaining the position of the film in an end-to-end bite.

4. Position the PID so that the central ray is directed through the midline of the arch toward the center of the film.

5. Position the PID so that the central ray is directed at −55 degrees toward the center of the film. The PID should be centered over the chin.

6. As recommended by the Eastman Kodak Company, use the following exposure factors for E-speed film: 65 kVp, 10 mA, 15 impulses, or 90 kVp, 10 mA, 5 impulses.

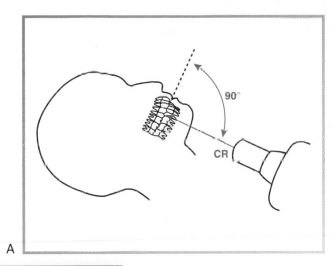

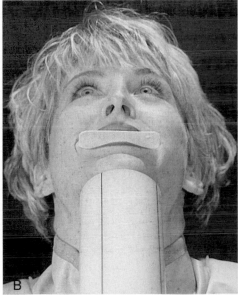

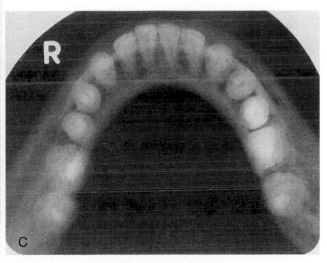

FIGURE 21–5. *A,* The central ray (CR) is perpendicular (90 degrees) to the plane of the film. *B,* Relationship of film and PID. *C,* Mandibular occlusal cross-sectional projection. (*A* and *C* reprinted courtesy of Eastman Kodak Company.)

PROCEDURE

Mandibular Cross-Sectional Occlusal Projection

1. Recline the patient and position the mandibular arch perpendicular to the floor.
2. Position a Size 4 film with the white side facing the mandible and the long edge in a side-to-side direction. Insert the film into the patient's mouth as far posteriorly as the anatomy of the patient permits.
3. Instruct the patient to bite gently on the film to retain the position of the film in an end to end bite.
4. Position the PID so that the central ray is directed through the midline of the arch toward the center of the film.

5. Position the PID so that the central ray is directed at 90 degrees toward the center of the film. The PID should be centered approximately 1 inch below the chin.
6. As recommended by the Eastman Kodak Company, use the following exposure factors for E-speed film: 65 kVp, 10 mA, 15 impulses, or 90 kVp, 10 mA, 5 impulses.

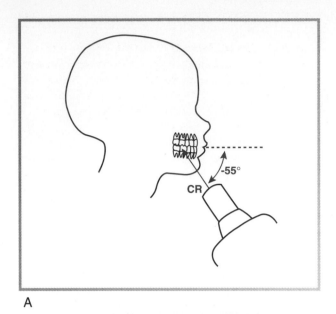

A

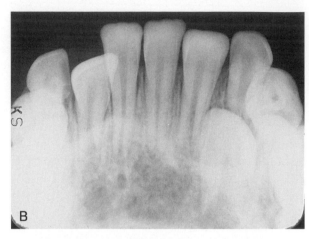

B

FIGURE 21–6. *A,* The central ray (CR) is directed at −55 degrees to the plane of the film. *B,* Mandibular occlusal pediatric projection.

PROCEDURE

Mandibular Pediatric Occlusal Projection

1. Position the mandibular arch parallel to the floor.
2. Position a Size 2 periapical film with the white side facing the maxilla and the long edge in a side-to-side directon. Insert the film into the child's mouth.
3. Instruct the child to bite gently on the film to retain the position of the film in an end-to-end bite.
4. Position the PID so that the central ray is di-

rected through the midline of the arch toward the center of the film.
5. Position the PID so that the central ray is directed at −55 degrees. The PID should be centered over the chin.
6. As recommended by the Eastman Kodak Company, use the following exposure factors for E-speed film: 65 kVp, 10 mA, 10 impulses, or 90 kVp, 10 mA, 3 impulses.

PEDIATRIC PROJECTION

The **mandibular pediatric occlusal projection** is used to examine the anterior teeth of the mandible and is recommended for use in children 5 years old or younger (Fig. 21–6). (See "Procedure: Mandibular Pediatric Occlusal Projection.")

The recommended vertical angulations for all maxillary and mandibular occlusal films are summarized in Table 21–1.

HELPFUL HINTS
For Exposing Occlusal Projections

➤ **DO** use exposure factors recommended by the film manufacturer.

➤ **DO** set all exposure factors (kilovoltage, milliamperage, time) before placing an occlusal film in the mouth.
➤ **DO** ask patients to remove all intraoral objects and eyeglasses prior to placing an occlusal film in the mouth.
➤ **DO** explain the radiographic procedure to be performed.
➤ **DO** instruct patients on how to close gently on the occlusal film and remain still during the exposure.
➤ **DO** position the patient's head before placing the occlusal film.
➤ **DO** position the occlusal film so that the white side faces the arch being exposed.
➤ **DO** position the film so that a minimal film edge extends beyond the teeth being exposed.
➤ **DO** center the occlusal film directly over the area of interest so that all necessary information can be recorded.
➤ **DO** set the vertical angulation for each occlusal projection as recommended in this chapter.

Projection	Vertical Angulation (degrees)
TABLE 21–1. Occlusal Projections and Corresponding Vertical Angulations	
Maxillary occlusal topographic	+65
Maxillary occlusal lateral (right or left)	+60
Maxillary occlusal pediatric	+60
Mandibular occlusal topographic	−55
Mandibular occlusal cross-sectional	90
Mandibular occlusal pediatric	−55

LOCALIZATION TECHNIQUES

A **localization technique** is a method used to locate the position of a tooth or object in the jaws. Before the dental radiographer can use localization techniques, a thorough understanding of basic concepts is necessary. In addition, a knowledge of step-by-step procedures is required.

Basic Concepts

PURPOSE AND USE

The dental radiograph is a two-dimensional picture of a three-dimensional object. A radiograph depicts an object in the superior-inferior and anterior-posterior relationships. The dental radiograph, however, does not depict the buccal-lingual relationship, or depth, of an object. There are times when it is necessary to establish the buccal-lingual position of a structure, such as a foreign object or impacted tooth, within the jaws. Localization techniques can be used to obtain this three-dimensional information. Localization techniques may be used to locate the following:

- foreign bodies
- impacted teeth
- unerupted teeth
- retained roots
- root positions
- salivary stones
- jaw fractures
- broken needles and instruments
- filling materials

TYPES

Two basic techniques are used to localize objects: the buccal object rule and the right-angle technique.

Buccal Object Rule. The **buccal object rule** is a rule governing the orientation of structures portrayed in two radiographs exposed at different angulations. One periapical or bite-wing film is exposed using proper technique and angulation. A second periapical or bite-wing film is then exposed after changing the direction of the x-ray beam; a different horizontal or vertical angulation is used. For example, a different *horizontal angulation* is used when trying to locate *vertically aligned* images (e.g., root canals), whereas a different *vertical angulation* is used when trying to locate a *horizontally aligned* image, such as the mandibular canal. After the two films have been exposed and processed, the radiographs are compared with each other.

When the dental structure or object seen in the second radiograph appears to have moved in the *same direction as the shift of the PID*, the structure or object in question is positioned to the *lingual* (Fig. 21–7).

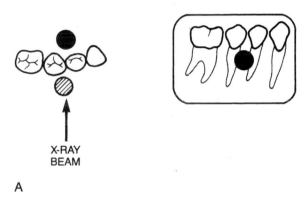

A

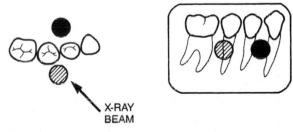

B

FIGURE 21–7. Buccal and lingual objects shift positions when the direction of the x-ray beam is changed. *A,* Buccal (cross-hatched circle) and lingual (black circle) are superimposed in the original radiograph. *B,* If the tubehead is shifted in a mesial direction, the buccal object moves distally and the lingual object moves mesially. (Same direction = lingual; opposite direction = buccal.) (From Haring JI, Lind LJ: Radiographic Interpretation for the Dental Hygienist. Philadelphia, WB Saunders, 1993.)

For example, if the horizontal angulation is changed by shifting the PID mesially, and the object in question moves mesially on the dental radiograph, then the object lies to the lingual (*same = lingual*).

Conversely, when the dental structure or object seen in the second radiograph appears to have moved in the *direction opposite the shift of the PID,* the structure or object in question is positioned to the *buccal* (Fig. 21–8). For example, if the horizontal angulation is changed by shifting the PID distally, and the object in question moves mesially on the dental radiograph, then the object lies to the buccal (*opposite = buccal*).

There is a mnemonic that can be used to remember the buccal object rule: SLOB.

SLOB stands for

Same = **L**ingual, **O**pposite = **B**uccal

In other words, when the two radiographs are compared, the object that lies to the *lingual* appears to have moved in the *same* direction as the PID, and the object that lies to the *buccal* appears to have moved in the *opposite* direction as the PID.

Right-Angle Technique. The **right-angle technique** is another rule for the orientation of structures seen in

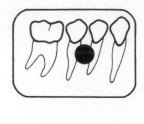
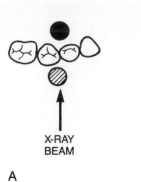
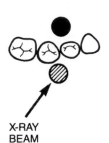
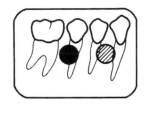

FIGURE 21–8. Buccal and lingual objects shift positions when the direction of the x-ray beam is changed. *A,* Buccal (cross-hatched circle) and lingual (black circle) objects are superimposed in the original radiograph. *B,* If the tubehead is shifted in a distal direction, the buccal object moves mesially and the lingual object moves distally. (Same direction = lingual; opposite direction = buccal.) (From Haring JI, Lind LJ: Radiographic Interpretation for the Dental Hygienist. Philadelphia, WB Saunders, 1993.)

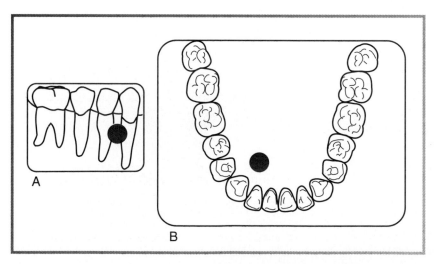

FIGURE 21–9. The right-angle technique. *A,* The object appears to be located in bone on the periapical radiograph. *B,* The occlusal radiograph reveals that the object is actually located in soft tissue lingual to the mandible.

two radiographs. One periapical film is exposed using the proper technique and angulation to show the position of the object in the superior-inferior and anterior-posterior relationships. Next, an occlusal film is exposed directing the central ray at a right angle, or perpendicular (90 degrees), to the film. The occlusal film shows the object in the buccal-lingual and anterior-posterior relationships. After the two films have been exposed and processed, the radiographs are compared with each other to locate the object in three dimensions (Fig. 21–9). This technique is primarily used for locating objects in the mandible.

Step-by-Step Procedures

Step-by-step procedures for localization techniques include patient and equipment preparations and film placements and comparisons.

PATIENT AND EQUIPMENT PREPARATIONS

Prior to exposing localization films, infection control procedures (as described in Chapter 15) must be carried out. In addition, patient and equipment preparations (described earlier in this chapter) must be completed.

FILM PLACEMENTS AND COMPARISONS

BUCCAL OBJECT RULE

EXAMPLE

The buccal object rule can be used to determine the position of a root canal filled with gutta percha (an endodontic filling material) in a maxillary second premolar (Fig 21–10)
1. *Position the maxillary arch parallel to the floor.*
2. *Expose one molar periapical film using proper technique and angulation.*
3. *Shift the PID in a mesial direction and expose a premolar periapical film.*
4. *In the second film, when the PID was moved in a mesial direction, the gutta percha moved in the opposite direction. Therefore, the gutta percha is in the root canal that lies to the buccal (opposite = buccal).*

EXAMPLE

The buccal object rule can be used to determine the location of an impacted supernumerary (extra) tooth (Fig. 21–11).
1. *Position the maxillary arch parallel to the floor.*
2. *Expose one central-lateral incisor periapical film using proper technique and angulation.*
3. *Shift the PID in a distal direction and expose the canine periapical film.*
4. *In the second film, when the PID was moved in a distal direction, the tooth moved in the same direction. Therefore, the tooth lies to the lingual (same = lingual).*

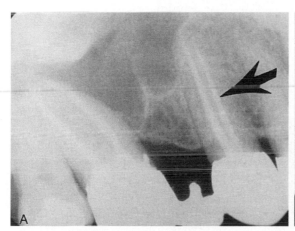
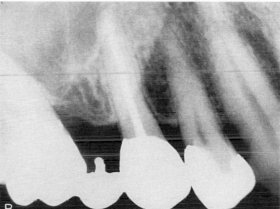

FIGURE 21–10. *A,* Notice the two canals filled with gutta percha in the maxillary second premolar (*arrow*). *B,* The tubehead was shifted in a mesial direction, and the gutta percha moved in a distal direction. The gutta percha is buccal. (Radiographs courtesy of Dr. Robert Jaynes, Assistant Professor, Oral Radiology Group, The Ohio State University College of Dentistry. Reprinted from Haring JI, Lind LJ: Radiographic Interpretation for the Dental Hygienist. Philadelphia, WB Saunders, 1993.)

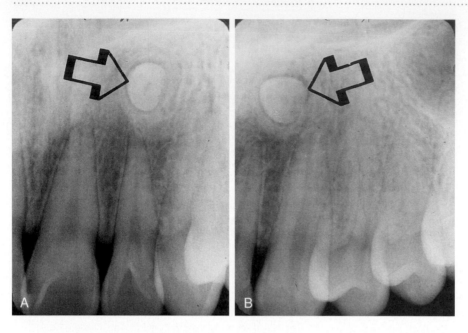

FIGURE 21–11. *A,* Notice the impacted tooth (*arrow*). *B,* The PID was shifted in a distal direction, and the tooth moved in a distal direction. The tooth is located lingual to the adjacent teeth. (Radiographs courtesy of Dr. Robert Jaynes, Assistant Professor, Oral Radiology Group, The Ohio State University College of Dentistry.)

RIGHT-ANGLE TECHNIQUE

EXAMPLE

The right-angle technique can be used to determine the position of a radiopaque object (Fig. 21–12).
1. Position the maxillary arch parallel with the floor.
2. Expose one periapical film using proper technique and angulation.

3. Expose an occlusal film and direct the central ray perpendicular to the film.
4. In the occlusal film, the radiopaque object is located buccal to the mandible.

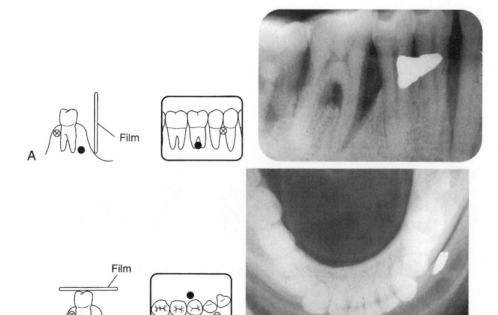

FIGURE 21–12. Right-angle localization technique. Two films are exposed at right angles to each other to identify the location of an object. The periapical radiograph (*A*) will demonstrate the superoinferior and anteroposterior positions of objects. A cross-sectional occlusal radiograph (*B*) will demonstrate the anteroposterior and buccal-lingual positions. These two radiographic views will demonstrate all three dimensions of an area, and the location of objects can be identified. (From Olson SS: Dental Radiography Laboratory Manual. Philadelphia, WB Saunders, 1995.)

SUMMARY

- The occlusal technique is a method used to examine large areas of the upper or lower jaw. The film is so named because the patient "occludes" or bites on the film.
- Size 4 intraoral film is used in the occlusal technique.
- The occlusal radiograph is preferred when the area of interest is larger than a periapical film or when the placement of periapical films is too difficult for the patient.
- Uses for occlusal radiographs include the following:
  - localization of roots, impacted teeth, unerupted teeth, foreign bodies, or salivary stones
  - evaluation of the size of lesions, the boundaries of the maxillary sinus, or jaw fractures
  - examination of patients who cannot open their mouths
  - measurement of changes in the size and shape of the jaws
- The principles of the occlusal technique are:
  - the film is positioned with the white side facing the arch being exposed
  - the film is placed in the mouth between the occlusal surfaces of the teeth
  - the film is stabilized when the patient gently bites on the surface of the film
- Prior to film exposure using the occlusal technique, the dental radiographer must complete infection control procedures, prepare the treatment area and supplies, seat the patient, explain the radiographic procedures to be performed, make the proper chair and headrest adjustments, place the lead apron, remove any intraoral objects and eyeglasses, and set the exposure factors.
- A localization technique is a method used to locate the position of a tooth or object in the jaws. A localization technique can be used to determine the buccal-lingual relationship of an object or to locate foreign bodies, impacted and unerupted teeth, retained roots, root positions, salivary stones, jaw fractures, broken needles and instruments, and filling materials.
- The buccal object rule, a rule for the orientation of structures seen in two radiographs exposed at different angles, can be used as a localization technique.
- The right-angle technique, another rule for the orientation of structures seen in two radiographs (one periapical, one occlusal), can also be used as a localization technique.

BIBLIOGRAPHY

Eastman Kodak Company: Intraoral—the bisecting technic (short cone). *In* X Rays in Dentistry. Rochester, NY, Eastman Kodak Company, 1985, pp. 40–51.

Frommer HH: Accessory radiographic techniques. *In* Radiology for Dental Auxiliaries, 6th edition. St. Louis, Mosby-Year Book, 1996, pp. 181–204.

Frommer HH: Patient management and special problems. *In* Radiology for Dental Auxiliaries, 6th edition. St. Louis, Mosby-Year Book, 1996, pp. 245–267.

Goaz PW, White SC: Projection geometry. *In* Oral Radiology: Principles of Interpretation, 3rd edition. St. Louis, Mosby-Year Book, 1994, pp. 102–105.

Goaz PW, White SC: Intraoral radiographic examinations. *In* Oral Radiology: Principles of Interpretation, 3rd edition. St. Louis, Mosby-Year Book, 1994, pp. 206–212.

Johnson ON, McNally MA, Essay CE: Preliminary interpretation of the radiographs. *In* Essentials of Dental Radiography for Dental Assistants and Hygienists, 6th edition. Norwalk, CT, Appleton and Lange, 1999, pp. 259–296.

Johnson ON, McNally MA, Essay CE: The occlusal examination. *In* Essentials of Dental Radiography for Dental Assistants and Hygienists, 6th edition. Norwalk, CT, Appleton and Lange, 1999, pp. 391–401.

Langland OE, Sippy FH, Langlais RP: Intraoral radiographic techniques. *In* Textbook of Dental Radiography, 2nd edition. Springfield, IL, Charles C Thomas, 1984, pp. 269–275.

Langland OE, Sippy FH, Langlais RP: Atlas of special technics in dental radiology. *In* Textbook of Dental Radiography, 2nd edition. Springfield, IL, Charles C Thomas, 1984, pp. 557–566.

Manson-Hing LR: Fast exposure and localization technics. *In* Fundamentals of Dental Radiography, 3rd edition. Philadelphia, Lea & Febiger, 1990, pp. 136–139.

Manson-Hing LR: Occlusal film and extraoral radiography. *In* Fundamentals of Dental Radiography, 3rd edition. Philadelphia, Lea & Febiger, 1990, pp. 140–144.

Miles DA, Van Dis ML, Jensen CW, Ferretti A: Accessory radiographic techniques and patient management. *In* Radiographic Imaging for Dental Auxiliaries, 3rd edition. Philadelphia, WB Saunders, 1999, pp. 129–148.

Quiz Questions ··

1. What does the term occlusal refer to?

   _____

2. What size film is recommended for use with the occlusal technique in the adult patient?

   _____

3. What size film is recommended for use with the occlusal technique in the child patient with a primary dentition?

   _____

4. How is the patient's head positioned prior to exposing a maxillary occlusal film?

   _____

5. What are the uses for the occlusal film?

   _____

6. State the vertical angulation used for the maxillary occlusal topographic projection.

   _____

7. State the vertical angulation used for the maxillary occlusal lateral projection.

   _____

8. State the vertical angulation used for the mandibular occlusal topographic projection.

   _____

9. State the vertical angulation used for the mandibular occlusal cross-sectional projection.

   _____

10. State the vertical angulations used for the maxillary and mandibular occlusal pediatric projections.

    _____

SHORT ANSWER

For questions 11 to 15, use the *buccal object rule* and refer to the appropriate figures.

11. In Figure 21–13, is the labeled amalgam pit buccal or lingual? Why?

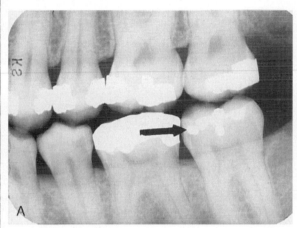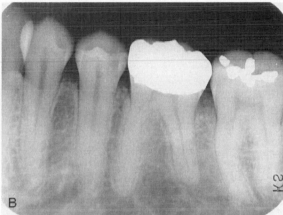

FIGURE 21–13. (Radiographs courtesy of Dr. Robert Jaynes, Assistant Professor, Oral Radiology Group, The Ohio State University College of Dentistry. Reprinted from Haring JI, Lind LJ: Radiographic Interpretation for the Dental Hygienist. Philadelphia, WB Saunders, 1993.)

12. In Figure 21–14, is the amalgam fragment between the maxillary second and third molars buccal or lingual? Why?

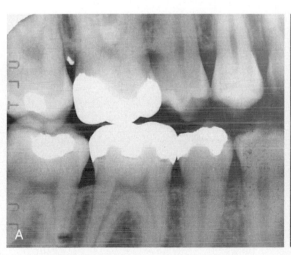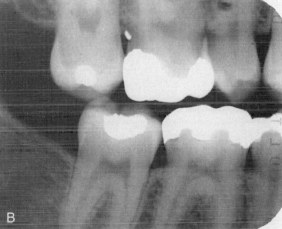

FIGURE 21–14. (Radiographs courtesy of Dr. Robert Jaynes, Assistant Professor, Oral Radiology Group, The Ohio State University College of Dentistry. Reprinted from Haring JI, Lind LJ: Radiographic Interpretation for the Dental Hygienist. Philadelphia, WB Saunders, 1993.)

13. In Figure 21–15, is the impacted canine located buccal or lingual to the adjacent teeth? Why?

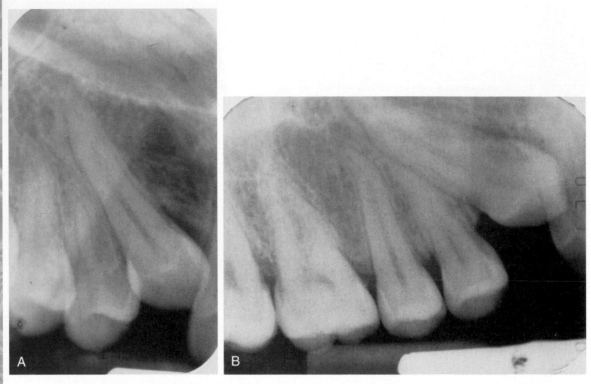

FIGURE 21–15. (Radiographs courtesy of Dr. Robert Jaynes, Assistant Professor, Oral Radiology Group, The Ohio State University College of Dentistry. Reprinted from Haring JI, Lind LJ: Radiographic Interpretation for the Dental Hygienist. Philadelphia, WB Saunders, 1993.)

14. In Figure 21–16, is the labeled canal with gutta percha located buccal or lingual? Why?

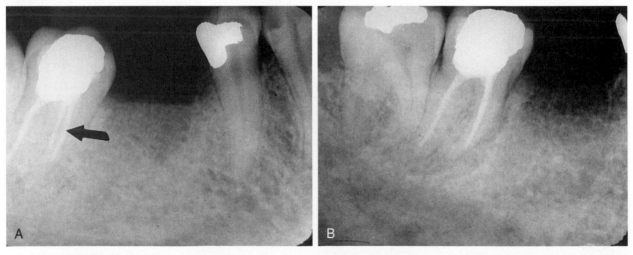

FIGURE 21–16. (Radiographs courtesy of Dr. Robert Jaynes, Assistant Professor, Oral Radiology Group, The Ohio State University College of Dentistry.)

15. In Figure 21-17, is the impacted canine located buccal or lingual to the adjacent teeth? Why?

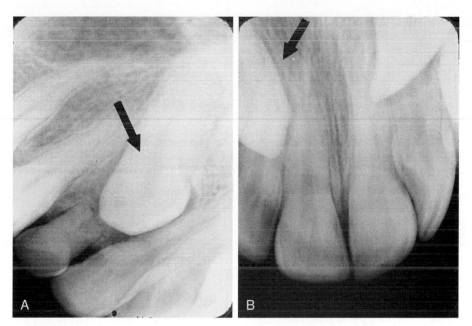

FIGURE 21-17. (Radiographs courtesy of Dr. Robert Jaynes, Assistant Professor, Oral Radiology Group, The Ohio State University College of Dentistry.)

Answers are supplied at the end of this book.

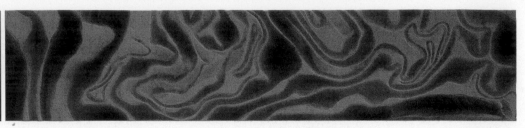

Panoramic Radiography

OBJECTIVES

After completion of this chapter, the student will be able to:

- *Define the key words.*
- *Describe the purpose and uses of panoramic radiography.*
- *Describe the fundamentals of panoramic radiography.*
- *Describe the equipment used in panoramic radiography.*
- *Describe the patient preparations, equipment preparations, and patient positioning procedures needed before exposing a panoramic film.*
- *Identify the patient preparation and positioning errors seen on panoramic radiographs.*
- *Discuss the causes of patient preparation and positioning errors and the necessary measures needed to correct such errors.*
- *Discuss the advantages and disadvantages of panoramic radiography.*

INTRODUCTION

It is often difficult, if not impossible, to obtain adequate diagnostic information from a series of intraoral films alone. Impacted third molar teeth, jaw fractures, and large lesions in the posterior mandible cannot always be seen well enough on intraoral films; in such cases, the panoramic radiograph is the film of choice. The panoramic radiograph allows the dental professional to view a large area of the maxilla and mandible on a single film.

The purpose of this chapter is to present basic concepts of panoramic radiography and to describe the patient preparation, equipment preparation, and patient positioning procedures needed to perform this procedure. In addition, this chapter describes the advantages and disadvantages of panoramic radiography and reviews helpful hints.

BASIC CONCEPTS

As the term **panoramic** suggests, a **panoramic film** shows a wide view of the upper and lower jaws (Fig. 22–1). **Panoramic radiography** is an extraoral radiographic technique that is used to examine the upper and lower jaws on a single film. As defined in Chapter 6, an extraoral film is one that is positioned *outside* the mouth during x-ray exposure. In panoramic radiography (also known as rotational panoramic radiography), both the film and the tubehead rotate around the patient, producing a series of individual images. When such images are combined on a single film, an overall view of the maxilla and mandible is created.

Purpose and Use

The panoramic film provides the dental radiographer with an overall image of the maxilla and mandible and is often used to supplement bite-wing and selected periapical films. The panoramic radiograph is typically used for the following purposes:

- to evaluate impacted teeth
- to evaluate eruption patterns, growth, and development
- to detect diseases, lesions, and conditions of the jaws
- to examine the extent of large lesions
- to evaluate trauma

The images on a panoramic film are not as defined or sharp as the images seen on intraoral films. Consequently, a panoramic film should not be used to evaluate and diagnose caries (see Chapter 30), periodontal disease (see Chapter 31), or periapical lesions (see Chapter 32). The panoramic radiograph should *not* be used as a substitute for intraoral films.

Fundamentals

When intraoral radiographs (e.g., periapical and bite-wing films) are exposed, the film and x-ray tubehead remain stationary. In panoramic radiography, the film and x-ray tubehead move around the patient. The x-ray tube rotates around the patient's head in one direction while the film rotates in the opposite direction (Fig. 22–2). The patient may stand or sit in a stationary position, depending on the type of panoramic x-ray machine that is used. The movement of the film and the tubehead produces an image through the process known as tomography. The term *tomo* means section; **tomography** is a radiographic technique that allows the imaging of one layer or section of the body while blurring images from structures in other planes. In panoramic radiography, this image conforms to the shape of the dental arches.

ROTATION CENTER

In panoramic radiography, the film or cassette carrier and x-ray tubehead are connected and rotate simultaneously around a patient during exposure. The pivotal point, or axis, around which the cassette carrier and x-ray tubehead rotate is termed a **rotation center**. Depending on the manufacturer, the number and location of the rotational centers differ. One of three basic rotation centers is used in panoramic x-ray machines (Fig. 22–3):

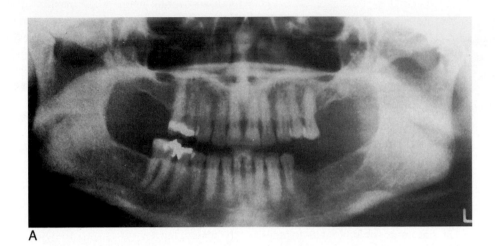

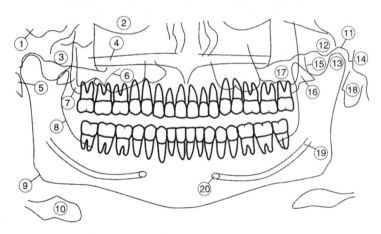

① Middle cranial fossa	⑪ Glenoid fossa
② Orbit	⑫ Articular eminence
③ Zygomatic arch	⑬ Mandibular condyle
④ Palate	⑭ Vertebra
⑤ Styloid process	⑮ Coronoid process
⑥ Septa in maxillary sinus	⑯ Pterygoid plates
⑦ Maxillary tuberosity	⑰ Maxillary sinus
⑧ External oblique line	⑱ Ear lobe
⑨ Angle of mandible	⑲ Mandibular canal
⑩ Hyoid bone	⑳ Mental foramen

FIGURE 22–1. *A,* Panoramic radiograph. (From Miles DA, Van Dis ML, Jensen CW, et al: Radiographic Imaging for Dental Auxiliaries, 2nd ed. WB Saunders, 1993.) *B,* Panoramic anatomy. (From Olson SS: Dental Radiography Laboratory Manual. Philadelphia, WB Saunders, 1995.)

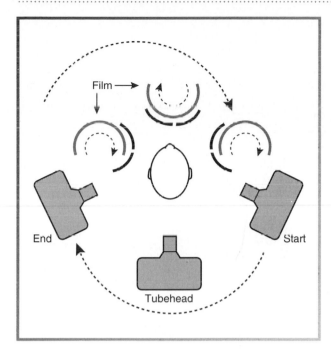

FIGURE 22–2. The film and x-ray tubehead move around the patient in opposite directions in panoramic radiography. (Courtesy of Dr. Robert M. Jaynes, Assistant Professor, Oral Radiology Group, The Ohio State University College of Dentistry.)

- the double-center rotation
- the triple-center rotation
- the moving-center rotation

In all cases, the center of rotation changes as the film and tubehead rotate around the patient. This rotational change allows the image layer to conform to the elliptical shape of the dental arches. The location and number of rotational centers influence the size and shape of the focal trough.

FOCAL TROUGH

In panoramic radiography, the focal trough is a theoretical concept used to determine where the dental arches must be positioned to achieve the clearest image (Fig. 22–4). The **focal trough** (also known as the image layer) can be defined as a three dimensional curved zone in which structures are clearly demonstrated on a panoramic radiograph. The structures located within the focal trough appear reasonably well defined on the resulting panoramic radiograph. The structures positioned inside or outside of the focal trough appear blurred or indistinct and are not readily visible on the panoramic film.

The size and shape of the focal trough vary with the manufacturer of the panoramic x-ray unit. The closer the rotation center is to the teeth, the narrower the focal trough. In most panoramic x-ray machines, the focal trough is narrow in the anterior region and wide in the posterior region.

Each panoramic x-ray unit has a focal trough that is designed to accommodate the average jaw. Each manufacturer provides specific instructions about patient positioning to ensure that the teeth are positioned within the focal trough. The quality of the resulting panoramic radiograph depends on the positioning of the patient's teeth within the focal trough and how closely the patient's jaws conform to the focal trough designed for the average jaw.

Equipment

In panoramic radiography, the use of special equipment, including a panoramic x-ray unit, screen film, intensifying screens, and cassette, is necessary.

PANORAMIC X-RAY UNITS

There are a number of different panoramic x-ray units; examples include the Orthopantomograph 10E (Siemens), the GX-Pan (Gendex Corporation), and the Cranex 3 Ceph (Soredex Medical Systems) (Fig. 22–5). Panoramic units may differ in the number of the rotation centers, the size and shape of the focal trough, and the type of film transport mechanism used. Although each manufacturer's panoramic unit is slightly different, all panoramic machines have similar components. The main components of the panoramic unit include (Fig. 22–6):

- x-ray tubehead
- head positioner
- exposure controls

The panoramic x-ray **tubehead** is very similar to an intraoral x-ray tubehead; each has a filament used to produce electrons and a target used to produce x-rays. The **collimator** used in the panoramic x-ray tubehead, however, differs from the collimator used in the intraoral x-ray tube head. As described in Chapter 5, the collimator used in the intraoral x-ray machine is a lead plate with a small round or rectangular opening in the middle. The function of the collimator is to restrict the size and shape of the x-ray beam. The collimator used in the panoramic x-ray machine is a lead plate with an opening in the shape of a narrow vertical slit (Fig. 22–7).

The x-ray beam emerges from the panoramic tubehead through the collimator as a narrow band. The

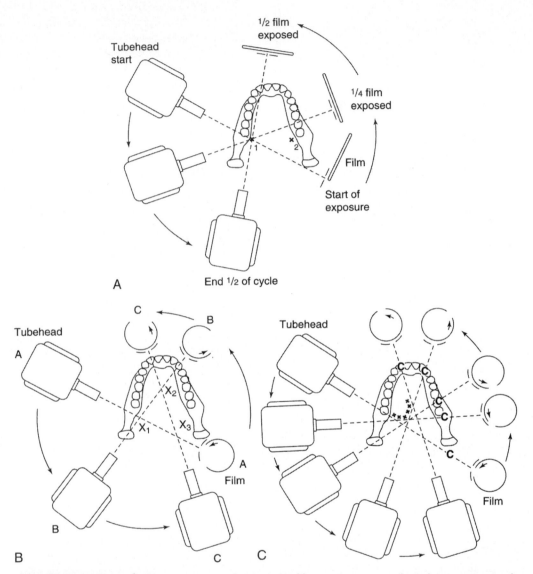

Tubehead
start

¹/₂ film
exposed

¹/₄ film
exposed

Film

Start of
exposure

End ¹/₂ of cycle

A

Tubehead

C   B

X₂

X₁   X₃

A
Film

B   C

B

Tubehead

Film

C

FIGURE 22-3. Types of panoramic x-ray machines. *A,* Double-center rotation machines have two rotational centers, one for the right and one for the left side of the jaws. *B,* Triple-center rotation machines have three centers of rotation and create an uninterrupted radiographic image of the jaws. *C,* Moving-center rotation machines rotate around a continuously moving center that is similar to the arches, creating an uninterrupted image of the jaws. (From Olson SS: Dental Radiography Laboratory Manual. Philadelphia, WB Saunders, 1995.)

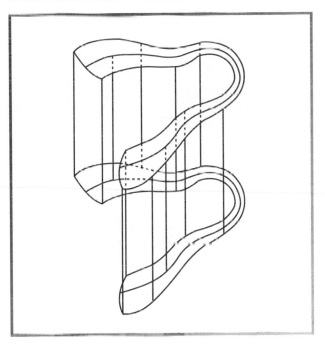

FIGURE 22–4. An example of an "image layer" or "focal trough." (Reprinted courtesy of Eastman Kodak Company.)

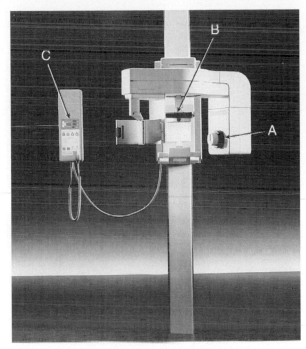

FIGURE 22–6. The main components of the panoramic unit include (A) the x-ray tubehead, (B) the head positioner, and (C) the exposure controls. (Courtesy of Siemens Company, Charlotte, NC.)

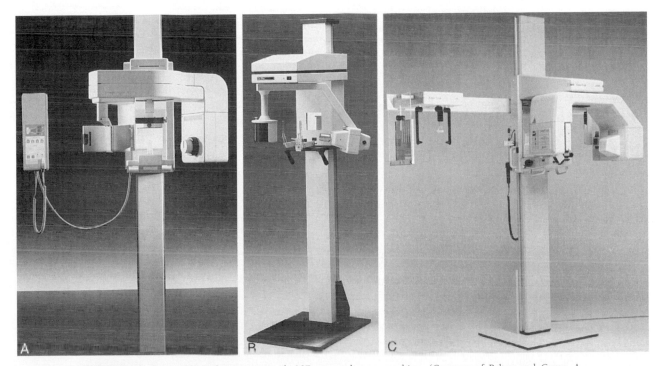

FIGURE 22–5. *A*, The Orthopantomograph 10E extraoral x-ray machine. (Courtesy of Pelton and Crane, A Siemens Company, Charlotte, NC.) *B*, The GX-Pan extraoral x-ray machine. (Courtesy of Gendex Corp., Des Plaines, IL.) *C*, The Cranex 3 Ceph extraoral x-ray machine. (Courtesy of Soredex Medical Systems, Conroe, TX.)

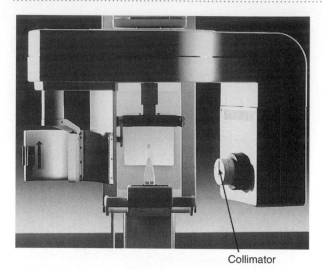

FIGURE 22–7. The collimator on a panoramic unit has a narrow slit opening. (Courtesy of Siemens Company, Charlotte, NC.)

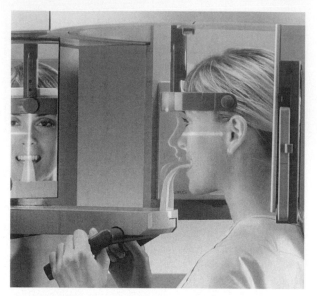

FIGURE 22–8. The head positioner (notched bite-block, forehead rest, and lateral head supports) is used to align the patient's teeth in the focal trough. (Courtesy of Siemens Company, Charlotte, NC.)

beam passes through the patient and then exposes the film through another vertical slit in the cassette carrier (the metal holder that supports the cassette). The narrow x-ray beam that emerges from the collimator minimizes patient exposure to x-radiation.

Unlike the intraoral tubehead, the vertical angulation of the panoramic tubehead is not varied. The tubehead of the panoramic unit is fixed in position so that the x-ray beam is directed slightly upward. In addition, the tubehead of the panoramic unit always rotates *behind* the patient's head as the film rotates in front of the patient.

Each panoramic unit has a head positioner used to align the patient's teeth as accurately as possible in the focal trough. The typical **head positioner** consists of a chin rest, notched bite-block, forehead rest, and lateral head supports or guides (Fig. 22–8). Each panoramic unit is different, and the operator must follow the manufacturer's instructions on how to position the patient in the focal trough.

Each panoramic unit has **exposure factors** that are determined by the manufacturer; suggested exposure factors (milliamperage and kilovoltage) are provided by the manufacturer in the x-ray machine instruction manual. The milliamperage and kilovoltage settings are adjustable and can be varied to accommodate patients of different sizes (Fig. 22–9). The exposure time, however, is fixed and cannot be changed.

FILM

Screen film is used in panoramic radiography; this film is sensitive to the light emitted from intensifying screens (see Chapter 7). A screen film is placed between two intensifying screens in a cassette holder. When the cassette holder is exposed to x-rays, the screens convert the x-ray energy into light, which in turn exposes the screen film. Some screen films are sensitive to green light (Kodak T-Mat G and Ortho G film), whereas, others are sensitive to blue light (Kodak X-Omat RP and Ektamat G films). Blue-sensitive film must be paired with screens that produce blue light, and green-sensitive film must be paired with screens that produce green light. The film used in panoramic radiography is available in two sizes: 5- × 12-inch and 6- × 12-inch.

INTENSIFYING SCREENS

There are two basic types of **intensifying screens:** calcium tungstate and rare earth (see Chapter 7). Calcium tungstate screens emit blue light, and the rare earth screens emit green light. Rare earth screens require less x-ray exposure than calcium tungstate screens and are considered "faster." Consequently, rare earth screens are recommended in panoramic radiography because there is less radiation exposure for the patient.

CASSETTE

The **cassette** is a device that is used to hold the extraoral film and intensifying screens (see Chapter 7). The cassette may be rigid or flexible, curved or

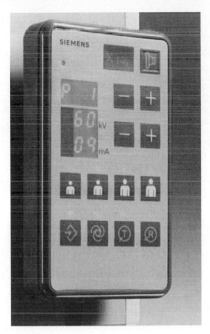

FIGURE 22–9. An example of an exposure control switch for a panoramic unit. (Courtesy of Siemens Company, Charlotte, NC.)

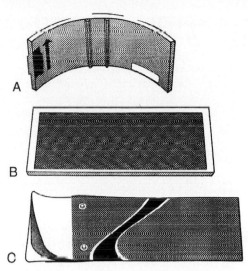

FIGURE 22–10. Film cassettes. *A* and *B* are rigid cassettes. In a rigid cassette, the intensifying screens are attached to the inside cover and base of the cassette. When the panoramic film is placed in the cassette, it lies in-between the screens. *C* shows a flexible cassette that has an opening at one end creating a pouch. The panoramic film is placed between two removable, flexible intensifying screens, which are then slid into the pouch. (Reprinted courtesy of Eastman Kodak Company.)

straight, depending on the panoramic x-ray unit (Fig. 22–10). All cassettes must be light-tight to protect the film from exposure. One intensifying screen is placed on each side of the film and held in place when the cassette is closed.

The cassette must be marked to orient the finished radiograph. Prior to exposure, a metal letter R can be attached to the front of the cassette to indicate the patient's right side; the letter L is used to identify the patient's left side (Fig. 22–11). Special labeling may also be attached to indicate the patient's name,

the dentist's name, and the date. If the cassette is not labeled prior to exposure, the film must be labeled immediately after processing; a marking pen or adhesive label can be used to label the radiograph.

STEP-BY-STEP PROCEDURES

Step-by-step procedures for the exposure of a panoramic film include equipment preparation, patient

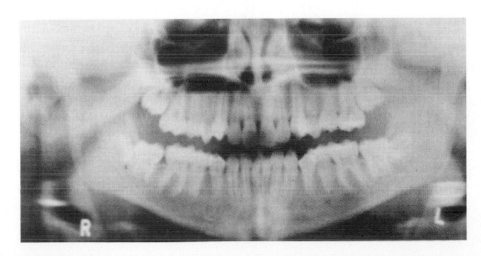

FIGURE 22–11. This panoramic film is labeled with two metal letters indicating the patient's right and left sides.

PROCEDURE

Equipment Preparation

1. Load the panoramic cassette in the darkroom under safelight conditions. One extraoral film and two intensifying screens must be placed in the cassette, and the cassette must be securely closed.

2. Cover the bite-block with a disposable plastic coverslip. If the bite-block is not covered with an impervious material (e.g., plastic coverslip), it must be sterilized between patients.

3. Set the exposure factors (kilovoltage, milliamperage) according to the manufacturer's recommendations. Adjust the machine to accommodate the height of the patient and align all movable parts properly. The cassette must be loaded in the cassette carrier of the panoramic unit.

preparation, and patient positioning. Prior to exposing a panoramic film, infection control procedures (as described in Chapter 15) must be completed.

Equipment Preparation

The dental radiographer must complete equipment preparations prior to preparing a patient for the exposure of a panoramic film (see "Procedure: Equipment Preparation").

Patient Preparation

After preparing the panoramic equipment, the dental radiographer must prepare the patient for the procedure (see "Procedure: Patient Preparation").

PROCEDURE

Patient Preparation

1. Explain the radiographic procedures about to be performed.

2. Place a lead apron, *without* a thyroid collar, on the patient and secure it. A double-sided lead apron (one that protects the front and back of the patient) is recommended (Fig. 22–12). The lead apron must be placed low around the neck so that it does not block the x-ray beam. A thyroid collar is *not* recommended for panoramic radiography because it blocks part of the beam and obscures important diagnostic information.

3. Remove all objects from the head and neck area that may interfere with film exposure. The patient must remove eyeglasses, earrings, necklaces, napkin chains, hearing aids, hairpins, and complete and partial dentures.

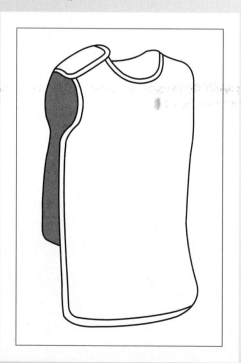

FIGURE 22–12. A double-sided lead apron is recommended for use during exposure of a panoramic film.

1. Instruct the patient to sit or stand "as tall as possible" with the back straight and erect. The vertebral column must be perfectly straight. The spinal column is very dense; if the spine is not straight, a white shadow appears over the middle of the radiograph and obscures diagnostic information.

2. Instruct the patient to bite on the plastic bite-block. The upper and lower front teeth must be placed in an end-to-end position in the groove (notch) that is found on the bite-block (Fig. 22–13). This groove is used to align the teeth in the focal trough. (In a patient without teeth, the radiographer must align the upper and lower ridges over the notched area on the bite-block. Cotton rolls can be placed on each side of the bite-block to provide stabilization for the patient.)

3. Position the **midsagittal plane** (an imaginary line that divides the patient's face into right and left sides) perpendicular to the floor. (Fig. 22–14). The patient's head must not be tipped or tilted; if the midsagittal plane is not positioned perpendicular to the floor, a distorted image results on the panoramic radiograph.

4. Position the **Frankfort plane** (an imaginary plane that passes through the top of the ear canal and the bottom of the eye socket) parallel with the floor (Fig. 22–15). When the Frankfort plane is parallel to the floor, the occlusal plane is positioned at the correct angle.

5. Instruct the patient to position the tongue on the roof of the mouth. The radiographer may suggest

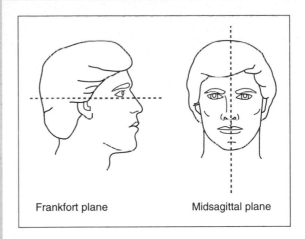

FIGURE 22–14. Frankfort and midsagittal planes. The Frankfort plane passes through the floor of the orbit and the external auditory meatus. The midsagittal plane divides the body in half into right and left sides. (From Olson SS: Dental Radiography Laboratory Manual. Philadelphia, WB Saunders, 1995.)

that the patient "swallow and feel the tongue rise up to the roof of the mouth" and then instruct the patient to keep the tongue in that position during the exposure of the film. Also instruct the patient to close the lips around the bite-block.

6. After the patient has been positioned, instruct the patient to remain still while the machine is rotating during exposure.

7. Expose the film and proceed with film processing as described in Chapter 9.

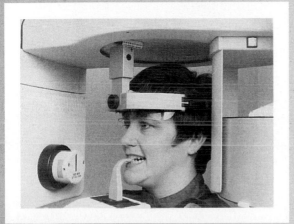

FIGURE 22–13. The patient's teeth must be positioned in the grooves on the bite-block. (From Haring JI, Lind LJ: Radiographic Interpretation for the Dental Hygienist. Philadelphia, WB Saunders, 1993.)

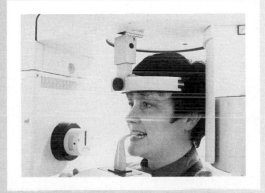

FIGURE 22–15. The patient's Frankfort plane must be positioned so that it is parallel to the floor. (From Haring JI, Lind LJ: Radiographic Interpretation for the Dental Hygienist. Philadelphia, WB Saunders, 1993.)

Patient Positioning

The dental radiographer must be familiar with the manufacturer's specific directions for patient positioning included in the instruction manual. Although each manufacturer's positioning and exposure procedures are slightly different, the following patient positioning steps are common to all panoramic machines (see "Procedure: Patient Positioning").

COMMON ERRORS

To produce a diagnostic panoramic radiograph and minimize patient exposure, mistakes must be avoided. The dental radiographer must be able to recognize common patient preparation and positioning errors and understand what steps are necessary to correct such errors.

Patient Preparation Errors

Proper patient preparation is critical in obtaining a diagnostic panoramic film. Two of the more common patient preparation errors include ghost images and the lead apron artifact.

GHOST IMAGES

Problem. If all metallic or radiodense objects (e.g., eyeglasses, earrings, necklaces, hairpins, removable partial dentures, complete dentures, orthodontic retainers, hearing aids, and napkin chains) are not removed before the exposure of a panoramic film, a ghost image results that obscures diagnostic information.

A **ghost image** is a radiopaque artifact seen on a panoramic film that is produced when a radiodense object is penetrated twice by the x-ray beam. A ghost image resembles its real counterpart and is found on the *opposite* side of the film; it appears indistinct, larger, and higher than its actual counterpart. For example, a ghost image of a hoop earring appears on the opposite side of the film as a radiopacity that is larger and higher than the real hoop earring. In addition, the ghost image of the hoop earring appears blurred in both a horizontal and vertical direction (Fig. 22–16).

Solution. To prevent such an artifact, the dental radiographer must instruct the patient to remove all radiodense objects in the head and neck region prior to positioning the patient for a panoramic film.

LEAD APRON ARTIFACT

Problem. If the lead apron is incorrectly placed, or if a lead apron with a thyroid collar is used during the exposure of a panoramic film, a radiopaque cone-shaped artifact results that obscures diagnostic information (Fig. 22–17).

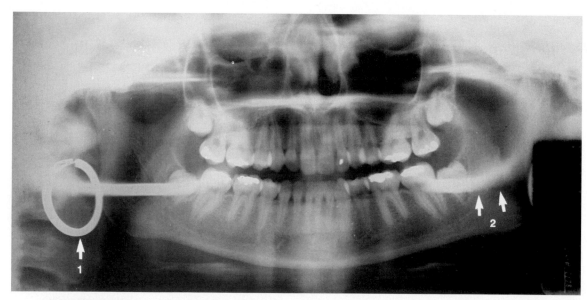

FIGURE 22–16. Large hoop earrings (1) and ghost images (2). The ghost image of the earring appears on the opposite side of the film and is enlarged and laterally distorted. (From Haring JI, Lind LJ: Radiographic Interpretation for the Dental Hygienist. Philadelphia, WB Saunders, 1993.)

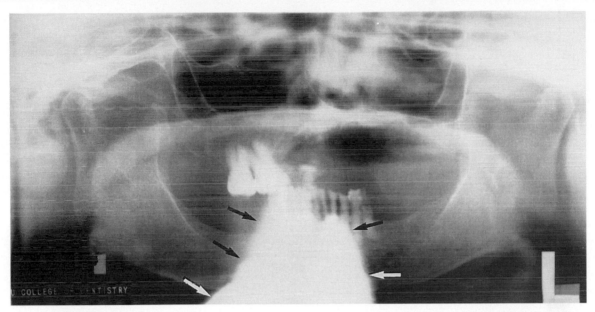

FIGURE 22–17. On a panoramic radiograph, a lead apron artifact appears as a large cone-shaped radiopacity obscuring the mandible. (From Haring JI, Lind LJ: Radiographic Interpretation for the Dental Hygienist. Philadelphia, WB Saunders, 1993.)

Solution. To prevent such an artifact, the dental radiographer must always use a lead apron without a thyroid collar when exposing a panoramic film. The lead apron must be placed low around the neck of the patient so that it does not block the x-ray beam.

Patient Positioning Errors

Patient positioning is of critical importance during exposure of a panoramic film. Because the panoramic image does not produce the fine anatomic detail seen on intraoral radiographs, even the smallest positioning error can create a distorted image.

POSITIONING OF THE LIPS AND TONGUE

Problem. If the patient's lips are not closed on the bite-block during the exposure of a panoramic film, a dark radiolucent shadow results that obscures the anterior teeth. If the tongue is not in contact with the palate during the exposure of a panoramic film, a dark radiolucent shadow results that obscures the apices of the maxillary teeth (Fig. 22–18).

Solution. To prevent such errors, the dental radiographer must instruct the patient to close the lips around the bite-block. The patient must also be instructed to swallow and then raise the tongue up to the palate during the exposure of the film.

POSITIONING OF THE FRANKFORT PLANE—UPWARD

Problem. If the patient's chin is positioned too high or is tipped up (Fig. 22–19), the Frankfort plane is angled upward, and the following results:

- the hard palate and floor of the nasal cavity appear superimposed over the roots of the maxillary teeth
- there is a loss of detail in the maxillary incisor region
- the maxillary incisors appear blurred and magnified
- a "reverse smile line" (curved downward) is apparent on the radiograph (Fig. 22–20)

Solution. To prevent such an error, the dental radiographer must carefully position the patient so that the Frankfort plane is parallel with the floor.

POSITIONING OF THE FRANKFORT PLANE—DOWNWARD

Problem. If the patient's chin is positioned too low or is tipped down (Fig. 22–21), the Frankfort plane is angled downward and the following results:

- the mandibular incisors appear blurred
- there is a loss of detail in the anterior apical regions
- the condyles may not be visible
- an "exaggerated smile line" (curved upward) is apparent on the radiograph (Fig. 22–22)

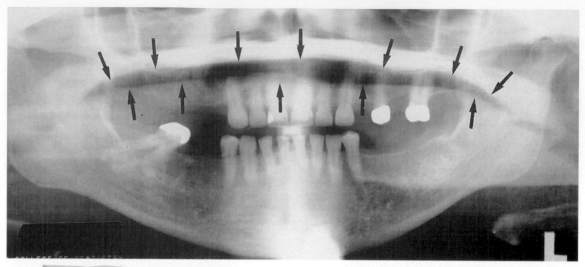

FIGURE 22–18. If the tongue is not placed on the roof of the mouth, a radiolucent shadow will be superimposed over the apices of the maxillary teeth. (From Haring JI, Lind LJ: Radiographic Interpretation for the Dental Hygienist. Philadelphia, WB Saunders, 1993.)

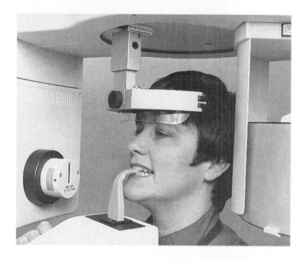

FIGURE 22–19. The patient's head is incorrectly positioned; the chin is tipped up. (From Haring JI, Lind LJ: Radiographic Interpretation for the Dental Hygienist. Philadelphia, WB Saunders, 1993.)

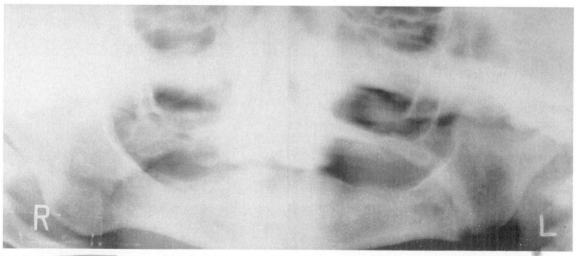

FIGURE 22–20. A "reverse smile line" is seen on a panoramic film when the patient's chin is tipped up. (From Haring JI, Lind LJ: Radiographic Interpretation for the Dental Hygienist. Philadelphia, WB Saunders, 1993.)

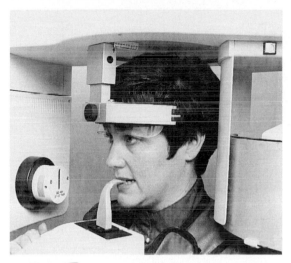

FIGURE 22–21. The patient's head is incorrectly positioned; the chin is tipped down. (From Haring JI, Lind LJ: Radiographic Interpretation for the Dental Hygienist. Philadelphia, WB Saunders, 1993.)

Solution. To prevent such an error, the dental radiographer must carefully position the patient so that the Frankfort plane is parallel with the floor.

POSITIONING OF TEETH—ANTERIOR TO THE FOCAL TROUGH

Problem. If the patient's anterior teeth are not positioned in the focal trough indicated by the groove in the bite-block, the teeth appear blurred. If the patient's teeth are positioned too far forward on the bite-block or anterior to the focal trough (Fig. 22–23), the anterior teeth appear "skinny" and out of focus on the radiograph (Fig. 22–24).

Solution. To prevent such an error, the dental radiographer must position the patient so that the anterior teeth are placed in an end to end position in the groove on the bite-block. The forehead support must then be adjusted to stabilize the patient's head position and prevent the patient from sliding forward on the bite-block.

POSITIONING OF TEETH—POSTERIOR TO THE FOCAL TROUGH

Problem. If the patient's anterior teeth are not positioned in the focal trough indicated by the groove in the bite-block, the teeth appear blurred. If the patient's teeth are positioned too far back on the bite-block or posterior to the focal trough (Fig. 22–25), the anterior teeth appear "fat" and out of focus on the radiograph (Fig. 22–26).

Solution. To prevent such an error, the dental radiographer must position the patient so that the anterior teeth are placed in an end-to-end position in the groove on the bite-block.

POSITIONING OF THE MIDSAGITTAL PLANE

Problem. If the patient's head is not centered (Fig. 22–27), the ramus and posterior teeth ap-

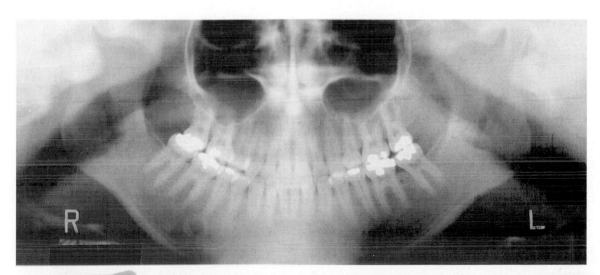

FIGURE 22–22. An "exaggerated smile" is seen on a panoramic film when the patient's chin is tipped down. (From Haring JI, Lind LJ: Radiographic Interpretation for the Dental Hygienist. Philadelphia, WB Saunders, 1993.)

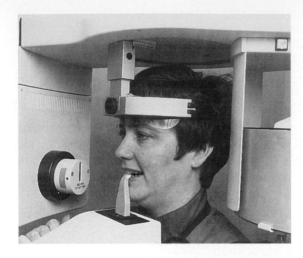

FIGURE 22–23. The patient is incorrectly positioned; the teeth are too far forward on the bite-block. (From Haring JI, Lind LJ: Radiographic Interpretation for the Dental Hygienist. Philadelphia, WB Saunders, 1993.)

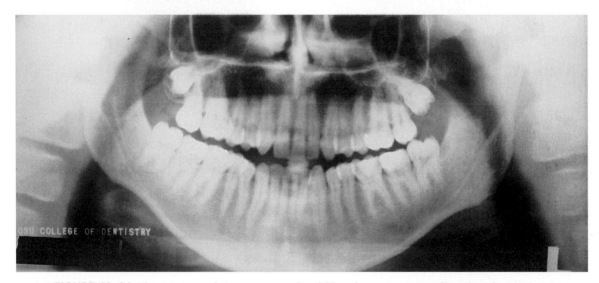

FIGURE 22–24. The anterior teeth appear narrowed and blurred on a panoramic film when the patient is positioned too far forward on the bite-block. (From Haring JI, Lind LJ: Radiographic Interpretation for the Dental Hygienist. Philadelphia, WB Saunders, 1993.)

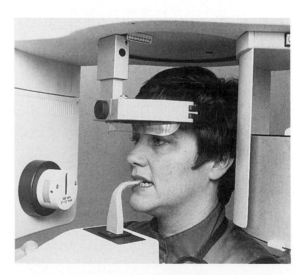

FIGURE 22–25. The patient is incorrectly positioned; the teeth are too far back and not on the bite-block. (From Haring JI, Lind LJ: Radiographic Interpretation for the Dental Hygienist. Philadelphia, WB Saunders, 1993.)

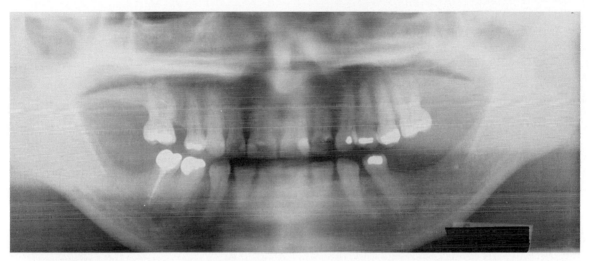

FIGURE 22–26. The anterior teeth appear widened and blurred on a panoramic film when the patient is positioned too far back on the bite-block. (From Haring JI, Lind LJ: Radiographic Interpretation for the Dental Hygienist. Philadelphia, WB Saunders, 1993.)

pear unequally magnified on the panoramic radiograph. The side farthest from the film appears magnified, and the side closest to the film appears smaller (Fig. 22–28).

Solution. To prevent such an error, the dental radiographer must position the patient's head so that the midsagittal plane is perpendicular to the floor while the midline is centered on the bite-stick. The lateral head supports must then be adjusted to stabilize the position of the patient's head.

POSITIONING OF THE SPINE

Problem. If the patient is not standing or sitting with a straight spine, the cervical spine appears as a radiopacity (Fig. 22–29) in the center of the film and obscures diagnostic information.

Solution. To prevent such an error, the dental radiographer must instruct the patient to stand or sit "as tall as possible" with a straight back.

ADVANTAGES AND DISADVANTAGES

As with all radiographic techniques, panoramic radiography has both advantages and disadvantages.

Advantages

- **Field size.** The panoramic radiograph includes coverage of the entire maxilla and mandible.

More anatomic structures can be viewed on a panoramic film than on a complete intraoral radiographic series. In addition, lesions and conditions of the jaws that may not be seen on intraoral films can be detected on a panoramic radiograph.

- **Simplicity.** Exposure of a panoramic radiograph is relatively simple and requires a minimal amount of time and training for the dental radiographer.

- **Patient cooperation.** The exposure of a panoramic radiograph is readily accepted by

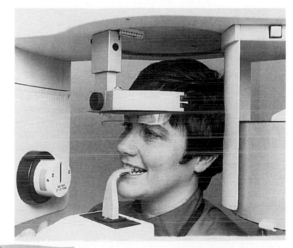

FIGURE 22–27. The patient is incorrectly positioned; the head is not centered. (From Haring JI, Lind LJ: Radiographic Interpretation for the Dental Hygienist. Philadelphia, WB Saunders, 1993.)

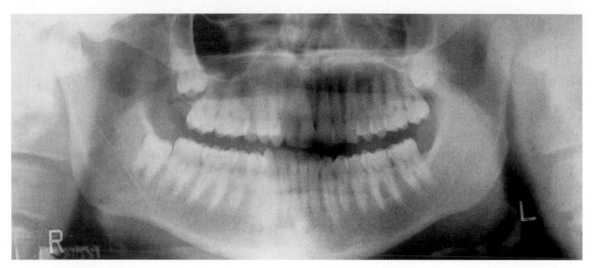

FIGURE 22–28. The patient's posterior teeth and ramus appear to be magnified on a panoramic film when the head is not centered. (From Haring JI, Lind LJ: Radiographic Interpretation for the Dental Hygienist. Philadelphia, WB Saunders, 1993.)

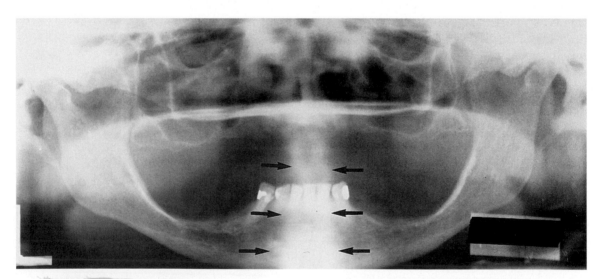

FIGURE 22–29. If the patient is not standing erect, superimposition of the cervical spine (*arrows*) may be seen on the center of the panoramic film. (From Haring JI, Lind LJ: Radiographic Interpretation for the Dental Hygienist. Philadelphia, WB Saunders, 1993.)

the patient because there is no discomfort involved.

- **Minimal exposure.** A panoramic radiograph results in minimal radiation exposure for the patient.

Disadvantages

- **Image quality.** The images seen on a panoramic radiograph are not as sharp as those on intraoral radiographs because of the intensifying screens. As a result, the panoramic radiograph cannot be used to evaluate dental caries, periodontal disease, or periapical lesions.
- **Focal trough limitations.** Objects of interest that are located outside the focal trough are not seen.
- **Distortion.** A certain amount of magnification, distortion, and overlapping is present on a panoramic radiograph, even when proper technique is used.
- **Equipment cost.** The cost of a panoramic x-ray unit, compared to the cost of an intraoral x-ray unit, is relatively high.

HELPFUL HINTS
For Exposing Panoramic Radiographs

- ➤ **DO** cover the bite-block with a disposable plastic coverslip prior to positioning the patient.
- ➤ **DO** choose the exposure factors (kilovoltage, milliamperage) according to the manufacturer's recommendations prior to positioning the patient.
- ➤ **DO** briefly explain to the patient the radiographic procedure that is about to be performed.
- ➤ **DO** place a lead apron without a thyroid collar on the patient and secure it.
- ➤ **DO** ask the patient to remove all radiodense objects from the head and neck area prior to positioning.
- ➤ **DO** instruct the patient to stand or sit "as straight and tall as possible."
- ➤ **DO** instruct the patient to place the front teeth in an end-to-end position in the deep groove on the bite-block.
- ➤ **DO** position the midsagittal plane of the patient perpendicular to the floor.
- ➤ **DO** position the Frankfort plane of the patient parallel with the floor.
- ➤ **DO** instruct the patient to close the lips on the bite-block and to swallow and place the tongue against the roof of the mouth. Instruct the patient to remain in that position during the exposure of the film.
- ➤ **DO** instruct the patient to remain still during the exposure of the film.

SUMMARY

- The panoramic radiograph allows the dental professional to view a large area of the maxilla and mandible on a single film.
- Uses of the panoramic radiograph include the following:
  - evaluation of impacted teeth
  - evaluation of eruption patterns and growth and development
  - detection of diseases, lesions, and conditions of the jaws
  - examination of the extent of large lesions
  - evaluation of trauma
- The panoramic radiograph is typically used to supplement bite-wing and periapical films and is not a substitute for intraoral films. The panoramic radiograph should not be used to evaluate caries, periodontal disease, and periapical lesions.
- In panoramic radiography, both the film and the tubehead are connected and rotate simultaneously around the patient during exposure. Rotational centers allow the image layer to conform to the elliptical shape of the dental arches. The number and location of the rotational centers influence the size and shape of the focal trough.
- The focal trough is a three-dimensional curved zone in which structures are clearly demonstrated on a panoramic radiograph; the structures located within the focal trough appear reasonably well defined, whereas structures outside of the focal trough appear blurred.
- The use of special equipment including a panoramic x-ray unit, screen film, intensifying screens, and cassette is necessary in panoramic radiography.
- Prior to preparing the patient for exposure of a panoramic film, the following tasks must be completed: preparation of the cassette, infection control procedures, selection of exposure factors, adjustment of the panoramic machine for patient height and proper alignment of movable parts, and loading of the cassette into the cassette carrier.
- After preparing the equipment, the dental radiographer must prepare the patient by explaining the radiographic procedure to the patient, placing the lead apron on the patient, and removing all radiodense objects from the head and neck region.
- The patient must then be positioned according to the manufacturer's recommendations for the positioning of the spine, teeth, midsagittal plane, Frankfort plane, lips, and tongue.
- The dental radiographer must be able to identify patient preparation and positioning errors and know what steps to take to correct such errors.
- The advantages of panoramic radiography include field size, simplicity of use, patient cooperation, and minimal patient exposure to x-radiation.
- The disadvantages of panoramic radiography include image quality, focal trough limitation, distortion, and the cost of equipment.

BIBLIOGRAPHY

Chomenko AG: Plane-in-focus and area of sharpness. *In* Atlas for Maxillofacial Pantomographic Interpretation. Chicago, Quintessence Publishing, 1985, pp. 14–23.

Eastman Kodak Company: Panoramic radiography. *In* Successful Panoramic Radiography. Rochester, Eastman Kodak Company, 1990, pp. 3–25.

Frommer HH: Panoramic radiography, new imaging systems. *In* Radiology for Dental Auxiliaries, 6th edition. St. Louis, Mosby-Year Book, 1996, pp. 223–243.

Goaz PW, White SC: Panoramic radiography. *In* Oral Radiology: Principles of Interpretation, 3rd edition. St. Louis, Mosby-Year Book, 1994, pp. 242–253.

Johnson ON, McNally MA, Essay CE: Panoramic radiography. *In* Essentials of Dental Radiography for Dental Assistants and Hygienists, 6th edition. Norwalk, CT, Appleton and Lange, 1999, pp. 451–474.

Langland OE, Langlais RP, McDavid WD, et al: Theory of rotational panoramic radiography. *In* Panoramic Radiology, 2nd edition. Philadelphia, Lea & Febiger, 1989, pp. 38–68.

Manson-Hing LR: Panoramic radiography. *In* Fundamentals of Dental Radiography, 3rd edition. Philadelphia, Lea & Febiger, 1990, pp. 160–185.

Miles DA, Van Dis ML, Jensen CW, Ferretti A: Panoramic radiography. *In* Radiographic Imaging for Dental Auxiliaries, 3rd edition. Philadelphia, WB Saunders, 1999, pp. 165–180.

Miles DA, Van Dis ML, Razmus TF: Plain film extraoral radiographic techniques. *In* Basic Principles of Oral and Maxillofacial Radiology. Philadelphia, WB Saunders, 1992, pp. 124–133.

Olson SS: Auxiliary radiographic techniques. *In* Dental Radiography Laboratory Manual. Philadelphia, WB Saunders, 1995, pp. 189–200.

Quiz Questions ··

MULTIPLE CHOICE

_____ 1. Which of the following describes a use of a panoramic film?

    a. diagnosis of caries
    b. evaluation of periodontal disease
    c. evaluation of impacted molars
    d. evaluation of periapical disease

_____ 2. The zone in which structures are clearly demonstrated on a panoramic radiograph is termed the:

    a. focal trough
    b. rotation center
    c. ghost image
    d. midsagittal plane

_____ 3. Rare earth intensifying screens are recommended in panoramic radiography because:

    a. rare earth screens emit a blue light
    b. rare earth screens provide a more diagnostic image
    c. rare earth screens require less x-ray exposure for the patient
    d. the images convert faster in automatic processors

_____ 4. A thyroid collar is _not_ recommended in panoramic radiography because:

    a. it blocks the x-ray beam and obscures information
    b. there is a relatively low dose of radiation to the thyroid gland in panoramic radiography
    c. it is impossible to sterilize the thyroid collar
    d. all of the above

_____ 5. The imaginary line that passes from the bottom of the eye socket through the top of the ear canal is termed the:

    a. midsagittal plane
    b. Frankfort plane
    c. vertebral plane
    d. orbital plane

MATCHING

For questions 6 to 20, match the following types of procedures with the statements given below.

    a. panoramic radiography
    b. intraoral radiography
    c. both panoramic and intraoral radiography

_____ 6. The film and tubehead rotate around the patient.

_____ 7. This type of radiograph is used to examine the extent of large lesions.

_____ 8. The dental arches must be positioned in a focal trough.

_____ 9. The tubehead contains a filament used to produce electrons and a target used to produce x-rays.

_____ 10. The collimator is a lead plate with an opening in the shape of a narrow vertical slit.

_____ 11. The collimator is a lead plate with a small round or rectangular opening.

_____ 12. The vertical angulation of the tubehead is variable.

_____ 13. A head positioner is used to position the patient's head.

_____ 14. Screen film is used.

_____ 15. A cassette holder with two intensifying screens is used.

_____ 16. The x-ray film must be loaded into a cassette in a darkroom under safelight conditions.

_____ 17. A lead apron with a thyroid collar must be placed on the patient.

_____ 18. All jewelry (earrings and necklaces) must be removed prior to the exposure of films.

_____ 19. The midsagittal plane must be positioned perpendicular to the floor.

_____ 20. The vertebral column must be perfectly straight.

ESSAY

21. Discuss the equipment preparations necessary prior to the exposure of a panoramic film.

22. Discuss the patient preparations necessary prior to the exposure of a panoramic film.

23. Discuss the patient positioning steps necessary prior to the exposure of a panoramic film.

24. Give examples of Frankfort plane positioning errors and discuss what steps can be taken to correct such errors.

25. Discuss the advantages and disadvantages of panoramic radiography.

_____

Answers are supplied at the end of this book.

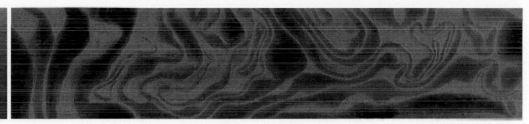

Extraoral Radiography

OBJECTIVES

After completion of this chapter, the student will be able to:

- *Define the key words.*
- *Describe the purpose and uses of extraoral radiography.*
- *Describe the equipment used in extraoral radiography.*
- *Detail the equipment and patient preparations necessary prior to exposing an extraoral film.*
- *Identify the specific purpose of each of the extraoral film projections.*
- *Describe the head position, film placement, and beam alignment for each of the following extraoral films: lateral jaw projection—body of the mandible, lateral jaw projection—ramus of the mandible, lateral cephalometric projection, posteroanterior projection, Waters projection, submentovertex projection, reverse Towne projection, and transcranial projection.*

INTRODUCTION

As discussed in Chapter 22, it is not always possible to obtain adequate diagnostic information from a series of intraoral radiographs. Jaw fractures, impacted teeth, and large lesions cannot always be seen well enough on intraoral films; in such cases, extraoral radiographs can be used to view large areas of teeth and bone. The extraoral radiograph allows the dental professional to view a large area of the jaws and skull on a single film.

The purpose of this chapter is to present the basic concepts of and describe the patient and equipment preparations needed for extraoral radiography. In addition, this chapter introduces a number of extraoral projection techniques and describes the film placement, patient positioning, and beam alignment for such projections.

BASIC CONCEPTS

As the term **extraoral** suggests, an **extraoral radiograph** is one that is placed *outside the mouth* during x-ray exposure. **Extraoral radiography** is used to image large areas of the skull or jaws. Many types of extraoral films exist; such films are primarily used in orthodontics and oral surgery. The most common ex-

traoral film is the panoramic radiograph (see Chapter 22).

Purpose and Use

The extraoral radiograph shows an overall image of the skull and jaws. The extraoral film is typically used for the following purposes:

- to evaluate large areas of the skull and jaws
- to evaluate growth and development
- to evaluate impacted teeth
- to detect diseases, lesions, and conditions of the jaws
- to examine the extent of large lesions
- to evaluate trauma
- to evaluate the temporomandibular joint area

In some instances, an extraoral film is used because the patient has swelling or discomfort and is unable to tolerate the placement of intraoral films. Extraoral radiographs may be used alone or in conjunction with intraoral films. As in the panoramic radiograph, the images seen on an extraoral film are not as defined or sharp as the images seen on an intraoral radiograph.

Equipment

X-RAY UNIT

A standard intraoral x-ray machine (see Chapter 6) may be used for a variety of extraoral projections (e.g., transcranial and lateral jaw projections). To aid in patient positioning and alignment of the x-ray beam, special head positioning and beam alignment devices can be added to the intraoral x-ray machine (Fig. 23–1). Some panoramic x-ray units (see Chapter 22) may also be used for extraoral projections. In such cases, the panoramic x-ray tubehead is used in conjunction with a special extension arm and a device known as a **cephalostat,** or craniostat (Fig. 23–2). The cephalostat includes a film holder and head positioner that allow the dental radiographer to position both film and patient easily.

FILM

Most extraoral exposures are made with screen film placed in a cassette with intensifying screens. **Screen film** is sensitive to the light emitted from intensifying screens (see Chapter 7). The use of screen film and intensifying screens minimizes the x-ray exposure necessary to produce a diagnostic radiograph. As previously discussed in Chapters 7 and 22, some screen

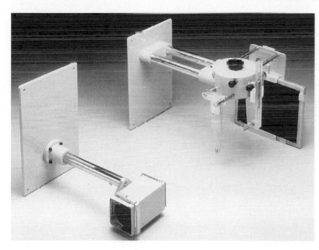

FIGURE 23–1. This unit can be used with most intraoral x-ray tubeheads. It is equipped with a collimator to allow accurate beam alignment and a head positioner to allow for proper patient positioning. (Courtesy of Wehmer Corporation, Addison, IL.)

films are sensitive to green light (Kodak T-Mat G, T-Mat L, Ortho G, and Ortho L), whereas others are sensitive to blue light (Kodak X-Omat RP and Ektamat G). Blue-sensitive film must be paired with screens that produce blue light, and green-sensitive film must be paired with screens that produce green light. Extraoral film size varies; the sizes most often used are 5- × 7-inch and 8- × 10-inch.

An occlusal film (size 4) may be used for some extraoral radiographs (e.g., lateral jaw or transcranial projection). An occlusal film is a **nonscreen film** and does not require the use of screens for exposure. As discussed earlier in Chapter 7, a nonscreen film requires more exposure time than a screen film. As a result, the occlusal film used extraorally requires more radiation exposure than a screen film. In addition, the occlusal film used extraorally does not cover as large an area as a screen film.

INTENSIFYING SCREENS

An **intensifying screen** is a device that converts x-ray energy into visible light; the light, in turn, exposes the screen film. As discussed in Chapters 7 and 22, calcium tungstate screens emit blue light, and rare earth screens emit green light. The screen film must be compatible with the light emitted from the screen, blue-sensitive film must be paired with screens that emit blue light, and green-sensitive film must be paired with screens that emit green light. Rare earth screens require less exposure than calcium tungstate screens. To minimize patient exposure, the fastest film and screen combination that provides a diagnostic image should be used.

CASSETTE

The purpose of the **cassette** is to hold the film in tight contact with the intensifying screen and to protect the film from exposure to light (see Chapter 7). Extraoral cassettes, with the exception of some panoramic cassettes, are rigid and are constructed of metal and plastic.

The cassette must be labeled prior to exposure to orient the finished radiograph; a metallic **R** or **L** can be used to identify the patient's right or left side. These metallic letters must always be placed on the front of the cassette. The front side of the cassette is typically constructed of plastic and permits the passage of the x-ray beam, whereas the back side is made of metal to reduce scatter radiation. The front side is also known as the tube side, or the side that faces the x-ray beam. The front side of the cassette must always face the patient during exposure.

GRID

A **grid** is a device used to reduce the amount of scatter radiation that reaches an extraoral film during exposure. As previously discussed, scatter radiation causes film fog and reduces film contrast. A grid can be used to decrease film fog and increase the contrast of the radiographic image.

A grid is composed of a series of thin lead strips embedded in a material (e.g., plastic) that permits the passage of the x-ray beam. The grid is placed between the patient's head and the film. During exposure, the grid permits the passage of the x-ray beam between the lead strips. When some of the x-rays interact with the patient's tissues, scatter radiation is produced; this scatter radiation is then directed at the grid and film at an angle. As a result, scatter radiation is absorbed by the lead strips and does not reach the surface of the film to cause film fog (Fig. 23–3). To compensate for the lead strips found in the grid, an increased exposure time must be used to expose a film. Because of this increase in exposure time, a grid should be used only when improved image quality and high contrast are necessary.

■ STEP-BY-STEP PROCEDURES

Step-by-step procedures for the exposure of an extraoral film include equipment preparation, patient

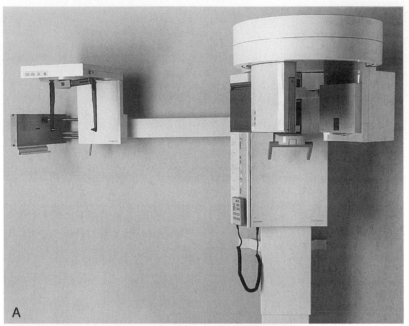

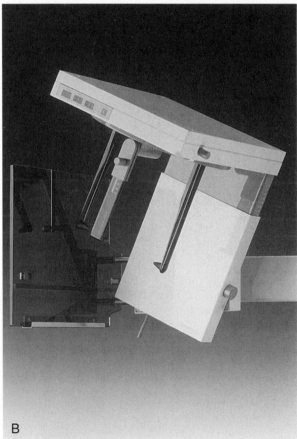

FIGURE 23–2. *A,* An extraoral radiographic unit with a cephalostat. *B,* An example of a cephalostat. (Reprinted with permission from Siemens Company.)

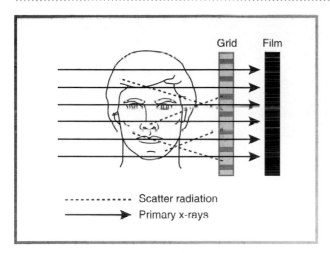

Grid   Film

‑ ‑ ‑ ‑ ‑ ‑ ‑ ‑ Scatter radiation
⟶ Primary x-rays

FIGURE 23–3. A grid decreases the amount of scatter radiation that reaches the extraoral film. (Courtesy of Dr. Robert M. Jaynes, Assistant Professor, Oral Radiology Group, The Ohio State University College of Dentistry.)

preparation, and patient positioning. Prior to exposing an extraoral film, infection control procedures (as described in Chapter 15) must be completed. If an extraoral x-ray unit with cephalostat is used, the ear rods must be wiped with a disinfectant between patients.

Equipment Preparation

The dental radiographer must prepare the equipment before preparing a patient for the exposure of an extraoral film (see "Procedure: Equipment Preparation").

PROCEDURE

Equipment Preparation

1. Load the extraoral cassette in the darkroom under safelight conditions. Place one extraoral film between two intensifying screens and securely close the cassette.

2. Set the exposure factors (kilovoltage, milliamperage, time) according to the manufacturer's recommendations. Load the cassette into the cassette carrier.

Patient Preparation

After preparing the equipment, the dental radiographer must prepare the patient (see "Procedure: Patient Preparation").

Patient Positioning

Patient positioning varies with each extraoral radiographic projection and is discussed in the next section on specific extraoral projection techniques.

▇ EXTRAORAL PROJECTION TECHNIQUES

A variety of projection techniques are used in extraoral radiography (Table 23–1). The purpose, film placement, head position, beam alignment, and exposure factors differ for each projection used in lateral jaw radiography, skull radiography, and temporomandibular joint radiography.

Lateral Jaw Radiography

Lateral jaw radiography is used to examine the posterior region of the mandible and is valuable for use in

PROCEDURE

Patient Preparation

1. Explain to the patient the radiographic procedure about to be performed.

2. Place a lead apron *without* a thyroid collar over the patient and secure it. A doublesided lead apron is recommended (see Chapter 22). The lead apron must be placed low around the back of the neck so that it does not block the x-ray beam. A thyroid collar is not recommended for extraoral radiography because it blocks part of the beam and obscures important diagnostic information.

3. Remove all objects from the head and neck region that may interfere with film exposure. The patient must remove eyeglasses, earrings, necklaces, napkin chains, hearing aids, hairpins, and complete and partial dentures.

TABLE 23–1. Extraoral Projection Techniques

Projection	Film Placement	Head Position	X-Ray Beam Point of Entry
lateral jaw, body (mandible)	flat against cheek centered over body of mandible	tipped 15 degrees toward side being imaged chin extended and elevated	below inferior border of mandible vertical angulation −15 to −20 degrees ⊥ to horizontal plane of cassette
lateral jaw, ramus (mandible)	flat against cheek centered over ramus of mandible	tipped 15 degrees toward side being imaged chin extended and elevated	posterior to third molar area vertical angulation −15 to −20 degrees ⊥ to horizontal plane of cassette
lateral cephalometric	cassette ⊥ to floor long axis horizontal	left side near cassette MSP ⊥ to floor FP ‖ to floor	center of cassette ⊥ to cassette
posteroanterior	cassette ⊥ to floor long axis vertical	forehead and nose touch cassette MSP ⊥ to floor FP ‖ to floor	center of cassette ⊥ to cassette
Waters	cassette ⊥ to floor long axis vertical	chin touches cassette tip of nose 1–2 inches from cassette MSP ⊥ to floor	center of cassette ⊥ to cassette
submentovertex	cassette ⊥ to floor long axis vertical	head tipped back top of head touches cassette MSP and FP ⊥ to floor	center of cassette ⊥ to cassette
reverse Towne	cassette ⊥ to floor long axis vertical	head tipped down mouth open top of forehead touches cassette MSP ⊥ to floor	center of cassette ⊥ to cassette
transcranial	flat against ear centered over TMJ	MSP ⊥ to floor	2 inches above and 0.5 inch below the ear canal opening vertical angulation +25 degrees horizontal angulation 20 degrees

Abbreviations: FP, Frankfort plane; MSP, midsagittal plane; TMJ, temporomandibular joint; ⊥, perpendicular; ‖, parallel.

children, in patients with limited jaw opening due to a fracture or swelling, and in patients who have difficulty in stabilizing or tolerating intraoral film placement. Although lateral jaw radiography is useful, it is important to note that a panoramic radiograph is preferred to the lateral jaw radiograph because more diagnostic information is obtained.

As the term lateral jaw radiography suggests, the film in this extraoral projection technique is positioned lateral to the jaw during exposure. Lateral jaw radiography does not require the use of a special x-ray unit; a standard intraoral x-ray machine can be used. Two **lateral jaw projection** techniques are used:

- body of mandible projection
- ramus of mandible projection

BODY OF MANDIBLE

Purpose. The purpose of this film is to evaluate impacted teeth, fractures, and lesions located in the body of the mandible. This projection demonstrates the mandibular premolar and molar regions as well as the inferior border of the mandible (Fig. 23–4).

Film Placement. The cassette is placed flat against the patient's cheek and is centered over the body of the mandible. The cassette must also be positioned parallel with the body of the mandible. The patient must hold the cassette in position with the thumb placed under the edge of the cassette and the palm against the outer surface of the cassette.

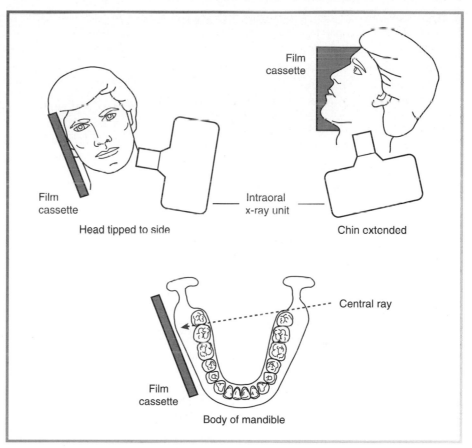

A

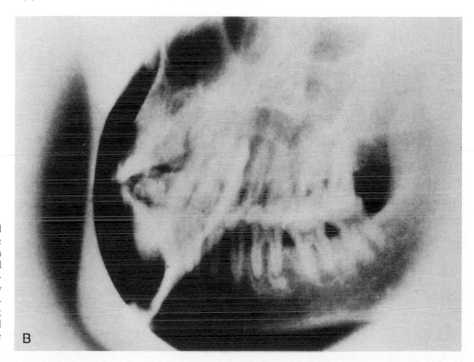

B

FIGURE 23–4. *A,* For the lateral jaw projection of the body of the mandible, proper patient and film positioning is shown as viewed from the front and side of the patient. *B,* An example of a lateral jaw radiograph: the body of the mandible. (*A* and *B* courtesy of Dr. Robert M. Jaynes, Assistant Professor, Oral Radiology Group, The Ohio State University College of Dentistry.)

Head Position. The head is tipped approximately 15 degrees toward the side being imaged. The chin is extended and elevated slightly.

Beam Alignment. The central ray is directed to a point just below the inferior border of the mandible on the side *opposite* the cassette. The beam is directed upward (−15 to −20 degrees) and centered on the body of the mandible. The beam must be directed perpendicular to the horizontal plane of the film.

Exposure Factors. The exposure factors for this projection vary with the film, intensifying screens, and equipment used.

RAMUS OF MANDIBLE

Purpose. The purpose of this film is to evaluate impacted third molars, large lesions, and fractures that extend into the ramus of the mandible. This projection demonstrates a view of the ramus from the angle of the mandible to the condyle (Fig. 23–5).

Film Placement. The cassette is placed flat against the patient's cheek and is centered over the ramus of the mandible. The cassette is also positioned parallel with the ramus of the mandible. The patient must hold the cassette in position with the thumb placed under the edge of the cassette and the palm placed against the outer surface of the cassette.

Head Position. The head is tipped approximately 15 degrees toward the side being imaged. The chin is extended and elevated slightly.

Beam Alignment. The central ray is directed to a point posterior to the third molar region on the side *opposite* the cassette. The beam is directed upward (−15 to −20 degrees) and centered on the ramus of the mandible. The beam must be directed perpendicular to the horizontal plane of the film.

Exposure Factors. The exposure factors for this projection vary with the film, intensifying screens, and equipment used.

Skull Radiography

Skull radiography is used to examine the bones of the face and skull and is most often used in oral surgery and orthodontics. Although some skull films can be exposed using a standard intraoral x-ray machine, most require the use of an extraoral unit and cephalostat.

Radiographs of the skull may be difficult to interpret because of the numerous anatomic structures that exist in a very small area; these structures often appear superimposed over each other. In many instances, multiple exposures may be necessary to obtain a clear view of the area in question. The most common skull radiographs used in dentistry include:

- **lateral cephalometric projection**
- **posteroanterior projection**
- **Waters projection**
- **submentovertex projection**
- **reverse Towne projection**

LATERAL CEPHALOMETRIC PROJECTION

Purpose. The purpose of this film is to evaluate facial growth and development, trauma, and disease and developmental abnormalities. This projection demonstrates the bones of the face and skull as well as the soft tissue profile of the face (Fig. 23–6).

The soft tissue outline of the face is more readily seen on the resulting radiograph when a filter is used. A filter is placed at the x-ray source, or between the patient and the film, and serves to remove some of the x-rays that pass through the soft tissue of the face, thus enhancing the image of the soft tissue profile of the face.

Film Placement. The cassette is placed perpendicular to the floor in a cassette-holding device. The long axis of the cassette is positioned *horizontally*.

Head Position. The *left* side of the patient's head is positioned adjacent to the cassette. The midsagittal plane (an imaginary line that divides the face in half) must be positioned perpendicular to the floor and parallel with the cassette. The Frankfort plane (a line extending from the top of the ear canal to the bottom of the eye socket) is positioned parallel with the floor. The head is centered over the cassette.

Beam Alignment. The central ray is directed through the center of the cassette and perpendicular to the cassette.

Exposure Factors. The exposure factors for this projection vary with the film, intensifying screens, and equipment used.

POSTEROANTERIOR PROJECTION

Purpose. The purpose of this film is to evaluate facial growth and development, trauma, and disease and developmental abnormalities. This projection also demonstrates the frontal and ethmoid sinuses, the orbits, and the nasal cavity (Fig. 23–7).

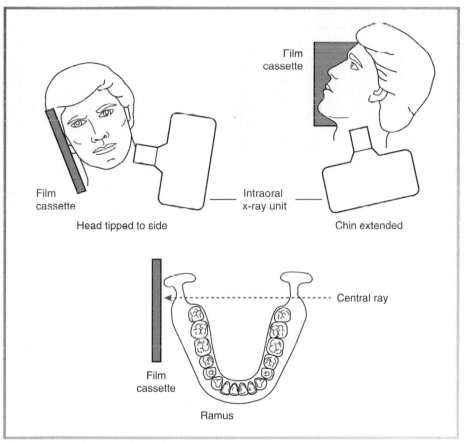

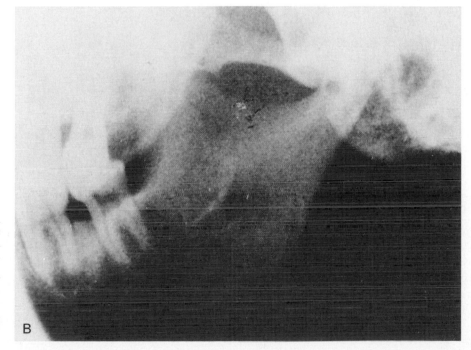

A

B

FIGURE 23–5. *A,* For the lateral jaw projection of the ramus of the mandible, proper patient and film positioning is shown as viewed from the front and side of the patient. *B,* An example of a lateral jaw radiograph: the ramus of the mandible. *(A* and *B* courtesy of Dr. Robert M. Jaynes, Assistant Professor, Oral Radiology Group, The Ohio State University College of Dentistry.)

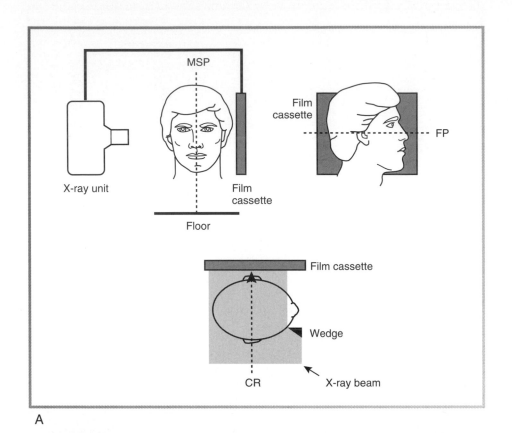

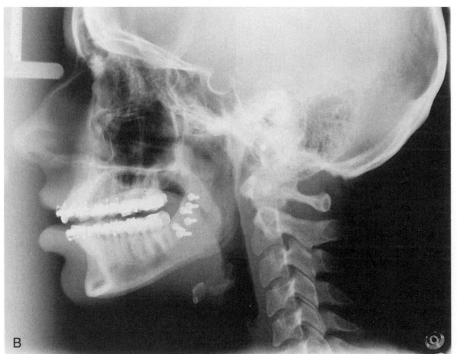

FIGURE 23–6. *A,* For the lateral cephalometric projection, proper patient and film positioning is shown as viewed from the front, side, and top of the patient (MSP, midsagittal plane; FP, Frankfort plane; CR, central ray). *B,* An example of a lateral cephalometric radiograph. (*A* and *B* courtesy of Dr. Robert M. Jaynes, Assistant Professor, Oral Radiology Group, The Ohio State University College of Dentistry.)

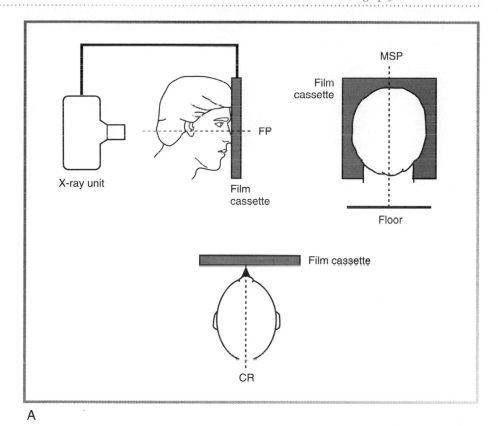

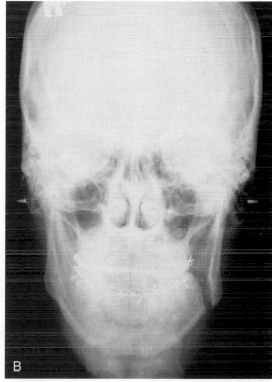

FIGURE 23–7. *A,* For the posteroanterior skull projection, proper patient and film positioning is shown as viewed from the side, back, and top of the patient (MSP, midsagittal plane; FP, Frankfort plane, CR, central ray). *B,* An example of a posteroanterior skull radiograph. (*A* and *B* courtesy of Dr. Robert M. Jaynes, Assistant Professor, Oral Radiology Group, The Ohio State University College of Dentistry.)

Film Placement. The cassette is placed perpendicular to the floor in a cassette-holding device. The long axis of the cassette is positioned *vertically*.

Head Position. The patient faces the cassette; the forehead and nose both touch the cassette. The midsagittal plane is positioned perpendicular to the floor, and the Frankfort plane is positioned parallel with the floor. The head is centered over the cassette.

Beam Alignment. The central ray is directed through the center of the head and perpendicular to the cassette.

Exposure Factors. The exposure factors for this projection vary with the film, intensifying screens, and equipment used.

WATERS PROJECTION

Purpose. The purpose of this film is to evaluate the maxillary sinus area. This projection also demonstrates the frontal and ethmoid sinuses, the orbits, and the nasal cavity (Fig. 23–8).

Film Placement. The cassette is placed perpendicular to the floor in a cassette-holding device. The long axis of the cassette is placed *vertically*.

Head Position. The patient faces the cassette and elevates the chin; the chin touches the cassette, and the tip of the nose is positioned 1/2 to 1 inch away from the cassette. The midsagittal plane must be positioned perpendicular to the floor, and the head is centered over the cassette.

Beam Alignment. The central ray is directed through the center of the head and perpendicular to the cassette.

Exposure Factors. The exposure factors for this projection vary with the film, intensifying screens, and equipment used.

SUBMENTOVERTEX PROJECTION

Purpose. The purpose of this film is to identify the position of the condyles, demonstrate the base of the skull, and evaluate fractures of the zygomatic arch. This projection also demonstrates the sphenoid and ethmoid sinuses and the lateral wall of the maxillary sinus (Fig. 23–9).

Film Placement. The cassette is placed perpendicular to the floor in a cassette-holding device. The long axis of the cassette is placed *vertically*.

Head Position. The patient's head and neck are tipped back as far as possible; the vertex (top) of the skull touches the cassette. Both the midsagittal plane and the Frankfort plane are positioned perpendicular to the floor. The head is centered on the cassette.

Beam Alignment. The central ray is directed through the center of the head and perpendicular to the cassette.

Exposure Factors. The exposure factors for this projection vary with the film, intensifying screens, and equipment used. If the zygomatic arch is the area of interest, the exposure time is reduced to approximately one-third the normal exposure time for a submentovertex projection.

REVERSE TOWNE PROJECTION

Purpose. The purpose of this film is to identify fractures of the condylar neck and ramus area (Fig. 23–10).

Film Placement. The cassette is placed perpendicular to the floor in a cassette-holding device. The long axis of the cassette is placed *vertically*.

Head Position. The patient faces the cassette with the head tipped down and the mouth open as wide as possible; the chin rests on the chest, while the top of the forehead touches the cassette. The midsagittal plane must be positioned perpendicular to the floor, and the head is centered on the cassette.

Beam Alignment. The central ray is directed through the center of the head and perpendicular to the cassette.

Exposure Factors. The exposure factors for this projection vary with the film, intensifying screens, and equipment used.

Temporomandibular Joint Radiography

The **temporomandibular joint (TMJ)** is the jaw joint. As the term temporomandibular suggests, this joint includes the temporal bone and the mandible. The glenoid fossa and articular eminence of the temporal bone, the condyle of the mandible, and the articular disk between the bones comprise the TMJ area. This area can be very difficult to examine radiographically because of the multiple adjacent bony structures.

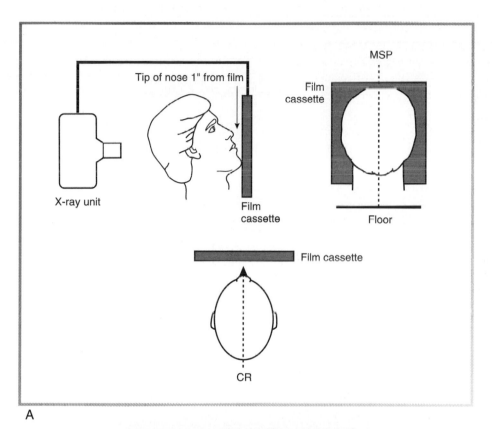

A

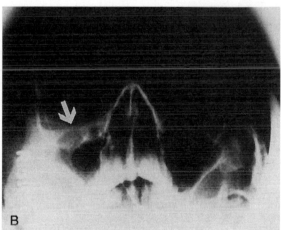

B

FIGURE 23–8. *A,* For the Waters projection, proper patient and film positioning is shown as viewed from the side, back, and top of the patient (MSP, midsagittal plane; CR, central ray). *B,* This instance of chronic maxillary sinusitis secondary to an oroantral fistula is represented by thickening of the lining membrane *(arrow)* (Waters view). (*A* courtesy of Dr. Robert M. Jaynes, Assistant Professor, Oral Radiology Group, The Ohio State University College of Dentistry; *B* from Pedersen GW: Oral Surgery. Philadelphia, WB Saunders, 1988.)

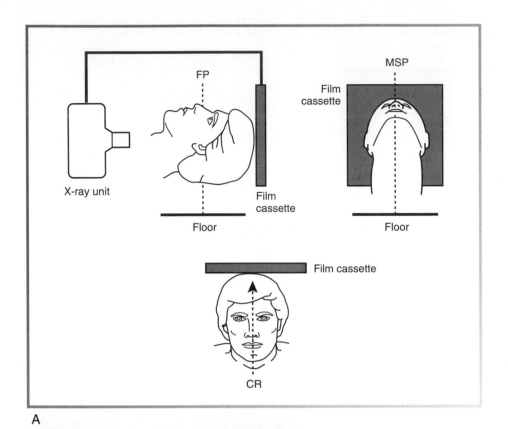

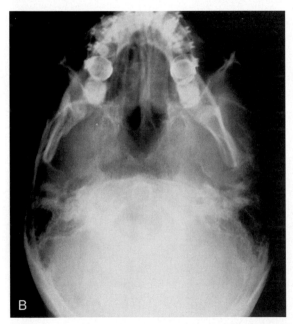

FIGURE 23–9. *A,* For the submentovertex projection, proper patient and film positioning is shown as viewed from the side, front, and top of the patient (MSP, midsagittal plane; FP, Frankfort plane; CR, central ray). *B,* An example of a submentovertex radiograph. (*A* and *B* courtesy of Dr. Robert M. Jaynes, Assistant Professor, Oral Radiology Group, The Ohio State University College of Dentistry.)

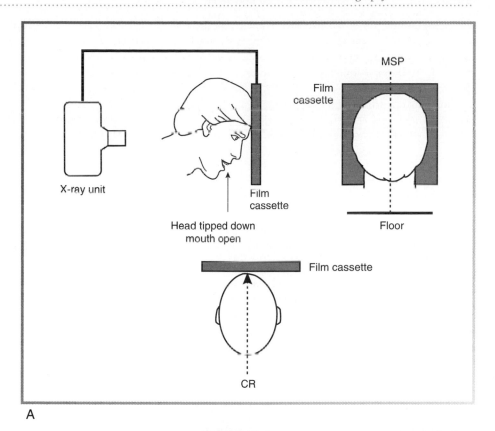

A

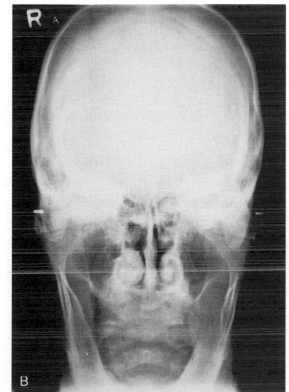

B

FIGURE 23-10. *A,* For the reverse Towne projection, proper patient and film positioning is shown as viewed from the side, back, and top of the patient (MSP, midsagittal plane; CR, central ray). *B,* An example of a reverse Towne radiograph. (*A* and *B* courtesy of Dr. Robert M. Jaynes, Assistant Professor, Oral Radiology Group, The Ohio State University College of Dentistry.)

Radiography cannot be used to examine the articular disk and other soft tissue areas of the TMJ; instead, specialized imaging techniques (e.g., arthrography and magnetic resonance imaging) must be used. Radiography, however, can be used to show the bone and the relationship of the joint components. For instance, changes in bone (e.g., erosions or bony deposits) can be seen on TMJ radiographs. Two projection techniques are used in TMJ radiography:

- **transcranial projection**
- **temporomandibular joint tomography**

TRANSCRANIAL PROJECTION (LINDBLOM TECHNIQUE)

Purpose. The purpose of this film is to evaluate the superior surface of the condyle and the articular eminence (Fig. 23–11). This projection can also be used to evaluate movement of the condyle when the mouth is opened and to compare the joint spaces (right versus left).

Film Placement. The cassette is placed flat against the patient's ear and is centered over the TMJ.

Head Position. The midsagittal plane must be positioned perpendicular to the floor and parallel with the cassette.

Beam Alignment. The central ray is directed toward a point 2 inches above and 0.5 inches behind the opening of the ear canal. The beam is directed downward (+25 degrees) and forward (20 degrees) and is centered on the TMJ that is being imaged.

Exposure Factors. The exposure factors for this projection vary with the film, intensifying screens, and equipment used.

The intraoral x-ray unit can be used in the exposure of a transcranial projection. There are special positioning devices that can be used to coordinate the alignment of the film, the patient's head, and the beam to obtain an accurate transcranial film. Such devices are also used to reproduce the same patient positioning in subsequent exposures, thereby permitting comparison of images.

TEMPOROMANDIBULAR JOINT TOMOGRAPHY

Temporomandibular joint tomography is a radiographic technique that is used to examine the temporomandibular joint. Tomography, as defined in Chapter 22, is a radiographic technique used to show structures located within a selected plane of tissue while blurring structures outside of the selected plane. In TMJ tomography, this is accomplished by moving the film and x-ray tubehead in opposite directions around a fixed rotation point; the location of this rotation point determines what plane of the head will be imaged (Fig. 23–12).

TMJ tomography provides the most definitive imaging of the bony components of the temporomandibular joint; as a result, the condyle, articular eminence, and glenoid fossa can all be examined on a radiograph known as the **tomogram.** In addition, the tomogram can be used to estimate joint space and evaluate the extent of movement of the condyle when the mouth is open.

A special tomographic x-ray unit, such as the Quint Sectograph (Denar Corporation, Los Angeles, CA), is required for TMJ tomography. Most dental practitioners do not purchase such specialized equipment because of the prohibitive cost. As a result, dental patients who require TMJ tomography are usually referred to a specialized radiographic imaging facility. Further discussion about the specifics of TMJ tomography is beyond the scope of this text.

▨ SUMMARY

- The extraoral film is a film that is placed outside of the mouth during x-ray exposure.
- Uses of extraoral film include the following:
  - evaluation of large areas of the skull and jaws
  - evaluation of growth and development
  - evaluation of impacted teeth
  - detection of diseases, lesions, and conditions of the jaws
  - examination of the extent of large lesions
  - evaluation of trauma
  - evaluation of the temporomandibular joint area
- The use of special equipment, including an x-ray unit, screen film, intensifying screens, grid, and cassette, is necessary in extraoral radiography.
- Prior to preparing the patient for exposure of an extraoral film, the cassette must be prepared, infection control procedures must be finished, and exposure factors must be selected.
- After preparing the equipment, the dental radiographer must explain the radiographic procedures to the patient, place the lead apron, and remove all radiodense objects from the head and neck region.
- A variety of projection techniques are used in extraoral radiography depending on what information is needed.

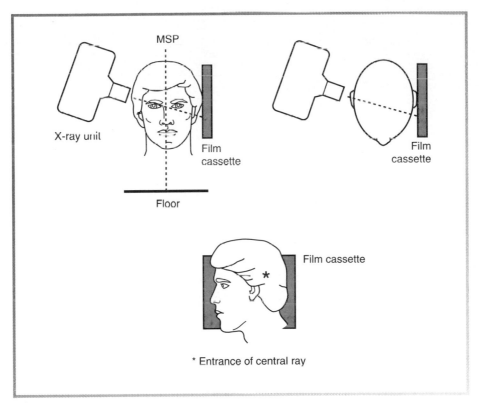

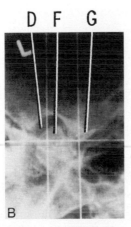

FIGURE 23–11. *A,* For the transcranial projection, proper patient and film positioning is shown as viewed from the front, top, and side of the patient (MSP, midsagittal plane). *B,* Transcranial view of the temporomandibular joint in the rest position (D, glenoid fossa; F, head of the mandibular condyle; G, articular eminence). (*A* courtesy of Dr. Robert M. Jaynes, Assistant Professor, Oral Radiology Group, The Ohio State University College of Dentistry; *B* from Kasle MJ: An Atlas of Dental Radiographic Anatomy, 4th ed. Philadelphia, WB Saunders, 1994.)

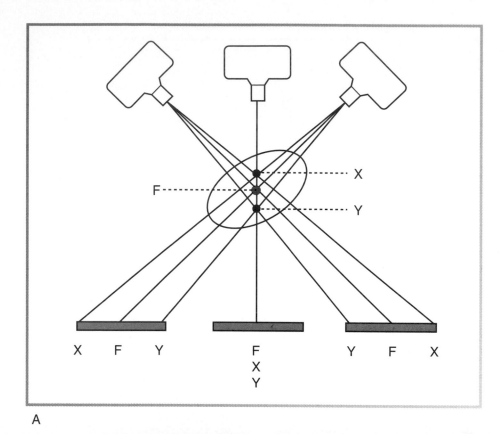

A

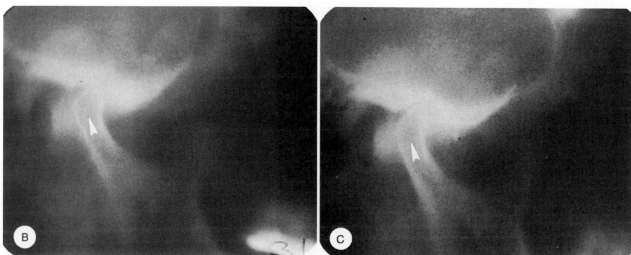

FIGURE 23–12. *A,* As the tubehead and film move in opposite directions around the patient, objects in the image layer (F) appear sharp on the film. Objects on either side of the image layer (X, Y) are blurred. *B* and *C,* Corrected axis tomograms showing decreased joint space and posterior positioning of the left condyle (*arrowheads*) due to the anteriorly placed meniscus. (*A* courtesy of Dr. Robert M. Jaynes, Assistant Professor, Oral Radiology Group, The Ohio State University College of Dentistry; *B* and *C* from Kasle MJ: An Atlas of Dental Radiographic Anatomy, 4th ed. Philadelphia, WB Saunders, 1994.)

BIBLIOGRAPHY

Frommer HH: Accessory radiographic techniques. *In* Radiology for Dental Auxiliaries, 6th edition. St. Louis, Mosby-Year Book, 1996, pp. 181–204.

Goaz PW, White SC: Extraoral radiographic examinations. *In* Oral Radiology: Principles of Interpretation, 3rd edition. St. Louis, Mosby-Year Book, 1994, pp. 227–211.

Johnson ON, McNally MA, Essay CE: Extraoral radiography. *In* Essentials of Dental Radiography for Dental Assistants and Hygienists, 6th edition. Norwalk, CT, Appleton and Lange, 1999, pp. 433–449.

Manson-Hing LR: Occlusal film and extraoral radiography. *In* Fundamentals of Dental Radiography, 3rd edition. Philadelphia, Lea & Febiger, 1990, pp. 144–154.

Miles DA, Van Dis ML, Jensen CW, Ferretti A: Extraoral radiography. *In* Radiographic Imaging for Dental Auxiliaries, 3rd edition. Philadelphia, WB Saunders, 1999, pp. 181–197.

Miles DA, Van Dis ML, Razmus TF: Plain film extraoral radiographic techniques. *In* Basic Principles of Oral and Maxillofacial Radiology. Philadelphia, WB Saunders, 1992, pp. 133–141.

Olson SS: Auxiliary radiographic techniques. *In* Dental Radiography Laboratory Manual. Philadelphia, WB Saunders, 1995, pp. 200–206.

Quiz Questions ···

_____ 14. Which of the following projections is best for examination of fractures of the mandibular body?

   a. lateral cephalometric projection
   b. submentovertex projection
   c. lateral jaw projection
   d. transcranial projection

_____ 15. Which of the following projections is best for examination of a large lesion in the ramus?

   a. posteroanterior projection
   b. Waters projection
   c. lateral cephalometric projection
   d. lateral jaw projection

Answers are supplied at the end of this book.

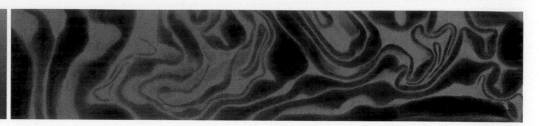

Digital Radiography

OBJECTIVES

After completion of this chapter, the student will be able to:

- *Define the key words.*
- *Describe the purpose and use of digital radiography.*
- *Discuss the fundamentals of digital radiography.*
- *List and describe the equipment used in digital radiography.*
- *List and describe the three types of digital imaging.*
- *Describe the patient and equipment preparations required for digital radiography.*
- *List and discuss the advantages and disadvantages of digital radiography.*

KEY WORDS

Charge-coupled device (CCD)	Indirect digital imaging
Digital radiography	Pixel
Digital subtraction	Sensor
Digitize	Storage phosphor imaging
Direct digital imaging	

INTRODUCTION

Recent technologic advances have produced a significant impact on the field of dental radiography; such advances in computer technology have resulted in a unique "filmless" imaging system known as **digital radiography.** Since its introduction to dentistry in 1987, digital radiography has influenced both how dental disease is recognized and how it is diagnosed. Before the dental radiographer can use this very specialized technology, an understanding of the basic concepts, which include terminology, purpose, use, and fundamentals, is necessary. In addition, the dental radiographer must have a working knowledge of the equipment used in digital radiography.

The purpose of this chapter is to present the basic concepts of digital radiography, to introduce the types of digital imaging, and to discuss the advantages and disadvantages of digital radiography.

BASIC CONCEPTS

Digital radiography is used to record radiographic images. Unlike conventional dental radiography techniques discussed in the previous chapters on technique, *no* film or processing chemistry is used. Instead, digital radiography uses an electronic sensor and computerized imaging system that produces x-ray images almost instantly on a computer monitor. Before the dental radiographer can use this technique competently, a thorough understanding of the terminology and fundamentals of digital radiography is necessary. A knowledge of radiation exposure, equipment, and types of digital imaging is also required.

Terminology

Charge-coupled device (CCD): A solid state detector used in many devices (e.g., fax machine, home video camera); in digital radiography, a CCD is an image receptor found in the intraoral sensor.

Digital radiography: A filmless imaging system; a method of capturing a radiographic image using a sensor, breaking it into electronic pieces, and, presenting and storing the image using a computer.

Digital subtraction: One feature of digital radiography; a method of reversing the gray-scale as an image is viewed; radiolucent images (normally black) appear white and radiopaque images (normally white) appear black.

Digitize: In digital radiography, to convert an image into a digital form that, in turn, can be processed by a computer.

Direct digital imaging: A method of obtaining a digital image in which an intraoral sensor is exposed to x-rays to capture a radiographic image that can be viewed on a computer monitor.

Indirect digital imaging: A method of obtaining a digital image in which an existing radiograph is scanned and converted into a digital form using a CCD camera.

Pixel: A discrete unit of information. In digital electronic images, digital information is contained in, and presented as, discrete units of information (also termed *picture element*).

Sensor: In digital radiography, a small detector that is placed intraorally to capture a radiographic image.

Storage phosphor imaging: A method of obtaining a digital image in which the image is recorded on phosphor-coated plates and then placed into an electronic processor where a laser scans the plate and produces an image on a computer screen.

Purpose and Use

The purpose of digital radiography is to generate images that can be used in the diagnosis and assessment of dental disease. The images produced are diagnostically equivalent to film-based imaging and enable the dental radiographer to identify many conditions that may otherwise go undetected and to see conditions that cannot be identified clinically. Like film-based radiographic procedures, digital radiography allows the radiographer to obtain a wealth of information about the teeth and supporting structures. Digital radiography is used for the following:

- to detect lesions, diseases and conditions of the teeth and surrounding structures
- to confirm or classify suspected disease
- to provide information during dental procedures (e.g., root canal therapy instrumentation and surgical placement of implants)
- to evaluate growth and development
- to illustrate changes secondary to caries, periodontal disease, or trauma
- to document the condition of a patient at a specific point in time

Fundamentals

The term **digital radiography** refers to a method of capturing a radiographic image using a sensor, breaking it into electronic pieces, and presenting and storing the image using a computer. In digital radiography, the patient is exposed to x-radiation similar to that used in conventional radiography; however, the resulting image is displayed on a computer screen rather than on film that must be processed in a darkroom. The source of x-radiation is activated and a detector, or sensor, is placed inside the patient's mouth to receive the image information of the exposed area. A computer stores the image and displays it within moments of exposure. With digital radiography, the term *image* (*not* radiograph or x-ray film) is used to describe the pictures that are produced (Fig. 24–1).

In digital radiography, a **sensor,** or small detector, is placed inside the mouth of the patient to capture the radiographic image. The sensor is used *instead of* intraoral dental film. As in conventional radiography, the x-ray beam is aimed to strike the sensor. An electronic charge is produced on the surface of the sensor; this electronic signal is **digitized,** or converted into "digital" form. The digital sensor in turn transmits this information to a computer. After the image has been digitized by the sensor, it is processed by a computer. Software is used to store the image electronically. The image is displayed within seconds and may be readily manipulated to enhance the appearance for interpretation and diagnosis.

Digital radiography systems are not limited to intraoral images; panoramic and cephalometric images may also be obtained (Fig. 24–2). For example, the extraoral film traditionally used in panoramic radiography is replaced with an electronic sensor that delivers the image information to a computer for storage in digital format. As with intraoral radiography, the images are displayed on a computer monitor and may be stored for future use.

Radiation Exposure

Digital radiography requires *less* x-radiation than conventional radiography. Why? Less x-radiation is necessary to form a digital image on the sensor because the

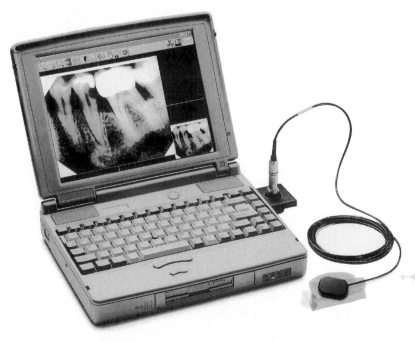

FIGURE 24–1. The radiographic image on the computer monitor is displayed as a normal periapical and a magnified version of the same image. (Photo courtesy of DEXIS Digital Radiography, Garden City, NY.)

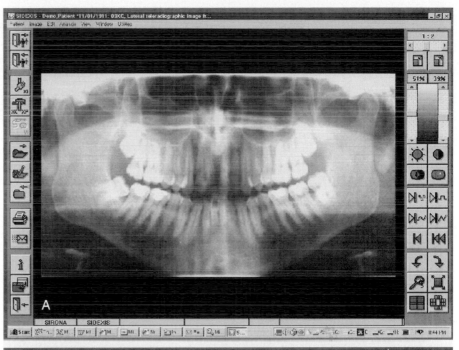

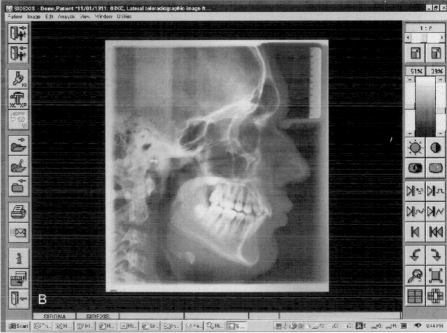

FIGURE 24–2. Computer monitors illustrating (*A*) panoramic and (*B*) cephalometric images. (Photo courtesy of Sirona USA.)

typical sensor is *more* sensitive to x-rays than conventional film. Exposure times for digital radiography are 50 to 80% less than that required for conventional radiography using E-speed film. For example, the typical exposure time required to produce an image for digital radiography is three impulses (3/60 second or 0.05 seconds). This exposure time is far less than the 12 impulses (12/60 second or 0.2 seconds) required for E-speed intraoral film used in conventional film-based radiography. With less radiation exposure, the absorbed dose to the patient is significantly lower.

Equipment

In digital radiography, the use of specialized equipment is necessary. The essential components of a direct digital imaging system include: **x-radiation source, intraoral sensor,** and **computer.**

X-RADIATION SOURCE

Most digital radiography systems use a conventional dental x-ray unit as the x-radiation source. The conventional x-radiation source is compatible with the digital imaging system; however, the x-ray unit timer must be adapted to allow exposures in a time frame of 1/100 of a second. A standard x-ray unit that is adapted for digital radiography can still be functional for conventional radiography.

INTRAORAL SENSOR

As previously defined, the sensor is a small detector that is placed in the mouth of the patient and used to capture the radiographic image. Intraoral sensors used in digital radiography systems may be wired or wireless. *Wired* refers to the fact that the imaging sensor is *linked by a fiber optic cable* to a computer that records the generated signal (Fig. 24–3). With wired systems, the cable varies in length from 8 to 35 feet; the shorter the cable, the more limited the range of motion will be. *Wireless* refers to the fact that the imaging sensor, a phosphor-coated plate, is *not linked by a cable.*

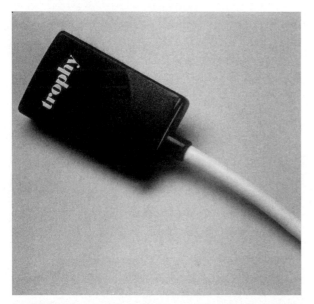

FIGURE 24–3. A wired intraoral sensor. (Photo courtesy of TREX Trophy, Dental Division, Danbury, CT.)

Currently, three types of direct sensor technologies exist: (1) **charge-coupled device** or **CCD**, (2) **complementary metal oxide semiconductor/active pixel sensor** or **CMOS/APS,** and (3) **charge injection device** or **CID.**

CHARGE-COUPLED DEVICE

At the time of printing, the **charge-coupled device (CCD)** is the most common image receptor used in dental digital radiography. The CCD technology used in digital radiography relies on a specialized fabrication process that is expensive to manufacture.

The CCD is not a new technology; it was first developed in the 1960s. Currently CCD technology is used in many devices; some examples include fax machines, home video cameras, microscopes, and telescopes. The CCD is a solid-state detector that contains a silicon chip with an electronic circuit embedded in it. This silicon chip is sensitive to x-rays or light.

The electrons that make up the silicon CCD can be visualized as being divided into an arrangement of blocks or picture elements known as *pixels.* A **pixel** is a small box or "well" into which the electrons produced by the x-ray exposure are deposited. A pixel is the digital equivalent of a silver crystal used in conventional radiography. As opposed to a film emulsion that contains a *random* arrangement of silver crystals, a pixel is structured in an *ordered* arrangement. The CCD is 640 × 480 individual pixels in size. Consequently, the CCD contains 307,200 pixels and functions to sense transmitted light and translate it into an electronic message.

The x-ray photons that come into contact with the CCD cause electrons to be released from the silicon and produce a corresponding electronic charge. Consequently, each pixel arrangement, or *electron potential well,* contains an electronic charge proportional to the number of electrons that reacted within the well. Furthermore, each electronic well corresponds to a specific area on the linked computer screen. When x-rays activate electrons and produce such electronic charges, an electronic latent image is produced; the latent image is then transmitted and stored in a computer and can be converted to a visible image on screen or printed on paper.

COMPLEMENTARY METAL OXIDE SEMICONDUCTOR/ACTIVE PIXEL SENSOR

Another sensor technology that is used in digital radiography is the complementary metal oxide semiconductor/active pixel sensor or **CMOS/APS.** Although the CMOS process is the standard in the making of semiconductor chips, it was not until APS was developed that CMOS became useful as a sensor in dental digital radiography. At this time, one digital radiography manufacturer, Schick Technologies, uses a CMOS/APS sensor instead of a CCD and claims for it a 25% greater resolution. Additional advantages of the CMOS/APS technology are that the chip is less expensive to produce and offers greater durability than the CCD.

CHARGE INJECTION DEVICE

The charge injection device or **CID** is another sensor technology used in dental digital radiography. A CID is a silicon-based solid-state imaging receptor much like the CCD. Structurally, however, the CID differs from the CCD. One manufacturer, Welch Allyn, introduced this technology to be used with its Reveal intraoral video camera platform. No computer is required to process the images. This system features a CID x-ray sensor, cord, and plug that are inserted into the Reveal light source on the camera platform; digital images are seen on the system monitor within seconds. The CID sensor uses the same docking platform as the Reveal intraoral camera. The images can be printed with a color video printer and saved as a computer file or onto a video disk recorder.

COMPUTER

A computer is used to store the incoming electronic signal. The computer is responsible for converting the electronic signal from the sensor into a shade of gray that is viewed on the computer monitor. Each pixel is represented numerically in the computer by location and level of color of gray. The range of numbers for a pixel varies from 0 to 255, which creates 256 shades of gray (referred to as a *pixel's gray-scale resolution*). In comparison, the human eye can only appreciate 32 shades of gray. This technology allows the dental professional to manipulate the image to enhance contrast and density without additional x-ray exposure of the patient (Fig. 24–4).

The computer digitizes, processes, and stores information received from the sensor. The computer monitor allows for immediate viewing of this exposure. An image is recorded on a computer monitor in 0.5 to 120 seconds, markedly less time than is required for conventional film processing. This speed of image recording is extremely useful during certain dental pro-

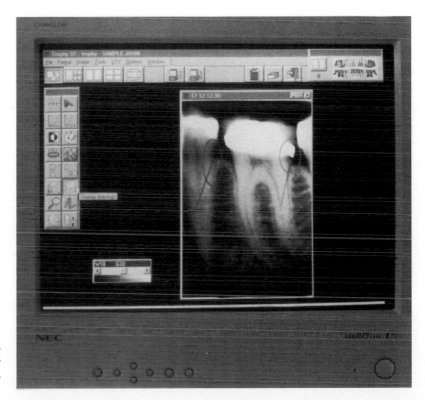

FIGURE 24–4. The image on the computer monitor can be manipulated to enhance density and contrast. (Photo courtesy of TREX Trophy, Dental Division, Danbury, CT.)

cedures, such as the placement of surgical implants or during root canal therapy instrumentation. The image may be stored permanently in the computer, printed on a hard copy for the patient record, or transmitted electronically to insurance companies or referring dental specialists.

Various computer viewing features are available with digital radiography systems. Digital systems feature split screen technology that allows the operator to view and compare multiple images on the same screen (Fig. 24–5). This feature is helpful in the comparison and evaluation of disease progression involving caries or periodontal disease. For example, caries progression can be evaluated by comparing successive bite-wing images. Digital systems also provide a feature that allows specific images to be magnified up to four times their original size. This feature is helpful when evaluating the apical area of a tooth. Linear and angular measurements can also be obtained, a feature that is helpful in measuring the length of a root.

TYPES OF DIGITAL IMAGING

Three methods of obtaining a digital image currently exist: direct digital imaging, indirect digital imaging, and storage phosphor imaging.

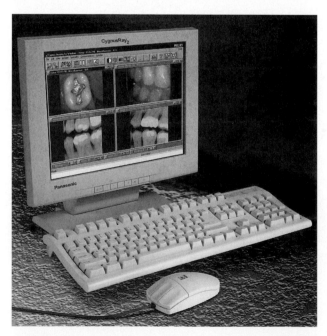

FIGURE 24–5. The image on the computer monitor reveals split screen technology; two clinical views and two radiographic views are simultaneously displayed. (Photo courtesy of Cygnus Imaging, Scottsdale, AZ.)

Direct Digital Imaging

The essential components of a **direct digital imaging** system include an x-ray machine, an intraoral sensor, and computer monitor. A sensor is placed into the mouth of the patient and exposed to x-rays. The sensor captures the radiographic image and then transmits the image to a computer monitor. Within seconds of exposing the sensor to x-rays, an image appears on the computer screen. Software is then used to enhance and store the image.

Indirect Digital Imaging

The essential components of an **indirect digital imaging system** include a CCD camera and computer. In this method, an existing x-ray film is "digitized" using a CCD camera. The CCD camera scans the image, digitizes or converts the image, and then displays it on the computer monitor. This concept is similar in theory to scanning an image, such as a photograph, to a computer screen. Indirect digital imaging is inferior to direct digital imaging because the resultant image is similar to a "copy" of the image versus the "original."

Storage Phosphor Imaging

A third method of obtaining a digital image is **storage phosphor imaging,** a *wireless* digital radiography system. In this system, a reusable imaging plate coated with phosphors is used *instead of* a sensor with a fiber optic cable. The phosphor-coated plates are flexible and fit into the mouth much like an intraoral film. A phosphor-coated plate is similar to an intensifying screen used to expose an extraoral film in that it converts x-ray energy into light.

Storage phosphor imaging records diagnostic data on plates following exposure to the x-ray source and then uses a high-speed scanner to convert the information into electronic files. After exposure, the plate is removed from the mouth and placed into an electronic processor where a laser scans the plate and produces an image that is transferred to a computer screen. No chemicals are used in this "processing." Because of the laser scanning step, this type of digital imaging is less rapid than direct digital imaging.

STEP-BY-STEP PROCEDURES

Step-by-step procedures for the use of digital radiography imaging systems vary by manufacturer. *It is critical to refer to the manufacturer-provided instruction booklet for information concerning the operation of the system, equipment preparation, patient preparation, and exposure.* Only very general guidelines concerning sensor preparation and placement are included here.

Sensor Preparation

Digital radiography involves placement of the intraoral sensor in the mouth of the patient, similar to the technique used in conventional film placement. Although the number and size of the sensor vary with different manufacturers, each sensor is sealed and waterproofed. For infection control purposes, the sensor *must* be covered with a disposable barrier because it cannot be sterilized.

Sensor Placement

The sensor is held in the mouth by bite-block attachments or devices that aim the beam and sensor accurately (Fig. 24–6). The paralleling technique is the preferred exposure method because of the dimensional accuracy of images and the ease of standardizing such images. Paralleling technique film holders must be used to stabilize the sensor in the mouth. As with conventional intraoral film, the sensor is centered over the area of interest.

ADVANTAGES AND DISADVANTAGES

As with any intraoral radiographic technique, digital radiography has both advantages and disadvantages.

Advantages

Advantages of digital radiography include the following: superior gray-scale resolution, reduced exposure to x-radiation, increased speed of image viewing, overall decreased cost of equipment and film, increased efficiency, and the capability to enhance images. It also serves as an effective tool that can be used to educate patients.

- **Superior gray-scale resolution.** A primary advantage to digital radiography is the superior gray-scale resolution that results. Digital radiography uses up to 256 colors of gray compared to

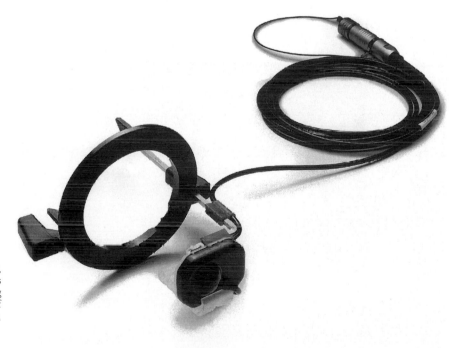

FIGURE 24–6. The intraoral sensor, held by the film holding device, allows the radiographer to utilize the paralleling technique for exposure. (Photo courtesy of DEXIS Digital Radiography Garden City, NY.)

the 16 to 25 shades of gray differentiated on a conventional film. The gray-scale resolution advantage is critical because diagnosis is often based on contrast discrimination. The ability to manipulate the density and contrast of the radiographic image without additional exposure to the patient is also an important advantage. (Fig. 24–7).

- **Reduced exposure to x-radiation.** Another primary advantage of the digital radiography imaging system is the reduction in patient exposure to x-radiation. Decreased exposure results from the sensitivity of the CCD. The radiation exposure for digital imaging systems is 50 to 80% less than what is required for E-speed film used in conventional radiography.

- **Increased speed of image viewing.** Dental professionals and patients are able to view the digital images instantaneously, thus allowing for immediate interpretation and evaluation. Speed of image viewing continues to be a compelling reason for the growing popularity of this technology.

- **Lower equipment and film cost.** Digital radiography eliminates the need for purchasing conventional film, costly processing equipment, and processing solutions. With digital radiography, a darkroom is not necessary and there is no need for processing solutions. Also, environmental problems are reduced because there is no disposal of processing chemicals and lead foil sheets.

The elimination of darkroom processing errors is also an advantage.

- **Increased efficiency.** Dental personnel can be more productive because digital radiography does not interrupt patient treatment or care. Both image storage and communication are easier with digital networking. The digital image can be incorporated into the electronic record of the patient and hard copies of the radiographic image can be printed when needed. Digital radiographs can also be electronically transmitted to referring dentists, insurance companies, or consultants.

- **Enhancement of diagnostic image.** Features such as colorization and zoom allow users to highlight conditions, such as bone resorption caused by periodontal disease or to help detect small areas of decay. Another feature that can be used to enhance a diagnostic image is **digital subtraction.** With digital subtraction, the gray-scale is reversed so that radiolucent images (normally black) appear white and radiopaque images (normally white) appear black (Fig. 24–8). Digital subtraction also eliminates distracting background information. For example, this feature permits the operator to remove all anatomic structures that have not changed between radiographic examinations for ease in identifying changes in diagnostic information.

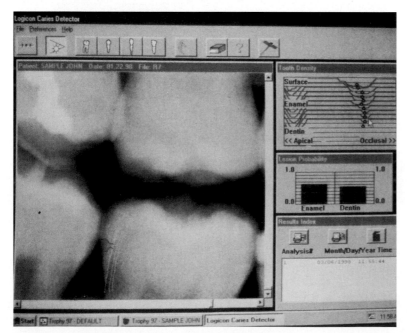

FIGURE 24–7. An image seen on the computer monitor reveals interproximal caries. (Photo courtesy of TREX Trophy, Dental Division, Danbury, CT.)

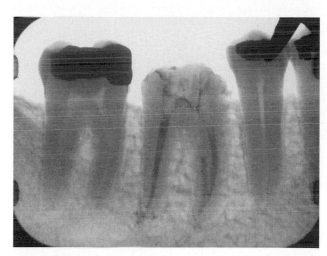

FIGURE 24–8. An image displays the feature of digital subtraction; the gray-scale is reversed. (Photo courtesy of Dentsply Gendex Digital Imaging System, Des Plaines, IL.)

• **Effective patient education tool.** Viewing digital images is an effective tool for patient education and interaction. Patients can view radiographic images with the operator, thus facilitating dialogue and rapport. Such visualization can increase a patient's understanding of the disease process and acceptance of treatment modalities. In addition, the size of the digitized image on the 15- or 17-inch computer screen (compared with a 2-inch piece of film) makes it attractive as a patient education tool.

Disadvantages

Disadvantages of digital radiography include the following: initial set-up costs, overall image quality, sensor size, infection control issues, and legal issues.

• **Initial set-up costs.** The initial cost of purchasing a digital imaging system is a significant disadvantage. The range of cost depends on the manufacturer, the level of computer equipment currently in the office, and auxiliary features, such as an intraoral camera. Service and maintenance for any repairs must also be considered. At the time of printing, typical start-up costs for one digital imaging system in the dental office is estimated at $10,000.

• **Image quality.** At this time, image quality continues to be a source of debate. The resolution of an image is defined as the number of line pairs per millimeter (lp/mm). Conventional dental x-ray film has a resolution of 12 to 20 lp/mm. A digital imaging system using a CCD has a resolution closer to 10 lp/mm. Given that the human eye can only resolve 8 to 10 lp/mm, a CCD system appears to be adequate for diagnosis of dental disease.

• **Sensor size.** Sensors are thicker than intraoral film. Patients may complain of the bulky nature of the sensor; the sensor may be uncomfortable or elicit the gag reflex.

• **Infection control.** The digital sensor cannot withstand heat sterilization. Therefore, the sensor requires complete coverage with disposable plastic sleeves that must be changed with each patient to prevent patient-to-patient cross-contamination.

• **Legal issues.** Because the original digital image can be manipulated, it is questionable whether digital radiographs can be used as evidence in lawsuits. To address this concern, manufacturers such as Kodak, with its Digital Science Dental Scanning System, have included a warning feature that appears if the original image is not comparable with the image displayed on the monitor.

SUMMARY

• Digital radiography is a method of capturing a radiographic image and displaying it on a computer screen; no film is used and no film processing is required.

• A conventional dental x-ray unit is used as the radiation source. A sensor or small detector is placed inside the mouth of the patient and the x-ray beam is aimed to strike the sensor. The electronic charge produced on the sensor is digitized (or converted into digital form) and can be viewed on a computer monitor.

• The advantages of digital radiography include: superior gray-scale resolution, reduced patient exposure to x-rays, increased speed of image viewing, lower equipment and film costs, increased time efficiency, improved patient education, and many viewing options to enhance the diagnostic information of the image.

• The disadvantages of digital radiography include: initial set-up costs of the digital system, image quality, size of the intraoral sensor, legal issues, and the inability to heat sterilize the sensor.

BIBLIOGRAPHY

Frommer HH: Panoramic radiography, new imaging systems. *In* Radiology for Dental Auxiliaries, 6th edition. St. Louis, Mosby-Year Book, 1996, pp. 223–243.

Goaz PW, White SC: Specialized radiographic techniques. *In* Oral Radiology: Principles and Interpretation, 3rd edition. St. Louis, Mosby-Year Book, 1994, pp. 266–290.

Langland OE, Langlais RP: Special radiographic techniques. *In* Principles of Dental Imaging. Baltimore, Williams & Wilkins, 1997, pp. 265–287.

Levato C: Are you ready for digital radiography? Dental Practice & Finance 7:17–24, May/June 1999.

Lusk LT: Comparison of film-based and digital radiography. J Practical Hygiene 7:45–50, 1998.

Miles DA, Van Dis ML, Jensen CW, Ferretti A: Digital imaging. *In* Radiographic Imaging for Dental Auxiliaries, 3rd edition. Philadelphia, WB Saunders, 1999, pp. 149–163.

Miles DA: Imaging using solid-state detectors. Dental Clinics of North America 37:531–539, 1993.

Razmus TF, Williamson GF: An overview of oral and maxillofacial imaging. *In* Current Oral and Maxillofacial Imaging. Philadelphia, WB Saunders, 1996, pp. 1–22.

Tyndall DA, Ludlow JB, Platin E, et al: A comparison of Kodak Ektaspeed Plus film and the Siemens Sidexis digital imaging system for caries detection using receiver operating characteristic analysis. Oral Surgery Oral Medicine Oral Pathology Oral Radiology and Endodontics 85:113–118, 1998.

Quiz Questions

MATCHING

For questions 1 to 9, match each term with its corresponding definition.

       a. charge-coupled device
       b. digital radiography
       c. digital subtraction
       d. digitize
       e. direct digital imaging
       f. indirect digital imaging
       g. pixel
       h. sensor
       i. storage phosphor imaging

_____ **1.** A small detector that is placed intraorally to capture the radiographic image.

_____ **2.** An image receptor found in the intraoral sensor.

_____ **3.** A method of obtaining a digital image in which the image is recorded on phosphor-coated plates and then placed into an electronic processor where a laser scans the plate and produces an image on a computer screen.

_____ **4.** To convert an image into digital form that, in turn, can be processed by a computer.

_____ **5.** A method of obtaining a digital image in which an intraoral sensor is exposed to x-rays to capture a radiographic image that can be viewed on a computer monitor.

_____ **6.** A discrete unit of information; a picture element.

_____ **7.** A method of obtaining a digital image in which an existing radiograph is scanned and converted into a digital form using a CCD camera.

_____ **8.** A method of reversing the gray-scale as a digital image is viewed.

_____ **9.** A filmless imaging system; a method of capturing a radiographic image using a sensor, breaking it into electronic pieces, and presenting and storing the image using a computer.

TRUE OR FALSE

_____ **10.** In digital radiography, the term used to describe the picture that is produced is _radiograph_.

_____ **11.** Digital radiography requires more x-radiation than conventional radiography.

_____ **12.** The x-radiation source used in most digital radiography systems is a conventional dental x-ray unit.

_____ **13.** Compared with film emulsion, the pixels used in digital radiography are structured in an orderly arrangement.

_____ **14.** Intraoral sensors can be heat sterilized after use.

_____ **15.** The preferred exposure method for intraoral digital radiography is the paralleling technique.

_____ **16.** One advantage of a digital radiography system is the superior gray-scale resolution that results.

_____ **17.** Digital subtraction is an advantage in digital radiography because it eliminates distracting background information from the image.

_____ **18.** The manipulation of the original digital images can be considered a legal issue.

MULTIPLE CHOICE

_____ **19.** Digital radiography was introduced to dentistry in:

a. 1967
b. 1977
c. 1987
d. 1997

_____ **20.** Digital radiography can be used for:

a. detecting conditions of the teeth and surrounding structures
b. evaluating growth and development of the jaws
c. confirmation of suspected disease
d. all of the above

_____ **21.** Digital radiography requires less radiation than conventional radiography because:

a. the sensor is larger
b. the sensor is more sensitive to x-rays
c. the exposure time is increased
d. the pixels sense transmitted light quickly

_____ **22.** The method of obtaining a digital image similar to scanning a photograph to a computer screen is termed:

a. direct digital imaging
b. indirect digital imaging
c. storage phosphor imaging
d. CMOS/APS

_____ **23.** The image receptor found in the intraoral sensor is termed:

a. CCD
b. pixel
c. semiconductor chip
d. software

_____ **24.** Digital radiography systems can be used for which of the following?

a. bite-wing images
b. panoramic images
c. cephalometric images
d. all of the above

_____ **25.** All of the following are advantages of digital radiography except:

a. digital subtraction
b. the ability to enhance the image
c. size of the intraoral sensor
d. patient education

Answers are supplied at the end of this book.

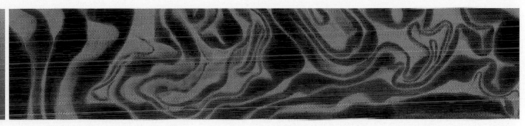

Radiography of Patients with Special Needs

OBJECTIVES

After completion of this chapter, the student will be able to:

- *Define the key words.*
- *List the areas of the oral cavity that are most likely to elicit the gag reflex when stimulated.*
- *List two precipitating factors responsible for initiating the gag reflex.*
- *Describe how to control the gag reflex using operator attitude, patient and equipment preparations, exposure sequencing, film placement and technique, and helpful hints.*
- *Describe common physical disabilities and what modifications in technique may be necessary during the radiographic examination.*
- *Describe common developmental disabilities and what modifications in technique may be necessary during the radiographic examination.*
- *List helpful hints that can be used when treating a person with a disability.*
- *Describe the prescribing of dental radiographs, patient and equipment preparations, recommended techniques, and patient management as they pertain to the pediatric dental patient.*
- *Describe the use of the dental radiograph, film placement modifications, and recommended periapical technique during root canal procedures.*
- *Describe the purposes of the radiographic examination in the edentulous patient.*
- *List and describe the three types of radiographic examination that may be used for the edentulous patient.*

KEY WORDS

Disability	Endodontics
Disability,	Gag reflex
developmental	Gagging
Disability, physical	Pediatric
Edentulous	Pediatric patient
Edentulous patient	Pediatrics
Endodontia	Stimuli, psychogenic
Endodontic patient	Stimuli, tactile

INTRODUCTION

Not all dental radiographic techniques can be successfully performed on all patients. Radiographic examination techniques must often be modified to accommodate patients with special needs. The dental radiographer must be competent in altering radiographic techniques to meet the specific diagnostic needs of individual patients.

The purpose of this chapter is to introduce the dental radiographer to the problems encountered in dealing with patients with special needs. In addition, this chapter also provides specific information on how to manage patients with a hypersensitive gag reflex, patients with physical or developmental disabilities, pediatric patients, endodontic patients, and edentulous patients.

PATIENTS WITH THE GAG REFLEX

The term **gagging** (also called retching) refers to the strong involuntary effort to vomit. The **gag reflex** (also called the pharyngeal reflex) can be defined as retching that is elicited by stimulation of the sensitive tissues of the soft palate region. The gag reflex is a protective mechanism of the body that serves to clear the airway of obstruction. All patients have gag reflexes, although some are more sensitive than others. In dental radiography, a hypersensitive gag reflex is a common problem.

The areas that are most likely to elicit the gag reflex when stimulated include the soft palate and the lateral posterior third of the tongue. Prior to the gag reflex, two reactions occur:

- cessation of respiration
- contraction of the muscles in the throat and abdomen

The precipitating factors that are responsible for initiating the gag reflex include **psychogenic stimuli** (stimuli originating in the mind) and **tactile stimuli** (stimuli originating from touch). To suppress the gag reflex, the dental radiographer must eliminate or lessen these precipitating factors.

Patient Management

To effectively manage the patient with a hypersensitive gag reflex, the dental radiographer must be aware of the following:

- operator attitude
- patient and equipment preparations
- exposure sequencing
- film placement and technique
- helpful hints for preventing the gag reflex

OPERATOR ATTITUDE

To prevent the gag reflex, the dental radiographer must convey a confident attitude. The patient must be confident of the radiographer's ability to perform radiographic procedures and must feel sure that there is no chance that the film will slip and lodge in the throat. If the dental radiographer does not appear to be in complete control of the procedures, the patient interprets this as a lack of confidence. This lack of confidence may act as a psychogenic stimulus and elicit the gag reflex.

In addition, the dental radiographer must also convey patience, tolerance, and understanding. Every effort should be made to relax and reassure the patient with a hypersensitive gag reflex. The dental radiographer should explain the radiographic procedures about to be performed and then compliment the patient as each exposure is completed. As the patient becomes comfortable with the radiographic procedures, he or she becomes more confident and, as a result, is less likely to gag.

PATIENT AND EQUIPMENT PREPARATIONS

Patient and equipment preparations (see Chapters 17, 18, and 19) can be used to prevent the gag reflex. In the patient with a hypersensitive gag reflex, every effort should be made to limit the amount of time that a film remains in the mouth. The longer a film stays in the mouth, the more likely the patient is to gag. When patient and equipment preparations are completed *prior* to film placement, valuable time is saved, and there is less likelihood of stimulating the gag reflex.

EXPOSURE SEQUENCING

Exposure sequencing plays an important role in preventing the gag reflex. As discussed in Chapters 17 to 19, the dental radiographer should always start with the anterior exposures. Anterior films are easier for the patient to tolerate and are less likely to elicit the gag reflex. With posterior film placements, the dental radiographer should always expose the premolar film before the molar film. Of all the film placements, *the maxillary molar film is the most likely to elicit the gag reflex*. In the patient with a hypersensitive gag reflex, the exposure sequence should be altered so that the maxillary molar films are exposed last.

FILM PLACEMENT AND TECHNIQUE

Film placement and technique also play an important role in preventing the gag reflex. To avoid stimulating the gag reflex, *each film must be placed and exposed as quickly as possible*. Placement and technique modifications include the following:

Avoid the palate. When placing films in the maxillary posterior areas, do not slide the film along the palate. Sliding the film along the palate stimulates this sensitive area and causes the gag reflex. Instead, position the film lingual to the teeth and then firmly bring the film into contact with the palatal tissues using one decisive motion.

Demonstrate film placement. In the areas that are most likely to elicit the gag reflex, rub a finger along the tissues near the intended area of film placement, while telling the patient, "This is where the film will be positioned." Then quickly place the film. This technique demonstrates where the film will be placed and desensitizes the tissues in the area.

Extreme Cases of the Gag Reflex

Occasionally, the dental radiographer encounters a patient with a gag reflex that is uncontrollable. In such a patient, intraoral films are impossible to obtain. Instead, the dental radiographer must use extraoral films such as panoramic or lateral jaw radiographs to obtain diagnostic information.

HELPFUL HINTS
to Reduce the Gag Reflex

➤ **NEVER** suggest gagging. The dental radiographer must never bring up the subject of gagging or ask the patient such questions as "Are you a gagger?" or "Do you gag?" The power of suggestion can act as a strong psychogenic stimulus and can in turn elicit the gag reflex. When the patient brings up the subject of gagging, the dental radiographer must refrain from using the terms gag, gagging, and gagger; instead, the radiographer should refer to the gag reflex as "a tickle in the back of the throat" when discussing the topic with the patient.

➤ **DO** reassure the patient. If the patient gags, the dental radiographer must remove the film *as quickly as possible* and then reassure the patient. The patient with a hypersensitive gag reflex must be reassured that such a response is not unusual. Some patients are very embarrassed, and others may even cry. The dental radiographer must always maintain control of the situation while remaining calm and understanding.

➤ **DO** suggest breathing. The dental radiographer should instruct the patient to "breathe deeply" through the nose during film placement and exposure. The breathing should be audible to the operator, who should demonstrate it to the patient. As previously stated, for the gag reflex to take place, respiration must cease; therefore, if the patient is breathing, the gag reflex cannot occur.

➤ **DO** try to distract the patient. Distraction often helps to suppress the gag reflex. The dental radiographer can instruct the patient to do one of the following during film placement and exposure: (1) bite as hard as possible on the film holder or film tab, or (2) suspend a leg or arm in the air. These acts help to divert the patient's attention and lessen the likelihood of eliciting the gag reflex.

➤ **DO** try to reduce tactile stimuli. Reducing tactile stimuli helps to prevent the gag reflex. The dental radiographer can try one of the following techniques before placing and exposing the film: (1) giving the patient a cup of ice water to drink, or (2) placing a small amount of ordinary table salt on the tip of the tongue. These techniques help to confuse the sensory nerve endings and lessen the likelihood of stimulating the gag reflex.

➤ **DO** use a topical anesthetic. In the patient with a severe hypersensitive gag reflex, a topical anesthetic spray may be used. The spray is used to numb the areas that elicit the gag reflex. The dental radiographer should instruct the patient to exhale while the anesthetic is sprayed on the soft palate and posterior tongue. Caution must be used to ensure that the patient does not inhale the spray; in such cases, an inflammation of the lungs may occur. The topical anesthetic spray takes effect after 1 minute and lasts for approximately 20 minutes. Topical anesthetic sprays should not be used in patients who are allergic to benzocaine.

PATIENTS WITH DISABILITIES

A **disability** can be defined as a "physical or mental impairment that substantially limits one or more of an individual's major life activities." In the dental office, persons with both physical and developmental disabilities are encountered. The dental radiographer must be prepared to modify radiographic techniques to accommodate persons with disabilities.

Physical Disabilities

A person with a **physical disability** may have problems with vision, hearing, or mobility. The dental radiographer must make every effort to meet the individual needs of such patients. In many cases, the person with a physical disability is accompanied to the dental office by a family member or caretaker; caretakers can be asked to assist the dental radiographer with communication or with the physical needs of the patient. The dental radiographer must be aware of the following common physical disabilities and the modifications necessary to deal with patients who have such problems:

Vision impairment. If a person is blind or visually impaired, the dental radiographer must communicate using clear verbal explanations. The dental radiographer must keep the patient informed of what is being done and explain each procedure before performing it. The dental radiographer must never gesture to another person in the presence of a person who is blind. Blind persons are sensitive to this kind of communication and perceive that the dental radiographer is "talking behind their back."

Hearing impairment. If a person is deaf or hearing impaired, the dental radiographer has several options. The radiographer may ask the caretaker to act as an interpreter, use gestures, or use written instructions. When the patient can read lips, the dental radiographer must face the patient and speak clearly and slowly.

Mobility impairment. If a person is in a wheelchair and does not have use of the lower limbs, the dental radiographer may offer to assist the patient in transferring to the dental chair or ask the caretaker to assist in the chair transfer. If a chair transfer is not possible, the dental radiographer may attempt to perform the necessary radiographic procedures with the patient seated in the wheelchair.

If a person does not have use of the upper limbs and a holder cannot be used to stabilize film placement, the dental radiographer may ask the caretaker to assist with film holding. In such cases, the caretaker must wear a lead apron and thyroid collar during exposure of the films. In addition, the caretaker must be given specific instructions on how to hold the film or the patient. As stated in previous chapters, the dental radiographer must *never* hold a film for a patient during an x-ray exposure.

Developmental Disabilities

A **developmental disability** is "a substantial impairment of mental or physical functioning that occurs before the age of 22 and is of indefinite duration." Examples include autism, cerebral palsy, epilepsy and other neuropathies, and mental retardation. The dental radiographer must make every effort to meet the individual needs of the patient with a developmental disability.

A person with a developmental disability may have problems with coordination or comprehension of instructions. As a result, the dental radiographer may experience difficulties in obtaining intraoral films. If coordination is a problem, mild sedation may be useful. If comprehension is a problem and the patient cannot hold a film, the caretaker may be asked to assist with film holding.

It is important that the dental radiographer recognize situations in which the patient cannot tolerate intraoral film exposure. In such instances, *no intraoral films must be exposed;* such exposure results only in nondiagnostic films and needless radiation exposure of the patient. In patients who cannot tolerate intraoral film exposure, extraoral films (e.g., lateral jaw and panoramic radiographs) may be used.

 HELPFUL HINTS • • • • • • • • • • • • • • • • •
For Treating a Patient with a Disability

➤ **DO NOT** ask personal questions about a disability; such questions are inappropriate for the dental radiographer.
➤ **DO** offer assistance to a person with a disability. For example, offer to push a wheelchair or to guide a person who is blind. The person with a disability will indicate whether help is needed and is often specific about how to provide assistance. For example, a person who is blind may prefer to hold the arm of a person offering guidance rather than having an arm held.
➤ **DO** talk directly to the person with a disability. It is inappropriate to talk to the caretaker instead of to the

patient. For example, instead of asking the caretaker "Can he [or she] transfer out of the wheelchair?" the radiographer should speak directly to the patient in the wheelchair. In addition, it is inappropriate to talk to the caretaker about a person with a disability as if that person were not present; the same is also true when an interpreter accompanies a deaf person.

PATIENTS WITH SPECIFIC DENTAL NEEDS

Different patients have different diagnostic dental requirements based on specific needs. Radiographic examination techniques must often be modified to accommodate patients with specific dental needs, including pediatric, endodontic, and edentulous patients.

Pediatric Patients

A **pediatric patient** is a child; the term **pediatric** is derived from the Greek word *pedia* meaning child. **Pediatrics** is the branch of dentistry dealing with the diagnosis and treatment of dental diseases in children. In children, dental radiographs are useful for detecting lesions and conditions of the teeth and bones, for showing changes secondary to caries and trauma, and for evaluating growth and development. When treating pediatric patients, the dental radiographer must be aware of the following:

- the prescribing of dental radiographs
- patient and equipment preparations
- recommended techniques
- patient management

PRESCRIBING OF DENTAL RADIOGRAPHS

As described in Chapter 5, the prescribing of dental radiographs is based on the individual needs of the patient. The *Guidelines for Prescribing Dental Radiographs* (see Table 5–1) include recommendations for both children and adults. For the pediatric patient, the prescribed number and type of dental films depends not only on the individual needs of the child but also on the age of the child and his or her ability to cooperate with the procedures.

PATIENT AND EQUIPMENT PREPARATIONS

Patient and equipment preparations for the pediatric patient are identical to those described for the adult patient (see Chapters 17, 18, 19). With the

pediatric patient, however, special attention must be devoted to the following preparations:

Explanation of procedure. The radiographic procedures that are to be performed must be explained to the child in terms that are easily understood. For example, the dental radiographer can refer to the tubehead as a camera, the lead apron as a coat, and the radiograph as a picture.

Lead apron. The growing tissues of a child are particularly susceptible to the effects of ionizing radiation and must be protected. As a result, a lead apron and thyroid collar must be placed on a child prior to x-ray exposure.

Exposure factors. Exposure factors (milliamperage, kilovoltage, time) must be reduced because of the size of the pediatric patient. A reduced exposure time is preferred; the shorter exposure time will reduce the chance of a blurred film should the child move. All exposure factors should be set according to the recommendations of the film manufacturer.

Film size. As described in Chapter 7, Size 0 film is recommended for use in the pediatric patient with a primary dentition because of the small mouth size. In the child with a transitional dentition, Size 1 or 2 film is recommended. As described in Chapter 20, Size 2 film is preferred for maxillary and mandibular occlusal pediatric projections.

RECOMMENDED TECHNIQUES

The techniques used to expose intraoral films in pediatric patients are basically the same as those used in adults. With periapical films, either the bisecting or the paralleling technique can be used (see Chapters 17 and 18). In children with a primary or transitional dentition, the bisecting technique is preferred because the small size of the mouth precludes the placement of a film beyond the apical regions of the teeth. The bitewing and occlusal techniques are also used in pediatric patients (see Chapters 19 and 21). Typical examinations of the primary and transitional dentitions using these techniques are described in Table 25–1.

PATIENT MANAGEMENT

Management of children requires that the dental radiographer be confident, patient, and understanding. The dental radiographer can use the following helpful hints in managing the pediatric patient:

TABLE 25–1. Radiographic Examination of the Pediatric Patient

Dentition	Number of Films	Type of Projection	Film Size
primary (3–6 years)	1	occlusal: maxillary	2
	1	occlusal: mandibular	2
	2	bite-wing	0
	2	periapical: maxillary molar	0
	2	periapical: mandibular molar	0
transitional (7–12 years)	3	periapical: maxillary anterior	1
	3	periapical: mandibular anterior	1
	2	bite-wing	1 or 2
	2	periapical: maxillary molar	1 or 2
	2	periapical: mandibular molar	1 or 2

HELPFUL HINTS
For Managing a Pediatric Patient

➤ **BE CONFIDENT.** Most children react favorably to the authority of a confident and capable operator. The dental radiographer must secure the child's confidence, trust, and cooperation. In addition, the dental radiographer must be patient and must not rush the radiographic procedures.

➤ **SHOW AND TELL.** The typical child is curious. The dental radiographer can use a "show and tell" approach to prepare the patient for radiographic procedures. Prior to making any x-ray exposures, the dental radiographer can show the child the equipment and materials that will be used and then tell him or her what will happen. The child should be encouraged to touch the tubehead, film, film holder, and lead apron.

➤ **REASSURE THE PATIENT.** The typical child has a fear of the unknown. Because a frightened child is not a cooperative one, the dental radiographer must reassure the child and allay any fears he or she may have about the procedures.

➤ **DEMONSTRATE BEHAVIOR.** With the pediatric patient, the dental radiographer can demonstrate the desired behavior to show the child exactly what to do. For example, the radiographer can demonstrate "how to hold still" and then ask the child to do the same thing.

➤ **REQUEST ASSISTANCE.** If a child cannot hold still or stabilize the film, the dental radiographer can ask the parent or accompanying adult to provide assistance. The adult can hold the film or the child during the x-ray exposure while wearing a lead apron and thyroid collar.

➤ **POSTPONE THE EXAMINATION.** Only in emergencies should a child be forced to undergo a radiographic examination. It is much better to postpone the examination until the second or third visit rather than instill a fear of visiting the dental office.

Endodontic Patients

The term **endodontia** is derived from two Greek words, *endon,* meaning within, and *odontos,* meaning tooth. **Endodontics** is the branch of dentistry concerned with the diagnosis and treatment of diseases of the dental pulp within the tooth. Endodontic treatment usually involves removal of the dental pulp (nerve tissue) from the pulp chamber and canals within the tooth, and then filling the empty pulp chamber and canals with a material such as gutta percha or silver points. This treatment is often referred to as a root canal procedure or root canal therapy. The **endodontic patient** is one who has undergone root canal therapy.

The dental radiograph is indispensable during root canal procedures and essential for diagnosing and managing pulpal problems. During a root canal procedure, a series of films is typically exposed of the same tooth; this series of exposures is used to evaluate the tooth before, during, and after treatment.

FILM PLACEMENT

The dental radiographer must modify film placement in the endodontic patient. During a root canal procedure, film placement is difficult because of the poor visibility of the tooth. The equipment used during a root canal procedure makes it difficult for the dental radiographer to see as well as position and stabilize the film. Equipment used during a root canal procedure includes a rubber dam, rubber dam clamp, root canal instruments (files, reamers, broaches), and root canal filling materials (gutta percha and silver points).

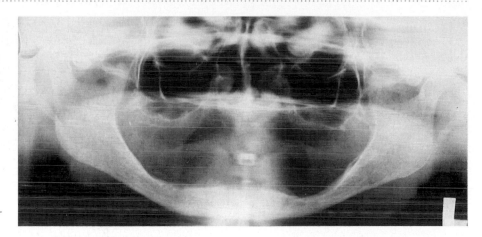

FIGURE 25–1. An edentulous panoramic radiograph.

The EndoRay film holder (see Chapter 6) can be used to aid in positioning the film during a root canal procedure; this holder fits around a rubber dam clamp and allows space for root canal instruments and filling materials to protrude from the tooth. A hemostat or a wooden tongue depressor may also be used to hold the film.

RECOMMENDED TECHNIQUE

During a root canal procedure, the length of the pulp canals must be accurately measured without distortion (elongation or foreshortening). To avoid distortion, the paralleling technique (see Chapter 17) should be used whenever possible; the use of the bisecting technique (see Chapter 18) may result in elongated or foreshortened images. With the paralleling technique, the use of a film holder (e.g., EndoRay, hemostat, tongue depressor) is strongly recommended.

Edentulous Patients

Edentulous means "without teeth." The **edentulous patient,** or patient without teeth, requires a dental radiographic examination for the following reasons:

- to detect the presence of root tips, impacted teeth, and lesions (cysts, tumors)
- to identify objects embedded in bone
- to establish the position of normal anatomic landmarks (e.g., mental foramen) relative to the crest of the alveolar ridge
- to observe the quantity and quality of bone that is present

The radiographic examination of the edentulous patient may include a panoramic radiograph, periapical radiographs, or a combination of occlusal and periapical radiographs.

PANORAMIC EXAMINATION

A panoramic radiograph (see Chapter 22) is the most common way of examining the edentulous jaw (Fig. 25–1). The panoramic examination is quick and easy for the patient and requires only one film. If a panoramic radiograph reveals any root tips, impacted teeth, foreign bodies, or lesions in the jaws, a periapical film of that specific area must be exposed. The periapical radiograph has more definition and permits the area in question to be examined in greater detail.

PERIAPICAL EXAMINATION

If a panoramic x-ray machine is not available, 14 periapical films (six anterior and eight posterior) can be use to examine the edentulous arches (Fig. 25–2). Size 2 film is typically used for the edentulous examination. Either the paralleling technique (see Chapter 17) or the bisecting technique (see Chapter 18) can be used for this periapical examination. If the paralleling technique is used, cotton rolls must be placed on both sides of the bite-block to take the place of the missing teeth (see Chapter 17). If the bisecting technique is used, the edentulous ridge and the film form the angle to be bisected (Fig. 25–3). The film should be positioned so that approximately one-third of it extends beyond the edentulous ridge. If the alveolar ridges of the patient are severely resorbed, the bisecting technique is recommended.

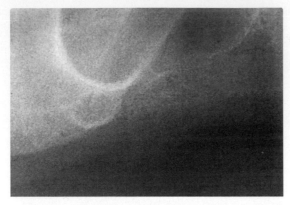

FIGURE 25–2. Radiographs must be exposed in all teeth-bearing areas of the mouth whether or not teeth are present. (From Olson SS: Dental Radiography Laboratory Manual. Philadelpia, WB Saunders, 1995.)

FIGURE 25–3. For the edentulous patient, the bisecting angle is formed by the ridge of bone and the film. The central ray (CR) is directed perpendicular to the imaginary bisector. Approximately one-third of the film should extend beyond the edentulous ridge. PID, position-indicating device.

OCCLUSAL AND PERIAPICAL EXAMINATION

Some practitioners prefer to use both occlusal and periapical radiographs to examine the edentulous patient. The mixed occlusal and periapical examination consists of a total of six films (Fig. 25–4), one maxillary topographic occlusal projection (Size 4 film), one mandibular cross-sectional occlusal projection (Size 4 film), and four standard molar periapical films (Size 2 film). As with the panoramic radiograph, if an object is identified on an occlusal film, a periapical film of that specific area should be exposed.

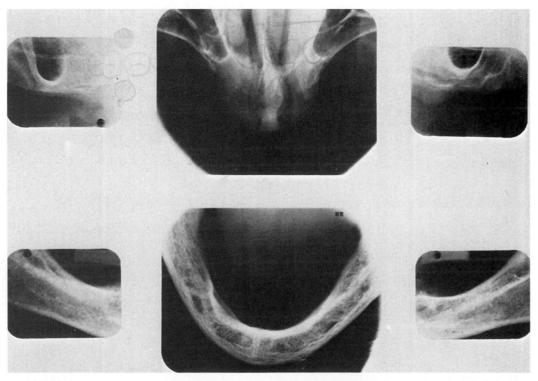

FIGURE 25–4. Mixed occlusal-periapical edentulous survey. (From Langland OE, Sippy FH, Langlais RP: Textbook of Dental Radiology, 2nd edition, 1984. Courtesy of Charles C Thomas, Springfield, Illinois.)

SUMMARY

- Radiographic techniques must often be modified to accommodate patients with special needs, including patients with a hypersensitive gag reflex, patients with physical or developmental disabilities, pediatric patients, endodontic patients, and edentulous patients.
- In dental radiography, the hypersensitive gag reflex is a common problem. The areas most likely to elicit the gag reflex when stimulated include the soft palate and the posterior third of the tongue.
- The dental radiographer can effectively manage the patient with a hypersensitive gag reflex by conveying a confident attitude, completing all patient and equipment preparations prior to film placement, using proper exposure sequencing, placing and exposing films as quickly as possible, and using modifications in technique as necessary.
- The following helpful hints can be used to prevent gagging: never suggest gagging, reassure the patient, suggest breathing, distract the patient, reduce tactile stimuli, and use a topical anesthetic.
- If the patient has an uncontrollable gag reflex, extraoral films (e.g., panoramic or lateral jaw radiographs) can be used to obtain diagnostic information.
- The dental radiographer must be aware of common physical disabilities (e.g., problems with vision, hearing, or mobility) and know what modifications in radiographic technique are necessary to accommodate a person with a disability.
- The dental radiographer must also be aware of patients with specific dental needs (e.g., pediatric patients, endodontic patients, and edentulous patients) and know what modifications in radiographic technique are necessary to accommodate such patients.
- With the pediatric patient, special attention must be paid to the prescribing of dental radiographs, patient and equipment preparations, recommended techniques, and patient management.
- With the endodontic patient, the dental radiographer must be able to modify film placement and, at the same time, accurately measure the length of the pulp canals without distortion.
- With the edentulous patient, the dental radiographer must also be able to modify film placements. A radiographic examination is used in the edentulous patient to detect lesions, root tips, impacted teeth, and objects embedded in bone, and to observe the quantity of bone present.

BIBLIOGRAPHY

Frommer HH: Patient management and special problems. *In* Radiology for Dental Auxiliaries, 6th edition. St. Louis, Mosby-Year Book, 1996, pp. 245–267.

Goaz PW, White SC: Intraoral radiographic examinations. *In* Oral Radiology: Principles of Interpretation, 3rd edition. St. Louis, Mosby-Year Book, 1994, pp. 213–218.

Johnson ON, McNally MA, Essay CE: Radiography for the edentulous patient. *In* Essentials of Dental Radiography for Dental Assistants and Hygienists, 6th edition. Norwalk, CT, Appleton and Lange, 1999, pp. 421–432.

Johnson ON, McNally MA, Essay CE: Radiography for children. *In* Essentials of Dental Radiography for Dental Assistants and Hygienists, 6th edition. Norwalk, CT, Appleton and Lange, 1999, pp. 403–419.

Ingersoll BD: The child patient. *In* Patient Management Skills for Dental Assistants and Hygienists. Norwalk, CT, Appleton-Century-Crofts, 1986, pp. 98–120.

Ingersoll BD: The handicapped patient. *In* Patient Management Skills for Dental Assistants and Hygienists. Norwalk, CT, Appleton-Century-Crofts, 1986, pp. 136–158.

Langland OE, Sippy FH, Langlais RP: Intraoral radiographic techniques. *In* Textbook of Dental Radiography, 2nd edition. Springfield, IL, Charles C Thomas, 1984, pp. 275–278.

Manson-Hing LR: Radiography of special patients. *In* Fundamentals of Dental Radiography, 3rd edition. Philadelphia, Lea & Febiger, 1990, pp. 186–200.

Miles DA, Van Dis ML, Jensen CW, Ferretti A: Accessory radiographic techniques and patient management. *In* Radiographic Imaging for Dental Auxiliaries, 3rd edition. Philadelphia, WB Saunders, 1999, pp. 129–148.

Miles DA, Van Dis ML, Razmus TF: Intraoral radiographic techniques. *In* Basic Principles of Oral and Maxillofacial Radiology. Philadelphia, WB Saunders, 1992, pp. 99–104.

Ohio Governor's Council on People with Disabilities: Ten Do's and Dont's When You Meet a Person with a Disability. Columbus, OH, Catalog No. G-16, 1990.

Normal Anatomy and Film Mounting Basics

CHAPTER 26

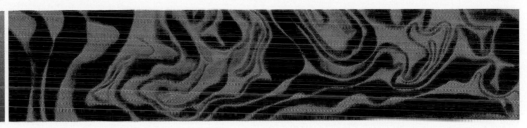

Normal Anatomy—Intraoral Films

OBJECTIVES

After completion of this chapter, the student will be able to:

- *Define the key words.*
- *State the difference between cortical and cancellous bone.*
- *Define the general terms that describe prominences, spaces, and depressions in bone.*
- *Identify and describe the normal anatomic landmarks of the maxilla on a human skull.*
- *Identify and describe the normal anatomic landmarks of the maxilla on dental radiographs.*
- *Identify and describe the normal anatomic landmarks of the mandible on a human skull.*
- *Identify and describe the normal anatomic landmarks of the mandible on dental radiographs.*
- *Identify and describe the radiographic appearance of tooth anatomy.*
- *Identify each normal radiographic landmark of the maxilla and mandible as either radiolucent or radiopaque.*
- *Identify each normal anatomic landmark of a tooth as radiolucent or radiopaque.*

INTRODUCTION

The dental radiographer must be able to recognize the normal anatomic landmarks on intraoral radiographs. Recognition of such normal anatomic landmarks enables the radiographer to mount and interpret intraoral films accurately. Without a working knowledge of normal anatomy, the dental radiographer may incorrectly mount dental radiographs or mistake normal anatomic structures for pathologic conditions.

Before dental radiographs can be interpreted and normal anatomic landmarks identified, the dental radiographer must first have a thorough knowledge of the anatomy of the maxilla and mandible. Each normal anatomic landmark seen on a periapical radiograph corresponds to that seen on the human skull. If the dental radiographer knows the anatomy of the maxilla and mandible as viewed on the human skull, he or she can identify the normal anatomy on a radiograph.

The purpose of this chapter is to review the normal anatomy of the maxilla and mandible as viewed on the skull and to describe the normal anatomic landmarks seen on intraoral radiographs.

DEFINITIONS OF GENERAL TERMS

A number of general terms are used to describe the anatomy of the bones of the skull. Terms describing types of bone, bony prominences, and bony spaces and depressions can be used to characterize areas of the maxilla and mandible normally seen on periapical radiographs. These general terms can be used by the dental radiographer to describe areas of normal anatomy viewed on intraoral radiographs.

Types of Bone

The composition of bone in the human body can be described as either cortical or cancellous.

CORTICAL BONE

The term **cortical** is derived from the Latin word *cortex* and means outer layer. Cortical bone, also referred to as compact bone, is the dense outer layer of bone (Fig. 26–1). Cortical bone resists the passage of the x-ray beam and appears radiopaque on a radiograph. The inferior border of the mandible is composed of cortical bone and appears radiopaque (Fig. 26–2).

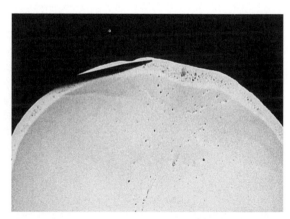

FIGURE 26–1. Cortical bone is dense and compact. (From Haring JI, Lind LJ: Radiographic Interpretation for the Dental Hygienist. Philadelphia, WB Saunders, 1993.)

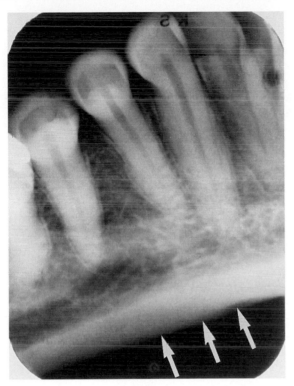

FIGURE 26–2. Cortical bone appears very radiopaque on a dental radiograph. (From Haring JI, Lind LJ: Radiographic Interpretation for the Dental Hygienist. Philadelphia, WB Saunders, 1993.)

CANCELLOUS BONE

The term **cancellous** is also derived from Latin and means "arranged like a lattice." Cancellous bone is the soft spongy bone located between two layers of dense cortical bone (Fig. 26–3). Cancellous bone is com-

posed of numerous bony trabeculae that form a lattice-like network of intercommunicating spaces filled with bone marrow. The trabeculae, actual pieces of bone, resist the passage of the x-ray beam and appear radiopaque; in contrast, the marrow spaces permit the passage of the x-ray beam and appear radiolucent. The larger the trabeculations, the more radiolucent the area of cancellous bone appears. Cancellous bone appears predominantly radiolucent (Fig. 26–4).

Prominences of Bone

Prominences of bone are composed of dense cortical bone and appear radiopaque on dental radiographs. Five terms can be used to describe the bony prominences seen in maxillary and mandibular periapical radiographs: process, ridge, spine, tubercle, and tuberosity.

> **Process:** A marked prominence or projection of bone; an example is the coronoid process of the mandible (Fig. 26–5).
>
> **Ridge:** A linear prominence or projection of bone; an example is the internal oblique ridge of the mandible (Fig. 26–6).
>
> **Spine:** A sharp, thorn-like projection of bone; an example is the anterior nasal spine of the maxilla (Fig. 26–7).
>
> **Tubercle:** A small bump or nodule of bone; an example is the genial tubercles of the mandible (Fig. 26–8).
>
> **Tuberosity:** A rounded prominence of bone; an example is the maxillary tuberosity (Fig. 26–9).

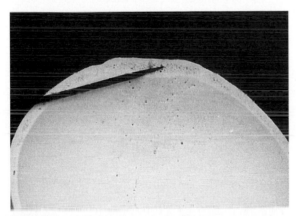

FIGURE 26–3. Cancellous or spongy bone is composed of numerous trabecular spaces. (From Haring JI, Lind LJ: Radiographic Interpretation for the Dental Hygienist. Philadelphia, WB Saunders, 1993.)

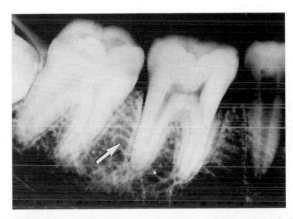

FIGURE 26–4. Cancellous bone appears predominantly radiolucent. (From Haring JI, Lind LJ: Radiographic Interpretation for the Dental Hygienist. Philadelphia, WB Saunders, 1993.)

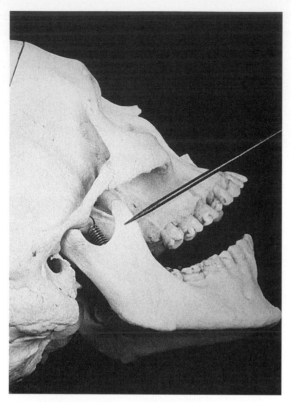

FIGURE 26–5. A process is a marked projection of bone. (From Haring JI, Lind LJ: Radiographic Interpretation for the Dental Hygienist. Philadelphia, WB Saunders, 1993.)

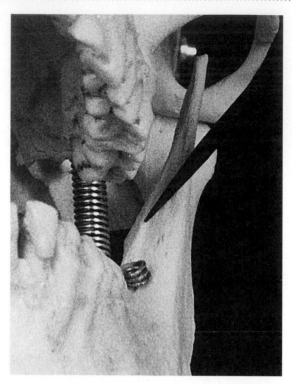

FIGURE 26–6. A ridge is a linear prominence of bone. (From Haring JI, Lind LJ: Radiographic Interpretation for the Dental Hygienist. Philadelphia, WB Saunders, 1993.)

Spaces and Depressions in Bone

Spaces and depressions in bone do not resist the passage of the x-ray beam and appear radiolucent on dental radiographs. Four terms can be used to describe the spaces and depressions in bone viewed in maxillary and mandibular periapical radiographs: canal, foramen, fossa, and sinus.

> **Canal:** A tube-like passageway through bone that contains nerves and blood vessels; an example is the mandibular canal (Fig. 26–10).
>
> **Foramen:** An opening or hole in bone that permits the passage of nerves and blood vessels; an example is the mental foramen of the mandible (Fig. 26–11).
>
> **Fossa:** A broad, shallow, scooped-out or depressed area of bone; an example is the submandibular fossa of the mandible (Fig. 26–12).
>
> **Sinus:** A hollow space, cavity, or recess in bone; an example is the maxillary sinus (Fig. 26–13).

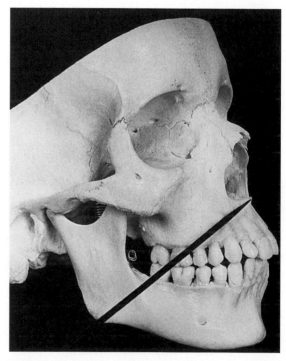

FIGURE 26–7. A spine is a sharp projection of bone. (From Haring JI, Lind LJ: Radiographic Interpretation for the Dental Hygienist. Philadelphia, WB Saunders, 1993.)

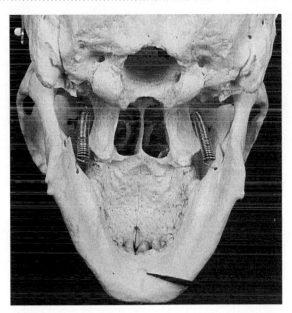

FIGURE 26–8. A tubercle is a tiny bump of bone. (From Haring JI, Lind LJ: Radiographic Interpretation for the Dental Hygienist. Philadelphia, WB Saunders, 1993.)

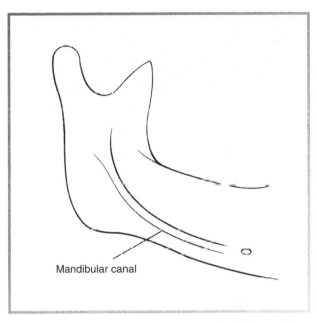

Mandibular canal

FIGURE 26–10. A canal is a passageway through bone. (From Haring JI, Lind LJ: Radiographic Interpretation for the Dental Hygienist. Philadelphia, WB Saunders, 1993.)

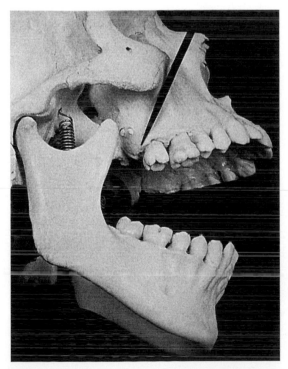

FIGURE 26–9. A tuberosity is a rounded prominence of bone. (From Haring JI, Lind LJ: Radiographic Interpretation for the Dental Hygienist. Philadelphia, WB Saunders, 1993.)

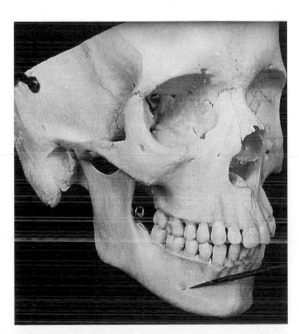

FIGURE 26–11. A foramen is a hole in bone. (From Haring JI, Lind LJ: Radiographic Interpretation for the Dental Hygienist. Philadelphia, WB Saunders, 1993.)

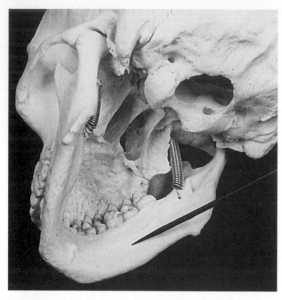

FIGURE 26–12. A fossa is a scooped-out or depressed area of bone. (From Haring JI, Lind LJ: Radiographic Interpretation for the Dental Hygienist. Philadelphia, WB Saunders, 1993.)

Miscellaneous Terms

Two other general terms that can be used to describe normal radiographic landmarks are septum and suture.

> **Septum:** A bony wall or partition that divides two spaces or cavities. A septum may be present within the space of a fossa or sinus. A bony septum appears radiopaque, in contrast to a space or cavity, which appears radiolucent. An example is the nasal septum (Fig. 26–14).
>
> **Suture:** An immovable joint that represents a line of union between adjoining bones of the skull. Sutures are found only in the skull. On dental radiographs, a suture appears as a thin radiolucent line. An example is the median palatal suture of the maxilla (Fig. 26–15).

NORMAL ANATOMIC LANDMARKS

Bony Landmarks of the Maxilla

The upper jaw is composed of two paired bones, the maxillae (Fig. 26–16). The paired maxillae meet at the midline of the face and are often referred to as a single

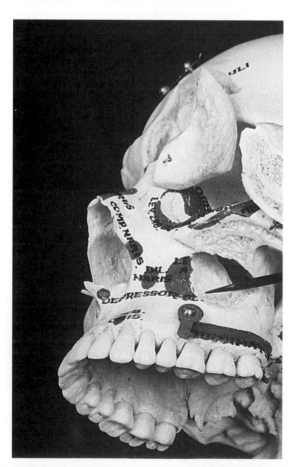

FIGURE 26–13. A sinus is a hollow cavity in bone. (From Haring JI, Lind LJ: Radiographic Interpretation for the Dental Hygienist. Philadelphia, WB Saunders, 1993.)

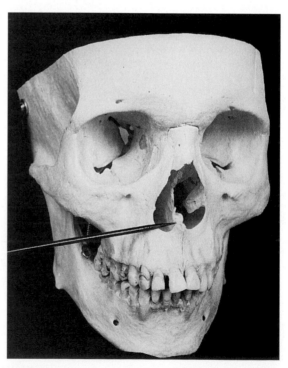

FIGURE 26–14. A septum is a bony partition. (From Haring JI, Lind LJ: Radiographic Interpretation for the Dental Hygienist. Philadelphia, WB Saunders, 1993.)

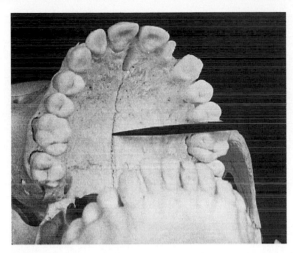

FIGURE 26–15. A suture is an immovable joint found in the skull. (From Haring JI, Lind LJ: Radiographic Interpretation for the Dental Hygienist. Philadelphia, WB Saunders, 1993.)

bone, the maxilla. The maxilla has been described as the architectural cornerstone of the face. All of the bones of the face articulate with the maxilla, with the exception of the mandible. The maxilla forms the floor of the orbit of the eyes, the sides and floor of the nasal cavities, and the hard palate. The lower border of the maxilla supports the upper teeth. This portion of this chapter reviews the bony landmarks that frequently appear in maxillary periapical radiographs.

INCISIVE FORAMEN

Description. The **incisive foramen** (also known as the nasopalatine foramen) is an opening or hole in bone that is located at the midline of the anterior portion of the hard palate directly posterior to the maxillary central incisors (Fig. 26–17). The nasopalatine nerve exits the maxilla through the incisive foramen.

Radiographic Appearance. On a maxillary periapical radiograph the incisive foramen appears as a small ovoid or round radiolucent area located between the roots of the maxillary central incisors (Fig. 26–18).

SUPERIOR FORAMINA OF THE INCISIVE CANAL

Description. The **superior foramina of the incisive canal** are two tiny openings or holes in bone that are located on the floor of the nasal cavity (foramina is the plural of foramen) (Fig. 26–19). The superior foramina are the openings of two small canals that extend downward and medially from the floor of the nasal cavity. These two small canals join together to form the incisive canal and share a common exit, the incisive foramen. The nasopalatine nerve enters the maxilla through the superior foramina, travels through the incisive canal, and exits at the incisive foramen.

Radiographic Appearance. On a maxillary periapical radiograph the superior foramina appear as two

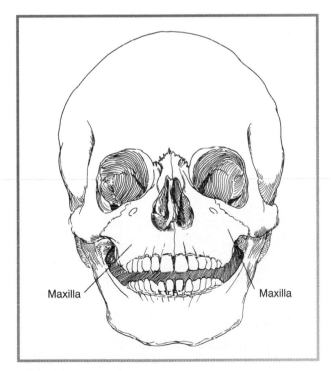

FIGURE 26–16. The paired bones of the maxilla. (From Haring JI, Lind LJ: Radiographic Interpretation for the Dental Hygienist. Philadelphia, WB Saunders, 1993.)

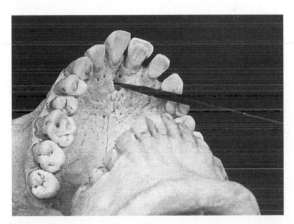

FIGURE 26–17. The incisive foramen is seen posterior to the maxillary central incisors. (From Haring JI, Lind LJ: Radiographic Interpretation for the Dental Hygienist. Philadelphia, WB Saunders, 1993.)

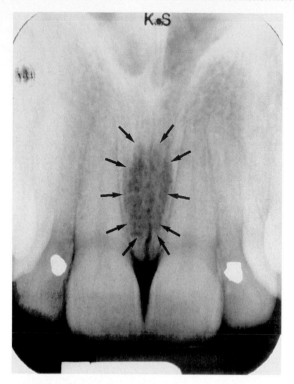

FIGURE 26–18. The incisive foramen appears radiolucent. (From Haring JI, Lind LJ: Radiographic Interpretation for the Dental Hygienist. Philadelphia, WB Saunders, 1993.)

small round radiolucencies located superior to the apices of the maxillary central incisors (Fig. 26–20).

MEDIAN PALATAL SUTURE

Description. The **median palatal suture** is the immovable joint between the two palatine processes of the maxilla. (The palatine processes of the maxilla form the major portion of the hard palate.) The median palatal suture extends from the alveolar bone between the maxillary central incisors to the posterior hard palate (Fig. 26–21).

Radiographic Appearance. On a maxillary periapical radiograph the median palatal suture appears as a thin radiolucent line between the maxillary central incisors (Fig. 26–22). The median palatal suture is bounded on both sides by dense cortical bone that appears radiopaque. As the median palatal suture fuses with age, it may become less distinct radiographically.

LATERAL FOSSA

Description. The **lateral fossa** (also known as the canine fossa) is a smooth, depressed area of the maxilla located just inferior and medial to the infraorbital

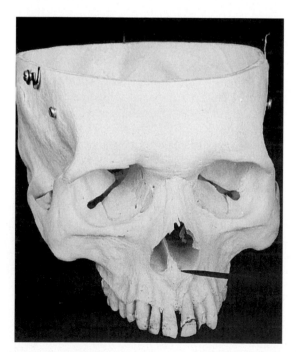

FIGURE 26–19. The superior foramina of the incisive canal are found on the floor of the nasal cavity. (From Haring JI, Lind LJ: Radiographic Interpretation for the Dental Hygienist. Philadelphia, WB Saunders, 1993.)

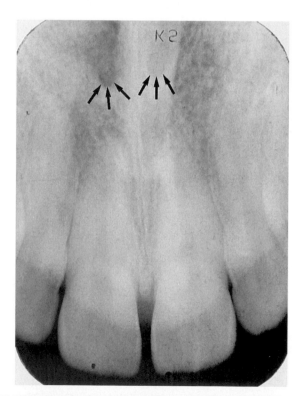

FIGURE 26–20. The superior foramina of the incisive canal appear as two small round radiolucencies. (From Haring JI, Lind LJ: Radiographic Interpretation for the Dental Hygienist. Philadelphia, WB Saunders, 1993.)

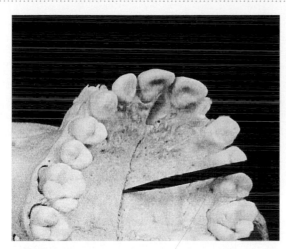

FIGURE 26–21. The median palatal suture is found between the two palatine processes of the maxilla. (From Haring JI, Lind LJ: Radiographic Interpretation for the Dental Hygienist. Philadelphia, WB Saunders, 1993.)

foramen between the canine and lateral incisors (Fig. 26–23).

Radiographic Appearance. On a maxillary periapical radiograph the lateral fossa appears as a radiolucent area between the maxillary canine and lateral incisors

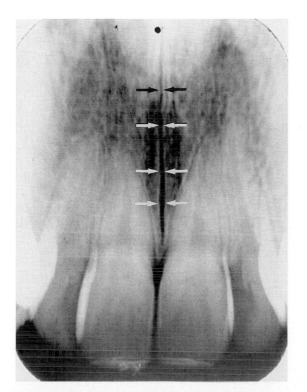

FIGURE 26–22. The median palatal suture appears as a thin radiolucent line. (From Haring JI, Lind LJ: Radiographic Interpretation for the Dental Hygienist. Philadelphia, WB Saunders, 1993.)

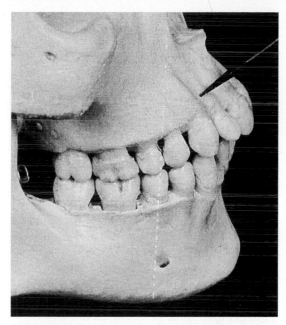

FIGURE 26–23. The lateral fossa is a depressed area of the maxilla found between the lateral incisor and the canine. (From Haring JI, Lind LJ: Radiographic Interpretation for the Dental Hygienist. Philadelphia, WB Saunders, 1993.)

(Fig. 26–24). In some periapical radiographs the lateral fossa may appear as a distinct radiolucency; in others it may appear to be absent. The radiographic appearance of the lateral fossa varies depending on the anatomy of the individual.

NASAL CAVITY

Description. The **nasal cavity** (also known as the nasal fossa) is a pear-shaped compartment of bone located superior to the maxilla (Fig. 26–25). The inferior portion, or floor, of the nasal cavity is formed by the palatal processes of the maxilla and the horizontal portions of the palatine bones. The lateral walls of the nasal cavity are formed by the ethmoid bone and the maxillae. The nasal cavity is divided by a bony partition, or wall, called the nasal septum.

Radiographic Appearance. On a maxillary periapical radiograph, the nasal cavity appears as a large radiolucent area above the maxillary incisors (Fig. 26–26).

NASAL SEPTUM

Description. The **nasal septum** is a vertical bony wall or partition that divides the nasal cavity into the right and left nasal fossae (fossae is the plural of fossa) (Fig. 26–27). The nasal septum is formed by two bones, the vomer and a portion of the ethmoid bone, and cartilage.

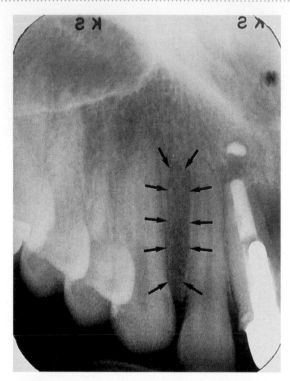

FIGURE 26–24. The lateral fossa appears as a radiolucent area between the lateral incisor and the canine. (From Haring JI, Lind LJ: Radiographic Interpretation for the Dental Hygienist. Philadelphia, WB Saunders, 1993.)

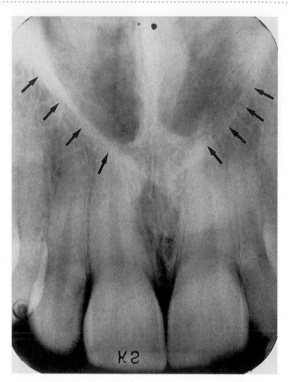

FIGURE 26–26. The nasal cavity appears as a large radiolucent area above the maxilla. (From Haring JI, Lind LJ: Radiographic Interpretation for the Dental Hygienist. Philadelphia, WB Saunders, 1993.)

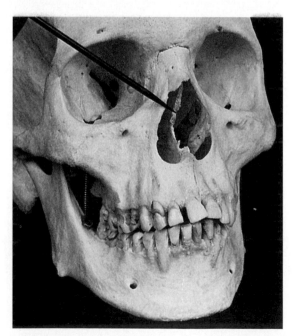

FIGURE 26–25. The nasal cavity is a pear-shaped opening of the skull above the maxilla. (From Haring JI, Lind LJ: Radiographic Interpretation for the Dental Hygienist. Philadelphia, WB Saunders, 1993.)

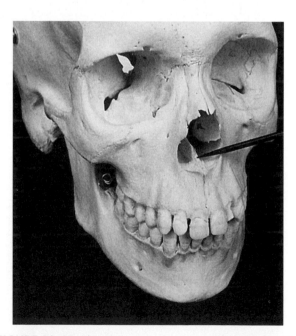

FIGURE 26–27. The nasal septum is a bony wall that divides the nasal cavity into two nasal fossae. (From Haring JI, Lind LJ: Radiographic Interpretation for the Dental Hygienist. Philadelphia, WB Saunders, 1993.)

Radiographic Appearance. On a maxillary periapical radiograph the nasal septum appears as a vertical radiopaque partition that divides the nasal cavity (Fig. 26–28). The nasal septum may be superimposed over the median palatal suture.

FLOOR OF THE NASAL CAVITY

Description. The **floor of the nasal cavity** is a bony wall formed by the palatal processes of the maxilla and the horizontal portions of the palatine bones (Fig. 26–29). The floor is composed of dense cortical bone and defines the inferior border of the nasal cavity.

Radiographic Appearance. On a maxillary periapical radiograph the floor of the nasal cavity appears as a dense radiopaque band of bone above the maxillary incisors (Fig. 26–30).

ANTERIOR NASAL SPINE

Description. The **anterior nasal spine** is a sharp projection of the maxilla located at the anterior and inferior portion of the nasal cavity (Fig. 26–31).

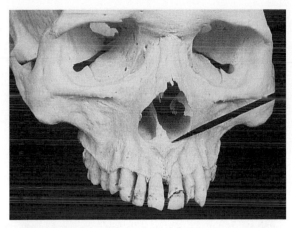

FIGURE 26–29. The floor of the nasal cavity is composed of dense cortical bone. (From Haring JI, Lind LJ: Radiographic Interpretation for the Dental Hygienist. Philadelphia, WB Saunders, 1993.)

Radiographic Appearance. On a maxillary periapical radiograph the anterior nasal spine appears as a V-shaped radiopaque area located at the intersection of the floor of the nasal cavity and the nasal septum (Fig. 26–32).

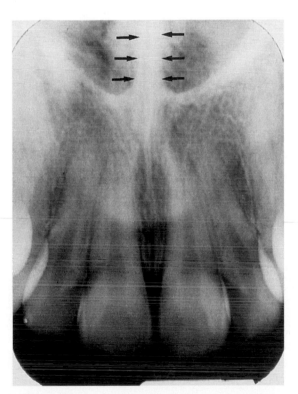

FIGURE 26–28. The nasal septum appears as a radiopaque partition that divides the nasal cavity. (From Haring JI, Lind LJ. Radiographic Interpretation for the Dental Hygienist. Philadelphia, WB Saunders, 1993.)

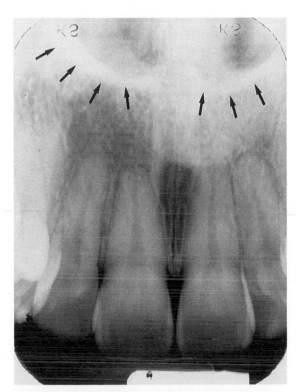

FIGURE 26–30. The floor of the nasal cavity appears as a radiopaque band. (From Haring JI, Lind LJ: Radiographic Interpretation for the Dental Hygienist. Philadelphia, WB Saunders, 1993.)

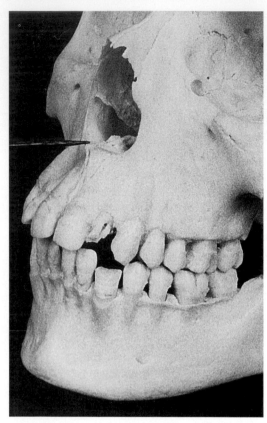

FIGURE 26–31. The anterior nasal spine is a sharp projection of bone located at the anterior inferior point of the nasal cavity. (From Haring JI, Lind LJ: Radiographic Interpretation for the Dental Hygienist. Philadelphia, WB Saunders, 1993.)

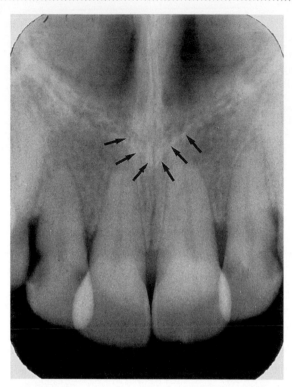

FIGURE 26–32. The anterior nasal spine appears as a **V**-shaped radiopacity at the midline of the floor of the nasal cavity. (From Haring JI, Lind LJ: Radiographic Interpretation for the Dental Hygienist. Philadelphia, WB Saunders, 1993.)

INFERIOR NASAL CONCHAE

Description. The **inferior nasal conchae** are wafer-thin, curved plates of bone that extend from the lateral walls of the nasal cavity (Fig. 26–33). The inferior nasal conchae are seen in the lower lateral portions of the nasal cavity. The term concha is derived from Latin and means shell-shaped or scroll-shaped.

Radiographic Appearance. On a maxillary periapical radiograph the inferior nasal conchae appear as a diffuse radiopaque mass or projection within the nasal cavity (Fig. 26–34).

MAXILLARY SINUS

Description. The **maxillary sinuses** are paired cavities or compartments of bone located within the maxilla (Fig. 26–35). The maxillary sinuses are located above the maxillary premolar and molar teeth. Rarely does the maxillary sinus extend anteriorly beyond the canine. At birth, the maxillary sinus is the size of a small pea. With growth, the maxillary sinus expands

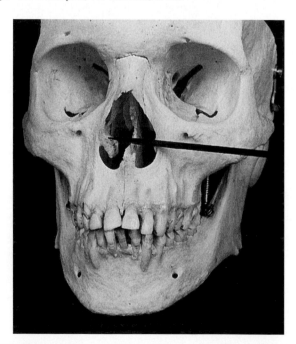

FIGURE 26–33. The inferior nasal conchae are scroll-shaped plates of bone that extend from the lateral wall of the nasal fossa. (From Haring JI, Lind LJ: Radiographic Interpretation for the Dental Hygienist. Philadelphia, WB Saunders, 1993.)

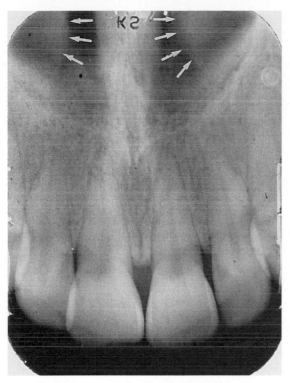

FIGURE 26–34. The inferior nasal conchae appear as diffuse radiopacities within the nasal cavity. (From Haring JI, Lind LJ: Radiographic Interpretation for the Dental Hygienist. Philadelphia, WB Saunders, 1993.)

and eventually occupies a large portion of the maxilla. The maxillary sinus may extend to include interdental bone, molar furcation areas, or the maxillary tuberosity region.

Radiographic Appearance. On a maxillary periapical radiograph, the maxillary sinus appears as a radiolucent area located above the apices of the maxillary premolars and molars (Fig. 26–36). The floor of the maxillary sinus is composed of dense cortical bone and appears as a radiopaque line.

SEPTA WITHIN THE MAXILLARY SINUS

Description. Bony **septa** (septa is the plural of septum) may be seen within the maxillary sinus. Septa are bony walls or partitions that appear to divide the maxillary sinus into compartments (Fig. 26–37).

Radiographic Appearance. On a maxillary periapical radiograph the septa appear as radiopaque lines within the maxillary sinus (Fig. 26–38). In some periapical radiographs the septa appear as distinct radiopaque lines; in others, no septa are present. The presence and number of bony septa within a maxillary sinus vary depending on the anatomy of the individual.

NUTRIENT CANALS WITHIN THE MAXILLARY SINUS

Description. **Nutrient canals** may be seen within the maxillary sinuses. Nutrient canals are tiny, tube-like passageways through bone that contain blood vessels and nerves that supply the maxillary teeth and interdental areas.

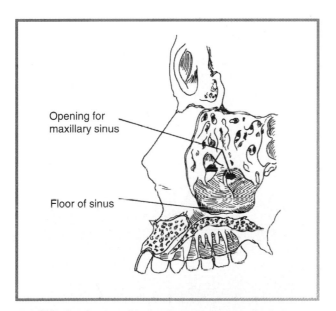

FIGURE 26–35. The maxillary sinuses are paired compartments or bone located above the maxillary posterior teeth. (From Haring JI, Lind LJ: Radiographic Interpretation for the Dental Hygienist. Philadelphia, WB Saunders, 1993.)

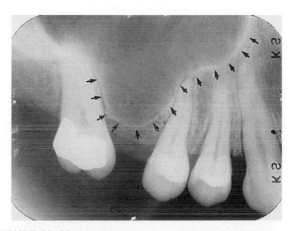

FIGURE 26–36. The maxillary sinus appears as a radiolucent area above the maxillary posterior teeth. (From Haring JI, Lind LJ: Radiographic Interpretation for the Dental Hygienist. Philadelphia, WB Saunders, 1993.)

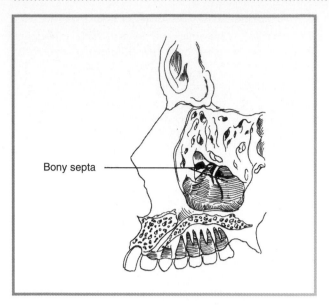

FIGURE 26–37. Septa are bony walls within the maxillary sinus. (From Haring JI, Lind LJ: Radiographic Interpretation for the Dental Hygienist. Philadelphia, WB Saunders, 1993.)

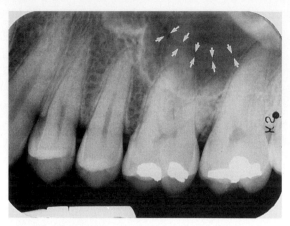

FIGURE 26–39. Nutrient canals appear as narrow radiolucent lines. (From Haring JI, Lind LJ: Radiographic Interpretation for the Dental Hygienist. Philadelphia, WB Saunders, 1993.)

Radiographic Appearance. On a maxillary periapical radiograph a nutrient canal appears as a narrow radiolucent band bounded by two thin radiopaque lines (Fig. 26–39). The radiopaque lines represent the cortical bone that comprises the walls of the canal.

INVERTED Y

Description. The **inverted** Y refers to the intersection of the maxillary sinus and the nasal cavity as viewed on a dental radiograph.

Radiographic Appearance. On a maxillary periapical radiograph, the inverted Y appears as a radiopaque upside-down Y formed by the intersection of the lat-

eral wall of the nasal fossa and the anterior border of the maxillary sinus (Fig. 26–40). Both the lateral wall of the nasal cavity and the anterior border of the maxillary sinus are composed of dense cortical bone and appear as a radiopaque line or band. The inverted Y is located above the maxillary canine.

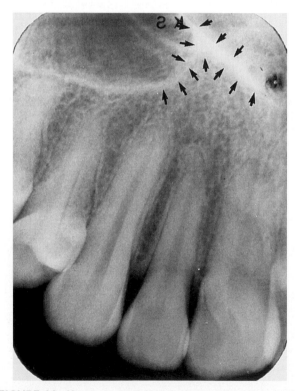

FIGURE 26–40. The inverted Y appears as a radiopaque upside-down Y. (From Haring JI, Lind LJ: Radiographic Interpretation for the Dental Hygienist. Philadelphia, WB Saunders, 1993.)

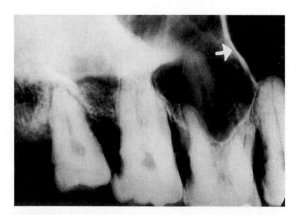

FIGURE 26–38. Septa within the maxillary sinus appear as radiopaque lines. (From Haring JI, Lind LJ: Radiographic Interpretation for the Dental Hygienist. Philadelphia, WB Saunders, 1993.)

MAXILLARY TUBEROSITY

Description. The **maxillary tuberosity** is a rounded prominence of bone that extends posterior to the third molar region (Fig. 26–41). Blood vessels and nerves enter the maxilla in this region and supply the posterior teeth.

Radiographic Appearance. On a maxillary periapical radiograph the maxillary tuberosity appears as a radiopaque bulge distal to the third molar region (Fig. 26–42).

HAMULUS

Description. The **hamulus** (also known as the hamular process) is a small hook-like projection of bone extending from the medial pterygoid plate of the sphenoid bone (Fig. 26–43). The hamulus is located posterior to the maxillary tuberosity region.

Radiographic Appearance. On a maxillary periapical radiograph the hamulus appears as a radiopaque hook-like projection posterior to the maxillary tuberosity area (Fig. 26–44). The radiographic appearance of the hamulus varies in length, shape, and density.

ZYGOMATIC PROCESS OF THE MAXILLA

Description. The **zygomatic process of the maxilla** is a bony projection of the maxilla that articulates with the zygoma or malar (cheek) bone (Fig. 26–45). The

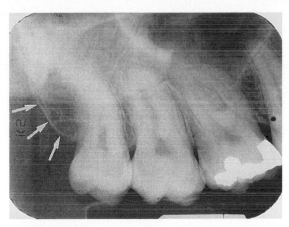

FIGURE 26–42. The maxillary tuberosity appears as a radiopaque bulge distal to the third molar region. (From Haring JI, Lind LJ: Radiographic Interpretation for the Dental Hygienist. Philadelphia, WB Saunders, 1993.)

zygomatic process of the maxilla is composed of dense cortical bone.

Radiographic Appearance. On a maxillary periapical radiograph the zygomatic process of the maxilla appears as a J- or U-shaped radiopacity located superior to the maxillary first molar region (Fig. 26–46).

ZYGOMA

Description. The **zygoma**, or cheek bone (also referred to as the malar or zygomatic bone) articulates

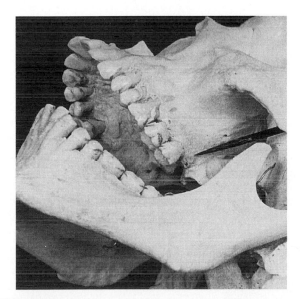

FIGURE 26–41. The maxillary tuberosity is a rounded prominence of bone posterior to the third molar region. (From Haring JI, Lind LJ: Radiographic Interpretation for the Dental Hygienist. Philadelphia, WB Saunders, 1993.)

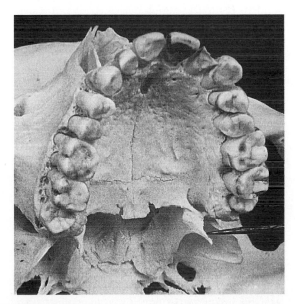

FIGURE 26–43. The hamulus is a hook-like projection of bone that extends from the medial pterygoid plate. (From Haring JI, Lind LJ: Radiographic Interpretation for the Dental Hygienist. Philadelphia, WB Saunders, 1993.)

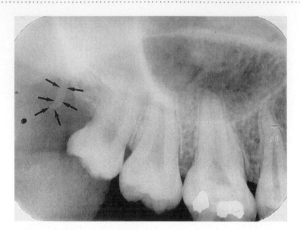

FIGURE 26–44. The hamulus appears as a hook-like radiopacity distal to the maxillary tuberosity area. (From Haring JI, Lind LJ: Radiographic Interpretation for the Dental Hygienist. Philadelphia, WB Saunders, 1993.)

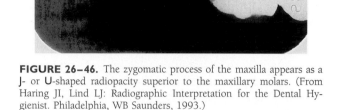
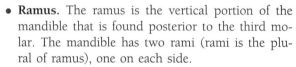

FIGURE 26–46. The zygomatic process of the maxilla appears as a J- or U-shaped radiopacity superior to the maxillary molars. (From Haring JI, Lind LJ: Radiographic Interpretation for the Dental Hygienist. Philadelphia, WB Saunders, 1993.)

with the zygomatic process of the maxilla (Fig. 26–47). The zygoma is composed of dense cortical bone.

Radiographic Appearance. On a maxillary periapical radiograph the zygoma appears as a diffuse, radiopaque band extending posteriorly from the zygomatic process of the maxilla (Fig. 26–48).

Bony Landmarks of the Mandible

The mandible, or lower jaw, is the largest and strongest bone of the face. The mandible can be divided into three main parts: the ramus, the body, and the alveolar process (Fig. 26–49).

- **Ramus.** The ramus is the vertical portion of the mandible that is found posterior to the third molar. The mandible has two rami (rami is the plural of ramus), one on each side.
- **Body.** The body of the mandible is the horizontal U-shaped portion that extends from ramus to ramus.
- **Alveolar process.** The alveolar process is the portion of the mandible that encases and supports the teeth.

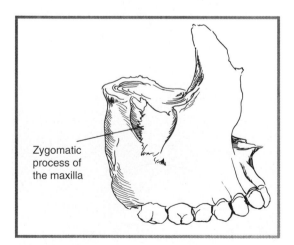

FIGURE 26–45. The zygomatic process of the maxilla is a small portion of the maxilla that articulates with the zygoma. (From Haring JI, Lind LJ: Radiographic Interpretation for the Dental Hygienist. Philadelphia, WB Saunders, 1993.)

Zygomatic process of the maxilla

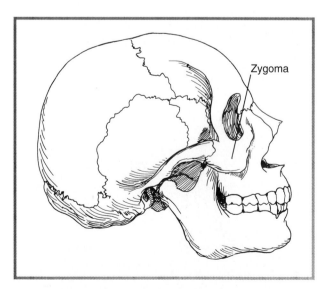

Zygoma

FIGURE 26–47. The zygoma (or cheekbone) articulates with the zygomatic process of the maxilla. (From Haring JI, Lind LJ: Radiographic Interpretation for the Dental Hygienist. Philadelphia, WB Saunders, 1993.)

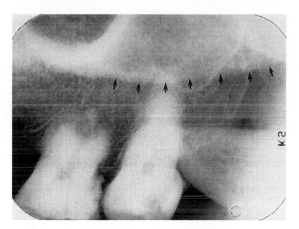

FIGURE 26-48. The zygoma appears as a diffuse radiopaque band that extends distally from the zygomatic process of the maxilla. (From Haring JI, Lind LJ: Radiographic Interpretation for the Dental Hygienist. Philadelphia, WB Saunders, 1993.)

This portion of the chapter reviews the bony landmarks that frequently appear in mandibular periapical radiographs.

GENIAL TUBERCLES

Description. The **genial tubercles** are tiny bumps of bone that serve as attachment sites for the genioglossus and geniohyoid muscles (Fig. 26-50). The genial tubercles are located on the lingual aspect of the mandible.

Radiographic Appearance. On a mandibular periapical radiograph the genial tubercles appear as a ring-shaped radiopacity below the apices of the mandibular incisors (Fig. 26-51).

LINGUAL FORAMEN

Description. The **lingual foramen** is a tiny opening or hole in bone located on the internal surface of the mandible (Fig. 26-52). The lingual foramen is located near the midline and is surrounded by the genial tubercles.

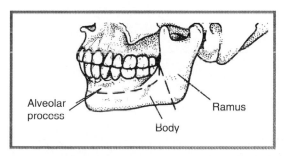

Alveolar process

Ramus

Body

FIGURE 26-49. The mandible. (From Haring JI, Lind LJ: Radiographic Interpretation for the Dental Hygienist. Philadelphia, WB Saunders, 1993.)

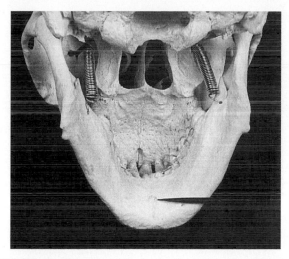

FIGURE 26-50. The genial tubercles are tiny bumps of bone at the midline on the lingual surface of the mandible. (From Haring JI, Lind. LJ: Radiographic Interpretation for the Dental Hygienist. Philadelphia, WB Saunders, 1993.)

Radiographic Appearance. On a mandibular periapical radiograph the lingual foramen appears as a small radiolucent dot located inferior to the apices of the mandibular incisors (Fig. 26-53). The lingual fora-

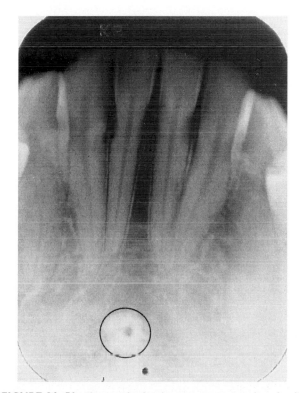

FIGURE 26-51. The genial tubercles appear as a ring-shaped radiopacity. (From Haring JI, Lind LJ: Radiographic Interpretation for the Dental Hygienist. Philadelphia, WB Saunders, 1993.)

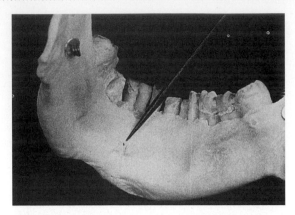

FIGURE 26-52. The lingual foramen is a small hole in bone seen at the midline on the lingual surface of the mandible. (From Haring JI, Lind LJ: Radiographic Interpretation for the Dental Hygienist. Philadelphia, WB Saunders, 1993.)

men is surrounded by the genial tubercles, which appear as a radiopaque ring.

NUTRIENT CANALS

Description. **Nutrient canals** are tube-like passageways through bone that contain nerves and blood vessels that supply the teeth. Interdental nutrient canals are most often seen in the anterior mandible, a region that typically has thin bone.

Radiographic Appearance. On a mandibular periapical radiograph nutrient canals appear as vertical radiolucent lines (Fig. 26-54). Radiographically, nutrient canals are readily seen in areas of thin bone. In the edentulous mandible, nutrient canals may be more prominent.

MENTAL RIDGE

Description. The **mental ridge** is a linear prominence of cortical bone located on the external surface of the anterior portion of the mandible (Fig. 26-55). The mental ridge extends from the premolar region to the midline and slopes slightly upward.

Radiographic Appearance. On a mandibular periapical radiograph the mental ridge appears as a thick radiopaque band that extends from the premolar region to the incisor region (Fig. 26-56). Radiographically, the mental ridge often appears superimposed over the mandibular anterior teeth.

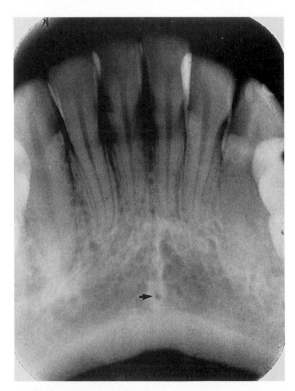

FIGURE 26-53. The lingual foramen appears as a small radiolucent dot. (From Haring JI, Lind LJ: Radiographic Interpretation for the Dental Hygienist. Philadelphia, WB Saunders, 1993.)

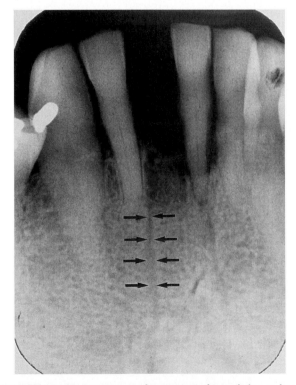

FIGURE 26-54. Nutrient canals appear as thin radiolucent lines. (From Haring JI, Lind LJ: Radiographic Interpretation for the Dental Hygienist. Philadelphia, WB Saunders, 1993.)

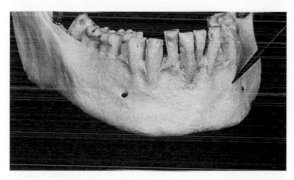

FIGURE 26–55. The mental ridge is a linear prominence of bone found on the external surface of the anterior mandible. (From Haring JI, Lind LJ: Radiographic Interpretation for the Dental Hygienist. Philadelphia, WB Saunders, 1993.)

MENTAL FOSSA

Description. The **mental fossa** is a scooped-out, depressed area of bone located on the external surface of the anterior mandible (Fig. 26–57). The mental fossa is located above the mental ridge in the mandibular incisor region.

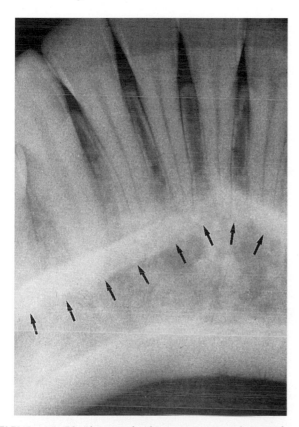

FIGURE 26–56. The mental ridge appears as a radiopaque band in the premolar and incisor region. (From Haring JI, Lind LJ: Radiographic Interpretation for the Dental Hygienist. Philadelphia, WB Saunders, 1993.)

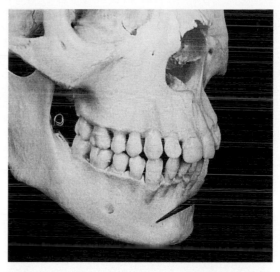

FIGURE 26–57. The mental fossa is a scooped-out or depressed area of the anterior mandible. (From Haring JI, Lind LJ: Radiographic Interpretation for the Dental Hygienist. Philadelphia, WB Saunders, 1993.)

Radiographic Appearance. On a mandibular periapical radiograph the mental fossa appears as a radiolucent area above the mental ridge (Fig. 26–58). The radiographic appearance of the mental fossa varies and is determined by the thickness of the bone in the anterior region of the mandible.

MENTAL FORAMEN

Description. The **mental foramen** is an opening or hole in bone located on the external surface of the mandible in the region of the mandibular premolars (Fig. 26–59). Blood vessels and nerves that supply the lower lip exit through the mental foramen.

Radiographic Appearance. On a mandibular periapical radiograph the mental foramen appears as a small ovoid or round radiolucent area located in the apical region of the mandibular premolars (Fig. 26–60). The mental foramen is frequently misdiagnosed as a periapical lesion (periapical cyst, granuloma, or abscess) because of its apical location.

MYLOHYOID RIDGE

Description. The **mylohyoid ridge** is a linear prominence of bone located on the internal surface of the mandible (Fig. 26–61). The mylohyoid ridge extends from the molar region downward and forward toward the lower border of the mandibular symphysis. The mylohyoid ridge serves as an attachment site for a muscle of the same name.

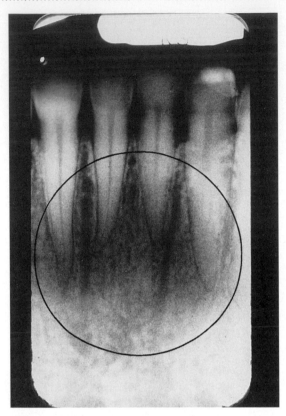

FIGURE 26-58. The mental fossa appears as a radiolucent area above the mental ridge. (From Haring JI, Lind LJ: Radiographic Interpretation for the Dental Hygienist. Philadelphia, WB Saunders, 1993.)

Radiographic Appearance. On a mandibular periapical radiograph the mylohyoid ridge appears as a dense radiopaque band that extends downward and forward from the molar region (Fig. 26-62). The mylohyoid ridge usually appears most prominent in the molar region and may be superimposed over the roots of the mandibular teeth. The mylohyoid ridge may appear to be continuous with the internal oblique ridge.

MANDIBULAR CANAL

Description. The **mandibular canal** is a tube-like passageway through bone that travels the length of the mandible. The mandibular canal extends from the mandibular foramen to the mental foramen and houses the inferior alveolar nerve and blood vessels.

Radiographic Appearance. On a mandibular periapical radiograph the mandibular canal appears as a radiolucent band (Fig. 26-63). The mandibular canal is outlined by two thin radiopaque lines that represent the cortical walls of the canal. The mandibular canal

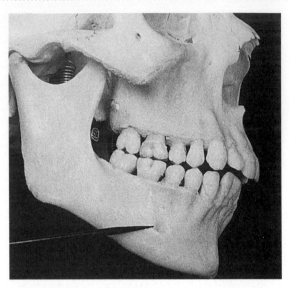

FIGURE 26-59. The mental foramen is a hole in bone located on the external surface of the mandible in the premolar area. (From Haring JI, Lind LJ: Radiographic Interpretation for the Dental Hygienist. Philadelphia, WB Saunders, 1993.)

appears below or superimposed over the apices of the mandibular molar teeth.

INTERNAL OBLIQUE RIDGE

Description. The **internal oblique ridge** (also known as the internal oblique line) is a linear prominence of bone located on the internal surface of the mandible that extends downward and forward from the ramus (Fig. 26-64). The internal oblique ridge may end in the region of the mandibular third molar, or it may continue on as the mylohyoid ridge.

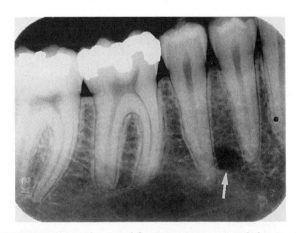

FIGURE 26-60. The mental foramen appears as a radiolucency in the mandibular premolar region. (From Haring JI, Lind LJ: Radiographic Interpretation for the Dental Hygienist. Philadelphia, WB Saunders, 1993.)

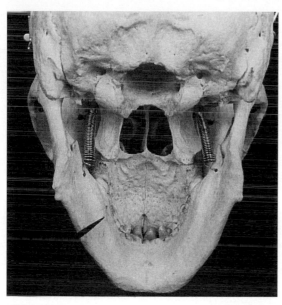

FIGURE 26–61. The mylohyoid ridge. (From Haring JI, Lind LJ: Radiographic Interpretation for the Dental Hygienist. Philadelphia, WB Saunders, 1993.)

Radiographic Appearance. On a mandibular periapical radiograph the internal oblique ridge appears as a radiopaque band that extends downward and forward from the ramus (Fig. 26–65). Depending on the radiographic technique used (bisecting versus paralleling technique), the internal and external oblique ridges may be superimposed on one another. When the ridges appear separate, the *superior* radiopaque band is the *external* oblique ridge, and the *inferior* radiopaque band is the *internal* oblique ridge.

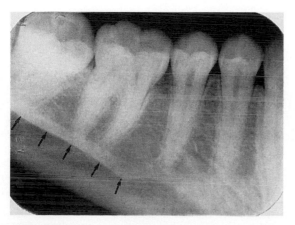

FIGURE 26–62. The mylohyoid ridge appears as a radiopaque band in the mandibular molar region. (From Haring JI, Lind LJ: Radiographic Interpretation for the Dental Hygienist. Philadelphia, WB Saunders, 1993.)

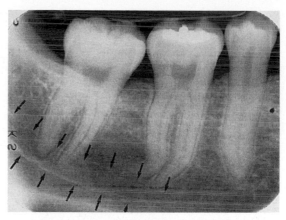

FIGURE 26–63. The mandibular canal appears as a radiolucent band outlined by two thin radiopaque lines. (From Haring JI, Lind LJ: Radiographic Interpretation for the Dental Hygienist. Philadelphia, WB Saunders, 1993.)

EXTERNAL OBLIQUE RIDGE

Description. The **external oblique ridge** (also known as the external oblique line) is a linear prominence of bone located on the external surface of the body of the mandible (Fig. 26–66). The anterior border of the ramus ends in the external oblique ridge.

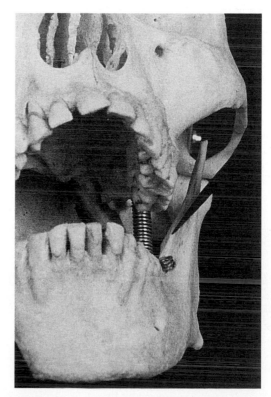

FIGURE 26–64. The internal oblique ridge is a linear prominence of bone located on the internal surface of the mandible. (From Haring JI, Lind LJ: Radiographic Interpretation for the Dental Hygienist. Philadelphia, WB Saunders, 1993.)

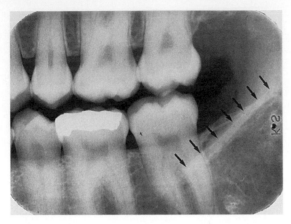

FIGURE 26–65. The internal oblique ridge appears as a radiopaque band. (From Haring JI, Lind LJ: Radiographic Interpretation for the Dental Hygienist. Philadelphia, WB Saunders, 1993.)

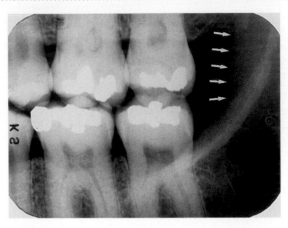

FIGURE 26–67. The external oblique ridge appears as a radiopaque band. (From Haring JI, Lind LJ: Radiographic Interpretation for the Dental Hygienist. Philadelphia, WB Saunders, 1993.)

Radiographic Appearance. On a mandibular periapical radiograph the external oblique ridge appears as a radiopaque band extending downward and forward from the anterior border of the ramus of the mandible (Fig. 26–67). The external oblique ridge typically ends in the mandibular third molar region.

SUBMANDIBULAR FOSSA

Description. The **submandibular fossa** (also known as the mandibular fossa or submaxillary fossa) is a scooped-out, depressed area of bone located on the internal surface of the mandible inferior to the mylohyoid ridge (Fig. 26–68). The submandibular salivary gland is found in the submandibular fossa.

Radiographic Appearance. On a mandibular periapical radiograph the submandibular fossa appears as a radiolucent area in the molar region below the mylohyoid ridge (Fig. 26–69). Few bony trabeculae are

usually seen in the region of the submandibular fossa. On some periapical radiographs the submandibular fossa may appear as a distinct radiolucency; in others, it may be slightly more radiolucent than the adjacent bone.

CORONOID PROCESS

Description. The **coronoid process** is a marked prominence of bone on the anterior ramus of the mandible (Fig. 26–70). The coronoid process serves as an attachment site for one of the muscles of mastication.

Radiographic Appearance. The coronoid process is not seen on a mandibular periapical radiograph but does appear on a maxillary molar periapical film. The coronoid process appears as a triangular radiopacity superimposed over, or inferior to, the maxillary tuberosity region (Fig. 26–71).

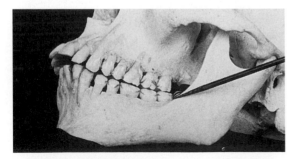

FIGURE 26–66. The external oblique ridge is a linear prominence of bone located on the external surface of the mandible. (From Haring JI, Lind LJ: Radiographic Interpretation for the Dental Hygienist. Philadelphia, WB Saunders, 1993.)

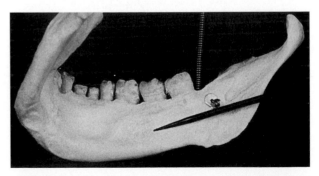

FIGURE 26–68. The submandibular fossa is a depressed area on the posterior internal surface of the mandible. (From Haring JI, Lind LJ: Radiographic Interpretation for the Dental Hygienist. Philadelphia, WB Saunders, 1993.)

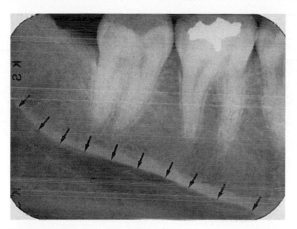

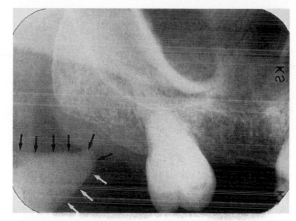

FIGURE 26–69. The submandibular fossa appears as a radiolucent area inferior to the mylohyoid ridge. (From Haring JI, Lind LJ: Radiographic Interpretation for the Dental Hygienist. Philadelphia, WB Saunders, 1993.)

FIGURE 26–71. The coronoid process appears as a triangular shaped radiopacity. (From Haring JI, Lind LJ: Radiographic Interpretation for the Dental Hygienist. Philadelphia, WB Saunders, 1993.)

▬ NORMAL TOOTH ANATOMY

Tooth Structure

Tooth structures that can be viewed on dental radiographs include the following: enamel, dentin, the dentinoenamel junction, and the pulp cavity (Fig. 26–72).

ENAMEL

Enamel is the densest structure found in the human body. Enamel is the outermost radiopaque layer of the crown of a tooth (Fig. 26–73).

DENTIN

Dentin is found beneath the enamel layer of a tooth and surrounds the pulp cavity (see Fig. 26–73). Den-

tin appears radiopaque and comprises most of the tooth structure. Dentin is not as radiopaque as enamel.

DENTINOENAMEL JUNCTION

The **dentinoenamel junction** (DEJ) is the junction between the dentin and the enamel of a tooth. The DEJ appears as a line where the enamel (very radiopaque) meets the dentin (less radiopaque) (see Fig. 26–73).

PULP CAVITY

The **pulp cavity** consists of a pulp chamber and pulp canals. It contains blood vessels, nerves, and lymphatics and appears relatively radiolucent on a dental radiograph (Fig. 26–74). When viewed on a dental

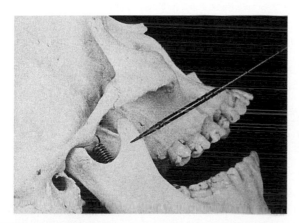

FIGURE 26–70. The coronoid process is a bony prominence on the anterior ramus of the mandible. (From Haring JI, Lind LJ: Radiographic Interpretation for the Dental Hygienist. Philadelphia, WB Saunders, 1993.)

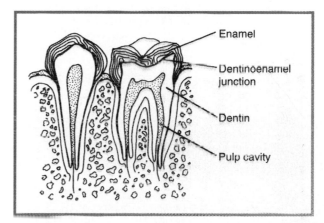

FIGURE 26–72. Tooth structures: enamel, dentin, dentinoenamel junction, and pulp cavity. (From Haring JI, Lind LJ: Radiographic Interpretation for the Dental Hygienist. Philadelphia, WB Saunders, 1993.)

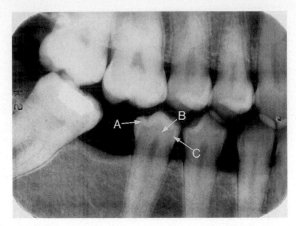

FIGURE 26–73. Tooth structures: (A) enamel, (B) dentin, and (C) dentinoenamel junction. (From Haring JI, Lind LJ: Radiographic Interpretation for the Dental Hygienist. Philadelphia, WB Saunders, 1993.)

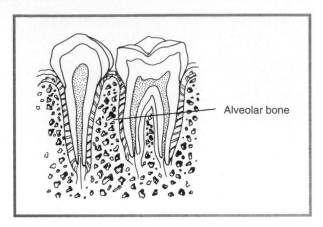

FIGURE 26–75. Alveolar bone. (From Haring JI, Lind LJ: Radiographic Interpretation for the Dental Hygienist. Philadelphia, WB Saunders, 1993.)

radiograph, the pulp cavity is generally larger in children than in adults because it decreases in size with age owing to the formation of secondary dentin. The size and shape of a pulp cavity vary with each tooth.

Supporting Structures

The alveolar process, or alveolar bone, serves as the supporting structure for the teeth of the jaws. The **alveolar bone** is the bone of the maxilla and mandible that supports and encases the roots of teeth (Fig. 26–75). Alveolar bone is composed of dense cortical bone and cancellous bone.

ANATOMY OF ALVEOLAR BONE

The anatomic landmarks of the alveolar process include the lamina dura, the alveolar crest, and the periodontal ligament space (Fig. 26–76).

LAMINA DURA

Description. The **lamina dura** is the wall of the tooth socket that surrounds the root of a tooth. The lamina dura is made up of dense cortical bone.

Radiographic Appearance. On a dental radiograph

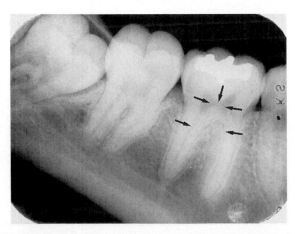

FIGURE 26–74. The pulp cavity. (From Haring JI, Lind LJ: Radiographic Interpretation for the Dental Hygienist. Philadelphia, WB Saunders, 1993.)

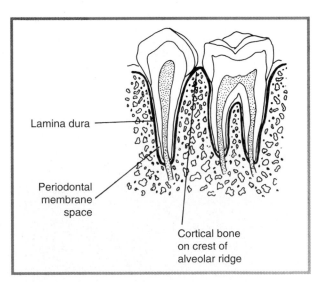

FIGURE 26–76. The alveolar process: lamina dura, alveolar crest, and periodontal ligament space. (From Haring JI, Lind LJ: Radiographic Interpretation for the Dental Hygienist. Philadelphia, WB Saunders, 1993.)

the lamina dura appears as a dense radiopaque line that surrounds the root of a tooth (Fig. 26–77).

ALVEOLAR CREST

Description. The **alveolar crest** is the most coronal portion of the alveolar bone found between the teeth. The alveolar crest is made up of dense cortical bone and is continuous with the lamina dura.

Radiographic Appearance. On a dental radiograph the alveolar crest appears radiopaque and is typically located 1.5 to 2.0 mm below the junction of the crown and the root surfaces (the cementoenamel junction) (Fig. 26–78).

PERIODONTAL LIGAMENT SPACE

Description. The **periodontal ligament space** (PDL) is the space between the root of the tooth and the lamina dura. The PDL space contains connective tissue fibers, blood vessels, and lymphatics.

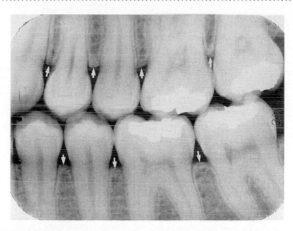

FIGURE 26–78. The alveolar crest typically appears 1.5 to 2.0 mm below the cementoenamel junction. (From Haring JI, Lind LJ: Radiographic Interpretation for the Dental Hygienist. Philadelphia, WB Saunders, 1993.)

Radiographic Appearance. On a dental radiograph the PDL space appears as a thin radiolucent line around the root of a tooth. In the healthy periodontium, the PDL space appears as a continuous radiolucent line of uniform thickness (Fig. 26–79).

SHAPE AND DENSITY OF ALVEOLAR BONE

The alveolar bone located between the roots of the teeth varies in shape and density.

Anterior Regions. Normal alveolar crest located in the anterior region appears pointed and sharp between the teeth (Fig. 26–80). The alveolar crest appears as a dense radiopaque line in the anterior regions.

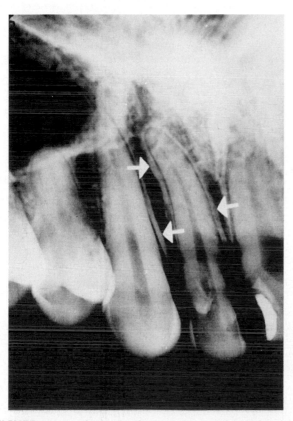

FIGURE 26–77. The lamina dura appears as a dense, thin radiopaque line around the root of a tooth. (From Haring JI, Lind LJ: Radiographic Interpretation for the Dental Hygienist. Philadelphia, WB Saunders, 1993.)

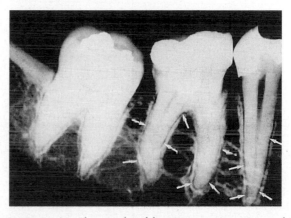

FIGURE 26–79. The periodontal ligament space appears as a thin radiolucent line around the root of the tooth. (From Haring JI, Lind LJ: Radiographic Interpretation for the Dental Hygienist. Philadelphia, WB Saunders, 1993.)

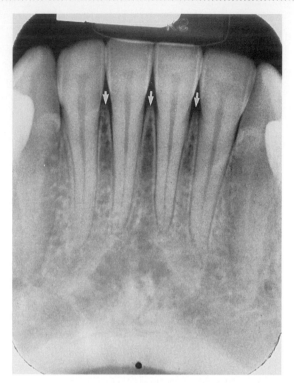

FIGURE 26–80. The anterior alveolar crest normally appears pointed and sharp. (From Haring JI, Lind LJ: Radiographic Interpretation for the Dental Hygienist. Philadelphia, WB Saunders, 1993.)

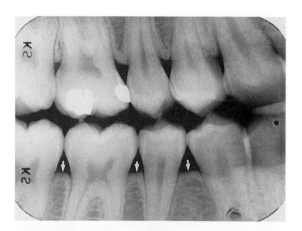

FIGURE 26–81. The posterior alveolar crest normally appears flat and smooth. (From Haring JI, Lind LJ: Radiographic Interpretation for the Dental Hygienist. Philadelphia, WB Saunders, 1993).

Posterior Regions. Normal alveolar crest located in the posterior region appears flat and smooth between the teeth (Fig. 26–81). The alveolar crest located in the posterior region tends to appear less dense and less radiopaque than the alveolar crest seen in the anterior region.

▌ SUMMARY

- The dental radiographer must have a thorough knowledge of the anatomy of the maxilla and mandible; each normal anatomic landmark seen on a periapical radiograph corresponds to that seen on the human skull. Knowledge of the anatomy of the maxilla and mandible as viewed on the human skull enables the dental radiographer to identify the normal anatomy seen on a radiograph.
- Recognition of normal anatomic landmarks enables the dental radiographer to distinguish between maxillary and mandibular radiographs and accurately mount dental films.
- Recognition of normal anatomic landmarks is also necessary for interpretation of dental radiographs. A knowledge of the normal anatomy seen on periapical radiographs is essential before the dental radiographer can begin to recognize abnormalities (e.g., diseases and lesions).
- Each normal anatomic landmark as viewed on a periapical radiograph is described in this chapter.

BIBLIOGRAPHY

Brand RW, Isselhard DE: Osteology of the skull. *In* Anatomy of Orofacial Structures, 4th edition. St. Louis, CV Mosby, 1990, pp. 117–133.

Dental Auxiliary Education Project: Normal Radiographic Landmarks. New York, Teachers College Press, 1982.

Frommer HH: Film mounting and radiographic anatomy. *In* Radiology for Dental Auxiliaries, 6th edition. St. Louis, Mosby-Year Book, 1996, pp. 269–298.

Goaz PW, White SC: Normal radiographic anatomy. *In* Oral Radiology: Principles of Interpretation, 3rd edition. St. Louis, Mosby-Year Book, 1994, pp. 126–149.

Haring JI, Lind LJ: Normal anatomy (periapical films). *In* Radiographic Interpretation for the Dental Hygienist. Philadelphia, WB Saunders, 1993, pp. 25–58.

Miles DA, Van Dis ML, Jensen CW, Ferretti A: Normal anatomy and film mounting. *In* Radiographic Imaging for Dental Auxiliaries, 3rd edition. Philadelphia, WB Saunders, 1999, pp. 211–230.

Quiz Questions

MATCHING

Match the following terms with the proper definitions.

a. hole or opening in bone
b. broad, shallow depression in bone
c. cavity, recess, or hollow space in bone
d. passageway through bone
e. sponge-like bone
f. bony partition that separates two spaces
g. immovable joint between bones
h. hard or compact bone

_b___ **1.** fossa

_d___ **2.** canal

_a___ **3.** foramen

_c___ **4.** sinus

_f___ **5.** septum

_g___ **6.** suture

_h___ **7.** cortical

_e___ **8.** cancellous

IDENTIFICATION

For questions 9 to 16, refer to Figures 26–82 to 26–89. Identify the labeled normal anatomic landmarks as required.

9. Identify the normal anatomic landmark labeled in Figure 26–82.

10. Identify the normal anatomic landmark labeled in Figure 26–83.

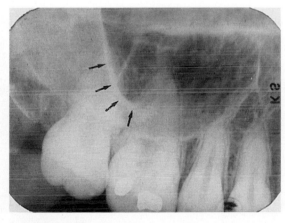

FIGURE 26–82

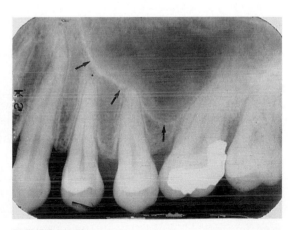

FIGURE 26–83

11. Identify the normal anatomic landmark labeled in Figure 26–84.
12. Identify the normal anatomic landmark labeled in Figure 26–85.
13. Identify the normal anatomic landmark labeled in Figure 26–86.
14. Identify the normal anatomic landmark labeled in Figure 26–87.

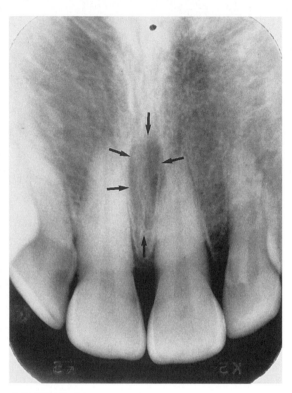

FIGURE 26–84

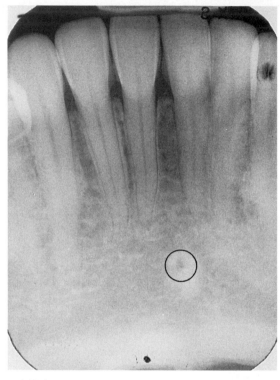

FIGURE 26–86

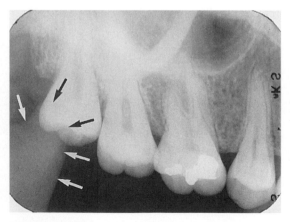

FIGURE 26–85

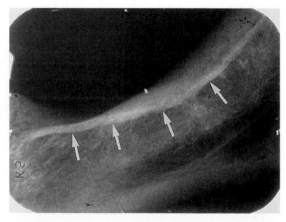

FIGURE 26–87

15. Identify the normal anatomic landmark labeled in Figure 26–88.

16. Identify the normal anatomic landmark labeled in Figure 26–89.

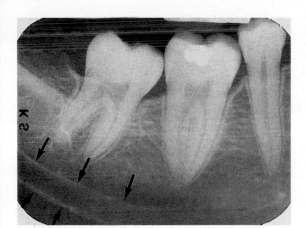

FIGURE 26–88

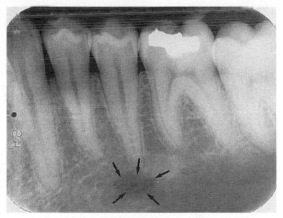

FIGURE 26–89

Answers are supplied at the end of this book.

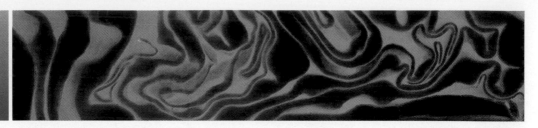

CHAPTER 27

Film Mounting and Film Viewing

OBJECTIVES

After completion of this chapter, the student will be able to:

- *Define the key words.*
- *List the individuals who are qualified to mount and view dental radiographs.*
- *Describe when and where films are mounted.*
- *List five reasons to use a film mount.*
- *Describe what information is placed on a film mount.*
- *Discuss the importance of normal anatomy in film mounting.*
- *Describe how the identification dot is used to determine film orientation.*
- *List and describe two methods of film mounting and identify the preferred method.*
- *List and describe the step-by-step procedures for film mounting.*
- *List and describe the necessary equipment for film viewing.*
- *Discuss the importance of masking extraneous viewbox light seen around a film mount.*
- *Describe optimal viewing conditions, and when and where films should be viewed.*
- *Explain the importance of examining films in an established viewing sequence.*
- *List and describe the step-by-step procedures for film viewing.*
- *Explain why multiple viewings of dental radiographs are necessary, and list the areas, diseases, and abnormalities that must be included in the examinations.*

INTRODUCTION

Film mounting is an essential step in the interpretation of dental radiographs. The dental radiographer must be able to mount dental radiographs in correct anatomic order. To mount dental radiographs properly, the radiographer must have a thorough knowledge of the normal anatomy of the maxilla, mandible, and related structures (see Chapter 26). Film viewing is also essential in the interpretation of dental radiographs; the dental radiographer must understand the importance of examining films under optimal viewing conditions.

The purpose of this chapter is to present the basic concepts of film mounting and film viewing and to describe the step-by-step procedures that must be followed to prepare for the interpretation of radiographs.

FILM MOUNTING

Mounted radiographs, or radiographs placed in a film holder in anatomic order, are invaluable to the dental professional. A series of mounted radiographs can be viewed more efficiently than individual films and are easier to interpret.

Basic Concepts

The term **mount** can be defined as "to place in an appropriate setting, as for display or study." In dental radiography, **film mounting** is the placement of radiographs in a supporting structure or holder.

WHAT IS A FILM MOUNT?

A **film mount** is a cardboard, plastic, or vinyl holder that is used to support and arrange dental radiographs in anatomic order (Fig. 27–1). **Anatomic order** refers to how the teeth are arranged within the dental arches. Each film mount has a number of windows or frames in which the individual radiographs are placed or "mounted." A film mount may be opaque or clear (Fig. 27–2). An opaque film mount is preferred because it masks the light around each radiograph. Subtle changes in density and contrast are easier to detect when extraneous light is eliminated. To minimize extraneous viewbox light, each window of a film mount should contain a radiograph. When all of the windows are not filled with radiographs, black opaque paper can be placed in the unused frames.

Film mounts are commercially available in many sizes and configurations. Film mounts accommodate any number of films; mounts are available for single films, bite-wings, a complete mouth radiographic series of films, and endless other combinations of films (Fig. 27–3). The overall size and shape of the film mounts are designed to fit a variety of viewboxes found in the dental office; the size of the film mount should correspond to the size of the viewbox.

WHO MOUNTS FILMS?

Any trained dental professional (dentist, dental hygienist, dental assistant) with a knowledge of the normal anatomic landmarks of the maxilla, mandible, and re-

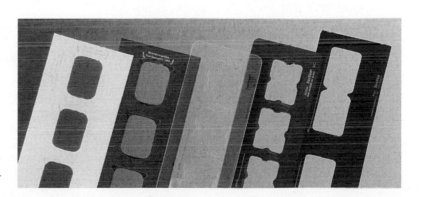

FIGURE 27–1. Examples of various film mounts. (Courtesy of Rinn Corporation, Elgin, IL.)

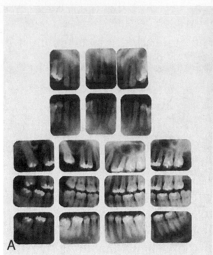
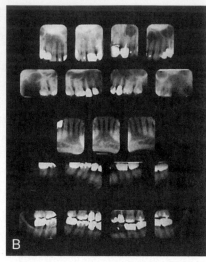

FIGURE 27–2. Full-mouth series mounted in (*A*) clear celluloid, and (*B*) opaque mounts. (From Frommer HH: Radiology for Dental Auxiliaries, 5th ed. St. Louis, Mosby-Year Book, 1992.)

lated structures is qualified to mount dental radiographs. In most dental offices, mounting films is the responsibility of the dental radiographer.

WHEN AND WHERE ARE FILMS MOUNTED?

The dental radiographer should always mount films immediately after processing. Films should be mounted in an area designated for film mounting. This area should consist of a clean, dry, light-colored work surface in front of an illuminator or viewbox.

WHY USE A FILM MOUNT?

The use of a film mount is strongly recommended for the following reasons:

- Mounted radiographs are quicker and easier to view and interpret.
- Mounted radiographs are easily stored in the patient record and are readily accessible for interpretation.
- Film mounts decrease the chances of error in determining the patient's right and left sides because each film is mounted in anatomic order.
- Film mounts decrease the handling of individual films and prevent damage to the emulsion (e.g., fingerprint marks and scratches).
- Film mounts mask illumination immediately adjacent to individual radiographs and aid in interpretation.

WHAT INFORMATION IS PLACED ON A FILM MOUNT?

The dental radiographer should label the film mount *before* the films are mounted. A special marking pencil designed to write on paper, plastic, or vinyl can be used to label film mounts. Radiographs are easily identified when the film mount has been clearly and legibly labeled with the following information:

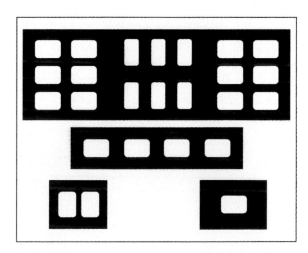

FIGURE 27–3. A variety of film mounts are available in many sizes and film combinations. (From Haring JI, Lind LJ: Radiographic Interpretation for the Dental Hygienist. Philadelphia, WB Saunders, 1993.)

- patient's full name
- date of exposure
- dentist's name
- radiographer's name

The patient's name and date of exposure are essential, the dentist's name is useful if the radiographs are sent to a third party (e.g., insurance company), and the radiographer's name is important if any questions should arise about the exposure of the films.

Normal Anatomy and Film Mounting

As stressed in Chapter 26, a knowledge of normal anatomy is necessary to mount dental radiographs properly. The dental radiographer must be familiar with the characteristic anatomic landmarks seen in each region of the jaws. Identification of landmarks aids in distinguishing maxillary periapical films from mandibular periapical films (Table 27–1).

Film Mounting Methods

There are two methods that can be used to mount films. Both methods rely on identification of the embossed dot found on the film. As described in Chapter 7, a small raised bump known as the **identification dot** is seen in one corner of each intraoral film packet; the dot on the packet indicates the location of the embossed identification dot on the radiograph (Fig. 27–4). The film is positioned in the packet so that the raised side of the dot faces the x-ray beam during exposure.

The identification dot is used to determine film orientation. After the films are processed, they should be placed in the film mount so that all the embossed dots are either raised (labial mounting) or depressed (lingual mounting); all of the embossed dots must face in the same direction. The dental radiographer can then distinguish between the right and left sides of the patient. Either labial or lingual mounting can be used.

LABIAL MOUNTING

Labial mounting is the preferred method of mounting dental radiographs and is recommended by the American Dental Association. In the **labial mounting** method, radiographs are placed in the film mount with the *raised* (convex) side of the identification dot *facing the viewer* (dental radiographer). The radiographs are then viewed from the labial aspect (hence the term labial mounting). With this method, the radiographs are viewed as if the viewer is looking directly at the patient; the patient's left side is on the viewer's right

Area	Maxillary Landmarks	Mandibular Landmarks
Incisor	Incisive foramen	Mental ridge
	Median palatal suture	Mental fossa
	Nasal cavity	Lingual foramen
	Inferior nasal conchae	Genial tubercles
		Nutrient canals
	Anterior nasal spine	
Canine	Lateral fossa	
	Inverted Y	
Premolar	Maxillary sinus	Mental foramen
		Mylohyoid ridge
Molar	Maxillary sinus	External oblique ridge
	Maxillary tuberosity	
	Hamulus	Internal oblique ridge
	Zygomatic process of maxilla	Submandibular fossa
	Zygoma	Mandibular canal
	Coronoid process of mandible	

TABLE 27–1. Landmarks Distinguishing Maxillary Periapical Films from Mandibular Periapical Films

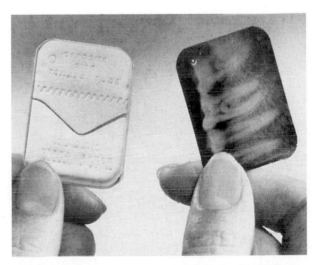

FIGURE 27–4. The dot on the packet indicates the relative location of the embossed identifying dot on the radiograph. (Reprinted courtesy of Eastman Kodak Company.)

and the patient's right side is on the viewer's left (Fig. 27–5). The images of the teeth are mounted in anatomic order and have the same relationship to the viewer as they do when facing the patient.

LINGUAL MOUNTING

Lingual mounting can be used as an alternative method. Although some practitioners still use lingual mounting, this system of film mounting is not recommended. In the **lingual mounting** method, radiographs are placed in the film mount with the *depressed* (concave) side of the identification dot *facing the viewer*. The dental radiographer then views the radiographs from the lingual aspect (hence the term lingual mounting). With this method, the radiographs are viewed as if the dental radiographer is inside the patient's mouth and looking out; the patient's left side is on the viewer's left and the patient's right side is on the viewer's right (Fig. 27–6).

Step-by-Step Procedures

The following step-by-step film mounting procedures are recommended for the dental radiographer who is in training. As the mounting skills of the radiographer improve, simpler and faster techniques may be used instead (see "Procedure: Mounting Dental Radiographs").

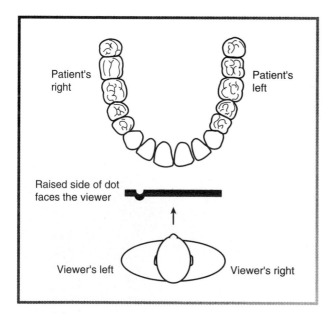

FIGURE 27–5. With the labial mounting method, the radiographs are viewed as if the dental radiographer were looking directly at the patient.

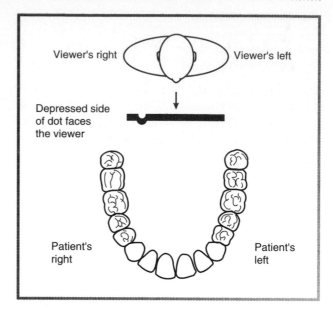

FIGURE 27–6. With the lingual mounting method, the radiographs are viewed as if the dental radiographer were inside the patient's mouth and looking out.

 HELPFUL HINTS • • • • • • • • • • • • • • • • •
For Mounting Radiographs

➤ **DO** master the normal anatomy of the maxilla, mandible, and adjacent structures. A working knowledge of normal anatomy is necessary to mount films.

➤ **DO** label and date the film mount *prior* to mounting the films; always include the patient's full name, date of exposure, dentist's name, and radiographer's name.

➤ **DO** mount films immediately after processing.

➤ **DO** mount radiographs in a designated area; use a light-colored working surface in front of a viewbox.

➤ **DO** use an opaque film mount to block out extraneous light around each film.

➤ **DO** use clean dry hands to mount radiographs, and handle each radiograph by the edges only.

➤ **DO** identify the embossed dot on each film; always mount radiographs with the raised side of the dot facing the same direction. For labial mounting, all of the raised dots must face the viewer.

➤ **DO** sort radiographs before mounting.

➤ **DO** use normal anatomic landmarks to distinguish maxillary films from mandibular films.

➤ **DO** use the order of the teeth to distinguish the right from the left side.

➤ **DO** use a definite order for mounting films. For example, start with maxillary anterior periapicals, proceed to mandibular anterior periapicals and bite-wings, and then finish with maxillary posterior periapicals and mandibular posterior periapicals.

➤ **DO** mount bite-wing radiographs with the curve of Spee (occlusal plane between the maxillary and mandibular teeth) directed upward toward the distal.

PROCEDURE

Mounting Dental Radiographs

1. Prepare for film mounting. Place a clean, light-colored paper towel over the work surface in front of the viewbox.

2. Turn on the viewbox.

3. Label and date the film mount (Fig. 27–7).

4. Wash and dry the hands.

5. Examine each radiograph, identify the embossed dot, and then place each radiograph on the work surface with the raised side of the dot facing up (for labial mounting, as recommended by the American Dental Association). All radiographs must be mounted with the raised side of the dot facing in the same direction. Handle radiographs by the edges only (Fig. 27–8).

6. Sort the radiographs into three groups—bitewings, anterior periapicals, and posterior periapicals. Bite-wing films can be distinguished from periapical films because the crowns of both the upper and lower teeth are seen on the film (Fig. 27–9). Anterior periapical films can be distinguished from posterior periapical films because of the orientation of the film: in anterior periapical films the long axis of the film is oriented vertically, and in posterior periapical films the long axis is oriented horizontally (Fig. 27–10).

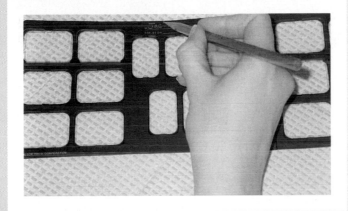

FIGURE 27–7. The dental radiographer must label and date the film mount before mounting the films.

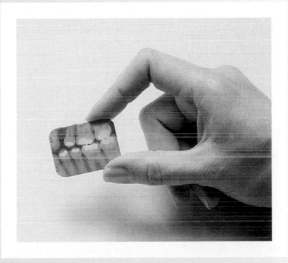

FIGURE 27–8. The dental radiographer should handle radiographs by the edges only.

Procedure continued on following page

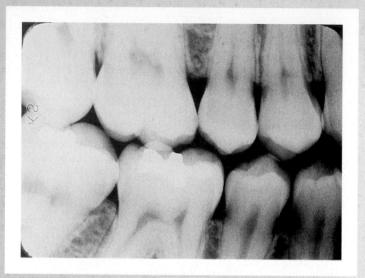

FIGURE 27-9. A bite-wing film shows the crowns of both the upper and lower teeth on one film.

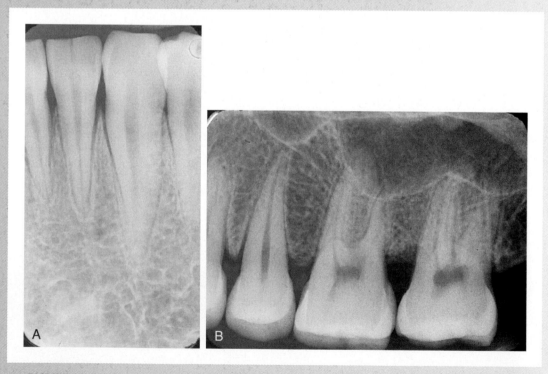

FIGURE 27-10. *A,* An anterior periapical film is oriented vertically. *B,* A posterior periapical film is oriented horizontally.

7. Arrange the radiographs on the work surface in anatomic order. The normal anatomic landmarks can be used to distinguished maxillary films from mandibular films. In addition, all maxillary radiographs must be oriented with the roots of the teeth pointing upward, and all mandibular radiographs must be oriented with the roots pointing downward (Fig. 27–11). The order of the teeth can be used to distinguish the right from the left (Fig. 27–12).

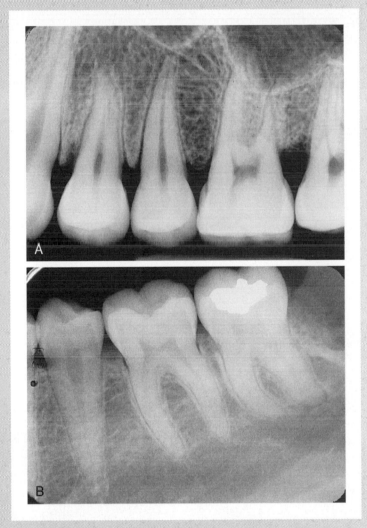

FIGURE 27–11. *A,* A maxillary periapical film is mounted with the roots pointing upward. *B,* A mandibular periapical film is mounted with the roots pointing downward.

Procedure continued on following page

PROCEDURE

Mounting Dental Radiographs CONTINUED

8. Place each film in the corresponding frame of the film mount and secure it (Fig. 27–13). The following order for film mounting is suggested:
1. maxillary anterior periapicals
2. mandibular anterior periapicals
3. bite-wings
4. maxillary posterior periapicals
5. mandibular posterior periapicals

9. Check radiographs by verifying the following:
- all embossed dots are oriented correctly
- all films are properly arranged in anatomic order
- all films are mounted securely
- the film mount is properly labeled and dated

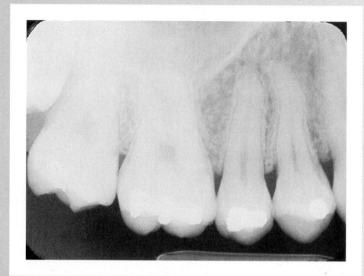

FIGURE 27–12. The order of the teeth can be used to distinguish right from left; the premolars are located in front of the molars; therefore, this is a maxillary right periapical.

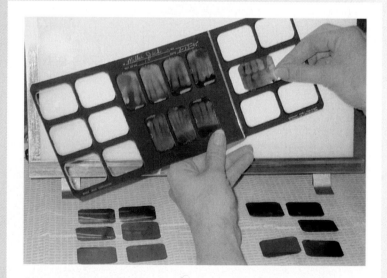

FIGURE 27–13. After the films have been arranged in proper order, the dental radiographer can place each film in the corresponding frame of the film mount.

➤ **DO** recognize the differences between maxillary and mandibular teeth (e.g., maxillary anterior teeth have larger crowns and longer roots than mandibular anterior teeth)

➤ **DO** remember that most mandibular molars have two roots, whereas most maxillary molars have three.

➤ **DO** recognize that most roots curve toward the distal.

➤ **DO** verify the following points after mounting radiographs: all of the embossed dots are oriented correctly, the radiographs are arranged in anatomic order, the radiographs are mounted securely, and the film mount is labeled and dated.

➤ **DO** file mounted radiographs in the patient record as soon as possible to eliminate the possibility of loss or mix-up.

FILM VIEWING

Film viewing is essential in the interpretation of dental radiographs. The dental radiographer must be knowledgeable about optimal film viewing conditions and the recommended evaluation sequence for film viewing.

Basic Concepts

The term **viewing** means "examining or inspecting." In dental radiography, **film viewing** is the examination of dental radiographs.

WHO VIEWS FILMS?

Any trained dental professional (dentist, dental hygienist, dental assistant) with a knowledge of the normal anatomic landmarks of the maxilla, mandible, and related structures is qualified to view dental radiographs. Although all members of the dental team may interpret dental radiographs, it is the responsibility of the dentist to establish a final or definitive interpretation and diagnosis. **Interpretation,** or the explanation of what is viewed on a dental radiograph, is discussed in Chapter 29.

WHAT EQUIPMENT IS REQUIRED FOR FILM VIEWING?

An adequate light source and magnification are required for optimal film viewing; both a viewbox and a magnifying glass are necessary.

Light Source: A light source known as a **viewbox,** or illuminator (see Chapter 10), is required to view dental radiographs accurately and assist in the interpretation of images (Fig. 27–14). The viewing area of the illuminator should be large enough to accommodate a variety of mounted films as well as unmounted extraoral films. The light from the viewbox should be of uniform intensity and evenly diffused. If the screen of the viewbox is not completely covered by the mounted radiographs, the harsh light around the mounted films must be masked to reduce glare and intensify the detail and contrast of the radiographic images (Fig. 27–15).

Magnification: The use of a pocket-sized magnifying glass is useful in interpretation. Magnification aids the viewer in evaluating slight changes in density and contrast in radiographic images (Fig. 27–16).

WHEN AND WHERE ARE FILMS VIEWED? *immediately cud in view box*

Radiographs should be viewed by the dental radiographer immediately after mounting. Immediate film viewing is necessary to verify the correct arrangement of the films in the mount.

Films are best viewed by the dental radiographer on

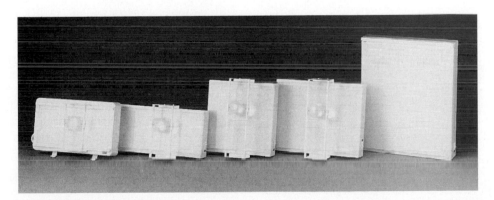

FIGURE 27–14. Examples of various viewboxes. (Courtesy of Rinn Corporation, Elgin, IL.)

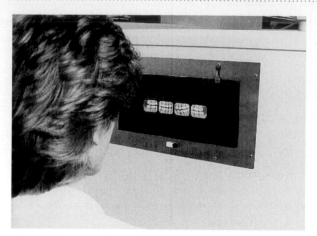

FIGURE 27–15. Extraneous light should be masked to reduce glare and intensify the contrast of the radiographic image. (From Haring JI, Lind LJ: Radiographic Interpretation for the Dental Hygienist. Philadelphia, WB Saunders, 1993.)

FIGURE 27–16. A magnifying glass aids the viewer in evaluation of subtle changes in density and contrast. (From Haring JI, Lind LJ: Radiographic Interpretation for the Dental Hygienist. Philadelphia, WB Saunders, 1993.)

a viewbox in a room with dimmed lighting. When interpreting dental radiographs, an area free of distractions with subdued lighting provides optimal film viewing conditions. Because such viewing conditions are typically present only in a medical facility, most films are examined on the viewbox at chairside in the dental setting.

Step-by-Step Procedures

Mounted radiographs must be viewed in sequential order. The dental radiographer must have an established viewing sequence to prevent errors in interpretation. The step-by-step procedures shown in "Procedure: Viewing Mounted Radiographs" can be used to examine a CMRS of dental radiographs (Fig. 27–17).

The dental radiographer must use this recommended viewing sequence to examine films for each of the following:

- unerupted, missing, and impacted teeth
- dental caries and the size and shape of the pulp cavities
- bony changes, the level of alveolar bone, and calculus
- roots and periapical areas
- all areas not previously examined (e.g., remaining areas of the jaws, sinuses, and so on)

Many examinations of dental radiographs are necessary to check for all the problems listed. For example,

the dental radiographer should first view the films quickly for evidence of unerupted, bony, or impacted teeth. Next, the examination sequence should be repeated for caries, pulp size, and pulp shape. The sequence must be repeated as many times as necessary to evaluate all surfaces of the teeth and supporting structures for evidence of disease and abnormalities.

PROCEDURE

Viewing Mounted Radiographs

1. Start with the right maxillary teeth (the maxillary periapical films on the upper left side of the film mount).

2. Move horizontally across to the left maxillary teeth (the maxillary periapical films on the upper right side of the mount).

3. Move down to the left mandibular teeth (the mandibular periapical films on the lower right side of the mount).

4. Move horizontally across to the right mandibular teeth (the mandibular periapical films on the lower left side of the mount).

5. Move up to bite-wing films. View bite-wings on the left side of the mount and then move to the bite-wings on the right side of the mount.

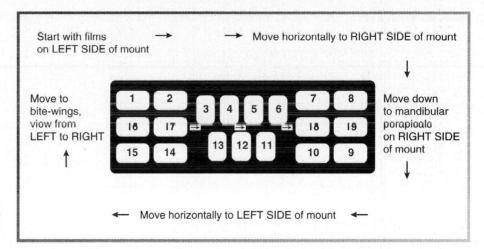

FIGURE 27–17. The dental radiographer must use a definite order for viewing radiographs. The sequence illustrated is recommended.

Following film viewing, the dental professional must note any findings in the patient record. A standard diagram is included in the patient record and can be used to record significant findings (Fig. 27–18). Although all dental professionals may note significant findings, it is important to remember that the final interpretation and diagnosis is the responsibility of the dentist.

HELPFUL HINTS
For Viewing Radiographs

➤ **DO** use a viewbox to examine radiographs; avoid holding mounted films "up to the light" to view.

➤ **DO** block out the harsh light on a viewbox that occurs around the edges of the film mount; harsh light must be masked to reduce glare.

➤ **DO** use a magnifying glass to evaluate slight changes in density and contrast in radiographic images.

➤ **DO** view films immediately after mounting.

➤ **DO** view films under optimal viewing conditions whenever possible; use an area free of distractions with dimmed lighting.

➤ **DO** use a definite order for film viewing. To view a CMRS, start with the films on the upper left side of the mount, move horizontally to the upper right, down to the lower right, across the lower left, up to the bite-wings, and then view the bite-wings from left to right.

➤ **DO** examine radiographs using the recommended viewing sequence as many times as necessary to evaluate them for the following entities: (1) unerupted, impacted, and missing teeth; (2) dental caries, pulp size, and pulp shape; (3) bony changes, level of alveolar bone, and calculus; (4) roots and periapical areas; and (5) all areas not previously examined.

➤ **DO** record all radiographic findings in the patient record.

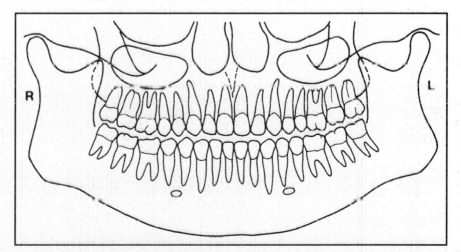

FIGURE 27–18. Standard diagram for recording radiologic findings. This one is used for panoramic and intraoral radiographs, but a similar arrangement can be used for other projections. In the form of rubber stamps, these diagrams can be placed anywhere in the patient's notes. (From Goaz PW, White SC: Oral Radiology: Principles and Interpretation, 3rd ed. St. Louis, Mosby-Year Book, 1994.)

▓ SUMMARY

- Film mounting is the placement of radiographs in a supporting structure or holder.
- A film mount is a plastic or cardboard holder used to arrange radiographs in anatomic order (i.e., the order in which teeth are arranged in the dental arches).
- Any trained dental professional with a knowledge of normal anatomy is qualified to mount dental radiographs. In most offices, the dental radiographer is responsible for the mounting of films.
- Dental radiographs should always be mounted immediately after processing in an area designated for film mounting.
- Mounted radiographs are quicker and easier to view and interpret, and more easily stored in the patient record. Mounted radiographs also decrease the chances of error in determining the patient's right and left sides, and they decrease the handling of films.
- A film mount should be labeled prior to mounting the films. The label includes the following information: patient's full name, date of exposure, dentist's name, and radiographer's name.
- Based on the orientation of the embossed dot, there are two methods of mounting radiographs: labial mounting and lingual mounting. The labial mounting method is recommended by the American Dental Association. Recommended step-by-step procedures for mounting films are described in this chapter.
- After films are mounted, the following must be verified: all embossed dots are oriented correctly, all films are arranged in anatomic order, all films are mounted securely, and the film mount is properly labeled and dated.
- Film viewing is the examination of radiographs. Films are best viewed on a viewbox (light source) in a room with dimmed lighting. Radiographs can be viewed by any trained dental professional and should be viewed immediately after mounting.
- Radiographs should be viewed in a sequential order as many times as necessary, and should be examined for each of the following: (1) unerupted, impacted, and missing teeth; (2) dental caries, pulp size, and pulp shape; (3) bony changes, level of alveolar bone, and calculus; (4) roots and periapical areas; and (5) all areas not previously examined.
- Following film viewing, all significant findings must be noted in the patient record.

BIBLIOGRAPHY

Eastman Kodak Company: Film processing/mounting and viewing. *In* X-Rays in Dentistry. Rochester, Eastman Kodak Company, 1985, p. 107.

Frommer, HH: Film mounting and radiographic anatomy. *In* Radiology for Dental Auxiliaries, 6th edition. St. Louis, Mosby-Year Book, 1996, pp. 269–298.

Goaz PW, White SC: Processing x-ray film. *In* Oral Radiology: Principles of Interpretation, 3rd edition. St. Louis, Mosby-Year Book, 1994, pp. 123–125.

Goaz PW, White SC: Principles of image interpretation. *In* Oral Radiology: Principles of Interpretation, 3rd edition. St. Louis, Mosby-Year Book, 1994, pp. 292–295.

Haring JI, Lind LJ: The importance of dental radiographs and interpretation. *In* Radiographic Interpretation for the Dental Hygienist. Philadelphia, WB Saunders, 1993, pp. 9–10.

Johnson ON, McNally MA, Essay CE: Identification of anatomical landmarks for mounting radiographs. *In* Essentials of Dental Radiography for Dental Assistants and Hygienists, 6th edition. Norwalk, CT, Appleton and Lange, 1999, pp. 227–258.

Langland OE, Sippy FH, Langlais RP: Film processing and duplication. *In* Textbook of Dental Radiography, 2nd edition. Springfield, IL, Charles C Thomas, 1984, pp. 308–314.

Manson-Hing LR: Intraoral radiographic anatomy and film mounting. *In* Fundamentals of Dental Radiography, 3rd edition. Philadelphia, Lea & Febiger, 1990, pp. 102, 106–107.

Matteson SR, Whaley C, Secrist VC: The film and the darkroom. *In* Dental Radiology, 4th edition. Chapel Hill, University of North Carolina Press, 1988, pp. 74–75.

Miles DA, Van Dis ML, Jensen CW, Ferretti A: Film processing and quality assurance. *In* Radiographic Imaging for Dental Auxiliaries, 3rd edition. Philadelphia, WB Saunders, 1999, pp. 49–71.

Miles DA, Van Dis ML, Jensen CW, Ferretti A: Normal anatomy and film mounting. *In* Radiographic Imaging for Dental Auxiliaries, 3rd edition. Philadelphia, WB Saunders, 1999, pp. 211–230.

Miles DA, Van Dis ML, Razmus TF: Radiographic processing and processing quality assurance. *In* Basic Principles of Oral and Maxillofacial Radiology. Philadelphia, WB Saunders, 1992, pp. 165, 167.

Quiz Questions

TRUE OR FALSE

_T_ 1. Anatomic order refers to how the teeth are arranged in the dental arches.

_F_ 2. A clear film mount is preferred (instead of an opaque film mount) to enhance interpretation of radiographs.

_F_ 3. Only the dentist is qualified to mount dental radiographs.

_F_ 4. Films may be mounted at any time after processing.

_T_ 5. Mounted films are quicker and easier to view and interpret.

_T_ 6. Mounted films decrease the chances of error in distinguishing the patient's right and left sides.

_T_ 7. Film mounts decrease the handling of individual films and prevent damage to the emulsion.

_T_ 8. In the labial film mounting method, all of the embossed identification dots are placed in the film mount with the raised (convex) side facing the viewer.

_F_ 9. The lingual mounting method is widely used and is recommended by the American Dental Association.

_F_ 10. Bite-wing radiographs must be mounted with the curve of Spee directed downward toward the distal.

_F_ 11. Film viewing refers to the placing of films in a supporting structure.

_T_ 12. Although all members of the dental team may view films, it is the responsibility of the dentist to establish a final or definitive interpretation and diagnosis.

_F_ 13. Mounted radiographs may be adequately viewed by holding the film mount up to the room light.

_T_ 14. If the viewbox screen is not completely covered by the mounted radiographs, the harsh light around the mounted films must be masked to reduce glare and enhance interpretation.

_T_ 15. When interpreting dental radiographs, an area free of distractions with dimmed room lighting provides optimum viewing conditions.

_F_ 16. Optimal viewing conditions are typically present in the dental setting.

_T_ 17. Mounted radiographs must be viewed in an established sequence to prevent errors in interpretation.

_T_ 18. The dental radiographer must examine mounted radiographs many times to check for the presence of disease and abnormalities.

_T_ 19. Following film viewing, all positive findings must be noted in the patient record.

_F_ 20. A viewbox is not necessary to examine dental radiographs adequately.

SHORT ANSWER

21. List five reasons for using a film mount.

22. List and describe the two methods of film mounting.

_____

23. List and describe the step-by-step procedures for film mounting.

_____

24. List and describe the necessary equipment for film viewing.

_____

25. List and describe the step-by-step procedures for film viewing.

_____

_____

Answers are supplied at the end of this book.

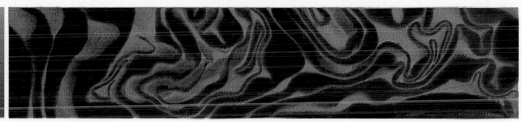

Normal Anatomy—Panoramic Films

OBJECTIVES

After completion of this chapter, the student will be able to:

- *Define the key words.*
- *Identify and describe the bony landmarks of the maxilla and surrounding structures as viewed on the panoramic radiograph.*
- *Identify and describe the bony landmarks of the mandible and surrounding structures as viewed on the panoramic radiograph.*
- *Identify air space images as viewed on the panoramic radiograph.*
- *Identify soft tissue images as viewed on the panoramic radiograph.*

INTRODUCTION

A panoramic radiograph allows the dental professional to view a large area of the mandible and maxilla on a single film. Just as dental professionals must be able to recognize normal anatomic landmarks on periapical films, they must also be able to recognize normal anatomic structures viewed on panoramic radiographs. The recognition of radiographic landmarks enables dental professionals to interpret panoramic films accurately. Without a working knowledge of anatomy, they may mistake normal anatomic structures for pathologic conditions.

To interpret the panoramic radiograph and identify normal anatomic landmarks, dental professionals must have a thorough knowledge of the anatomy of the maxilla and mandible. Each normal anatomic landmark seen on a panoramic radiograph corresponds to what is seen on the human skull. If dental professionals are familiar with the anatomy of the human skull, they can identify the normal anatomy viewed on a panoramic radiograph.

The purpose of this chapter is to review the normal anatomy of the maxilla and mandible as viewed on a panoramic radiograph. In addition to the normal anatomic landmarks, air space images and soft tissue images are also presented in this chapter.

NORMAL ANATOMIC LANDMARKS

Bony Landmarks of the Maxilla and Surrounding Structures

The maxilla forms the floor of the orbit of the eyes, the sides and floor of the nasal cavity, and the hard palate. The lower border of the maxilla supports the maxillary teeth. This portion of the chapter reviews the bony landmarks of the maxilla and surrounding structures that can be viewed on a panoramic radiograph.

Each of the following bony landmarks of the maxilla and surrounding structures can be found labeled on Figure 28–1.

MASTOID PROCESS

Description. The **mastoid process** is a marked prominence of bone located posterior and inferior to the temporomandibular joint (TMJ). The mastoid process is part of the temporal bone.

Radiographic Appearance. On a panoramic radiograph, the mastoid process appears as a rounded *radiopacity* located posterior and inferior to the TMJ area. The mastoid process is *not* seen on periapical radiographs.

STYLOID PROCESS

Description. The **styloid process** is a long, pointed, and sharp projection of bone that extends downward from the inferior surface of the temporal bone. The styloid process is located anterior to the mastoid process.

Radiographic Appearance. On a panoramic radiograph, the styloid process appears as a long *radiopaque* spine that extends from the temporal bone anterior to the mastoid process. The styloid process is *not* seen on periapical radiographs.

EXTERNAL AUDITORY MEATUS

Description. The **external auditory meatus** (also known as the external acoustic meatus) is a hole or

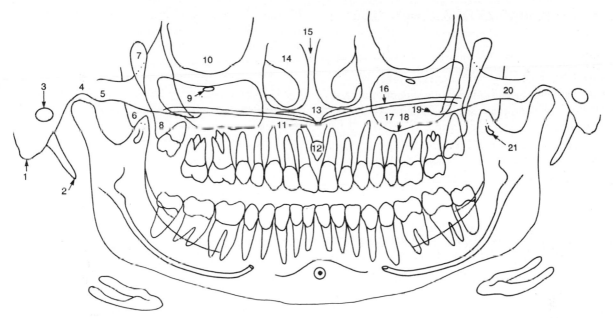

FIGURE 28–1. Normal anatomic landmarks of the maxilla and surrounding structures: *1,* mastoid process; *2,* styloid process; *3,* external auditory meatus; *4,* glenoid fossa; *5,* articular eminence; *6,* lateral pterygoid plate; *7,* pterygomaxillary fissure; *8,* maxillary tuberosity; *9,* infraorbital foramen; *10,* orbit; *11,* incisive canal; *12,* incisive foramen; *13,* anterior nasal spine; *14,* nasal cavity and conchae; *15,* nasal septum; *16,* hard palate; *17,* maxillary sinus; *18,* floor of maxillary sinus; *19,* zygomatic process of maxilla; *20,* zygomatic arch; *21,* hamulus. (Modified from Dental Auxiliary Education Projects: Normal Radiographic Landmarks. New York, Teachers College Press, © 1982 by Teachers College, Columbia University. All rights reserved.)

opening in the temporal bone located superior and anterior to the mastoid process.

Radiographic Appearance. On a panoramic radiograph, the external auditory meatus appears as a round-to-ovoid *radiolucency* anterior and superior to the mastoid process. The external auditory meatus is *not* seen on periapical radiographs.

GLENOID FOSSA

Description. The **glenoid fossa** (also known as the mandibular fossa) is a concave, depressed area of the temporal bone. The mandibular condyle rests in the glenoid fossa. The glenoid fossa is located anterior to the mastoid process and the external auditory meatus.

Radiographic Appearance. On a panoramic radiograph, the glenoid fossa appears as a concave *radiopacity* superior to the mandibular condyle. The glenoid fossa is *not* seen on periapical radiographs.

ARTICULAR EMINENCE

Description. The **articular eminence** (also known as the articular tubercle) is a rounded projection of the temporal bone located anterior to the glenoid fossa.

Radiographic Appearance. On a panoramic radiograph, the articular eminence appears as a rounded *radiopaque* projection of the bone located anterior to the glenoid fossa. The articular eminence is *not* seen on periapical radiographs.

LATERAL PTERYGOID PLATE

Description. The **lateral pterygoid plate** is a wing-shaped bony projection of the sphenoid bone located distal to the maxillary tuberosity region.

Radiographic Appearance. On a panoramic radiograph, the lateral pterygoid plate appears as a *radiopaque* projection of bone distal to the maxillary tuberosity region. The lateral pterygoid plate is *not* seen on periapical radiographs.

PTERYGOMAXILLARY FISSURE

Description. The **pterygomaxillary fissure** is a narrow space or cleft that separates the lateral pterygoid plate and the maxilla.

Radiographic Appearance. On a panoramic radiograph, the pterygomaxillary fissure appears as a *radiolucent* area between the lateral pterygoid plate and the maxilla. The zygoma is often superimposed on this region and obscures the pterygomaxillary fissure. The pterygomaxillary fissure is *not* seen on periapical radiographs.

MAXILLARY TUBEROSITY

Description. The **maxillary tuberosity** is a rounded prominence of bone that extends posterior to the third molar region.

Radiographic Appearance. On a panoramic radiograph, the maxillary tuberosity appears as a *radiopaque* bulge distal to the third molar region.

INFRAORBITAL FORAMEN

Description. The **infraorbital foramen** is a hole or opening in bone found inferior to the border of the orbit.

Radiographic Appearance. On a panoramic radiograph, the infraorbital foramen appears as a round or ovoid *radiolucency* inferior to the orbit. The infraorbital foramen may be superimposed over the maxillary sinus. The infraorbital foramen is *not* seen on periapical radiographs.

ORBIT

Description. The **orbit** is the bony cavity that contains the eyeball.

Radiographic Appearance. On a panoramic radiograph, the orbit appears as a round *radiolucent* compartment with radiopaque borders located superior to the maxillary sinuses. On most panoramic radiographs, only the inferior border of the orbit is visible, where it appears as a radiopaque line.

INCISIVE CANAL

Description. The **incisive canal** (also known as the nasopalatine canal) is a passageway through bone that extends from the superior foramina of the incisive canal (located on the floor of the nasal cavity) to the incisive foramen (located on the anterior hard palate).

Radiographic Appearance. On a panoramic radiograph, the incisive canal appears as a tube-like *radiolucent* area with radiopaque borders. The incisive canal is located between the maxillary central incisors.

INCISIVE FORAMEN

Description. The **incisive foramen** (also known as the nasopalatine foramen) is an opening or hole in bone that is located at the midline of the anterior portion of the hard palate directly posterior to the maxillary central incisors.

Radiographic Appearance. On a panoramic radiograph, the incisive foramen appears as a small ovoid or round *radiolucency* located between the roots of the maxillary central incisors.

ANTERIOR NASAL SPINE

Description. The **anterior nasal spine** is a sharp bony projection of the maxilla located at the anterior and inferior portion of the nasal cavity.

Radiographic Appearance. On a panoramic radiograph, the anterior nasal spine appears as a **V**-shaped *radiopaque* area located at the intersection of the floor of the nasal cavity and the nasal septum.

NASAL CAVITY

Description. The **nasal cavity** (also known as the nasal fossa) is a pear-shaped compartment of bone located superior to the maxilla.

Radiographic Appearance. On a panoramic radiograph, the nasal cavity appears as a large *radiolucent* area above the maxillary incisors.

NASAL SEPTUM

Description. The **nasal septum** is a vertical bony wall or partition that divides the nasal cavity into the right and left nasal fossae.

Radiographic Appearance. On a panoramic radiograph, the nasal septum appears as a vertical *radiopaque* partition that divides the nasal cavity.

HARD PALATE

Description. The **hard palate** is the bony wall that separates the nasal cavity from the oral cavity.

Radiographic Appearance. On a panoramic radiograph, the hard palate appears as a horizontal *radiopaque* band superior to the apices of the maxillary teeth.

MAXILLARY SINUS AND FLOOR OF THE MAXILLARY SINUS

Description. The **maxillary sinuses** are paired cavities or compartments of bone located within the maxilla and are located above the maxillary premolar and molar teeth.

Radiographic Appearance. On a panoramic radiograph, the maxillary sinuses appear as paired *radiolucent* located above the apices of the maxillary premolars and molars. The floor of the maxillary sinus is composed of dense cortical bone and appears as a *radiopaque* line.

ZYGOMATIC PROCESS OF THE MAXILLA

Description. The **zygomatic process of the maxilla** is a bony projection of the maxilla that articulates with the zygoma or malar (cheek) bone.

Radiographic Appearance. On a panoramic radiograph, the zygomatic process of the maxilla appears as a J- or U-shaped *radiopacity* located superior to the maxillary first molar region.

ZYGOMA

Description. The **zygoma** (also known as the malar or zygomatic bone) is the cheek bone and articulates with the zygomatic process of the maxilla.

Radiographic Appearance. On a panoramic radiograph, the zygoma appears as a *radiopaque band* that extends posteriorly from the zygomatic process of the maxilla.

HAMULUS

Description. The **hamulus** (also known as the hamular process) is a small hook-like projection of bone that extends from the medial pterygoid plate of the sphenoid bone. The hamulus is located posterior to the maxillary tuberosity.

Radiographic Appearance. On a panoramic radiograph, the hamulus appears as a *radiopaque* hook-like projection posterior to the maxillary tuberosity area.

Figures 28–2, 28–3, and 28–4 illustrate the normal anatomic landmarks of the maxilla and surrounding structures that can be viewed on a panoramic radiograph.

Bony Landmarks of the Mandible and Surrounding Structures

This portion of Chapter 28 reviews the bony landmarks of the mandible and surrounding structures that can be viewed on a panoramic radiograph. Each of the following bony landmarks of the mandible and surrounding structures can be found labeled on Figure 28–5.

MANDIBULAR CONDYLE

Description. The **mandibular condyle** is a rounded projection of bone extending from the posterior superior border of the ramus of the mandible. The mandibular condyle articulates with the glenoid fossa of the temporal bone.

Radiographic Appearance. On a panoramic radiograph, the mandibular condyle appears as a bony, rounded *radiopaque* projection extending from the posterior border of the ramus of the mandible. The mandibular condyle is *not* seen on periapical radiographs.

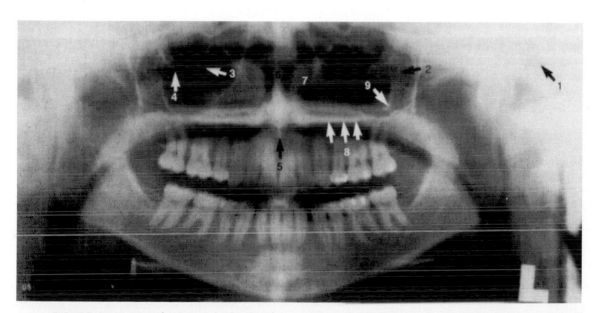

FIGURE 28–2. Normal anatomic landmarks of the maxilla and surrounding structures seen on panoramic films: *1,* external auditory meatus; *2,* pterygomaxillary fissure; *3,* infraorbital foramen; *4,* orbit; *5,* anterior nasal spine; *6,* nasal septum; *7,* nasal conchae; *8,* hard palate; *9,* zygomatic process of the maxilla. (From Haring JI, Lind IJ: Radiographic Interpretation for the Dental Hygienist. Philadelphia, WB Saunders, 1993.)

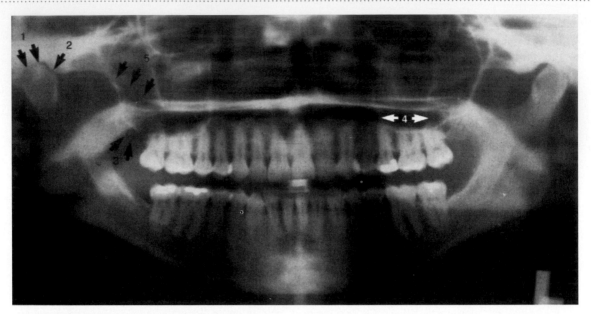

FIGURE 28–3. Normal anatomic landmarks of the maxilla and surrounding structures seen on panoramic films: *1,* glenoid fossa; *2,* articular eminence; *3,* maxillary tuberosity; *4,* maxillary sinus; *5,* zygoma. (From Haring JI, Lind LJ: Radiographic Interpretation for the Dental Hygienist. Philadelphia, WB Saunders, 1993.)

CORONOID NOTCH

Description. The **coronoid notch** is a scooped-out concavity of bone located distal to the coronoid process of the mandible.

Radiographic Appearance. On a panoramic radiograph, the coronoid notch appears as a *radiopaque* concavity located distal to the coronoid process on the superior border of the ramus. The coronoid notch is *not* seen on periapical radiographs.

CORONOID PROCESS

Description. The **coronoid process** is a marked prominence of bone found on the anterior superior ramus of the mandible.

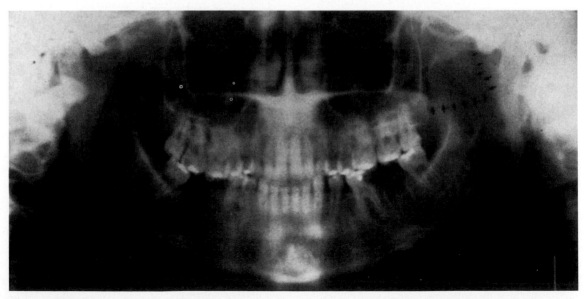

FIGURE 28–4. Lateral pterygoid plate. (From Haring JI, Lind LJ: Radiographic Interpretation for the Dental Hygienist. Philadelphia, WB Saunders, 1993.)

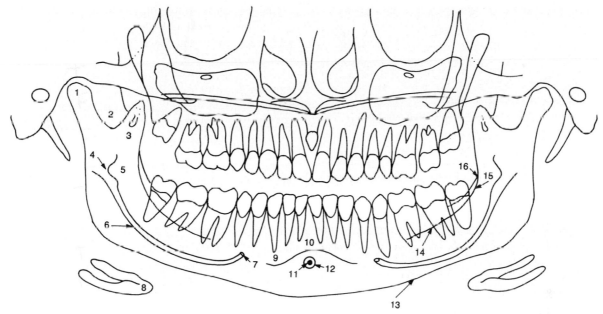

FIGURE 28–5. Normal anatomic landmarks of the mandible and surrounding structures: *1,* condyle; *2,* coronoid notch; *3,* coronoid process; *4,* mandibular foramen; *5,* lingula; *6,* mandibular canal; *7,* mental foramen; *8,* hyoid bone; *9,* mental ridge; *10,* mental fossa; *11,* lingual foramen; *12,* genial tubercles; *13,* inferior border of mandible; *14,* mylohyoid ridge; *15,* internal oblique ridge; *16,* external oblique ridge. (Modified from Dental Auxiliary Education Project: Normal Radiographic Landmarks. New York, Teachers College Press, © 1982 by Teachers College, Columbia University. All rights reserved.)

Radiographic Appearance. On a panoramic radiograph, the coronoid process appears as a triangular *radiopacity* posterior to the maxillary tuberosity region.

MANDIBULAR FORAMEN

Description. The **mandibular foramen** is a round or ovoid hole in bone on the lingual aspect of the ramus of the mandible.

Radiographic Appearance. On a panoramic radiograph, the mandibular foramen appears as a round or ovoid *radiolucency* centered within the ramus of the mandible. The mandibular foramen is *not* seen on periapical radiographs.

LINGULA

Description. The **lingula** is a small tongue-shaped projection of bone seen adjacent to the mandibular foramen.

Radiographic Appearance. On a panoramic radiograph, the lingula appears as an indistinct *radiopacity* anterior to the mandibular foramen. The lingula is *not* seen on periapical radiographs.

MANDIBULAR CANAL

Description. The **mandibular canal** is a tube-like passageway through bone that travels the length of the mandible. The mandibular canal extends from the mandibular foramen to the mental foramen and houses the inferior alveolar nerve and blood vessels.

Radiographic Appearance. On a panoramic radiograph, the mandibular canal appears as a *radiolucent* band outlined by two thin radiopaque lines representing the cortical walls of the canal.

MENTAL FORAMEN

Description. The **mental foramen** is an opening or hole in bone located on the external surface of the mandible in the region of the mandibular premolars.

Radiographic Appearance. On a panoramic radiograph, the mental foramen appears as a small ovoid or round *radiolucency* located in the apical region of the mandibular premolars.

MENTAL RIDGE

Description. The **mental ridge** is a linear prominence of cortical bone located on the external surface of the anterior portion of the mandible that extends from the premolar region to the midline.

Radiographic Appearance. On a panoramic radiograph, the mental ridge appears as a thick *radiopaque* band that extends from the mandibular premolar region to the incisor region.

MENTAL FOSSA

Description. The **mental fossa** is a scooped-out depressed area of bone located on the external surface of the anterior mandible above the mental ridge in the mandibular incisor region.

Radiographic Appearance. On a panoramic radiograph, the mental fossa appears as a *radiolucent* area above the mental ridge.

LINGUAL FORAMEN

Description. The **lingual foramen** is a tiny opening or hole in bone located on the internal surface of the mandible near the midline.

Radiographic Appearance. On a panoramic radiograph, the lingual foramen appears as a small *radiolucent* dot located inferior to the apices of the mandibular incisors.

GENIAL TUBERCLES

Description. The **genial tubercles** are tiny bumps of bone located on the lingual aspect of the mandible.

Radiographic Appearance. On a panoramic radiograph, the genial tubercles appear as a ring-shaped *radiopacity* surrounding the lingual foramen.

INFERIOR BORDER OF THE MANDIBLE

Description. The **inferior border of the mandible** is a linear prominence of cortical bone that defines the lower border of the mandible.

Radiographic Appearance. On a panoramic radiograph, the inferior border of the mandible appears as a dense *radiopaque* band that outlines the lower border of the mandible.

MYLOHYOID RIDGE

Description. The **mylohyoid ridge** is a linear prominence of bone located on the internal surface of the mandible that extends from the molar region downward and forward toward the lower border of the mandibular symphysis.

Radiographic Appearance. On a panoramic radiograph, the mylohyoid ridge appears as a dense *radiopaque* band that extends downward and forward from the molar region.

INTERNAL OBLIQUE RIDGE

Description. The **internal oblique ridge** is a linear prominence of bone located on the internal surface of the mandible that extends downward and forward from the ramus.

Radiographic Appearance. On a panoramic radiograph, the internal oblique ridge appears as a dense *radiopaque* band that extends downward and forward from the ramus.

EXTERNAL OBLIQUE RIDGE

Description. The **external oblique ridge** is a linear prominence of bone located on the external surface of the body of the mandible.

Radiographic Appearance. On a panoramic radiograph, the external oblique ridge appears as a dense *radiopaque* band that extends downward and forward from the anterior border of the ramus of the mandible.

ANGLE OF THE MANDIBLE

Description. The **angle of the mandible** is the area of the mandible where the body meets the ramus.

Radiographic Appearance. On a panoramic radiograph, the angle of the mandible appears as a *radiopaque* bony structure where the ramus joins the body of the mandible.

Figures 28–6, 28–7, and 28–8 illustrate the normal anatomic landmarks of the mandible and surrounding structures that can be viewed on a panoramic radiograph.

◼ AIR SPACE IMAGES SEEN ON PANORAMIC RADIOGRAPHS

This section reviews the air space images that can be viewed on a panoramic radiograph. Each of the following air space images can be found labeled on Figure 28–9.

PALATOGLOSSAL AIR SPACE

Description. The **palatoglossal air space** refers to the space found between the palate (*palato*) and tongue (*glossal*).

Radiographic Appearance. On a panoramic radiograph, the palatoglossal air space appears as a horizontal *radiolucent* band located above the apices of the maxillary teeth.

NASOPHARYNGEAL AIR SPACE

Description. The **nasopharyngeal air space** refers to the portion of the pharynx (*pharyngeal*) located posterior to the nasal cavity (*naso*).

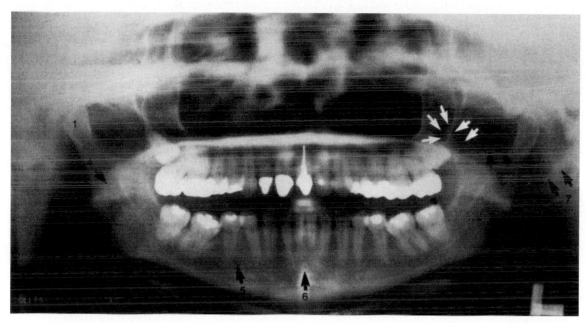

FIGURE 28–6. Normal anatomic landmarks of the mandible and surrounding structures seen on panoramic films: *1,* condyle; *2,* coronoid notch; *3,* coronoid process; *4,* mandibular foramen; *5,* mental foramen; *6,* genial tubercles; *7,* styloid process. (From Haring JI, Lind LJ: Radiographic Interpretation for the Dental Hygienist. Philadelphia, WB Saunders, 1993.)

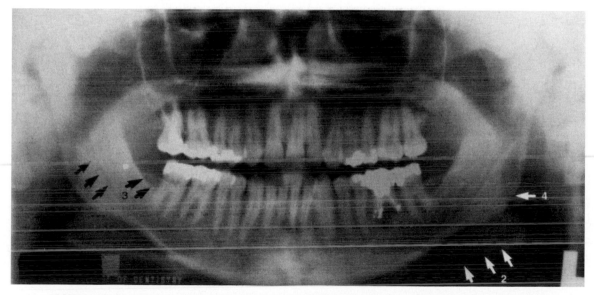

FIGURE 28–7. Normal anatomic landmarks of the mandible and surrounding structures seen on panoramic films: *1,* mandibular canal; *2,* hyoid; *3,* internal oblique ridge; *4,* angle of the mandible. (From Haring JI, Lind LJ: Radiographic Interpretation for the Dental Hygienist. Philadelphia, WB Saunders, 1993.)

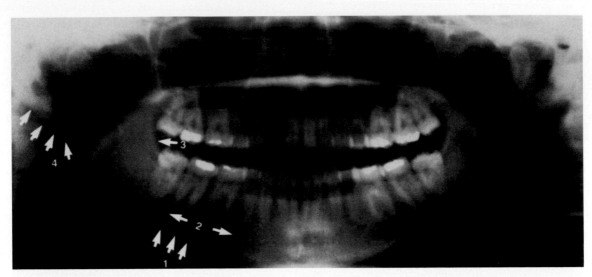

FIGURE 28–8. Normal anatomic landmarks of the mandible and surrounding structures as seen on panoramic films: *1,* inferior border of the mandible; *2,* submandibular fossa; *3,* external oblique ridge; *4,* soft tissue of the ear. (From Haring JI, Lind LJ: Radiographic Interpretation for the Dental Hygienist. Philadelphia, WB Saunders, 1993.)

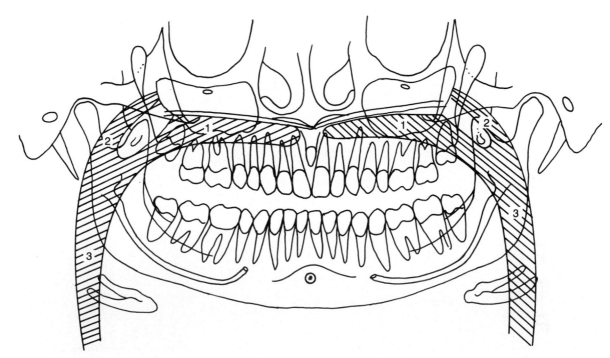

FIGURE 28–9. Air space images seen on panoramic films: *1,* palatoglossal air space; *2,* nasopharyngeal air space; *3,* glossopharyngeal air space. (Modified from Dental Auxiliary Education Project: Normal Radiographic Landmarks. New York, Teachers College Press, © 1982 by Teachers College, Columbia University. All rights reserved.)

Radiographic Appearance. On a panoramic radiograph, the nasopharyngeal air space appears as a diagonal *radiolucency* located superior to the radiopaque shadow of the soft palate and uvula.

GLOSSOPHARYNGEAL AIR SPACE

Description. The **glossopharyngeal air space** refers to the portion of the pharynx (*pharyngeal*) located posterior to the tongue (*glosso*) and oral cavity.

Radiographic Appearance. On a panoramic radiograph, the glossopharyngeal air space appears as a vertical *radiolucent* band superimposed over the ramus of the mandible. The glossopharyngeal air space is continuous with the nasopharyngeal air space superiorly and the palatoglossal air space inferiorly.

Figure 28–10 illustrates the air space images that can be viewed on a panoramic radiograph.

▨ SOFT TISSUE IMAGES SEEN ON PANORAMIC RADIOGRAPHS

This portion reviews the soft tissue images that can be viewed on a panoramic radiograph. Each of the following soft tissue images can be found labeled on Figure 28–11.

TONGUE

Description. The **tongue** is a movable muscular organ found attached to the floor of the mouth.

Radiographic Appearance. On a panoramic radiograph, the tongue appears as a *radiopaque* area superimposed over the maxillary posterior teeth.

SOFT PALATE AND UVULA

Description. The **soft palate and uvula** form a muscular curtain that separates the oral cavity from the nasal cavity.

Radiographic Appearance. On a panoramic radiograph, the soft palate and uvula appear as diagonal *radiopacity* projecting posteriorly and inferiorly from the maxillary tuberosity region.

LIPLINE

Description. The **lipline** is formed by the position of the patient's lips.

Radiographic Appearance. On a panoramic radiograph, the lipline is seen in the region of the anterior teeth. The areas of the teeth not covered by the lips appear more *radiolucent*; the areas covered by the lips appear more *radiopaque*.

EAR

Radiographic Appearance. On a panoramic radiograph, the **ear** appears as a *radiopaque* shadow that projects anteriorly and inferiorly from the mastoid process. The ear is viewed superimposed over the styloid process.

Figure 28–12 shows the soft tissue images that can be viewed on a panoramic radiograph.

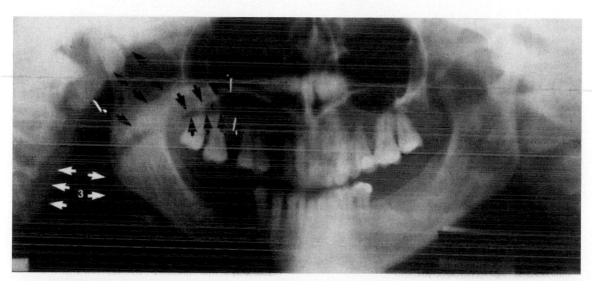

FIGURE 28–10. Air space images seen on panoramic films: *1*, palatoglossal air space; *2*, nasopharyngeal air space; *3*, glossopharyngeal air space. (From Haring JI, Lind LJ: Radiographic Interpretation for the Dental Hygienist. Philadelphia, WB Saunders, 1993.)

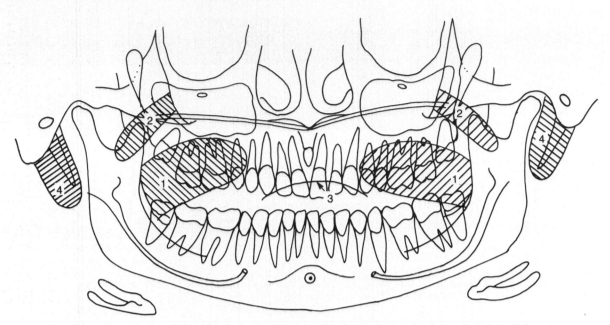

FIGURE 28–11. Soft tissue images seen on panoramic films: *1*, tongue; *2*, soft palate and uvula; *3*, lipline; *4*, ear. (Modified from Dental Auxiliary Education Project: Normal Radiographic Landmarks. New York, Teachers College Press, © 1982 by Teachers College, Columbia University. All rights reserved.)

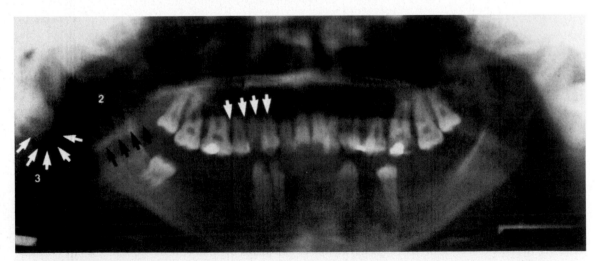

FIGURE 28–12. Soft tissue images seen on panoramic films: *1*, tongue; *2*, soft palate and uvula; *3*, ear. (From Haring JI, Lind LJ: Radiographic Interpretation for the Dental Hygienist. Philadelphia, WB Saunders, 1993.)

SUMMARY

- The panoramic radiograph allows the dental professional to view a large area of the maxilla and mandible on a single film.
- A knowledge of normal anatomic landmarks is necessary to interpret panoramic radiographs; each normal anatomic landmark seen on a panoramic film corresponds to that seen on a human skull. Knowledge of the anatomy of the maxilla, mandible, and adjacent bones as viewed on the human skull enables the dental radiographer to identify normal anatomy seen on a panoramic film.
- A knowledge of air space and soft tissue images is necessary to interpret panoramic radiographs.
- Each normal anatomic landmark, air space, and soft tissue image as viewed on a panoramic radiograph is described in this chapter.

BIBLIOGRAPHY

Brand RW, Isselhard DE: Osteology of the skull. *In* Anatomy of Orofacial Structures, 4th edition, St. Louis, CV Mosby, 1990, pp. 117–133.

Dental Auxiliary Education Project: Normal Radiographic Landmarks. New York, Teachers College Press, 1982.

Goaz PW, White SC: Panoramic radiography. *In* Oral Radiology: Principles of Interpretation, 3rd edition. St. Louis, Mosby-Year Book, 1994, pp. 747–765.

Haring JI, Lind LJ: Normal anatomy (panoramic films). *In* Radiographic Interpretation for the Dental Hygienist. Philadelphia, WB Saunders, 1993, pp. 59–81.

Langland OE, Langlis RP, McDavid WD, et al.: Panoramic Radiology, 2nd edition, Philadelphia, Lea & Febiger, 1989, pp. 224–271.

Quiz Questions ···

IDENTIFICATION

1. Identify the normal anatomic landmarks in Figure 28–13 labeled 1 to 15.

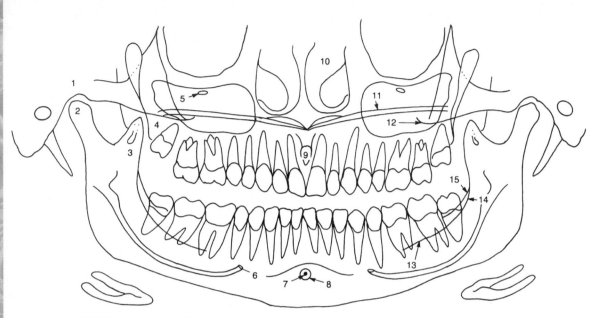

FIGURE 28–13. (From Haring JI, Lind LJ: Radiographic Interpretation for the Dental Hygienist. Philadelphia, WB Saunders, 1993.)

2. Identify the normal anatomic landmarks in Figure 28–14 labeled 1 to 16.

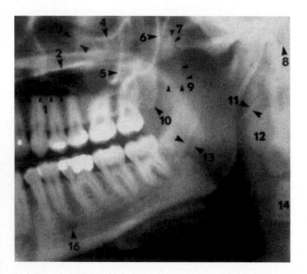

FIGURE 28–14. (From Haring JI, Lind LJ: Radiographic Interpretation for the Dental Hygienist. Philadelphia, WB Saunders, 1993.)

Radiographic Interpretation Basics

CHAPTER 29

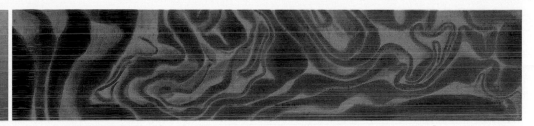

Introduction to Radiographic Interpretation

OBJECTIVES

After completion of this chapter, the student will be able to:

- *Define the key words.*
- *Summarize the importance of radiographic interpretation.*
- *Define the roles of the dentist and dental auxiliary in the interpretation of dental radiographs.*
- *Discuss the difference between interpretation and diagnosis.*
- *Describe who is able to interpret dental radiographs.*
- *Describe when and where dental radiographs are interpreted.*
- *Describe how radiographic interpretation can be used to educate the dental patient about the importance and use of dental radiographs.*

INTRODUCTION

Radiographic interpretation is an essential part of the diagnostic process. The ability to evaluate and recognize what is revealed by a radiograph enables the dental professional to play a vital role in the detection of diseases, lesions, and conditions of the jaws that cannot be identified clinically. In this section of the text, an overview of interpretation topics is presented. Detailed information on interpretation is beyond the scope of this text. For more complete information, the dental radiographer should refer to a text on radiographic interpretation. The purpose of this chapter is to present the basic concepts of radiographic interpretation and to review interpretation guidelines.

BASIC CONCEPTS

An explanation of what is viewed on a dental radiograph, or **radiographic interpretation,** is an important component of patient care. Before the dental radiographer can inspect dental radiographs adequately, a thorough understanding of the terminology and importance of radiographic interpretation is necessary.

Interpretation Terminology

Before the principles of radiographic interpretation are detailed, an explanation of basic terms is required.

Interpret: To offer an explanation.
Interpretation: An explanation.
Radiographic interpretation: An explanation of what is viewed on a dental radiograph; the ability to read what is revealed by a dental radiograph.
Diagnosis: The identification of a disease by examination or analysis. In the dental setting, the dentist is responsible for establishing a diagnosis. Other members of the dental team are restricted by law from rendering a diagnosis.

The Importance of Interpretation

In addition to understanding the importance of dental radiographs, the dental radiographer must also understand the importance of interpretation. As described in Chapter 11, dental radiographs are essential for diagnostic purposes. *All* dental radiographs must be carefully reviewed and interpreted. A great deal of information about the teeth and supporting bone is obtained from radiographic interpretation. Consequently, radiographic interpretation is of paramount importance to the dental professional. Radiographic interpretation enables the dental professional to play a vital role in the detection of diseases, lesions, and conditions of the teeth and jaws that cannot be identified clinically.

GUIDELINES

The dental radiographer must be familiar with who interprets radiographs, the difference between interpretation and diagnosis, when and where radiographs are interpreted, and how to use interpretation to educate the dental patient.

Who Interprets Radiographs?

Training is necessary to interpret dental radiographs. Any dental professional with training in interpretation can examine films. Both the dentist and the dental hygienist are trained to interpret radiographs; dental and dental hygiene curricula include instruction in radiographic interpretation. The dental assistant, however, may or may not be trained in the interpretation of radiographs. The amount and scope of training in dental radiography dictate whether radiographic interpretation can be performed by the dental assistant.

The dental radiographer plays an important role in the preliminary interpretation of dental radiographs. As an additional pair of eyes examining the films, the dental radiographer can direct the attention of the dentist to any areas of question or concern. To interpret films, the dental radiographer must be confident in the identification and recognition of the following:

- normal anatomy (see Chapters 26 and 28).
- dental caries (see Chapter 30).
- periodontal disease (see Chapter 31).
- traumatic injuries and periapical lesions (see Chapter 32).

Interpretation Versus Diagnosis

In the dental setting, the terms interpretation and diagnosis are often confused; it is important to note that these terms have very different meanings and should not be used synonymously. The term **interpretation** refers to an explanation of what is viewed on a radiograph, whereas the term **diagnosis** refers to the identification of disease by examination or analysis. In dentistry, a diagnosis is made by the dentist after a thorough review of the medical history, dental history, clinical examination, radiographic examination, and clinical or laboratory tests.

Although any dental professional with training in interpretation may examine radiographs, the final interpretation and diagnosis are the responsibilities of the dentist. Dental hygienists and dental assistants are restricted by law from rendering a diagnosis.

When and Where Are Radiographs Interpreted?

It is essential to remember that radiographs are taken to benefit the patient. To truly benefit the patient, radiographs must be taken at the beginning of the dental appointment, mounted, interpreted, and then used for diagnostic, therapeutic, and educational purposes. Ideally, dental radiographs should be reviewed and interpreted immediately after mounting in the presence of the patient. If any suspicious or questionable areas are seen on the films, the patient can be examined by the dentist or dental hygienist to obtain additional information or to confirm the problem that is suspected radiographically. If the patient is not present during the interpretation of radiographs, much needed clinical information is lacking.

Dental radiographs are best interpreted by the dental professional on a viewbox in a room with dimmed lighting, as described in Chapter 27. In the dental setting, most films are examined on the viewbox at chairside.

Interpretation and Patient Education

Interpretation of patient radiographs can be used as an educational tool in the dental setting. In addition to providing a preliminary interpretation, the dental radiographer can educate the patient by identifying and discussing what is normally found on a dental radiograph. Then the dentist can focus on specific problems or areas of concern. In this manner, all members of the dental team can work together using radiographic interpretation to educate patients about the importance and use of dental radiographs.

▬▬ SUMMARY

- Radiographic interpretation is the explanation of what is viewed on a dental radiograph.
- Radiographic interpretation is an important component of patient care and enables the dental professional to detect diseases, lesions, and conditions that cannot be identified clinically.
- Any dental professional with training in interpretation can examine films. To interpret dental radiographs, the dental radiographer must be confident in the identification and recognition of normal anatomy, dental caries, periodontal disease, traumatic injuries, and periapical lesions.
- Although any dental professional with training in interpretation may examine radiographs, final interpretation and diagnosis are the responsibilities of the dentist.
- Dental auxiliaries are restricted by law from rendering a diagnosis but can facilitate patient care by performing a preliminary radiographic interpretation.
- The dental radiographic examination should take place at the beginning of the appointment, and the radiographs should be interpreted in the presence of the patient.
- The dental professional can use radiographic interpretation to educate patients about the importance and use of dental radiographs.

BIBLIOGRAPHY

Goaz PW, White SC: Principles of image interpretation. *In* Oral Radiology: Principles of Interpretation, 3rd edition. St. Louis, Mosby-Year Book, 1994, pp. 291–294.

Haring JI, Lind LJ: The importance of dental radiographs and interpretation. *In* Radiographic Interpretation for the Dental Hygienist. Philadelphia, WB Saunders, 1993, pp. 1–12.

Johnson ON, McNally MA, Essay CE: Preliminary interpretation of the radiographs. *In* Essentials of Dental Radiography for Dental Assistants and Hygienists, 6th edition. Norwalk, CT, Appleton and Lange, 1999, pp. 259–296.

Manson-Hing LR: Interpretation and value of radiographs. *In* Fundamentals of Dental Radiography, 3rd edition. Philadelphia, Lea & Febiger, 1990, p. 201.

Miles DA, Van Dis ML, Jensen CW, Ferretti A: Interpretation: Normal versus abnormal and common radiographic presentation of lesions. *In* Radiographic Imaging for Dental Auxiliaries, 3rd edition. Philadelphia, WB Saunders, 1999, pp. 231–280.

Quiz Questions ··

SHORT ANSWER

1. Summarize the importance of radiographic interpretation.

_____

2. Define the roles of each member of the dental team in the interpretation of dental radiographs.

_____

3. Discuss the difference between interpretation and diagnosis.

_____

4. List the members of the dental team who may interpret dental radiographs.

_____

5. Describe when and where dental radiographs are interpreted.

_____

6. Describe how radiographic interpretation can be used to educate the patient about the importance and use of dental radiographs.

_____

TRUE OR FALSE

_____ 7. All radiographs must be carefully reviewed and interpreted.

_____ 8. Any dental professional with training in interpretation can examine films.

_____ 9. The amount and scope of training received dictate whether radiographic interpretation can be performed by the dental assistant.

_____ 10. The terms **interpretation** and **diagnosis** can be used synonymously.

_____ 11. Any dental professional can render a diagnosis.

_____ 12. Dental radiographs should not be interpreted in the presence of the patient.

_____ 13. There are no specific guidelines about when and where dental radiographs should be interpreted.

_____ 14. The dental radiographer can educate the patient by identifying and discussing what is normally found on a radiograph.

_____ 15. All members of the dental team can work together using radiographic interpretation to educate patients about the importance and use of dental radiographs.

_____

Answers are supplied at the end of the book.

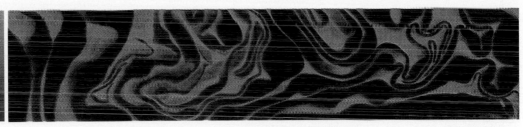

Interpretation of Dental Caries

OBJECTIVES

After completion of this chapter, the student will be able to:

- *Define the key words.*
- *Describe dental caries.*
- *Explain why caries appears radiolucent on a dental radiograph.*
- *Discuss interpretation tips for evaluating caries on a dental radiograph.*
- *Discuss the factors that may influence the radiographic interpretation of dental caries.*
- *Detail the radiographic classification of caries.*
- *Identify and describe the radiographic appearance of the following: incipient, moderate, advanced, and severe interproximal caries.*
- *Identify and describe the radiographic appearance of the following: incipient, moderate, and severe occlusal caries.*
- *Identify and describe the radiographic appearance of the following: buccal, lingual, root surface, recurrent, and rampant caries.*

INTRODUCTION

In the practice of dentistry, caries is probably the most frequent reason for taking dental radiographs. The dental radiographer must be confident about the identification and recognition of caries as viewed on a dental radiograph. An overview of the radiographic interpretation of caries is presented in this chapter. Detailed information about dental caries, however, is beyond the scope of this text. For more complete information on this topic, the dental radiographer should refer to a text on radiographic interpretation.

The purpose of this chapter is to describe dental caries and to describe caries detection. In addition, interpretation tips and factors that influence caries interpretation are presented, and an introduction to the radiographic classification of caries is included.

DESCRIPTION OF CARIES

Dental **caries**, or tooth decay, is the localized destruction of teeth by microorganisms. Normal mineralized tooth structure (enamel, dentin, cementum) is altered and destroyed by dental caries. The term caries comes from the Latin *cariosus,* which means rottenness. Caries literally refers to rotting of the teeth. A carious lesion, or an area of tooth decay, is often referred to as a **cavity.** In dentistry, the term cavity refers to a **cavita-**

tion, or hole, in a tooth that is the result of the caries process (Fig. 30–1).

DETECTION OF CARIES

To detect dental caries, both a careful clinical examination and a radiographic examination are necessary. A dental examination for caries cannot be considered complete without radiographs. Dental radiographs enable the dental professional to identify carious lesions that are not visible clinically. In addition, dental radiographs allow the dental professional to evaluate the extent and severity of carious lesions.

Clinical Examination

Some carious lesions can be detected by simply looking in the mouth, while others cannot. All teeth must be examined clinically for dental caries with a mirror and explorer. The mirror can be used to reflect light, to allow indirect vision, and to retract the tongue. The explorer can be used as a tactile device to detect the presence of any changes in consistency (e.g., catches or tug-back) in the pits, grooves, and fissures of the teeth.

A number of color changes may be seen with dental caries. Occlusal surfaces may show dark staining in the

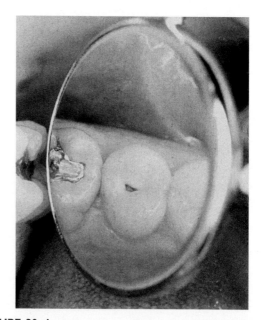

FIGURE 30–1. A cavitation is a hole in a tooth that results from the caries process.

fissures, pits, and grooves, or may show an obvious cavitation. Smooth surfaces may exhibit a chalky white spot or opacity, indicating demineralization. An interproximal ridge overlying a carious lesion may also appear discolored.

Some teeth with dental caries exhibit a discolored area or a cavitation (Fig. 30–2), whereas others have no visible changes. In addition, caries that occur between the teeth may be difficult or impossible to detect clinically. In such cases, radiographs play an important role. It is important to remember that a clinical examination alone is not adequate to detect dental caries; the clinical examination *must* be used in conjunction with a radiographic examination.

Radiographic Examination

Radiographs are useful in the detection of dental caries because of the nature of this disease process. Demineralization and destruction of the hard tooth structures result in a loss of tooth density in the area of the lesion. Decreased density allows greater penetration of x-rays in the carious area, so that the carious lesion appears **radiolucent** (dark or black) on a dental radiograph. Dental caries is the most frequently encountered radiolucent lesion on dental radiographs.

The bite-wing radiograph is the radiograph of choice for the evaluation of caries because it provides the dental professional with diagnostic information that cannot be obtained from any other source. A periapical radiograph using the paralleling technique can also be used for evaluation of dental caries.

■ INTERPRETATION OF CARIES

To recognize caries on a radiograph, the dental professional must be confident in the use of interpretation methods and must be able to identify factors that influence the radiographic interpretation of caries.

Interpretation Tips

As reviewed in Chapter 27, proper film mounting and viewing techniques are essential in the interpretation of dental radiographs, especially the evaluation of dental caries. All films must be properly mounted prior to interpretation. Mounted films should be viewed in a room with subdued lighting that is free of distractions. An illuminator or viewbox is required for accurate viewing of radiographs and assistance in the interpretation of images. If the screen of the viewbox is not completely covered by the mounted radiographs, the harsh light around the mounted films must be masked to reduce glare and intensify the detail and contrast of the radiographic images. The use of a pocket-sized magnifying glass is helpful in evaluating the radiographic appearance of dental caries and can be used to detect slight changes in density and contrast in radiographic images. Dental radiographs should be viewed in the presence of the patient (see Chapter 27).

Factors Influencing Caries Interpretation

A number of factors can influence the radiographic interpretation of dental caries. Radiographs must be of diagnostic quality to allow evaluation of dental caries. As described in Chapter 20, errors in technique may result in nondiagnostic films. For example, a bite-wing film used to detect dental caries must be free of overlapped contacts. Improper horizontal angulation causes overlapped contact areas and makes it impossible to interpret the interproximal regions for dental caries.

As discussed in Chapter 20, errors in exposure may also result in nondiagnostic films. For example, a dental radiograph used to detect dental caries must have proper contrast and density. Incorrect exposure factors result in films that are too dark or too light and thus are useless in the detection of caries.

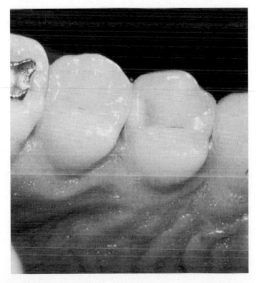

FIGURE 30–2. The discoloration on the distal of the maxillary first premolar represents dental caries.

RADIOGRAPHIC CLASSIFICATION OF CARIES

The radiographic appearance of dental caries can be classified according to the location of the caries on the tooth. Caries that involves the interproximal, occlusal, buccal, lingual, and root surfaces may be seen on a dental radiograph. In addition, recurrent and rampant caries may also be viewed on dental radiographs.

Interproximal Caries

The term **interproximal** means between two adjacent surfaces. Caries found between two teeth is termed **interproximal caries** (Fig. 30–3). On a dental radiograph, interproximal caries is typically seen at or just below (apical to) the contact point (Fig. 30–4). This area is difficult if not impossible to examine clinically with an explorer.

As caries progresses inward through the enamel of the tooth, it assumes a triangular configuration; the apex (or point) of the triangle is seen at the dentino-enamel junction (DEJ) (Fig. 30–5). As caries reaches the DEJ, it spreads laterally and continues into dentin. Another triangular configuration is seen in dentin; this time the base of the triangle is along the DEJ, and the apex is pointed toward the pulp chamber (Fig. 30–6).

Interproximal caries can be classified according to the depth of penetration of the lesion through the enamel and dentin. Interproximal carious lesions can be classified as incipient, moderate, advanced, and severe.

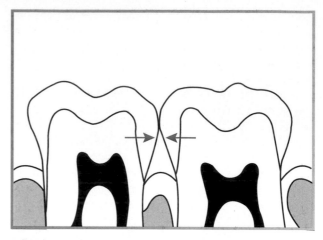

FIGURE 30–4. Caries is found at or just below the contact area. (From Haring JI, Lind LJ: Radiographic Interpretation for the Dental Hygienist. Philadelphia, WB Saunders, 1993.)

INCIPIENT INTERPROXIMAL CARIES

Incipient interproximal caries extends less than halfway through the thickness of enamel (Figs. 30–7 and 30–8). The term **incipient** means beginning to exist or appear. An incipient, or Class I, lesion is seen in enamel *only*.

MODERATE INTERPROXIMAL CARIES

Moderate interproximal caries extends more than halfway through the thickness of enamel but does not involve the DEJ (Figs. 30–9 and 30–10). A moderate, or Class II, lesion is seen in enamel *only*.

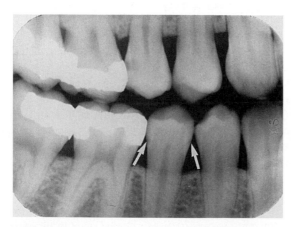

FIGURE 30–3. Interproximal caries is found at or just below the contact area. (From Haring JI, Lind LJ: Radiographic Interpretation for the Dental Hygienist. Philadelphia, WB Saunders, 1993.)

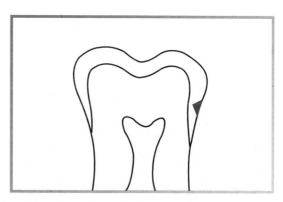

FIGURE 30–5. When confined to enamel, caries may exhibit a triangular configuration. (From Haring JI, Lind LJ: Radiographic Interpretation for the Dental Hygienist. Philadelphia, WB Saunders, 1993.)

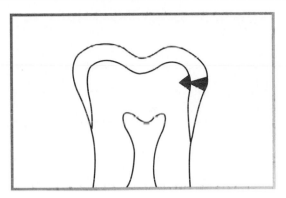

FIGURE 30–6. When caries reaches the dentinoenamel junction (DEJ), it spreads along the DEJ, and another triangular configuration results. (From Haring JI, Lind LJ: Radiographic Interpretation for the Dental Hygienist. Philadelphia, WB Saunders, 1993).

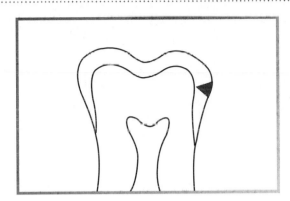

FIGURE 30–9. A moderate carious lesion extends more than halfway through the enamel but does not involve the DEJ. (From Haring JI, Lind LJ: Radiographic Interpretation for the Dental Hygienist. Philadelphia, WB Saunders, 1993.)

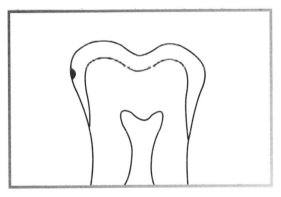

FIGURE 30–7. An incipient carious lesion extends less than halfway through the enamel. (From Haring JI, Lind LJ: Radiographic Interpretation for the Dental Hygienist. Philadelphia, WB Saunders, 1993.)

ADVANCED INTERPROXIMAL CARIES

Advanced interproximal caries extends to or through the DEJ and into dentin but does not extend through the dentin more than half the distance toward the pulp (Figs. 30–11 and 30–12). An advanced, or Class III, lesion affects *both* enamel and dentin.

SEVERE INTERPROXIMAL CARIES

Severe interproximal caries extends through enamel, through the dentin, and more than half the distance toward the pulp (Figs. 30–13 and 30–14). A severe, or Class IV, lesion involves *both* enamel and dentin and may appear clinically as a cavitation in the tooth.

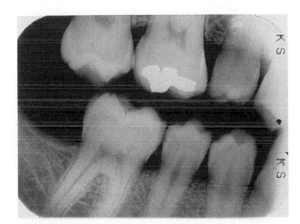

FIGURE 30–8. An incipient carious lesion on the distal of the mandibular second premolar. (From Haring JI, Lind LJ: Radiographic Interpretation for the Dental Hygienist. Philadelphia, WB Saunders, 1993.)

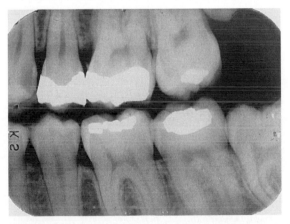

FIGURE 30–10. A moderate carious lesion on the distal of the mandibular second premolar. (From Haring JI, Lind LJ: Radiographic Interpretation for the Dental Hygienist. Philadelphia, WB Saunders, 1993.)

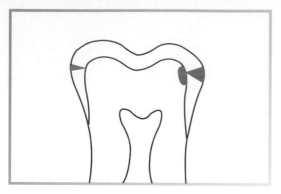

FIGURE 30–11. An advanced carious lesion extends through enamel and to or through the DEJ but does not extend through dentin more than half the distance to the pulp chamber. (From Haring JI, Lind LJ: Radiographic Interpretation for the Dental Hygienist. Philadelphia, WB Saunders, 1993.)

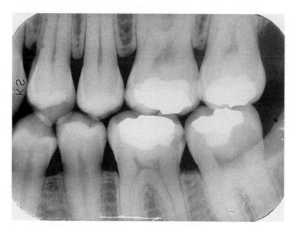

FIGURE 30–12. An advanced carious lesion that extends through the DEJ and into dentin is seen on the distal of the mandibular first molar. (From Haring JI, Lind LJ: Radiographic Interpretation for the Dental Hygienist. Philadelphia, WB Saunders, 1993.)

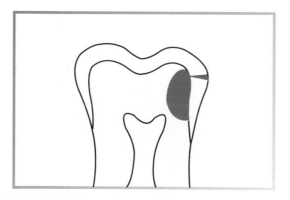

FIGURE 30–13. A severe carious lesion extends through enamel and dentin more than half the distance to the pulp chamber. (From Haring JI, Lind LJ: Radiographic Interpretation for the Dental Hygienist. Philadelphia, WB Saunders, 1993.)

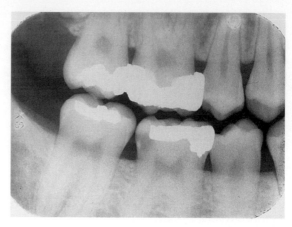

FIGURE 30–14. A severe carious lesion on the distal of the mandibular first molar. (From Haring JI, Lind LJ: Radiographic Interpretation for the Dental Hygienist. Philadelphia, WB Saunders, 1993.)

Occlusal Caries

The term **occlusal** refers to the chewing surfaces of teeth. Caries that involves the chewing surface of the posterior teeth is termed **occlusal caries**. A thorough clinical examination is the method of choice for the detection of occlusal caries. Because of the superimposition of the dense buccal and lingual enamel cusps, early occlusal caries is difficult to see on a dental radiograph; consequently, occlusal caries is not seen on a radiograph until there is involvement of the DEJ. Occlusal carious lesions can be classified as incipient, moderate, and severe.

INCIPIENT OCCLUSAL CARIES

Incipient occlusal caries cannot be seen on a dental radiograph and must be detected clinically with an explorer.

MODERATE OCCLUSAL CARIES

Moderate occlusal caries extends into dentin and appears as a very thin radiolucent line (Figs. 30–15 and 30–16). The radiolucency is located under the enamel of the occlusal surface of the tooth. Little if any radiographic change is noted in the enamel.

SEVERE OCCLUSAL CARIES

Severe occlusal caries extends into dentin and appears as a large radiolucency (Figs. 30–17 and 30–18). The radiolucency extends under the enamel of the occlusal surface of the tooth. Severe occlusal caries is apparent clinically and appears as a cavitation in a tooth.

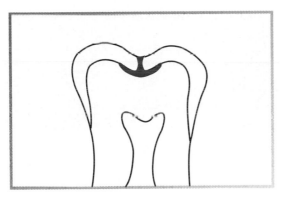

FIGURE 30–15. A moderate occlusal carious lesion extends through enamel and into dentin along the DEJ. (From Haring JI, Lind LJ: Radiographic Interpretation for the Dental Hygienist. Philadelphia, WB Saunders, 1993.)

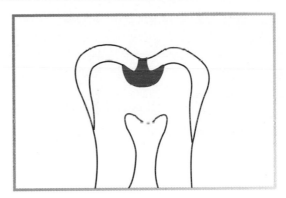

FIGURE 30–17. Severe occlusal caries extends through enamel and into dentin beyond the DEJ. (From Haring JI, Lind LJ: Radiographic Interpretation for the Dental Hygienist. Philadelphia, WB Saunders, 1993.)

Buccal and Lingual Caries

As the names suggest, **buccal caries** involves the buccal tooth surface, whereas **lingual caries** involves the lingual tooth surface. Because of the superimposition of the densities of normal tooth structure, buccal and lingual caries are difficult to detect on a dental radiograph and are best detected clinically. When viewed on a dental radiograph, caries that involves the buccal or lingual surface appears as a small, circular radiolucent area (Figs. 30–19 and 30–20). To determine the location of the lesion, a clinical examination with an explorer is necessary.

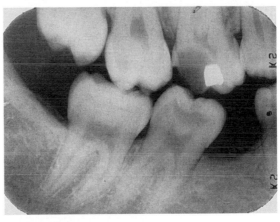

FIGURE 30–18. A severe occlusal carious lesion is seen as a large radiolucency in dentin on the mandibular first molar. (From Haring JI, Lind LJ: Radiographic Interpretation for the Dental Hygienist. Philadelphia, WB Saunders, 1993.)

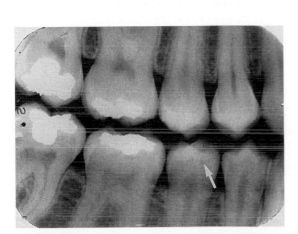

FIGURE 30–16. Occlusal caries appears as a tiny radiolucency just below the DEJ on the mandibular second premolar. (From Haring JI, Lind LJ: Radiographic Interpretation for the Dental Hygienist. Philadelphia, WB Saunders, 1993.)

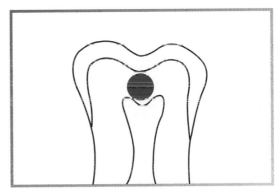

FIGURE 30–19. Buccal or lingual caries is seen as a round radiolucency on molars. (From Haring JI, Lind LJ: Radiographic Interpretation for the Dental Hygienist. Philadelphia, WB Saunders, 1993.)

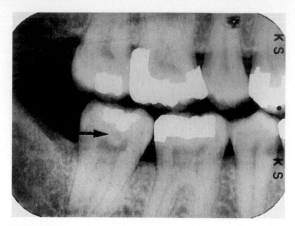

FIGURE 30–20. Buccal caries is seen as a small, circular radiolucency on the mandibular second molar. (From Haring JI, Lind LJ: Radiographic Interpretation for the Dental Hygienist. Philadelphia, WB Saunders, 1993.)

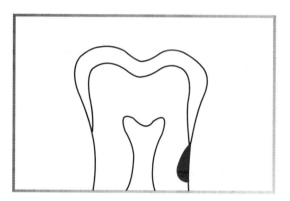

FIGURE 30–21. Root caries involves cementum and dentin only, not enamel. (From Haring JI, Lind LJ: Radiographic Interpretation for the Dental Hygienist. Philadelphia, WB Saunders, 1993.)

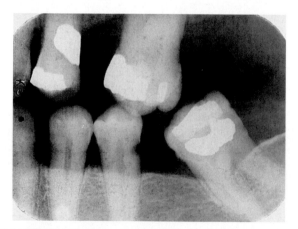

FIGURE 30–22. Root caries appears as a crater-shaped radiolucency just below the cementoenamel junction (CEJ) on the mandibular second premolar. (From Haring JI, Lind LJ: Radiographic Interpretation for the Dental Hygienist. Philadelphia, WB Saunders, 1993.)

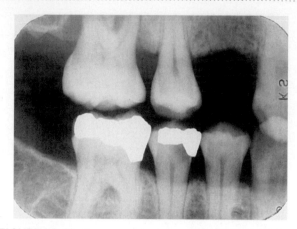

FIGURE 30–23. Recurrent caries is seen as a radiolucency below a two-surface amalgam restoration on the mandibular second premolar. (From Haring JI, Lind LJ: Radiographic Interpretation for the Dental Hygienist. Philadelphia, WB Saunders, 1993.)

Root Surface Caries

Root surface caries involves only the roots of teeth. The cementum and dentin located just below the cervical region or the tooth is involved (Figs. 30–21 and 30–22). No involvement of enamel occurs. Bone loss and corresponding gingival recession precede the caries process and result in exposed root surfaces.

Clinically, root surface caries is easily detected on exposed root surfaces. The most common locations include the exposed roots of the mandibular premolar and molar areas. On a dental radiograph, root surface caries appears as a cupped-out or crater-shaped radiolucency just below the cementoenamel junction (CEJ). Early lesions may be difficult to detect on a dental radiograph.

Recurrent Caries

Secondary or **recurrent caries** occurs adjacent to a preexisting restoration. Caries occurs in this region because of inadequate cavity preparation, defective margins, or incomplete removal of caries prior to the placement of the restoration. On a dental radiograph, recurrent caries appears as a radiolucent area just beneath a restoration (Fig. 30–23). Recurrent caries occurs most often beneath the interproximal margins of a restoration.

Rampant Caries

The term **rampant** means growing or spreading unchecked. **Rampant caries** is advanced and severe car-

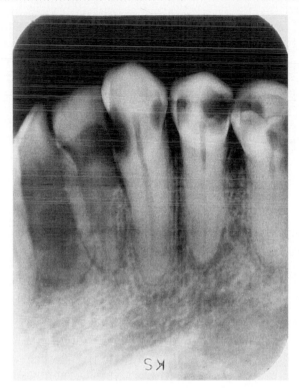

FIGURE 30–24. Rampant caries. (From Haring JI, Lind LJ: Radiographic Interpretation for the Dental Hygienist. Philadelphia, WB Saunders, 1993.)

ies that affects numerous teeth (Fig. 30–24). Rampant caries is typically seen in children with poor dietary habits or in adults with a decreased salivary flow.

SUMMARY

- Dental caries is a destructive process that causes decalcification of enamel, destruction of enamel and dentin, and cavitation of teeth.
- Careful clinical and radiographic examinations are necessary to detect dental caries.
- Dental radiographs allow the dental professional to identify carious lesions that are not visible clinically.
- Dental caries appears radiolucent on a radiograph. Of all the radiolucent lesions that can be seen on a dental radiograph, dental caries is seen most frequently.

- The dental professional must be confident in the use of interpretation methods to identify dental caries and the recognition of factors that influence caries interpretation (e.g., errors in technique and exposure).
- Dental caries may involve any surface of the tooth crown or root. The radiographic appearance of dental caries can be classified according to the location of the caries on the tooth. Caries involving the interproximal, occlusal, buccal, lingual, and root surfaces may all be seen on dental radiographs.
- The radiographic appearance of interproximal caries can be classified as incipient, moderate, advanced, or severe depending on the amount of enamel and dentin involved in the caries process. These classifications are described in this chapter.
- The radiographic appearance of occlusal caries can be classified as moderate or severe, depending on the amount of enamel and dentin involved in the caries process. These classifications are described in this chapter.
- Buccal and lingual carious lesions are difficult to detect on dental radiographs because of the superimposition of normal tooth structure; instead, these lesions are best detected on a clinical basis.
- Root surface caries involves cementum and dentin and is easily detected on a clinical basis. On a dental radiograph, root surface caries appears as a cupped-out radiolucency below the CEJ.
- Other radiographic appearances of dental caries include: recurrent caries, which appears as a radiolucency adjacent to an existing restoration, and rampant caries, which affects numerous teeth.

BIBLIOGRAPHY

Frommer HH: Radiographic interpretation: caries and periodontal disease. In Radiology for Dental Auxiliaries, 6th edition, St. Louis, Mosby-Year Book, 1996, pp. 299–318.

Goaz PW, White SC: Dental caries In Oral Radiology: Principles of Interpretation, 3rd edition St. Louis, Mosby-Year Book, 1994, pp. 306–326.

Haring JI, Lind LJ: Dental caries. In Radiographic Interpretation for the Dental Hygienist. Philadelphia, WB Saunders, 1993, pp. 105–118.

Johnson ON, McNally MA, Essay CE: Preliminary interpretation of the radiographs. In Essentials of Dental Radiography for Dental Assistants and Hygienists, 6th edition. Norwalk, CT, Appleton and Lange, 1999, pp. 259–296.

Langland OE, Sippy FH, Langlais RP: Radiologic interpretation of dental disease. In Textbook of Dental Radiography, 2nd edition. Springfield, IL, Charles C Thomas, 1984, pp. 432–451

Miles DA, Van Dis ML, Jensen CW, Ferretti A: Interpretation: Normal versus abnormal and common radiographic presentation of lesions. In Radiographic Imaging for Dental Auxiliaries, 3rd edition. Philadelphia, WB Saunders, 1999, pp. 231–280.

IDENTIFICATION

For questions 1 to 5, refer to Figures 30–25 through 30–29. Identify the radiographic classification of each carious lesion shown.

1. Figure 30–25

_____

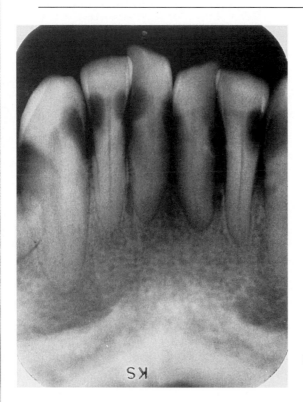

FIGURE 30–25. (From Haring JI, Lind LJ: Radiographic Interpretation for the Dental Hygienist. Philadelphia, WB Saunders, 1993.)

2. Figure 30–26

_____

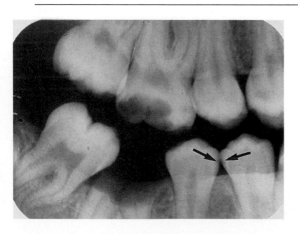

FIGURE 30–26. (From Haring JI, Lind LJ: Radiographic Interpretation for the Dental Hygienist. Philadelphia, WB Saunders, 1993.)

3. Figure 30–27

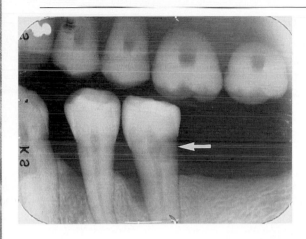

FIGURE 30–27. (From Haring JI, Lind LJ: Radiographic Interpretation for the Dental Hygienist. Philadelphia, WB Saunders, 1993.)

4. Figure 30–28

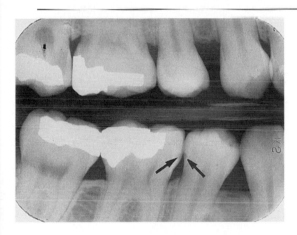

FIGURE 30–28. (From Haring JI, Lind LJ: Radiographic Interpretation for the Dental Hygienist. Philadelphia, WB Saunders, 1993.)

5. Figure 30–29

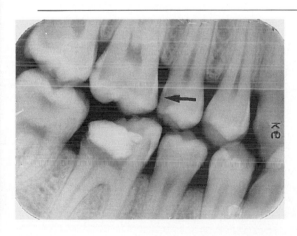

FIGURE 30–29. (From Haring JI, Lind LJ: Radiographic Interpretation for the Dental Hygienist. Philadelphia, WB Saunders, 1993.)

MATCHING

For questions 6 to 12, match the classification of radiographic caries with the appropriate description.

      a. caries that extends more than halfway through the enamel but does not involve the DEJ
      b. caries that extends to or through the DEJ but does not extend more than half the distance to the pulp
      c. caries that cannot be seen on a radiograph
      d. caries that extends through enamel, through dentin, and more than half the distance to the pulp
      e. caries that extends less than halfway through enamel
      f. caries seen as a large radiolucency in dentin under the enamel of the chewing surfaces of the teeth
      g. caries seen as a thin radiolucent line in dentin under the enamel of the chewing surfaces of the teeth
      h. none of the above

_____   **6.** incipient interproximal

_____   **7.** moderate interproximal

_____   **8.** advanced interproximal

_____   **9.** severe interproximal

_____   **10.** incipient occlusal

_____   **11.** moderate occlusal

_____   **12.** severe occlusal

SHORT ANSWER

13. Describe dental caries.

_____

14. Explain why caries appears radiolucent on a dental radiograph.

_____

15. List the radiographic classifications of interproximal caries.

_____

16. List the radiographic classifications of occlusal caries.

_____

17. Describe the radiographic appearance of root caries.

_____

18. Describe the radiographic appearance of recurrent caries.

_____

19. Describe the radiographic appearance of rampant caries.

_____

20. Discuss the factors that may influence the radiographic interpretation of dental caries.

_____

Answers are supplied at the end of this book.

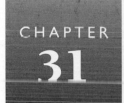

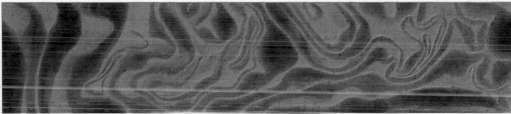

CHAPTER 31

Interpretation of Periodontal Disease

OBJECTIVES

After completion of this chapter, the student will be able to:

- *Define the key words.*
- *Describe the healthy periodontium.*
- *Briefly describe periodontal disease.*
- *Discuss the importance of the clinical and radiographic examinations in the diagnosis of periodontal disease.*
- *Describe the limitations of radiographs in the detection of periodontal disease.*
- *Describe the type of radiographs that should be used to document periodontal disease and the preferred exposure technique.*
- *State the difference between horizontal and vertical bone loss.*
- *State the difference between localized and generalized bone loss.*
- *State the difference between mild, moderate, and severe bone loss.*
- *List each of the four ADA Case Types and describe the corresponding radiographic appearance.*
- *Recognize each of the four ADA Case Types on dental radiographs.*
- *List two predisposing factors for periodontal disease.*
- *Recognize and describe the radiographic appearance of calculus.*

INTRODUCTION

Dental radiographs play an integral role in the assessment of periodontal disease. A radiographic examination is essential for diagnostic purposes because it enables the dental professional to obtain vital information about supporting bone that cannot be obtained clinically. Detailed information about periodontal disease is beyond the scope of this text. For more complete information on this topic, the dental radiographer should refer to a text on radiographic interpretation or periodontal disease.

The purpose of this chapter is to introduce the dental radiographer to the description and detection of periodontal disease. In addition, the radiographic interpretation of periodontal disease with an emphasis on a description of bone loss, ADA case types, and identification of predisposing factors is included.

DESCRIPTION OF THE PERIODONTIUM

The term **periodontium** refers to the tissues that invest and support the teeth such as the gingiva and alveolar bone. As described in Chapter 26, the normal anatomic landmarks of alveolar bone include the lamina dura, alveolar crest, and periodontal ligament space. The radiographic appearance of healthy alveolar bone can be described as follows:

 Lamina dura: In health, the lamina dura around the roots of the teeth appears as a dense radiopaque line (Fig. 31–1).
 Alveolar crest: The normal healthy alveolar crest is located approximately 1.5 to 2.0 mm apical to the cementoenamel junctions of adjacent teeth (see Fig. 31–1). The shape and density of the

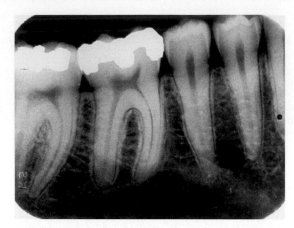

FIGURE 31–1. Healthy alveolar crest, normal lamina dura, and periodontal ligament space on a periapical radiograph. (From Haring JI, Lind LJ: Radiographic Interpretation for the Dental Hygienist. Philadelphia, WB Saunders, 1993.)

alveolar crest varies between the anterior and posterior regions of the mouth. In the anterior regions, the alveolar crest appears pointed and sharp and is normally very radiopaque (Fig. 31–2). In the posterior regions, the alveolar crest appears flat, smooth, and parallel to a line between adjacent cementoenamel junctions (Fig. 31–3). The alveolar crest in the posterior regions appears slightly less radiopaque than that in the anterior regions.
 Periodontal ligament space: The normal periodontal ligament space appears as a thin radiolucent line between the root of the tooth and the lamina dura. In health, the periodontal ligament space is continuous around the root structure and is of uniform thickness (see Fig. 31–1).

DESCRIPTION OF PERIODONTAL DISEASE

The term **periodontal** literally means around a tooth. **Periodontal disease** refers to a group of diseases that affects the tissues around the teeth. Periodontal disease may range from a superficial inflammation of the gingiva to the destruction of the supporting bone and periodontal ligament. With periodontal disease, the gingiva exhibits varying degrees of inflammation. The gingival tissues affected by periodontal disease do not appear stippled, pink, and firm. Instead, the gingiva

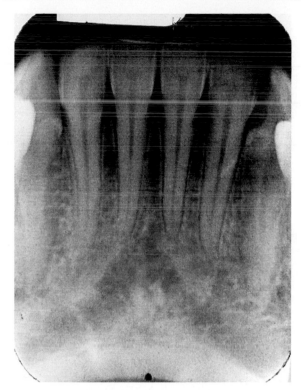

FIGURE 31–2. Healthy alveolar crest in the anterior region appears pointed and very radiopaque. (From Haring JI, Lind LJ: Radiographic Interpretation for the Dental Hygienist. Philadelphia, WB Saunders, 1993.)

appears swollen, red, and bleeding, and soft tissue pocket formation is seen.

The radiographic appearance of alveolar bone affected by periodontal disease differs from that of healthy alveolar bone. With periodontal disease, the

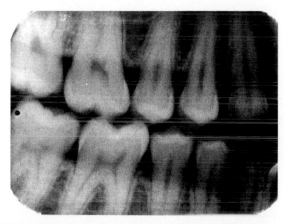

FIGURE 31–3. Healthy alveolar crest in the posterior region appears flat, smooth, and radiopaque. (From Haring JI, Lind LJ: Radiographic Interpretation for the Dental Hygienist. Philadelphia, WB Saunders, 1993.)

alveolar crest is no longer located 1.5 to 2.0 mm apical to the cementoenamel junctions and no longer appears radiopaque. Instead, the alveolar crest appears indistinct, and bone loss is seen. Periodontal disease may result in severe destruction of bone and loss of teeth.

■ DETECTION OF PERIODONTAL DISEASE

To detect periodontal disease, both clinical and radiographic examinations are necessary. Dental radiographs *must* be used in conjunction with a clinical examination. In general, what is seen clinically cannot be evaluated on dental radiographs, and what is viewed on dental radiographs cannot be evaluated clinically. The clinical examination provides information about the soft tissue, and radiographs permit the evaluation of bone.

Clinical Examination

The clinical examination must be performed by the dentist and dental hygienist and should include an evaluation of the soft tissues (gingiva) for signs of inflammation (e.g., redness, bleeding, swelling, pus). A thorough clinical assessment must include periodontal probing. Whenever there is clinical evidence of periodontal disease, radiographs must be taken to obtain maximum diagnostic information.

Radiographic Examination

Radiographs, along with the clinical examination, allow the dental professional to evaluate periodontal disease. Dental radiographs provide an overview of the amount of bone present and indicate the pattern, distribution, and severity of bone loss that has occurred as a result of periodontal disease. In addition, dental radiographs allow the dental professional to document periodontal disease.

The periapical radiograph is the film of choice for the evaluation of periodontal disease. The paralleling technique is the preferred periapical exposure method for the demonstration of the anatomic features of periodontal disease. With the paralleling technique, the height of crestal bone is accurately recorded in relation to the tooth root. If the bisecting technique is used to expose periapical radiographs, a dimensional distortion of bone is seen because of the vertical angulation used.

As a result, periapical films using the bisecting technique may appear to show more or less bone loss than is actually present. (Figs. 31–4 and 31–5).

The horizontal bite-wing should not be used to document periodontal disease. This film has limited use in the detection of periodontal disease; severe interproximal bone loss cannot be adequately visualized on horizontal bite-wing radiographs.

The vertical bite-wing radiograph can be used to examine bone levels in the mouth and is best used as a post-treatment or follow-up film. The panoramic film has little diagnostic value in the identification of periodontal disease and is not recommended to demonstrate the anatomic features of this condition.

Radiographs alone cannot be used to diagnose periodontal disease because they have limitations in detecting and diagnosing this condition; they must be used in conjunction with a thorough clinical examination. For example, radiographs do not provide information about the condition of the soft tissue or the early bony changes seen in periodontal disease. Because dental radiographs record two-dimensional images of three-dimensional structures, certain areas of teeth and bone are difficult if not impossible to examine radiographically. Buccal and lingual areas are particularly difficult to evaluate. For example, bone loss in a **furcation area,** the area between the roots of multirooted teeth, may not be detected on a dental radiograph because of the superimposition of buccal and lingual bone.

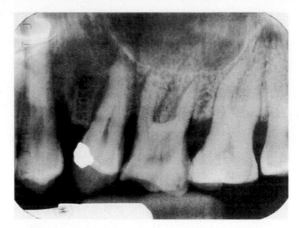

FIGURE 31–5. Paralleling technique used to examine the same area seen in Figure 31–4. Note the difference in bone level. With the paralleling technique, the height of crestal bone is accurately recorded in relation to the tooth root. (From Haring JI, Lind LJ: Radiographic Interpretation for the Dental Hygienist. Philadelphia, WB Saunders, 1993.)

■ RADIOGRAPHIC INTERPRETATION OF PERIODONTAL DISEASE

The dental radiographer must be familiar with the radiographic appearance of periodontal disease. All radiographs should be evaluated for bone loss and examined for other predisposing factors that may contribute to periodontal disease.

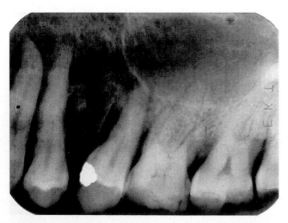

FIGURE 31–4. Because of the vertical angulation used, the bisecting technique may distort the level of bone present. (From Haring JI, Lind LJ: Radiographic Interpretation for the Dental Hygienist. Philadelphia, WB Saunders, 1993.)

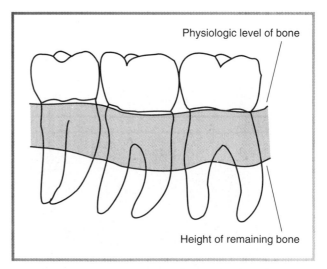

FIGURE 31–6. Bone loss is estimated as the difference between the physiologic level of bone and the height of the remaining bone. (From Haring JI, Lind LJ: Radiographic Interpretation for the Dental Hygienist. Philadelphia, WB Saunders, 1993.)

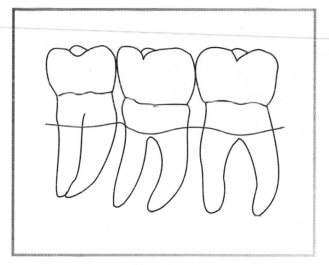

FIGURE 31–7. Horizontal bone loss occurs in a plane parallel to the cementoenamel junctions of adjacent teeth. (From Haring JI, Lind LJ: Radiographic Interpretation for the Dental Hygienist. Philadelphia, WB Saunders, 1993.)

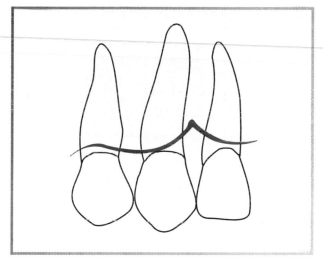

FIGURE 31–9. Vertical bone loss occurs in a plane that is not parallel to the cementoenamel junctions of adjacent teeth. (From Haring JI, Lind LJ: Radiographic Interpretation for the Dental Hygienist. Philadelphia, WB Saunders, 1993.)

Bone Loss

A radiograph allows the dental professional to view the amount of bone remaining rather than the amount of bone lost. However, in documenting bone levels, the amount of bone loss that has occurred is recorded rather than the amount of bone that remains. The amount of bone loss can be estimated as the difference between the physiologic bone level and the height of remaining bone (Fig. 31–6). Bone loss can be described in terms of the pattern, distribution, and severity of loss.

PATTERN

The pattern of bone loss viewed on a dental radiograph can be described as either horizontal or vertical. The cementoenamel junctions of adjacent teeth can be used as a plane of reference in determining the pattern of bone loss present. With **horizontal bone loss**, the bone loss occurs in a plane parallel to the cementoenamel junctions of adjacent teeth (Figs. 31–7 and 31–8). With **vertical bone loss** (also known as angular bone loss), the bone loss does not occur in a plane parallel to the cementoenamel junctions of adjacent teeth (Figs. 31–9 and 31–10).

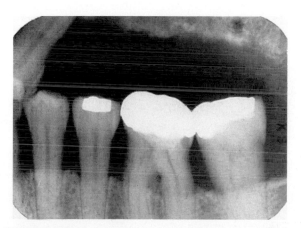

FIGURE 31–8. Horizontal bone loss. (From Haring JI, Lind LJ: Radiographic Interpretation for the Dental Hygienist. Philadelphia, WB Saunders, 1993.)

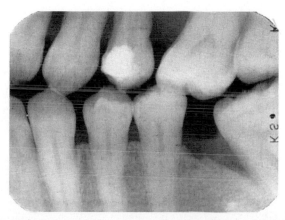

FIGURE 31–10. Vertical bone loss. (From Haring JI, Lind LJ: Radiographic Interpretation for the Dental Hygienist. Philadelphia, WB Saunders, 1993.)

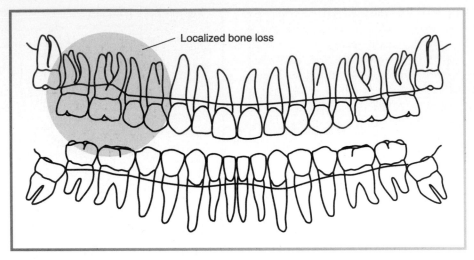

FIGURE 31–11. Localized bone loss occurs in isolated areas. (From Haring JI, Lind LJ: Radiographic Interpretation for the Dental Hygienist. Philadelphia, WB Saunders, 1993.)

DISTRIBUTION

The distribution of bone loss seen on a dental radiograph can be described as localized or generalized, depending on the areas involved. **Localized** bone loss occurs in isolated areas. (Fig. 31–11) **Generalized** bone loss occurs evenly throughout the dental arches (Fig. 31–12).

SEVERITY

Bone loss viewed on a dental radiograph can be classified as either mild, moderate, or severe. The severity of bone loss is measured as a percentage of loss of the normal amount of bone and can be defined as follows:

- mild bone loss: crestal changes
- moderate bone loss: bone loss of 10 to 33%
- severe bone loss: bone loss of 33% or more

Classification of Periodontal Disease

Radiographs can be used in the classification of periodontal disease. Based on the amount of bone loss,

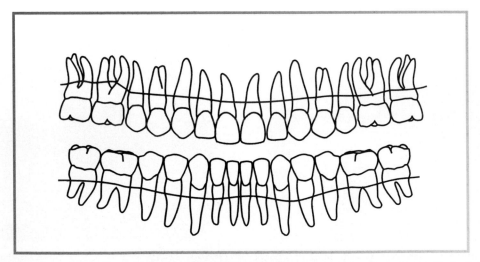

FIGURE 31–12. Generalized bone loss occurs throughout the dental arches. (From Haring JI, Lind LJ: Radiographic Interpretation for the Dental Hygienist. Philadelphia, WB Saunders, 1993.)

periodontal disease can be classified as follows: the American Dental Association (ADA) Case Type I (gingivitis), ADA Case Type II (early periodontitis), ADA Case Type III (moderate periodontitis), or ADA Case Type IV (advanced periodontitis). Each disease type has a specific radiographic appearance. Radiographs can also be used to detect the contributing factors of periodontal disease, such as calculus and defective restorations.

ADA CASE TYPE I

There is no bone loss associated with type I disease (gingivitis), and therefore, no radiographic change in the bone is seen.

ADA CASE TYPE II

The bone loss associated with type II disease (early periodontitis) is mild crestal changes (Fig. 31-13).

ADA CASE TYPE III

The bone loss associated with type III disease (moderate periodontitis) is moderate (10 to 33%) (Figs. 31-14 to 31-16). The pattern of bone loss may be horizontal or vertical; the distribution may be localized or generalized. Furcation involvement, or the extension of periodontal disease between the roots of multirooted teeth, may also be seen with type III disease. When

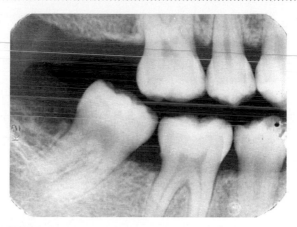

FIGURE 31-14. ADA Case Type III. (From Haring JI, Lind LJ: Radiographic Interpretation for the Dental Hygienist. Philadelphia, WB Saunders, 1993.)

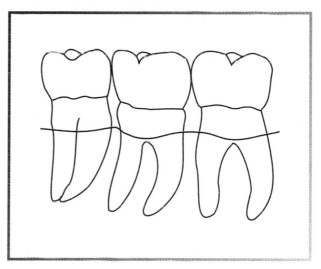

FIGURE 31-15. Moderate bone loss. (From Haring JI, Lind LJ: Radiographic Interpretation for the Dental Hygienist. Philadelphia, WB Saunders, 1993.)

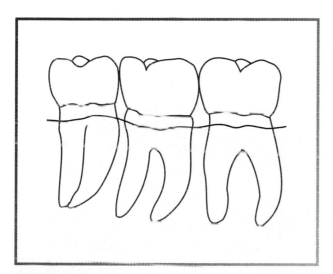

FIGURE 31-13. Mild bone loss. (From Haring JI, Lind LJ: Radiographic Interpretation for the Dental Hygienist. Philadelphia, WB Saunders, 1993.)

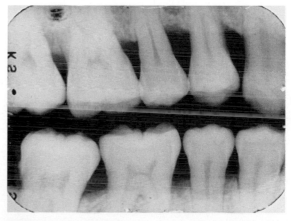

FIGURE 31-16. ADA Case Type III. (From Haring JI, Lind LJ: Radiographic Interpretation for the Dental Hygienist. Philadelphia, WB Saunders, 1993.)

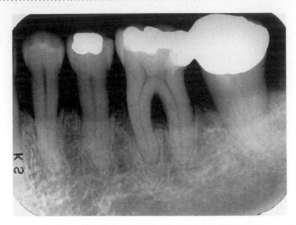

FIGURE 31–17. The furcation area of the mandibular first molar appears radiolucent. (From Haring JI, Lind LJ: Radiographic Interpretation for the Dental Hygienist. Philadelphia, WB Saunders, 1993.)

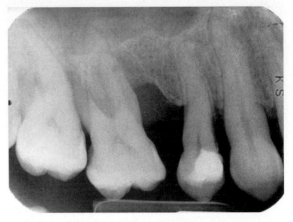

FIGURE 31–19. ADA Case Type IV. (From Haring JI, Lind LJ: Radiographic Interpretation for the Dental Hygienist. Philadelphia, WB Saunders, 1993.)

the bone in the furcation area is destroyed, a radiolucent area is evident on the dental radiograph (Fig. 31–17).

ADA CASE TYPE IV

The bone loss associated with type IV disease (advanced periodontitis) is severe (33% or more) (Figs. 31–18 and 31–19).

Predisposing Factors

A number of predisposing factors or local irritants contribute to periodontal disease. The identification, detection, and elimination of local irritants are important in the management and treatment of periodontal disease. Dental radiographs play a major role in the detection of local irritants such as calculus and defective restorations.

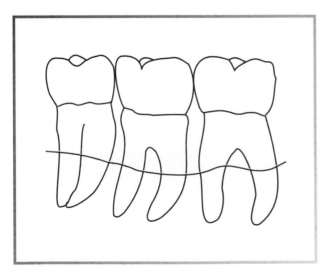

FIGURE 31–18. Severe bone loss. (From Haring JI, Lind LJ: Radiographic Interpretation for the Dental Hygienist. Philadelphia, WB Saunders, 1993.)

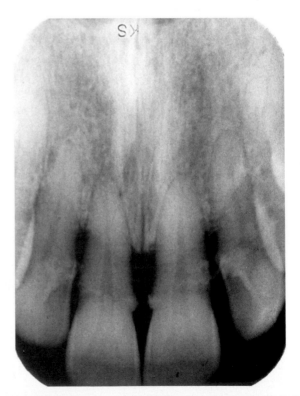

FIGURE 31–20. Subgingival calculus appears as irregular radiopaque projections in the maxillary anterior region. (From Haring JI, Lind LJ: Radiographic Interpretation for the Dental Hygienist. Philadelphia, WB Saunders, 1993.)

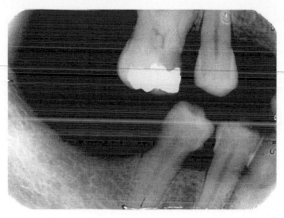

FIGURE 31–21. Calculus may appear as a sharp pointed radiopacity. (From Haring JI, Lind LJ: Radiographic Interpretation for the Dental Hygienist. Philadelphia, WB Saunders, 1993.)

CALCULUS

Calculus is a stone-like concretion that forms on the crowns and roots of teeth due to the calcification of bacterial plaque. Calculus acts as a contributing or predisposing factor to periodontal disease. Calculus appears radiopaque (white or light) on a dental radiograph (Fig. 31–20). Although calculus may have a variety of appearances on dental radiographs, it most often appears as pointed or irregular radiopaque projections extending from the proximal root surfaces (Fig. 31–21). Calculus may also appear as a ring-like radiopacity encircling the cervical portion of a tooth (Fig. 31–22), a nodular radiopaque projection (Fig. 31–23), or a smooth radiopacity on a root surface (Fig. 31–24).

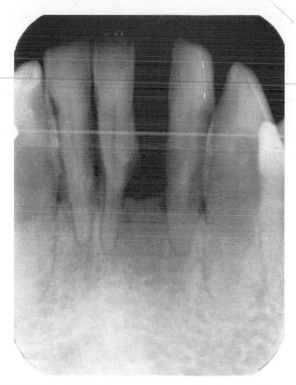

FIGURE 31–23. Calculus may appear nodular as seen here between two mandibular incisors. (From Haring JI, Lind LJ: Radiographic Interpretation for the Dental Hygienist. Philadelphia, WB Saunders, 1993.)

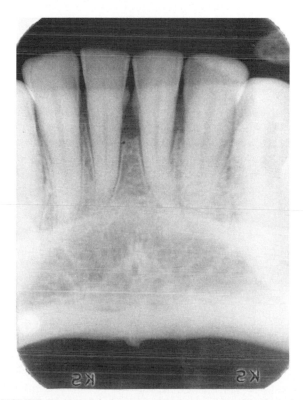

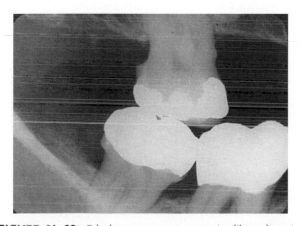

FIGURE 31–22. Calculus may appear as a ring-like radiopacity around the cervical region of a tooth. (From Haring JI, Lind LJ: Radiographic Interpretation for the Dental Hygienist. Philadelphia, WB Saunders, 1993.)

FIGURE 31–24. Calculus may appear as a smooth radiopacity. (From Haring JI, Lind LJ: Radiographic Interpretation for the Dental Hygienist. Philadelphia, WB Saunders, 1993.)

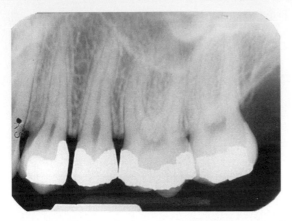

FIGURE 31–25. Open contact between maxillary premolars. (From Haring JI, Lind LJ: Radiographic Interpretation for the Dental Hygienist. Philadelphia, WB Saunders, 1993.)

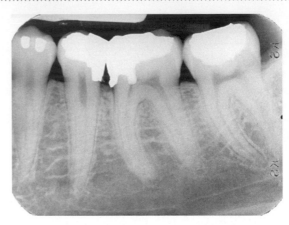

FIGURE 31–28. Amalgam overhang on the mesial of the mandibular first molar. (From Haring JI, Lind LJ: Radiographic Interpretation for the Dental Hygienist. Philadelphia, WB Saunders, 1993.)

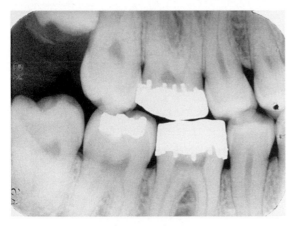

FIGURE 31–26. Poorly contoured crowns on maxillary and mandibular first molars. (From Haring JI, Lind LJ: Radiographic Interpretation for the Dental Hygienist. Philadelphia, WB Saunders, 1993.)

DEFECTIVE RESTORATIONS

Faulty dental restorations act as potential food traps and lead to the accumulation of food debris and bacterial deposits. Defective restorations act as contributing factors to periodontal disease; they can be detected both clinically and radiographically. Radiographs allow the dental professional to identify restorations with open or loose contacts (Fig. 31–25), poor contour (Fig. 31–26), uneven marginal ridges (Fig. 31–27), overhangs (Fig. 31–28), and inadequate margins (Fig. 31–29), all of which may contribute to periodontal disease.

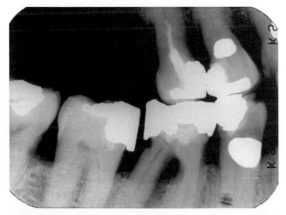

FIGURE 31–27. Uneven marginal ridges, open contacts, overhangs, and poorly contoured restorations on a bite-wing radiograph. (From Haring JI, Lind LJ: Radiographic Interpretation for the Dental Hygienist. Philadelphia, WB Saunders, 1993.)

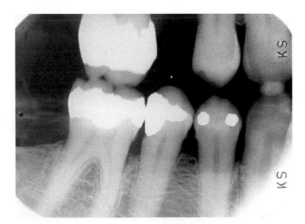

FIGURE 31–29. Inadequate margin on the distal of a mandibular second premolar. (From Haring JI, Lind LJ: Radiographic Interpretation for the Dental Hygienist. Philadelphia, WB Saunders, 1993.)

SUMMARY

- Periodontal disease refers to a group of diseases that affects the tissues found around the teeth.
- Thorough clinical and radiographic examinations are necessary to detect, evaluate, and diagnose periodontal disease. The clinical examination provides information about soft tissue, and the radiographic examination provides information about the supporting bone.
- Radiographs can be used to document periodontal disease and determine the success or failure of periodontal therapy.
- Interpretation of periodontal disease on dental radiographs should include an evaluation of the alveolar bone; bony changes can be described in terms of pattern (horizontal or vertical), distribution (localized or generalized), and severity (mild, moderate or severe).
- Radiographs can be used in the classification of periodontal disease. Based on the amount of bone loss, periodontal disease can be classified as follows: ADA Case Type I, ADA Case Type II, ADA Case Type III, and ADA Case Type IV. Each case type is described in this chapter.
- Radiographs can also be used to detect local irritants, such as calculus and defective restorations, that contribute to periodontal disease.

BIBLIOGRAPHY

Frommer HH: Radiographic interpretation: caries and periodontal disease. *In* Radiology for Dental Auxiliaries, 6th edition. St. Louis, Mosby-Year Book, 1996, pp. 299–318.

Goaz PW, White SC: Periodontal diseases. *In* Oral Radiology: Principles of Interpretation, 3rd edition. St. Louis, Mosby-Year Book, 1994, pp. 327–339.

Haring JI, Lind LJ: Periodontal disease. *In* Radiographic Interpretation for the Dental Hygienist. Philadelphia, WB Saunders, 1993, pp. 121–135.

Langland OE, Sippy FH, Langlais RP: Radiologic interpretation of dental disease. *In* Textbook of Dental Radiography, 2nd edition. Springfield, IL, Charles C Thomas, 1984, pp. 476–501.

Miles DA, Van Dis ML, Jensen CW, Ferretti A: Interpretation: Normal versus abnormal and common radiographic presentation of lesions. *In* Radiographic Imaging for Dental Auxiliaries, 3rd edition. Philadelphia, WB Saunders, 1999, pp. 231–280.

Quiz Questions ∙∙

IDENTIFICATION

For questions 1 to 5, identify the pattern and severity of bone loss, and the ADA Case Type represented by each radiograph.

1. Figure 31–30

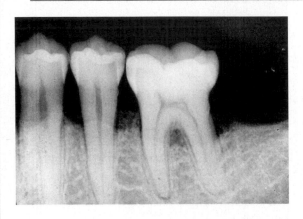

FIGURE 31–30. (From Haring JI, Lind LJ: Radiographic Interpretation for the Dental Hygienist. Philadelphia, WB Saunders, 1993.)

2. Figure 31–31

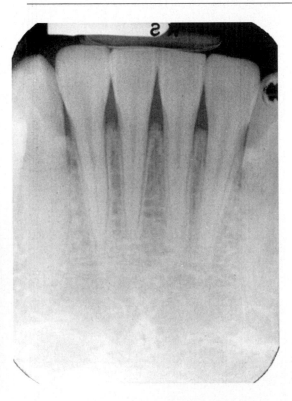

FIGURE 31–31. (From Haring JI, Lind LJ: Radiographic Interpretation for the Dental Hygienist. Philadelphia, WB Saunders, 1993.)

3. Figure 31–32

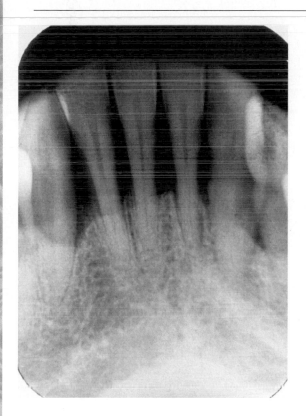

FIGURE 31–32. (From Haring JI, Lind LJ: Radiographic Interpretation for the Dental Hygienist. Philadelphia, WB Saunders, 1993.)

4. Figure 31–33

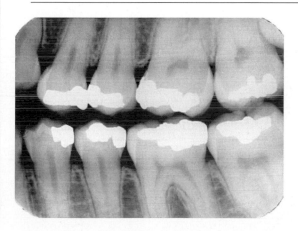

FIGURE 31–33. (From Haring JI, Lind LJ: Radiographic Interpretation for the Dental Hygienist. Philadelphia, WB Saunders, 1993.)

5. Figure 31–34

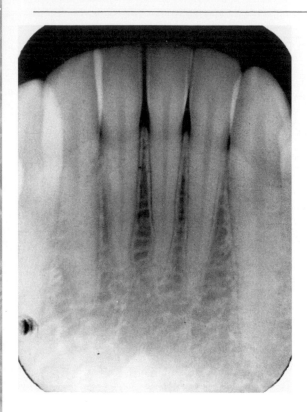

FIGURE 31–34. (From Haring JI, Lind LJ: Radiographic Interpretation for the Dental Hygienist. Philadelphia, WB Saunders, 1993.)

MATCHING

For questions 6 to 9, match each of the ADA Case Types with the appropriate radiographic description.

    a. Mild bone loss (crestal changes)
    b. Severe bone loss (33% or more)
    c. No bony change seen
    d. Moderate bone loss (10 to 33% loss)

_____ **6.** ADA Case Type I

_____ **7.** ADA Case Type II

_____ **8.** ADA Case Type III

_____ **9.** ADA Case Type IV

FILL IN THE BLANK

10. A term that refers to tissues that invest and support the teeth.

_____

11. A term that means "around a tooth."

_____

12. A term that refers to the area between the roots of multirooted teeth.

13. The film of choice for the evaluation of periodontal disease.

14. The preferred method of exposure for films documenting periodontal disease.

15. The term that describes bone loss that occurs in a plane parallel to the cementoenamel junctions of adjacent teeth.

16. The term that describes bone loss that does not occur in a plane parallel to the cementoenamel junctions of adjacent teeth.

17. The term that describes a group of diseases that affects the tissues found around the teeth.

18. The term that describes bone loss that occurs in isolated areas.

19. The term that describes bone loss that occurs evenly throughout the arches.

20. The term that describes a stone-like concretion that forms on the crowns and roots of teeth as the result of the calcification of plaque.

Answers are supplied at the end of this book.

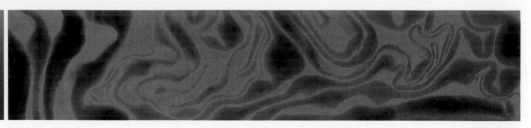

Interpretation of Trauma and Pulpal and Periapical Lesions

OBJECTIVES

After completion of this chapter, the student will be able to:

- *Define the key words.*
- *Describe and identify the radiographic appearance of crown, root, and jaw fractures.*
- *Describe and identify the radiographic appearance of an avulsion.*
- *Describe and identify the radiographic appearance of internal and external resorption.*
- *Describe and identify the radiographic appearance of pulpal sclerosis, pulpal obliteration, and pulp stones.*
- *Describe and identify the radiographic appearance of a periapical granuloma, cyst, and abscess.*
- *Describe and identify the radiographic appearance of condensing osteitis, sclerotic bone, and hypercementosis.*

INTRODUCTION

In many instances, the dental radiograph acts as a detector and shows change. Changes associated with trauma, resorption, and pulpal and periapical lesions can be seen on dental radiographs. Radiographs allow the dental professional to evaluate areas that cannot be examined clinically, such as the roots, pulp chambers, and periapical regions of the teeth. Detailed information about trauma and pulpal and periapical lesions is beyond the scope of this text. For more complete information on these topics, the dental radiographer should consult a text on radiographic interpretation.

The purpose of this chapter is to provide a brief overview of the common radiographic features of trauma and pulpal and periapical lesions.

RADIOGRAPHIC CHANGES DUE TO TRAUMA

Trauma can be defined as an injury produced by an external force. Trauma may affect the crowns and roots of teeth as well as alveolar bone. Trauma may result in fractures of teeth and bone and injuries such as intrusion, extrusion, and avulsion.

Fractures

A **fracture** can be defined as the breaking of a part. Fractures may affect the crowns and roots of teeth or the bones of the maxilla and mandible. Whenever a fracture is evident or suspected, radiographic examination of the injured area is necessary.

CROWN FRACTURES

Fractures that affect tooth crowns most often involve the anterior teeth. Most crown fractures result from an accident involving a fall or a motor vehicle. Crown fractures may involve the enamel only, the enamel and dentin, or the enamel, dentin, and pulp. The missing part of a crown caused by a fracture is evident on a dental radiograph (Fig. 32-1). The radiograph allows the dental professional to evaluate the proximity of the pulp chamber to the fracture and to examine the root for any additional fractures.

ROOT FRACTURES

Root fractures are less common than crown fractures and also result from an accident or traumatic blow. Root fractures occur most often in the maxillary central incisor region. Tooth roots may be fractured at any level along the root and may involve more than one root of a multirooted tooth. If the x-ray beam is parallel with the plane of the fracture, the root fracture appears as a sharp radiolucent line on a periapical radiograph (Fig. 32-2). If the x-ray beam is not parallel with the fracture, the adjacent areas of tooth struc-

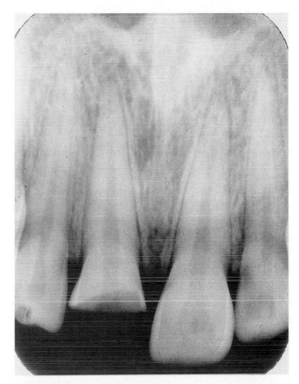

FIGURE 32-1. A fractured central incisor. (From Haring JI, Lind LJ: Radiographic Interpretation for the Dental Hygienist. Philadelphia, WB Saunders, 1993.)

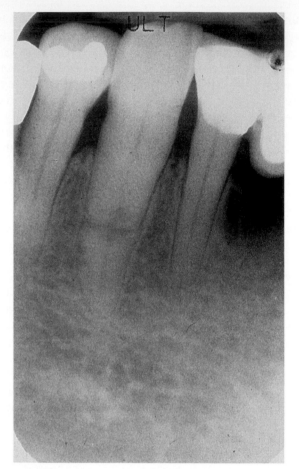

FIGURE 32–2. A root fracture on a mandibular canine. (From Haring JI, Lind LJ: Radiographic Interpretation for the Dental Hygienist. Philadelphia, WB Saunders, 1993.)

ture obscure the fracture site; as a result, the fracture cannot be seen on the dental radiograph. With time, root fractures have a tendency to enlarge due to displacement of root fragments, hemorrhage, or edema. Consequently, a root fracture that was initially overlooked may be identified on a later radiograph.

JAW FRACTURES

Fractures of the mandible occur more often than fractures of any other bone of the face and frequently result from assaults, accidents, and sports injuries. The panoramic radiograph is the film of choice for the evaluation of mandibular fractures. On a dental radiograph, a mandibular fracture appears as a radiolucent line at the site where the bone has separated (Fig. 32–3). Fractures of the maxilla occur less frequently than mandibular fractures and most often involve the ante-

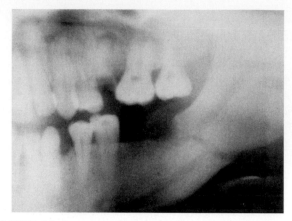

FIGURE 32–3. A fractured mandible. (From Haring JI, Lind LJ: Radiographic Interpretation for the Dental Hygienist. Philadelphia, WB Saunders, 1993.)

rior alveolar bone and teeth. Maxillary fractures are typically difficult to detect on a dental radiograph.

Injuries

In addition to fractures, trauma may result in the displacement of teeth. Radiographs allow the dental professional to evaluate dental structures after tooth displacement. Tooth displacement includes luxation (intrusion or extrusion) and avulsion.

LUXATION

Luxation is the abnormal displacement of teeth. Abnormal displacement of teeth can be categorized as either intrusion or extrusion. **Intrusion** refers to the abnormal displacement of teeth *into* bone (Fig. 32–4);

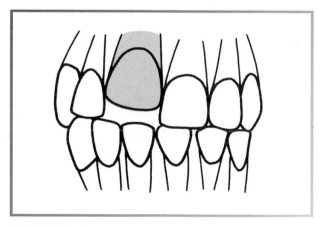

FIGURE 32–4. An intruded crown. (From Haring JI, Lind LJ: Radiographic Interpretation for the Dental Hygienist. Philadelphia, WB Saunders, 1993.)

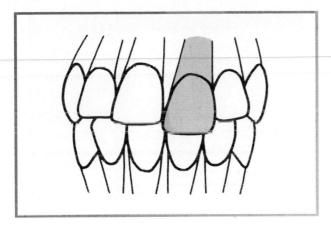

FIGURE 32–5. An extruded crown. (From Haring JI, Lind LJ: Radiographic Interpretation for the Dental Hygienist. Philadelphia, WB Saunders, 1993.)

extrusion refers to the abnormal displacement of teeth *out of* bone (Fig. 32–5). Teeth that have been luxated should be evaluated by a periapical radiograph and examined for root and adjacent alveolar bone fractures, damage to the periodontal ligament, and pulpal problems.

AVULSION

Avulsion is the complete displacement of a tooth from alveolar bone. Most avulsions result from trauma associated with an assault or accidental fall. An avulsed tooth is not seen on a dental radiograph; instead, a periapical radiograph shows a tooth socket without a tooth (Fig. 32–6). Dental radiographs are important in the evaluation of the socket area and should be used to examine the region for splintered bone.

RADIOGRAPHIC CHANGES DUE TO RESORPTION

Two types of resorption are associated with teeth: physiologic and pathologic.

Physiologic resorption is a process that is seen with the normal shedding of primary teeth. The roots of a primary tooth are resorbed as the permanent successor moves in an occlusal direction; the primary tooth is shed when resorption of the roots is complete (Fig. 32–7). **Pathologic resorption** is a regressive alteration of tooth structure that is observed when a tooth is subjected to abnormal stimuli. Resorption of teeth can be described as external or internal depending on the location of the resorption process.

External Resorption

External resorption is seen along the periphery of the root surface and is often associated with reimplanted teeth, abnormal mechanical forces, trauma, chronic inflammation, tumors and cysts, impacted teeth, or idiopathic causes. External resorption most often affects the apices of teeth; the apical region appears blunted, and the length of the root appears shorter than normal (Fig. 32–8). Both the lamina dura and bone around

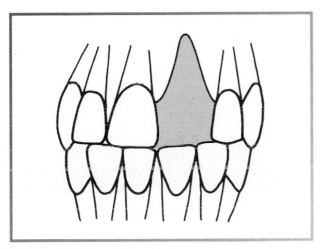

FIGURE 32–6. With avulsion, an empty tooth socket is seen on a dental radiograph. (From Haring JI, Lind LJ: Radiographic Interpretation for the Dental Hygienist. Philadelphia, WB Saunders, 1993.)

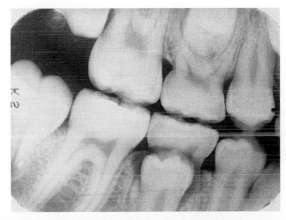

FIGURE 32–7. Physiologic resorption of a mandibular deciduous second molar. (From Haring JI, Lind LJ: Radiographic Interpretation for the Dental Hygienist. Philadelphia, WB Saunders, 1993.)

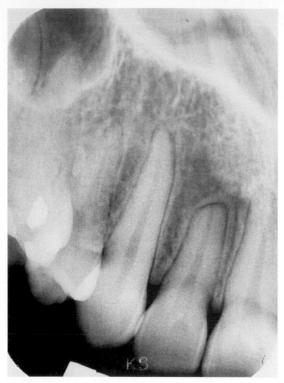

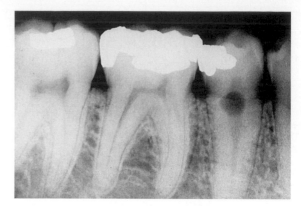

FIGURE 32–9. Internal resorption seen as a round radiolucency in the cervical region of a mandibular second premolar. (From Haring JI, Lind LJ: Radiographic Interpretation for the Dental Hygienist. Philadelphia, WB Saunders, 1993.)

FIGURE 32–8. External resorption of the apical region of a maxillary lateral incisor. (From Haring JI, Lind LJ: Radiographic Interpretation for the Dental Hygienist. Philadelphia, WB Saunders, 1993.)

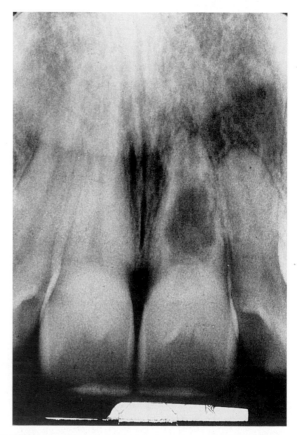

the blunted apex appear normal. External resorption is not associated with any signs or symptoms and is not detected clinically. Teeth that undergo external resorption do not exhibit mobility. There is no effective treatment for external resorption.

Internal Resorption

Internal resorption occurs within the crown or root of a tooth and involves the pulp chamber, pulp canals, and surrounding dentin. Precipitating factors such as trauma, pulp capping, and pulp polyps are believed to stimulate the internal resorption process. Internal resorption appears as a round-to-ovoid radiolucency in the midcrown or midroot portion of a tooth (Figs. 32–9 and 32–10). Internal resorption is generally asymptomatic. Treatment is variable; endodontic therapy may be used if the resorptive process has not physically weakened the tooth. If the tooth is weakened by the resorptive process, extraction is recommended.

FIGURE 32–10. Internal resorption seen as a radiolucency in the root of a maxillary central incisor. (From Haring JI, Lind LJ: Radiographic Interpretation for the Dental Hygienist. Philadelphia, WB Saunders, 1993.)

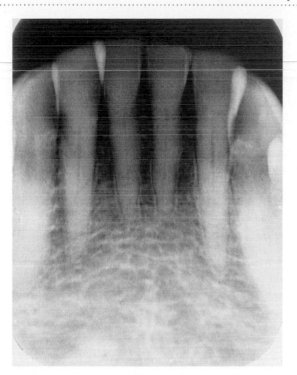

FIGURE 32–11. Thin atrophic pulp chambers in mandibular incisors. (From Haring JI, Lind LJ: Radiographic Interpretation for the Dental Hygienist. Philadelphia, WB Saunders, 1993.)

▇▇ RADIOGRAPHIC FEATURES OF PULPAL LESIONS

In many dental procedures, information about the size and location of the pulp cavity must be obtained before treatment. Without dental radiographs, examination of the pulp chambers and canals is impossible. Pulpal sclerosis, pulpal obliteration, and pulp stones are common conditions of the pulp cavity that can be seen on dental radiographs.

Pulpal Sclerosis

Pulpal sclerosis is a diffuse calcification of the pulp chamber and pulp canals of teeth that results in a pulp cavity of decreased size. For unknown reasons, pulpal sclerosis is associated with aging. Pulpal sclerosis appears as a pulp cavity that is reduced in size (Fig. 32–11). No clinical features are associated with pulpal sclerosis. Pulpal sclerosis is generally considered an incidental radiographic finding that is of little clinical significance unless endodontic therapy is indicated.

Pulpal Obliteration

Some conditions (e.g., attrition, abrasion, caries, dental restorations, trauma, and abnormal mechanical forces) may act as irritants to the pulp and stimulate the production of secondary dentin, which results in obliteration of the pulp cavity. On a dental radiograph, a tooth with **pulpal obliteration** does not appear to have a pulp chamber or pulp canals (Fig. 32–12). Teeth that exhibit pulpal obliteration are nonvital and do not require treatment.

Pulp Stones

Pulp stones are calcifications that are found in the pulp chamber or pulp canals of teeth. The cause of pulp stones is unknown. On a dental radiograph, pulp stones appear as round, ovoid, or cylindrical radiopacities; some pulp stones may conform to the shape of the pulp chamber or canal (Figs. 32–13 and 32–14). Pulp stones may vary in shape, size, and number. Pulp stones do not cause symptoms and do not require treatment.

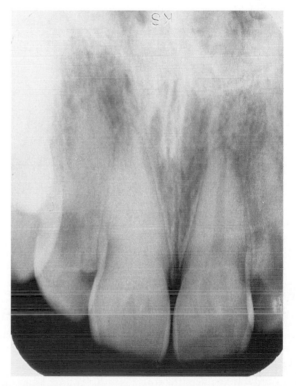

FIGURE 32–12. Pulpal obliteration in a maxillary central incisor. (From Haring JI, Lind LJ: Radiographic Interpretation for the Dental Hygienist. Philadelphia, WB Saunders, 1993.)

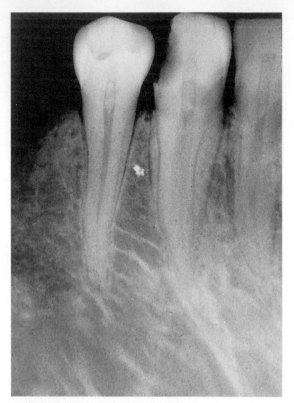

FIGURE 32–13. Cylindrical pulp stones in the mandibular canine and premolar. (From Haring JI, Lind LJ: Radiographic Interpretation for the Dental Hygienist. Philadelphia, WB Saunders, 1993.)

▮ RADIOGRAPHIC FEATURES OF PERIAPICAL LESIONS

A **periapical lesion** is a lesion that is located around the apex (tip of the root) of a tooth. The use of dental radiographs is particularly important in the identification of periapical problems. Periapical lesions cannot be evaluated on a clinical basis alone. On dental radiographs periapical lesions may appear either radiolucent (dark or black) or radiopaque (light or white).

Periapical Radiolucencies

Periapical granulomas, cysts, and abscesses are common periapical radiolucencies that can be seen on dental radiographs. These lesions cannot be diagnosed by their radiographic appearances alone; instead, diagnosis is based on the clinical features and radiographic and microscopic appearances. Because it is impossible to distinguish between these three periapical lesions based on their radiographic appearance, the dental radiographer should refer to these lesions simply as "periapical radiolucencies."

PERIAPICAL GRANULOMA

A **periapical granuloma** is a localized mass of chronically inflamed granulation tissue at the apex of a nonvital tooth. The periapical granuloma results from pulpal death and necrosis and is the most common sequela of pulpitis (inflammation of the pulp). A periapical granuloma may give rise to a periapical cyst or periapical abscess. A tooth with a periapical granuloma is typically asymptomatic but has a previous history of prolonged sensitivity to heat or cold. Treatment for a periapical granuloma may include endodontic therapy or removal of the tooth along with curettage of the apical region.

On a dental radiograph a periapical granuloma is initially seen as a widened periodontal ligament space

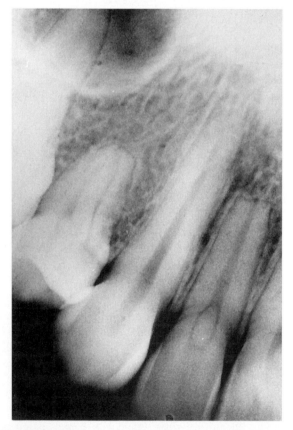

FIGURE 32–14. An ovoid pulp stone in a maxillary lateral incisor. (From Haring JI, Lind LJ: Radiographic Interpretation for the Dental Hygienist. Philadelphia, WB Saunders, 1993.)

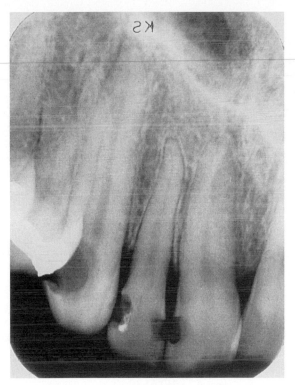

FIGURE 32–15. A widened periodontal ligament space at the apex of a maxillary lateral incisor. (From Haring JI, Lind LJ: Radiographic Interpretation for the Dental Hygienist. Philadelphia, WB Saunders, 1993.)

at the root apex (Fig. 32–15). With time, the widened periodontal ligament space enlarges and appears as a round or ovoid radiolucency (Fig. 32–16). The lamina dura is not visible between the root apex and the apical lesion.

PERIAPICAL CYST

A **periapical cyst** (also known as a radicular cyst) is a lesion that develops over a prolonged period of time; cystic degeneration takes place within a periapical granuloma and results in a periapical cyst. The periapical cyst results from pulpal death and necrosis. Periapical cysts are the most common of all tooth-related cysts and comprise 50 to 70% of all cysts in the oral region. Periapical cysts are typically asymptomatic. Treatment may include endodontic therapy or extraction of the tooth as well as curettage of the apical region. On a dental radiograph the typical periapical cyst appears as a round or ovoid radiolucency (Fig. 32–17).

PERIAPICAL ABSCESS

The **periapical abscess** is a localized collection of pus in the periapical region of a tooth that results from pulpal death. Periapical abscesses may be acute or chronic. An acute periapical abscess has features of an acute pus-producing process and inflammation. An acute abscess may result from an acute inflammation of the pulp or an area of chronic infection, such as a periapical granuloma. A chronic periapical abscess has features of a long-standing, low-grade, pus-producing process. A chronic abscess may develop from an acute abscess or a periapical granuloma.

An acute periapical abscess is painful—the pain may be intense, throbbing, and constant. The tooth is nonvital and is sensitive to pressure, percussion, and heat. Chronic periapical abscesses are usually asymptomatic because the pus drains through bone or the periodontal ligament space. Clinically, a gumboil may be seen in the apical region of the tooth at the site of

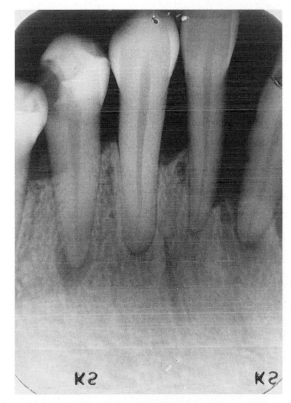

FIGURE 32–16. A periapical radiolucency associated with a mandibular premolar. (Note the lamina dura is not visible.) (From Haring JI, Lind LJ: Radiographic Interpretation for the Dental Hygienist. Philadelphia, WB Saunders, 1993.)

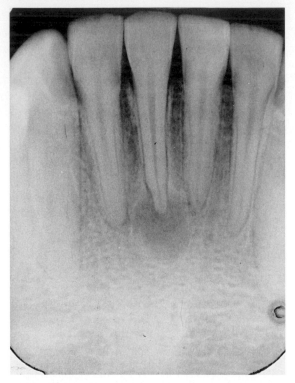

FIGURE 32–17. A well-defined round radiolucency seen at the apex of a mandibular central incisor. (From Haring JI, Lind LJ: Radiographic Interpretation for the Dental Hygienist. Philadelphia, WB Saunders, 1993.)

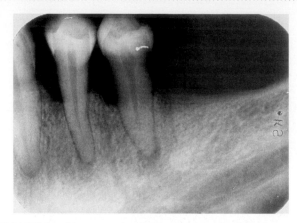

FIGURE 32–19. Periapical radiolucencies associated with the mandibular premolars. (From Haring JI, Lind LJ: Radiographic Interpretation for the Dental Hygienist. Philadelphia, WB Saunders, 1993.)

drainage. Treatment of the periapical abscess includes drainage and endodontic therapy or extraction.

With an acute periapical abscess, no radiographic change may be evident. Early radiographic changes include an increased widening of the periodontal ligament space (Fig. 32–18). A chronic periapical abscess appears as a round or ovoid apical radiolucency with poorly defined margins (Fig. 32–19). The lamina dura cannot be seen between the root apex and the radiolucent lesion.

Periapical Radiopacities

Condensing osteitis, sclerotic bone, and hypercementosis are a few of the common periapical radiopacities that can be seen on dental radiographs. Unlike periapical radiolucencies, periapical radiopacities can be diagnosed based on their radiographic appearance, clinical information, and patient history.

CONDENSING OSTEITIS

Condensing osteitis (also known as chronic focal sclerosing osteomyelitis) is a well-defined radiopacity that is seen below the apex of a nonvital tooth with a history of long-standing pulpitis (Fig. 32–20). The opacity represents a proliferation of periapical bone that is a result of a low-grade inflammation or mild irritation. The inflammation that stimulates condensing osteitis occurs in response to pulpal necrosis. Condensing osteitis may vary in size and shape and does not appear to be attached to the tooth root.

Condensing osteitis is the most common periapical radiopacity observed in adults. The tooth most fre-

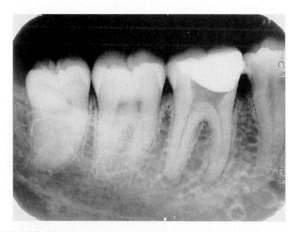

FIGURE 32–18. An increased widening of the periodontal ligament space is noted in the periapical region of the mandibular first molar. (From Haring JI, Lind LJ: Radiographic Interpretation for the Dental Hygienist. Philadelphia, WB Saunders, 1993.)

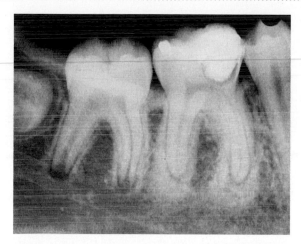

FIGURE 32–20. A diffuse radiopacity is noted along the roots a mandibular first molar. (From Haring JI, Lind LJ: Radiographic Interpretation for the Dental Hygienist. Philadelphia, WB Saunders, 1993.)

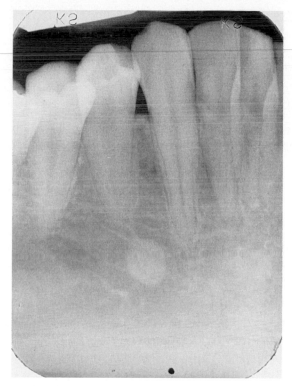

FIGURE 32–21. A well-defined radiopacity below the apex of a mandibular premolar. (From Haring JI, Lind LJ: Radiographic Interpretation for the Dental Hygienist. Philadelphia, WB Saunders, 1993.)

quently involved is the mandibular first molar. Teeth associated with condensing osteitis are nonvital and typically have a large carious lesion or large restoration. Because condensing osteitis is believed to represent a physiologic reaction of bone to inflammation, no treatment is necessary.

SCLEROTIC BONE

Sclerotic bone (also known as osteosclerosis or idiopathic periapical osteosclerosis) is a well-defined radiopacity that is seen below the apices of vital, noncarious teeth (Fig. 32–21). The cause of sclerotic bone is unknown; however, it is not believed to be associated with inflammation. The lesion is not attached to a tooth and varies in size and shape. The margins may appear smooth or irregular and diffuse. The borders are continuous with adjacent normal bone, and no radiolucent outline is seen. Sclerotic bone is asymptomatic and is usually discovered during routine radiographic examination.

HYPERCEMENTOSIS

Hypercementosis is the excess deposition of cementum on root surfaces. Hypercementosis results from supraeruption, inflammation, or trauma; sometimes there is no obvious cause. On dental radiographs hypercementosis is visible as an excess amount of cementum along all or part of a root surface (Fig. 32–22). The apical area is most often affected and appears enlarged and bulbous. Root areas affected by hypercementosis are separated from periapical bone by a nor-

mal appearing periodontal ligament space; the surrounding lamina dura appears normal as well.

No signs or symptoms are associated with hypercementosis; most cases are discovered during routine radiographic examination. Teeth affected by hypercementosis are vital and do not require treatment.

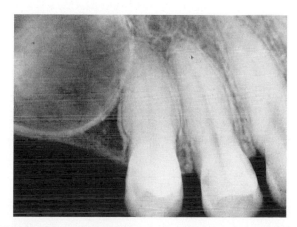

FIGURE 32–22. Hypercementosis of a maxillary premolar. (From Haring JI, Lind LJ: Radiographic Interpretation for the Dental Hygienist. Philadelphia, WB Saunders, 1993.)

SUMMARY

- Changes associated with trauma, resorption, and pulpal and periapical lesions can be viewed on dental radiographs.
- Radiographs allow the dental professional to evaluate the roots, pulp cavities, and periapical regions of the teeth—all of which are areas that cannot be examined clinically.
- Radiographic examinations are important in the evaluation of trauma and injury and can be used for diagnostic, treatment, and post-treatment purposes.
- Dental radiographs are useful in the evaluation of tooth and jaw fractures and tooth injuries that include intrusion, extrusion, and avulsion.
- Dental radiographs are useful in identifying regressive alterations of teeth, such as external and internal resorption; these regressive alterations are usually asymptomatic and are discovered only during radiographic examination.
- Dental radiographs are also useful in examining and obtaining information about the pulp cavity. Pulpal sclerosis, obliteration of the the pulp cavity, and pulp stones are common conditions that can be viewed on dental radiographs.

- Periapical lesions cannot be examined without dental radiographs; examples include periapical granulomas, periapical cysts, periapical abscesses, condensing osteitis, sclerotic bone, and hypercementosis.

BIBLIOGRAPHY

Frommer HH: Pulpal and periapical lesions. *In* Radiology for Dental Auxiliaries, 6th edition. St. Louis, Mosby-Year Book, 1996, pp. 319–331.

Goaz PW, White SC: Infection and inflammation of the jaws and facial bones. *In* Oral Radiology: Principles of Interpretation, 3rd edition. St. Louis, Mosby-Year Book, 1994, pp. 381–385.

Haring JI, Lind LJ: Trauma, pulpal and periapical lesions. *In* Radiographic Interpretation for the Dental Hygienist, Philadelphia, WB Saunders, 1993, pp. 140–155.

Johnson ON, McNally MA, Essay CE: Preliminary interpretation of the radiographs. *In* Essentials of Dental Radiography for Dental Assistants and Hygienists, 6th edition. Norwalk, CT, Appleton and Lange, 1999, pp. 259–296.

Manson-Hing LR: Interpretation and value of radiographs. *In* Fundamentals of Dental Radiography, 3rd edition. Philadelphia, Lea & Febiger, 1990, pp. 207–208.

Miles DA, Van Dis ML, Jensen CW, Ferretti, A: Interpretation: Normal versus abnormal and common radiographic presentation. *In* Radiographic Imaging for Dental Auxiliaries, 3rd edition. Philadelphia, WB Saunders, 1999, pp. 231–280.

Quiz Questions ••

MATCHING

For questions 1 to 6, match the terms with the appropriate definition.

a. abnormal displacement of teeth
b. an injury produced by an external force
c. complete displacement of a tooth from alveolar bone
d. abnormal displacement of teeth out of bone
e. the breaking of a part
f. abnormal displacement of teeth into bone

_____ 1. trauma

_____ 2. fracture

_____ 3. luxation

_____ 4. intrusion

_____ 5. extrusion

_____ 6. avulsion

IDENTIFICATION

For questions 7 to 12, refer to Figures 32–23 to 32–28. Identify or describe the periapical and pulpal lesions shown in each figure.

7. Figure 32–23

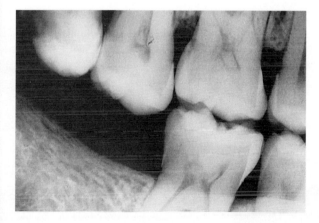

FIGURE 32–23. (From Haring JI, Lind LJ: Radiographic Interpretation for the Dental Hygienist. Philadelphia, WB Saunders, 1993.)

8. Figure 32–24

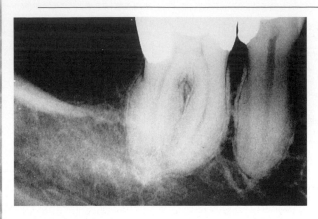

FIGURE 32–24. (From Haring JI, Lind LJ: Radiographic Interpretation for the Dental Hygienist. Philadelphia, WB Saunders, 1993.)

9. Figure 32–25

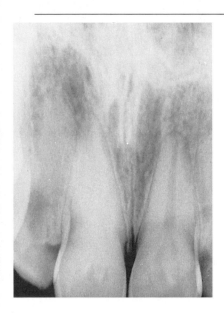

FIGURE 32–25. (From Haring JI, Lind LJ: Radiographic Interpretation for the Dental Hygienist. Philadelphia, WB Saunders, 1993.)

10. Figure 32–26

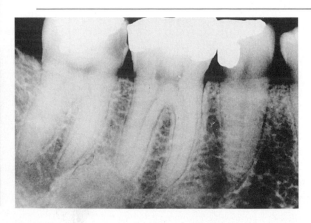

FIGURE 32–26. (From Haring JI, Lind LJ: Radiographic Interpretation for the Dental Hygienist. Philadelphia, WB Saunders, 1993.)

11. Figure 32-27

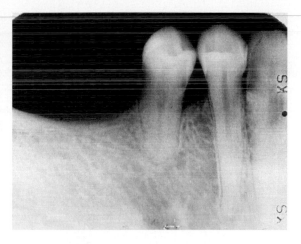

FIGURE 32-27. (From Haring JI, Lind LJ: Radiographic Interpretation for the Dental Hygienist. Philadelphia, WB Saunders, 1993.)

12. Figure 32-28

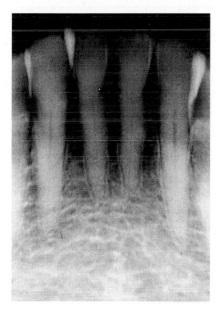

FIGURE 32-28. (From Haring JI, Lind LJ: Radiographic Interpretation for the Dental Hygienist. Philadelphia, WB Saunders, 1993.)

Answers are supplied at the end of this book.

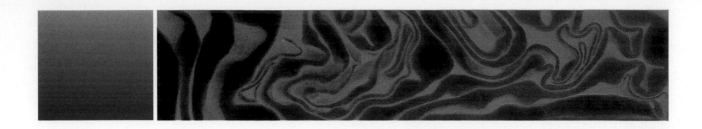

Self-Study Examination Questions

1. Identify which of the following processes occurs with ionization:

   a. cell death takes place
   b. photons penetrate matter
   c. radiant energy is converted to heat
   d. an electron is displaced from its orbit

2. Identify the term used to describe an atom that has lost an electron from its orbit:

   a. ion
   b. photon
   c. neutron
   d. particle

3. Identify which of the following is *not* a property of x-rays:

   a. the ability to penetrate organic matter
   b. the ability to fluoresce all materials
   c. the ability to produce ionization of matter
   d. the ability to produce a latent image

4. Identify which of the following element(s) is/are located within the x-ray tube:

   a. anode
   b. cathode
   c. focusing cup
   d. all of the above

5. Identify which of the following is *not* a type of particulate radiation:

   a. alpha particles
   b. beta particles
   c. protons
   d. nucleons

6. Identify which of the following is *not* a type of electromagnetic radiation:

   a. electrons
   b. radar waves
   c. microwaves
   d. x-rays

7. Identify which of the following is *false:*

    a. x rays cause ionization
    b. x-rays cannot be focused to a point
    c. x-rays have no charge
    d. x-rays travel at the speed of sound

8. Identify the part of the x-ray tube that contains the focal spot:

    a. anode
    b. cathode
    c. filament
    d. focusing cup

9. Identify the part of the x-ray tube where x-rays are produced:

    a. at the positively charged anode
    b. at the positively charged cathode
    c. at the negatively charged anode
    d. at the negatively charged cathode

10. Identify the unit of time used to measure x-ray exposure:

    a. amperes
    b. milliamperes
    c. volts
    d. impulses

11. Identify the function(s) of the milliamperage setting on the x-ray machine:

    a. controls quantity of x-rays produced
    b. controls heat of the tungsten filament
    c. controls quality of the x-rays produced
    d. a and b

12. Identify the characteristics of x-rays produced with a high kilovoltage:

    1. more penetrating
    2. less penetrating
    3. of longer wavelength
    4. of shorter wavelength
        a. 1 and 3
        b. 1 and 4
        c. 2 and 3
        d. 2 and 4

13. Identify the function of the kilovoltage setting on the x-ray machine:

    a. controls the quantity of x-rays produced
    b. controls the penetrating power of the x-ray beam
    c. controls the number of photons available
    d. all of the above

14. Identify the term used to describe the overall blackness or darkness of a film:

    a. contrast
    b. density
    c. overexposure
    d. intensity

15. Identify the exposure factor(s) that affect(s) contrast:

    a. milliamperage
    b. kilovoltage
    c. exposure time
    d. all of the above

16. Identify the density and contrast of a film produced using a high kilovoltage setting:

    a. increased density; low contrast
    b. increased density; high contrast
    c. decreased density; low contrast
    d. decreased density; high contrast

17. Identify which of the following results when a film is exposed with a high milliamperage setting:

    a. high contrast
    b. low contrast
    c. increased density
    d. decreased density

18. Identify the kilovoltage peak (kVp) setting that produces the greatest contrast among images on a radiograph:

    a. 65 kVp
    b. 75 kVp
    c. 80 kVp
    d. 90 kVp

19. Identify the reduction in exposure time when changing from D-speed film to E-speed film:

    a. reduce exposure time by 1/8
    b. reduce exposure time by 1/4
    c. reduce exposure time by 1/3
    d. reduce exposure time by 1/2

20. Identify the periapical film size used for a maxillary premolar exposure in an adult patient:

    a. size 1
    b. size 2
    c. size 3
    d. size 4

21. Identify the major advantage of using the paralleling technique versus the bisecting angle technique:

    a. decreased density
    b. increased density
    c. more contrast
    d. decreased distortion

22. Identify the positioning of the film in relation to the tooth when using the paralleling technique:

    a. the film is placed perpendicularly to the tooth
    b. the film is placed parallel to the tooth
    c. the film is placed in direct contact with the tooth
    d. the film is placed on the occlusal surface of the tooth

23. Identify which of the following is *not* an advantage of the paralleling technique:

    a. simplicity of use
    b. films are easily duplicated
    c. patient comfort
    d. films are easily placed in the mouth

24. Identify the benefit of using a long-cone (16") position-indicating device (PID) versus a short-cone (8") PID:

    a. increased distortion occurs
    b. less magnification occurs
    c. decreased definition occurs
    d. less resolution occurs

25. Identify the error that causes teeth to appear foreshortened on a radiograph:

    a. excessive vertical angulation
    b. insufficient vertical angulation
    c. excessive horizontal angulation
    d. insufficient horizontal angulation

26. Identify the angulation of the central ray when using the bisecting angle technique:

    a. 90 degrees to the imaginary bisector
    b. 90 degrees to the film
    c. 90 degrees to the long axis of the tooth
    d. 90 degrees to the contact area

27. Identify the result of using excessive finger pressure on the film with the bisecting angle technique:

    a. a herringbone pattern
    b. increased density
    c. increased image distortion
    d. a cone-cut

28. Identify a likely cause of gagging during radiographic exposure:

    a. exposure of bite-wing radiographs
    b. the film is held in place by the patient
    c. the film is moved across the soft palate
    d. the film impinges on the floor of the mouth

29. Identify the film that is used to detect both interproximal caries and crestal bone levels:

    a. occlusal
    b. bite-wing
    c. panoramic
    d. periapical

30. Identify the cause of overlapped contacts on a bite-wing radiograph.

    a. incorrect vertical angulation
    b. incorrect horizontal angulation
    c. increased vertical angulation
    d. decreased vertical angulation

31. Identify the vertical angulation required for exposing a bite-wing radiograph:

    a. +20 degrees
    b. +10 degrees
    c. −20 degrees
    d. −10 degrees

32. Identify the error that results when the central x-ray is not centered on the film:

    a. overlap
    b. distortion
    c. cone-cut
    d. elongation

33. Identify one use for the occlusal radiograph:

    a. localize foreign bodies
    b. diagnose dental caries
    c. evaluate periodontal conditions
    d. examine lesions of the mucosa

34. Identify the film size and vertical angulation required to expose a maxillary occlusal projection on a 5-year-old child:

    a. size 2 film; +60 degrees
    b. size 2 film; −60 degrees
    c. size 2 film; +90 degrees
    d. size 4 film; +90 degrees

35. Identify which instruction(s) should be given to the patient concerning exposure of a panoramic radiograph:

    a. swallow, then raise tongue to the roof of the mouth
    b. stand or sit as straight as possible
    c. remain still during the exposure
    d. all of the above

36. Identify the error that results when a patient is positioned for a panoramic exposure with the chin tipped up:

    a. a reverse smile line
    b. an exaggerated smile line
    c. excessive cervical spine on the film
    d. narrow, skinny mandibular incisors

37. Identify which of the following is *true* concerning intensifying screens:

    a. used to magnify the amount of radiation produced
    b. used to help to absorb scatter radiation
    c. found in extraoral and intraoral film packets
    d. emit light when struck by x-radiation

38. Identify the function of the intensifying screen:

    a. reduce exposure time
    b. increase exposure time
    c. increase processing time
    d. clarify periapical structures

39. Identify the cause of a herringbone pattern on a processed radiograph:

    a. film was underdeveloped
    b. exposure time was too short
    c. exposure time was too long
    d. film was placed backward in the mouth

40. Identify the appearance of a film exposed to light before processing:

    a. clear
    b. black
    c. fogged
    d. normal

41. Identify the likely cause of black lines on a processed film:

    a. dirty rollers
    b. exposure time was too long
    c. improper safelight
    d. overdevelopment

42. Identify the radiopaque anatomic landmark:

    a. maxillary sinus
    b. incisive foramen
    c. genial tubercles
    d. mandibular canal

43. Identify the radiolucent anatomic landmark:

    a. nasal septum
    b. canine fossa
    c. external oblique ridge
    d. maxillary tuberosity

44. Identify the film that includes the mental foramen:

    a. mandibular premolar
    b. mandibular molar
    c. maxillary premolar
    d. maxillary molar

45. Identify the film that includes the lingual foramen:

    a. mandibular incisor
    b. mandibular canine
    c. mandibular premolar
    d. maxillary canine

46. Identify the film that includes the canine fossa:

    a. maxillary incisor
    b. maxillary canine
    c. mandibular incisor
    d. mandibular canine

47. Identify which of the following affect(s) the life of the developer solution:

    a. size of films processed
    b. number of films processed
    c. cleanliness of processing tanks
    d. all of the above

48. Identify which of the following produce(s) a light radiographic image:

    a. developing in cool solutions
    b. processing with exhausted chemicals
    c. accidental overexposure
    d. a and b

49. Identify which of the following produce(s) yellow or brown stains on a film:

    a. exhausted developer solution
    b. exhausted fixer solution
    c. insufficient washing
    d. all of the above

50. Identify the appearance of a film left in the fixer for a long time:

    a. film becomes discolored
    b. film demonstrates a decrease in density
    c. film demonstrates an increase in density
    d. film demonstrates proper density

51. Identify the cause of light (white) spots on a processed radiograph:

    a. developer contacts film prior to processing
    b. fixer contacts film prior to processing
    c. static electricity created with opening of film packet
    d. processing solutions are too warm

52. Identify the cause of a radiograph that appears too dark:

    a. film remained in the fixer too long
    b. film was underexposed
    c. temperature of the developing solution is high
    d. insufficient washing

53. Identify which of the following results in film fog:

    1. improper safelighting
    2. film exposed to chemical fumes
    3. use of outdated film
    4. placing the film backward in the mouth
       a. 1, 2
       b. 1, 3
       c. 1, 2, 3
       d. 2, 3, 4

54. Identify the likely cause if one or two films of a complete series appear simply clear after processing:

    a. processing solutions are too cool
    b. overexposure of films
    c. films were not exposed to radiation
    d. incorrect processing

55. Identify the optimum temperature for the developer solution:

    a. 55°F
    b. 68°F
    c. 75°F
    d. 80°F

56. Identify the appearance of a radiograph processed with exhausted developer:

    a. dark radiographic image
    b. thin, faded radiographic image
    c. yellow-brown radiographic image
    d. black image

57. Identify the recommended distance between the safelight and work surface:

    a. a minimum of 1 foot
    b. a minimum of 2 feet
    c. a minimum of 3 feet
    d. a minimum of 4 feet

58. Identify the reason(s) film should not be stored in the darkroom:

    a. processing solutions may splash on the boxes of film
    b. chemical fumes may fog film
    c. unopened boxes of film should not be exposed to the safelight
    d. all of the above

59. Identify which of the following does *not* affect the life of the processing solutions:

    a. age of the processing solutions
    b. care in preparation of processing solutions
    c. type of safelight filter used
    d. number of films processed

60. Identify the error that results when a film is subjected to sudden temperature change (e.g., between developer solution and water bath):

    a. reticulation of emulsion
    b. yellow-brown stains
    c. fixer spots
    d. static electricity

For questions 61 to 64, identify the films placed in the following frames, using the labial mounting method.

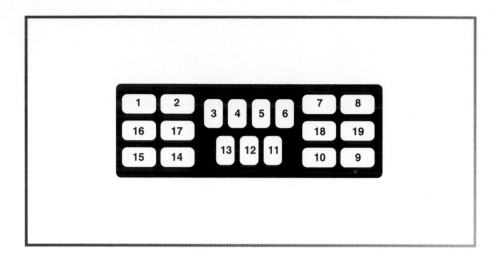

61. Frame #1:

    a. maxillary right molar periapical
    b. maxillary left molar periapical
    c. right molar bite-wing
    d. left molar bite-wing

62. Frame #7:

    a. maxillary right premolar periapical
    b. maxillary left premolar periapical
    c. right premolar bite-wing
    d. left premolar bite-wing

63. Frame #11:

    a. maxillary left canine periapical
    b. maxillary right canine periapical
    c. mandibular left canine periapical
    d. mandibular right canine periapical

64. Frame #17:

    a. maxillary right molar periapical
    b. maxillary left molar periapical
    c. right premolar bite-wing
    d. left molar bite-wing

65. Identify the information that should appear on every film mount:

    a. patient's name
    b. prescribing dentist's name
    c. date of exposure
    d. all of the above

66. Identify the maxillary anatomic landmark:

    a. mental foramen
    b. genial tubercles
    c. incisive foramen
    d. mylohyoid ridge

67. Identify the mandibular anatomic landmark:

    a. median palatal suture
    b. lingual foramen
    c. nasal fossa
    d. zygomatic process

68. Identify which of the following is *true* concerning labial mounting:

    a. the patient's left is on your left
    b. the patient's left is on your right
    c. the teeth are mounted in reverse anatomic order
    d. the radiographs are viewed as if the operator were inside the patient's mouth looking out

69. Identify which of the following is *true* regarding duplicating film:

    a. emulsion is on one side only
    b. exposure to light makes the film lighter
    c. exposure to light makes the film darker
    d. a and b

70. Identify which of the following is/are *true* regarding duplicating film:

    a. the emulsion on the duplicating film must contact the original radiographs
    b. the duplicating film is placed on the duplicator with the emulsion side up
    c. duplicating radiographs may be performed in the lab or operatory
    d. all of the above

71. The practicing clinician has primary custodial rights to the radiographs of patients. Patients have property rights to their radiographs and records.

    a. both statements are true
    b. both statements are false
    c. the first statement is true; the second statement is false
    d. the first statement is false; the second statement is true

72. Identify the best description of primary radiation:

    a. the beam that exits the tubehead
    b. the beam that is created when x-rays contact matter
    c. the beam that is deflected from its path by matter
    d. the beam that is less penetrating

73. Identify the radiation produced when matter is irradiated by x-rays:

    a. leakage radiation
    b. primary radiation
    c. diverging radiation
    d. secondary radiation

74. Identify the portion of the cell that is damaged when a genetic mutation results:

    a. lipids
    b. proteins
    c. DNA
    d. cytoplasm

75. Identify which of the following is *true* concerning radiation injury:

    a. all radiation injuries are evident immediately
    b. x-radiation only injures somatic cells
    c. acute injury due to x-radiation exposure is common
    d. cumulative effects of x-radiation exposure lead to health problems

76. Identify the x-rays that are most likely absorbed by the skin, thus causing x-ray injury:

    a. deep, penetrating x-rays
    b. aluminum-filtered x-rays
    c. long-wavelength x-rays
    d. short-wavelength x-rays

77. Identify an early clinical sign of excessive exposure to radiation:

    a. jaundice
    b. erythema
    c. bleeding
    d. loss of hair

78. Identify the most dangerous time for a fetus to be exposed to ionizing radiation:

    a. first trimester
    b. second trimester
    c. third trimester
    d. all of the above

79. Identify why a child's cells are more susceptible to damage from x-radiation than adult cells:

    a. more sensitive cell epithelium
    b. more rapid cell reproduction
    c. less rapid cellular repair
    d. less bone tissue

80. Identify the cells that are most sensitive to x-radiation:

    a. nerve cells
    b. muscle cells
    c. small lymphocytes
    d. cardiac cells

81. Identify which of the following are patient protection measures used to limit exposure to x-radiation:

    1. use of lead apron and thyroid collar
    2. use of film-holding devices
    3. following the ALARA concept
    4. use of E-speed film
       a. 1, 2, 3, 4
       b. 1, 2, 3
       c. 1, 2, 4
       d. 1, 3

82. Identify the maximum permissible dose (MPD) of an occupationally exposed person:

    a. 0.01 Sv/year (1.0 rem/year)
    b. 0.02 Sv/year (2.0 rem/year)
    c. 0.03 Sv/year (3.0 rem/year)
    d. 0.05 Sv/year (5.0 rem/year)

83. Identify the maximum permissible dose (MPD) of a nonoccupationally exposed person:

    a. 0.001 Sv/year (0.1 rem/year)
    b. 0.002 Sv/year (0.2 rem/year)
    c. 0.003 Sv/year (0.3 rem/year)
    d. 0.005 Sv/year (0.5 rem/year)

84. Identify the maximum diameter of the collimated x-ray beam as it exits the PID:

    a. 1.75 inches
    b. 2.25 inches
    c. 2.75 inches
    d. 3.25 inches

85. Identify the function of the collimator:

    a. to restrict the size and shape of the x-ray beam
    b. to remove the long wavelengths from the x-ray beam
    c. to remove the low energy x-rays from the beam
    d. to increase scatter radiation

86. Identify which of the following is used to make a collimator:

    a. aluminum
    b. copper
    c. lead
    d. tungsten

87. Identify the function of filtration:

    a. to restrict the size and shape of the x-ray beam
    b. to remove the long wavelengths from the x-ray beam
    c. to remove the low energy x-rays from the beam
    d. b and c

88. Identify which of the following is *not* a component of inherent filtration:

    a. oil
    b. unleaded glass window
    c. the lead-lined cone
    d. the tubehead seal

89. Identify which of the following is used to make a filter:

    a. aluminum
    b. copper
    c. lead
    d. tungsten

90. Identify the term used to describe the x-ray beam that exits the PID:

    a. primary radiation
    b. secondary radiation
    c. scatter radiation
    d. direct radiation

91. Identify which of the following is *true* concerning the use of E-speed film:

    a. requires a longer developing time than D-speed film
    b. requires a shorter developing time than D-speed film
    c. requires a longer exposure time than D-speed film
    d. requires a shorter exposure time than D-speed film

92. Identify the exposure factor adjustment used to produce a beam with greater penetrating power:

    a. increase the milliamperage
    b. increase the kilovoltage
    c. increase the time setting
    d. increase the target-film distance

93. Identify the intensity of the x-ray beam if the PID is increased from 8 inches to 16 inches:

    a. the beam will be 1/4 as intense
    b. the beam will be 1/2 as intense
    c. the beam will be twice as intense
    d. the beam will be four times as intense

94. Identify which of the following results in the greatest reduction of x-ray exposure:

    a. low kilovoltage
    b. E-speed film
    c. a short developing time
    d. a long PID

95. Identify which of the following is determined by the milliamperage and exposure time settings:

    a. energy of the radiation produced
    b. amount of film fog
    c. number of x-rays produced
    d. penetrating ability of the x-ray beam

96. Identify the radiation effects that occur in the exposed person, *not* in the reproductive cells:

    a. genetic effects
    b. somatic effects
    c. direct effects
    d. short-term effects

97. Identify which of the following is most effective in reducing x-radiation exposure:

    a. 8-inch, lead-lined, round PID
    b. 8-inch, lead-lined, rectangular PID
    c. 16-inch, lead-lined, round PID
    d. 16-inch, lead-lined, rectangular PID

98. Identify the purpose of a radiation film badge:

    a. to reduce the radiation exposure to the patient
    b. to protect the radiographer from radiation exposure
    c. to protect the radiology cubicle from overheating
    d. to monitor the radiation exposure to the radiographer

99. Identify which of the following is *false* concerning radiation film badges:

    a. each radiographer should have his or her own film badge
    b. the film badge should be worn at waist level
    c. the film badge may be stored in the x-ray area when not being worn
    d. the film badge should not be worn when the radiographer is undergoing x-ray exposure

100. Identify the potential sources of occupational exposure to x-radiation:

    a. primary radiation
    b. leakage radiation
    c. scattered radiation
    d. all of the above

101. Identify the recommended distance from the radiographer to the tubehead during x-ray exposure:

    a. at least 3 feet
    b. at least 6 feet
    c. at least 9 feet
    d. at least 12 feet

102. Identify the recommended positioning of the dental radiographer to the primary beam:

    a. 60 to 90 degrees
    b. 90 to 120 degrees
    c. 90 to 135 degrees
    d. 135 to 180 degrees

103. Identify which of the following statements is/are *true* concerning operator protection:

    a. it is acceptable for the radiographer to hold a film in place for a patient
    b. it is acceptable for the radiographer to hold the tubehead during x-ray exposure
    c. the radiographer should stand behind a protective barrier during exposure whenever possible
    d. all of the above are true

104. Identify the safest positioning for a radiographer during x-ray exposure:

    a. behind a lead barrier
    b. parallel to the tubehead
    c. at least 6 feet behind the patient's head
    d. at a 45-degree angle to the patient

105. Identify the safest positioning for a radiographer during an x-ray exposure in which no shielding is available:

    a. at a 45-degree angle to the patient
    b. at least 6 feet behind the tubehead
    c. at least 6 feet behind the patient's head
    d. none of the above

106. Identify the quality assurance procedures used in radiography:

    1. periodic monitoring of x-ray equipment and supplies
    2. monitoring of processing solutions
    3. use of kilovoltage settings of 90 and higher
    4. use of the lead apron by personnel during all exposures
        a. 1, 2
        b. 1, 2, 3
        c. 1, 2, 4
        d. all of the above

107. Identify the purpose of creating a reference radiograph:

    a. to determine the strength of the developer solution
    b. to determine the strength of the fixer solution
    c. to determine proper safelight distance and wattage
    d. to determine whether the darkroom is "light-tight"

108. Identify the purpose of the "coin test":

    a. to determine the strength of the developer solution
    b. to determine the strength of the fixer solution
    c. to determine the proper safelight distance and wattage
    d. to determine whether the darkroom is "light-tight"

109. Unopened boxes of radiographic film should not be stored in the darkroom. Chemical fumes from the processing solutions may fog the unopened film.

    a. both statements are true
    b. both statements are false
    c. the first statement is true; the second statement is false
    d. the first statement is false; the second statement is true

110. Identify the appearance of a radiograph if the film is exposed to a small light leak in the darkroom:

    a. underexposed
    b. fogged
    c. spotted
    d. all of the above

ANSWERS

1. d	29. b	57. d	84. c
2. a	30. b	58. b	85. a
3. b	31. b	59. c	86. c
4. d	32. c	60. a	87. d
5. d	33. a	61. a	88. c
6. a	34. a	62. b	89. a
7. d	35. d	63. c	90. a
8. a	36. a	64. c	91. d
9. a	37. d	65. d	92. b
10. d	38. a	66. c	93. a
11. d	39. d	67. b	94. b
12. b	40. b	68. b	95. c
13. b	41. a	69. d	96. b
14. b	42. c	70. a	97. d
15. b	43. b	71. a	98. d
16. a	44. a	72. a	99. c
17. c	45. a	73. d	100. d
18. a	46. b	74. c	101. b
19. d	47. d	75. d	102. c
20. b	48. d	76. c	103. c
21. d	49. d	77. b	104. a
22. b	50. b	78. a	105. b
23. c	51. b	79. b	106. c
24. b	52. c	80. c	107. a
25. a	53. c	81. a	108. c
26. a	54. c	82. d	109. a
27. c	55. b	83. d	110. b
28. c	56. b		

Glossary

Absorption The process through which x-radiation imparts some or all of its energy to the material through which it passes; absorption depends on the atomic structure of matter and the wavelength of the x-ray beam

Accelerator One of the basic ingredients of the developer solution that contains the chemical sodium carbonate; the accelerator activates and provides an alkaline environment for the developing agents and softens the film emulsion

Acetic acid A chemical found in the fixer solution that stops the action of the developer

Acidifier One of the basic ingredients of the fixer solution (e.g., acetic acid or sulfuric acid); the acidifier neutralizes the alkaline developer and stops further action of the developer

ADA Case Types The categorization of periodontal disease by the American Academy of Periodontology. Four categories have been described: ADA Case Types I, II, III, and IV

Adhesive layer A thin layer of adhesive material that covers both sides of the film base and attaches the emulsion to the base

Air bubbles A film handling error; white spots appear on a film as a result of trapped air that remains on the film surface after the film has been placed in the processing solution

ALARA concept A concept of radiation protection that states that all exposure to radiation must be kept to a minimum, or "*as low as reasonably achievable*"

Alignment, object-film One of the influencing factors for image distortion that refers to the alignment of the tooth and film; less image distortion results when the tooth and film are parallel to each other

Alpha particles A type of particulate radiation emitted from the nuclei of heavy metals; alpha particles contain two protons and two neutrons and are positively charged

Aluminum disks Disks or sheets of aluminum, usually 0.5 mm thick, that are placed in the path of the x-ray beam; filter out the nonpenetrating, longer-wavelength x-rays

Alveolar bone Bone that supports and encases the roots of the teeth; appears radiopaque

Alveolar crest The most coronal portion of alveolar bone found between the teeth; composed of dense cortical bone and appears radiopaque (also known as crestal bone)

Ammonium thiosulfate A chemical found in the fixing agent that clears the unexposed, undeveloped silver halide crystals from the film emulsion

Amperage The number of electrons that pass through a conductor; the strength of an electric current

Ampere (A) A unit of electrical current strength; the intensity of an electric current produced by 1 volt acting through a resistance of 1 ohm

Anatomic order The order in which the teeth are arranged within the dental arches

Angle In geometry, a figure formed by two lines diverging from a common point

Angle, right In geometry, an angle of 90 degrees formed by two lines perpendicular to each other

Angle of the mandible Area of the mandible where the body meets the ramus

Angulation The alignment of the central x-ray beam in the horizontal and vertical planes

Angulation, horizontal The positioning of the tube head and direction of the central ray in a side-to-side (horizontal) plane

Angulation, negative vertical The positioning of the position-indicating device (PID) below the occlusal plane that directs the central ray upward

Angulation, positive vertical The positioning of the PID above the occlusal plane that directs the central ray downward

Angulation, vertical The positioning of the tubehead and direction of the central ray in an up-and-down (vertical) plane

Anode The positive electrode in the x-ray tube; consists of a wafer-thin tungsten plate embedded in a solid copper rod; converts electrons into x-ray photons

Anterior nasal spine A sharp projection of the maxilla located at the anterior and inferior portion of the nasal cavity; appears radiopaque

Antiseptic   A substance that inhibits the growth of bacteria

Articular eminence   A rounded projection of the temporal bone located anterior to the glenoid fossa

Asepsis   The absence of pathogens or disease-causing microorganisms

Atom   A tiny, invisible particle that is the fundamental unit of matter; the smallest part of an element that has the properties of that element

Atom, neutral   An atom that contains an equal number of protons (positive charges) and electrons (negative charges)

Atomic number   Each atom has an atomic number that corresponds to the total number of protons in the nucleus

Atomic weight   The total number of protons and neutrons in the nucleus of an atom (also known as mass number)

Autotransformer   A voltage compensator that corrects for minor fluctuations in the current flowing through the x-ray machine

Avulsion   The complete displacement of a tooth from alveolar bone

Barrier envelope   A plastic shield that protects an intraoral film from saliva and is used to minimize contamination

Beam, primary   See *Radiation, primary*

Beam, useful   See *Radiation, primary*

Beam alignment device   A device used to align the position-indicating device (PID) in relation to the tooth and film

Beta particles   Fast-moving electrons emitted from the nucleus of radioactive atoms

Binding energy   The attraction between the positive nucleus and the negative electrons that maintains electrons in their orbits; determined by the distance between the nucleus and electrons (also known as electrostatic force or binding force)

Bisect   To divide into two equal parts

Bisecting technique   An intraoral radiographic technique used to expose periapical films, based on the following concepts: the film is placed along the lingual surface of the tooth; the central ray of the x-ray beam is directed perpendicular to the imaginary bisector formed by the film and the long axis of the tooth; a film holder or the patient's finger is used to stabilize the film

Bisector, imaginary   An imaginary plane that divides in half the angle formed by the film and the long axis of the tooth

Bite-wing, vertical   An intraoral film used to examine the level of alveolar bone in the mouth; this bite-wing is placed with the long portion of the film in a vertical direction

Bite-wing tab   A heavy paperboard loop or an adhesive paper tab used to stabilize a bite-wing film during exposure (also known as bite loop, bite tab)

Bite-wing technique   An intraoral radiographic technique in which the interproximal surfaces of the teeth are examined

Bloodborne pathogens   Microorganisms present in blood that cause disease in humans

Bone loss, generalized   Bone loss occurring evenly throughout the dental arches

Bone loss, horizontal   Bone loss that occurs in a plane parallel to the cementoenamel junctions of adjacent teeth

Bone loss, localized   Bone loss occurring in isolated areas

Bone loss, mild   Bone loss appearing as crestal changes

Bone loss, moderate   Bone loss measured on a dental radiograph of 10 to 33%

Bone loss, severe   Bone loss measured on a dental radiograph of 33% or more

Bone loss, vertical   Bone loss that does not occur in a plane parallel to the cementoenamel junctions of adjacent teeth (also known as angular bone loss)

Buccal object rule   A rule for the orientation of structures seen in two radiographs exposed at different angles; used to determine the buccal-lingual relationship of an object

Calculus   A stone-like concretion that forms on the crowns and roots of teeth as a result of the calcification of bacterial plaque; appears radiopaque

Canal   A tube-like passageway through bone that houses nerves and blood vessels; appears radiolucent

Cancellous   Refers to a latticelike structure; appears radiolucent

Caries   Tooth decay; appears radiolucent

Caries, buccal   Caries found on the buccal tooth surface

Caries, interproximal   Caries found between two adjacent teeth

Caries, interproximal advanced   Caries found between two teeth that extends to the DEJ or through the DEJ and into dentin but does not extend through the dentin more than half the distance toward the pulp

Caries, interproximal incipient   Caries found between two teeth that extends less than halfway through the thickness of enamel

Caries, interproximal moderate Caries found between two teeth that extends more than halfway through the thickness of enamel but does not involve the DEJ

Caries, interproximal severe Caries found between two teeth that extends through enamel, through dentin, and more than half the distance toward the pulp

Caries, lingual Caries found on the lingual tooth surface

Caries, occlusal Caries found on the chewing surface of posterior teeth

Caries, occlusal incipient Caries found on the chewing surface of posterior teeth; cannot be seen on a dental radiograph

Caries, occlusal moderate Caries found on the chewing surface of posterior teeth that extends into dentin; appears as a thin radiolucent line

Caries, occlusal severe Caries found on the chewing surface of posterior teeth that extends into dentin; appears as a large radiolucency

Caries, rampant Caries that affects numerous teeth in the dentition

Caries, recurrent Caries found adjacent to a preexisting restoration (also known as secondary caries)

Caries, root surface Caries found on the roots of teeth

Cassette A light-tight device used in extraoral radiography to hold film and intensifying screens

Cathode The negative electrode in the x-ray tube; consists of a tungsten wire filament in a molybdenum cup; supplies the electrons necessary to generate x-rays

Cathode ray A stream of high-speed electrons that originates from the cathode in an x-ray tube

Cavitation A hole or cavity in a tooth that results from the caries process; appears radiolucent

Cavity See *Cavitation*

Cell The basic structural unit of living organisms

Cell differentiation Individual characteristics of a cell that determine the response of the cell to radiation exposure (e.g., cells that are immature [not highly specialized] are more sensitive to radiation)

Cell metabolism The physical and chemical processes of a cell that determine the response of the cell to radiation exposure (e.g., cells with a high metabolic rate are more sensitive to radiation)

Central ray The central portion of the primary beam of x-radiation

Cephalostat In extraoral radiography, a device used to position and stabilize the film and the patient's head

Chairside manner The method in which a dental professional conducts himself or herself at the chairside of a patient

Charge-coupled device (CCD) A solid-state detector used in many devices (e.g., fax machine, home video camera); in digital radiography, a CCD is an image receptor found in the intraoral sensor

Circuit A path of electrical current

Circuit, filament The circuit that regulates the flow of electrical current to the filament of the x-ray tube; controlled by the milliampere settings (also known as low-voltage circuit)

Circuit, high-voltage The circuit that provides the high-voltage required to accelerate electrons and to generate x-rays in the x-ray tube; controlled by the kilovoltage settings

Circuit, low-voltage See *Circuit, filament*

CMRS (complete mouth radiographic series) An intraoral series of dental radiographs that shows all of the toothbearing areas of the upper and lower jaws (also known as a full mouth series or complete series)

Coherent scatter One of the interactions of x-radiation with matter in which the path of an x-ray photon is altered by matter without a change in energy (also known as unmodified scatter)

Collimating device See *Collimator*

Collimation The restriction of the size and shape of the x-ray beam

Collimator A diaphragm, usually lead, used to restrict the size and shape of the x-ray beam

Communication The process by which information is exchanged between two or more persons

Compartment, developer A component part of the automatic processor that holds the developer solution

Compartment, fixer A component part of the automatic processor that holds the fixer solution

Compartment, water A component part of the automatic processor that holds circulating water

Compton scatter One of the interactions of x-radiation with matter in which the x-ray photon is deflected from its path and loses energy

Condensing osteitis A well-defined radiopacity seen below the apex of a nonvital tooth that has a history of a long-standing pulpitis (also known as chronic focal sclerosing osteomyelitis); appears radiopaque

Cone-cut A clear, unexposed area on a dental radiograph that occurs when the PID is misaligned and the x-ray beam is not centered over the film

Confidential   Private; in dental radiography, information contained in the dental record is confidential

Contact areas   The area where adjacent tooth surfaces contact each other

Contacts, open   On a dental radiograph, open contacts appear as a thin radiolucent line between adjacent tooth surfaces

Contacts, overlapped   On a dental radiograph, the superimposition of adjacent tooth surfaces

Contrast   The difference in degrees of blackness between adjacent areas on a radiograph

Contrast, film   The characteristics of the film that influence radiographic contrast; characteristics include the inherent qualities of the film and film processing

Contrast, high   A term describing a radiograph with many black and white areas and few shades of gray

Contrast, long-scale   A term describing a radiograph with many densities, or many shades of gray; long-scale contrast results from the use of a higher kilovoltage range

Contrast, low   A term describing a radiograph with many shades of gray and few areas of black and white

Contrast, scale of   The range of useful densities seen on a dental radiograph

Contrast, short-scale   A term describing a radiograph with two densities, areas of black and white; short-scale contrast results from the use of a lower kilovoltage range

Contrast, subject   The characteristics of the subject that influence radiographic contrast; characteristics include thickness, density, and composition of the subject

Control devices   The components of the control panel of the x-ray machine that regulate the x-ray beam; includes the timer, kilovoltage, and milliamperage selectors

Control panel   A part of the dental x-ray machine that contains an on-off switch and an indicator light, an exposure button and indicator light, and control devices to regulate the x-ray beam

Copper stem   A portion of the anode that dissipates heat away from the tungsten target

Coronoid notch   A scooped-out area of bone located distal to the coronoid process on the ramus of the mandible

Coronoid process   A marked prominence of bone located on the anterior ramus of the mandible; appears radiopaque

Cortical   The outer layer of bone; appears radiopaque

Coulomb (C)   A unit of electrical charge; the quantity of electrical charge transferred by 1 ampere in 1 second

Coulombs per kilogram (C/kg)   The unit of measurement used to describe the number of electrical charges, or the number of ion pairs, in 1 kilogram of air

Critical organ   An organ that, if damaged, diminishes the quality of an individual's life (e.g., skin, thyroid gland, lens of the eye, bone marrow)

Cumulative effects   The additive effects of repeated radiation exposure

Current, alternating (AC)   A current in which electrons flow in opposite directions

Current, direct (DC)   A current in which electrons flow in one direction

Darkroom   A completely darkened room where x-ray film is handled and processed

Darkroom plumbing   Plumbing in the darkroom that includes hot and cold water and mixing valves to adjust water temperature

Darkroom storage space   An area in the darkroom used to store chemical processing solutions, film cassettes, and other miscellaneous supplies

Darkroom work space   A clean counter area where films can be unwrapped prior to processing

Daylight loader   A light-shielded compartment on an automatic film processor; films can be unwrapped in a daylight loader in a room with white light

Density   The overall darkness or blackness of a radiograph

Dentin   The tooth layer found beneath the enamel and surrounding the pulp cavity; appears radiopaque

Dentinoenamel junction (DEJ)   The junction between the dentin and enamel of a tooth

Dentulous   With teeth; areas that exhibit teeth

Developer cut-off   A film handling error; a straight white border appears on a film as a result of using too low a level of developer solution during processing

Developer solution   A chemical solution used in film processing that makes the latent image visible

Developer spots   A chemical contamination error; dark spots appear on the film because the developer solution has come in contact with the film before processing

Developing agent   One of the four basic ingredients of the developer solution; contains two chemicals, hydroquinone and elon, which reduce halides in the film emulsion to black metallic silver

Development The first step in film processing; the developer solution reduces the halides in the film emulsion to black metallic silver and softens the film emulsion

Diagnosis Identification of a disease by examination or analysis

Digital radiography A filmless imaging system; a method of capturing a radiographic image using a sensor, breaking it into electronic pieces, and presenting and storing the image using a computer

Digital subtraction One of the features of digital radiography; a method of reversing the gray scale as an image is viewed; radiolucent images (normally black) appear white and radiopaque images (normally white) appear black

Digitize In digital radiography, to convert an image into digital form that, in turn, can be processed by a computer

Direct digital imaging A method of obtaining a digital image in which an intraoral sensor is exposed to x-rays to capture a radiographic image that can be viewed on a computer monitor

Direct theory A theory that suggests that cell damage results when ionizing radiation hits critical areas directly within the cell

Disability A physical or mental impairment that substantially limits one or more of an individual's major life activities

Disability, developmental A substantial impairment of mental or physical functioning that occurs before age 22 and is of indefinite duration

Disability, physical A physical impairment involving vision, hearing, or mobility

Disclosure In dental radiography, the process of informing a patient about the particulars of exposing dental radiographs

Disinfect To inhibit or destroy disease-causing microorganisms through use of a chemical or physical procedure

Disinfectant, high-level Chemicals used to disinfect heat-sensitive, semicritical dental instruments

Disinfectant, intermediate-level EPA-registered chemical germicides labeled "hospital infectants" and "tuberculocidal"

Disinfectant, low-level EPA-registered chemical germicides labeled only as "hospital disinfectants"

Disinfection The act of disinfecting; see *Disinfect*

Distance, object-film One of the influencing factors of image magnification; refers to the distance between the object being radiographed (e.g., tooth) and the film; less image magnification results when the tooth and x-ray film are as close as possible

Distance, target-film One of the influencing factors of image magnification; refers to the distance between the source of x-rays and the film; less image magnification results when a longer PID is used

Distortion A geometric characteristic that refers to a variation in the true size and shape of the object being radiographed; radiographic distortion is influenced by object-film alignment and x-ray beam angulation

Dose The amount of energy absorbed by a tissue

Dose, total The quantity of radiation received, or the total amount of radiation energy absorbed

Dose equivalent A measurement used to compare the biologic effects of different types of radiation

Dose rate The dose of radiation received per unit of time

Dose-response curve A curve that demonstrates the dose, or amount, of radiation received and the response of, or damage to, tissues

Drying chamber A component part of the automatic processor in which heated air is used to dry the wet films

Ear the organ of hearing

Edentulous Without teeth; areas where teeth are no longer present

Edentulous patient A patient without teeth

Electric current The flow of electrons through a conductor; an electric current is used to produce x-rays

Electricity Electric current used as a source of power; the energy used to make x-rays

Electromagnetic spectrum Energies of electromagnetic radiation arranged in diagrammatic form on a chart

Electron A tiny negatively charged particle found in the atom

Electron, Compton An outer shell electron that is ejected from its orbit during Compton scatter; this electron carries a negative charge

Electron, recoil See *Electron, Compton*

Electron-volt The unit of measurement for the binding energies of orbital electrons

Electrostatic force The attraction between the positive nucleus and the negative electrons that maintains electrons in their orbits; determined by the distance between the nucleus and electrons (also known as binding energy or binding force)

Element A simple substance made up of atoms

Elon A chemical found in the developing agent that produces a visible radiographic image and generates many shades of gray

Elongated images On a dental radiograph, images of the teeth that appear long and distorted; see *Elongation*

Elongation A term used in radiography to describe images of the teeth that appear longer than the actual tooth; elongation is the result of insufficient vertical angulation

Enamel The outermost radiopaque layer of the crown of a tooth

Endodontia Within a tooth

Endodontic patient A patient who has undergone root canal therapy

Endodontics A branch of dentistry dealing with the diagnosis and treatment of diseases of the dental pulp

Energy The capacity for doing work

Erg A unit of energy equivalent to 1.0×10^{-7} joules or 2.4×10^{-8} calories

Exposure A measure of ionization produced in air by x- or gamma radiation

Exposure, occupational Contact with blood or other infectious materials involving the skin, eye, or mucous membranes that occurs as a result of procedures performed by the dental professional

Exposure, parenteral Contact with blood or other infectious materials that occurs as a result of piercing or puncturing the skin

Exposure button A component of the dental x-ray machine control panel; activates the dental x-ray machine to produce x-rays

Exposure factors Factors that influence the density of a radiograph (e.g., milliamperage, kilovoltage, and exposure time)

Exposure incident A specific incident involving contact with blood or other potentially infectious materials that results from procedures performed by the dental professional

Exposure light A component of the dental x-ray machine control panel; provides a visible signal when x-rays are produced

Exposure sequence A specific order for the placement and exposure of intraoral films

Exposure time The time interval during which x-rays are produced

Extension arm A part of the dental x-ray machine; suspends the x-ray tubehead and houses electrical wires that extend from the control panel to the tubehead

External auditory meatus A hole or opening in the temporal bone located superior and anterior to the mastoid process

External oblique ridge A linear prominence of bone located on the external surface of the body of the mandible; appears radiopaque

Extraoral Outside the mouth

Extraoral radiographic examination A radiographic inspection of large areas of the skull or jaws using film placed outside the mouth

Extraoral radiography See *Extraoral radiographic examination*

Extrusion The abnormal displacement of teeth out of bone

Facilitation skills Interpersonal skills used to ease communication and to develop a trusting relationship between the dental professional and the patient

Film, bite-wing An intraoral film used to examine the crowns of both the maxillary and mandibular teeth on one film

Film, blue-sensitive An extraoral film that requires the use of a screen for exposure and is sensitive to blue fluorescent light; this film must be paired with screens that produce blue light

Film, cephalometric An extraoral x-ray film used to view bony and soft tissue areas of the facial profile

Film, cleaning An extraoral-size film used to clean the rollers of the automatic processor

Film D-speed An intraoral film; the letter D identifies the film speed

Film, duplicating A special type of photographic film used to make an identical copy (duplicate) of an intraoral or extraoral radiograph; this film is not exposed to x-radiation

Film, E-speed An intraoral film; the letter E identifies the film speed

Film, extraoral A type of dental x-ray film that is placed outside the mouth during x-ray exposure; extraoral films are used to examine large areas of the skull or jaws

Film, fast A type of dental x-ray film that requires less radiation for exposure (e.g., D-speed film, E-speed film)

Film, fogged A processing error; fogged film appears gray and lacks detail and contrast; results from improper safelighting or light leaks in the darkroom

Film, green-sensitive An extraoral film that requires the use of a screen for exposure and is sensitive to green fluorescent light; this film must be paired with screens that produce green light

Film, intraoral A type of dental x-ray film placed inside the mouth during x-ray exposure; intraoral films are used to examine teeth and supporting structures

Film, nonscreen An extraoral film that does not require the use of a screen for exposure

Film, occlusal An intraoral film used to examine large areas of the maxilla or mandible; the patient "occludes" or bites on the entire film

Film, overdeveloped A processing error; an overdeveloped film appears dark; results from excessive development time, inaccurate timer, hot developer solution, inaccurate thermometer, or concentrated developer solution

Film, overexposed An exposure error that results in a dark film; results from excessive exposure time, kilovoltage, milliamperage, or a combination of these factors

Film, overlapped A film handling error; films that are overlapped during processing demonstrate white or dark areas where the overlap has occurred

Film, panoramic An extraoral film that shows a panoramic (wide) view of the upper and lower jaw on a single radiograph

Film, periapical An intraoral film used to examine the entire tooth and supporting bone

Film, scratched A film handling error; a scratched film exhibits white lines where the emulsion has been removed from the film base by a sharp object (e.g., a film clip or hanger)

Film, screen An extraoral film that requires the use of a screen for exposure

Film, standard See *Film, periapical*

Film, underdeveloped A processing error; an underdeveloped film appears light; results from inadequate development time, inaccurate timer, cool developer temperature, inaccurate thermometer, or depleted or contaminated developer solution

Film, underexposed An exposure error that results in a light film; results from inadequate exposure time, kilovoltage, milliamperage, or a combination of these factors

Film, x-ray An image receptor that consists of a film base, adhesive layer, film emulsion, and protective layer; an image is recorded when the film is exposed to x-rays

Film, yellow-brown A processing error; this film appears yellow-brown; results from exhausted developer or fixer, insufficient fixation time, or insufficient rinsing

Film badge A device used to measure and monitor radiation exposure; worn by persons frequently exposed to radiation

Film base A flexible piece of plastic that provides a stable support for the film emulsion as well as strength

Film composition The formulation of the film emulsion; depends on the size of the crystals in the film emulsion (e.g., the smaller the crystals, the sharper the radiographic image)

Film duplicator A light source used to expose duplicating film

Film emulsion A coating on radiographic film attached to the film base by an adhesive layer; a mixture of gelatin and silver halide crystals

Film feed slot An opening on the outside of the automatic processor housing; used to insert unwrapped films into the automatic processor

Film hangers A stainless steel device equipped with clips; used to hold films during manual processing

Film holder A device used to hold and align intraoral films in the mouth (also known as film-holding devices)

Film holder, EEZEE-Grip A type of film-holding device used to stabilize film (formerly known as Snap-A-Ray)

Film holder, hemostat A small surgical clamp inserted through a rubber bite-block and used to stabilize film

Film holder, precision A type of film-holding device that includes a metal collimating shield to restrict the size of the x-ray beam

Film holder, Stabe A disposable film holder designed for one-time use only

Film-holding device See *Film holder*

Film mount A cardboard, plastic, or vinyl holder used to support and arrange dental radiographs in anatomic order

Film mounting The placement of radiographs in a supporting structure or holder

Film placement The specific area where a film is positioned prior to exposure

Film recovery slot An opening on the outside of the automatic processor housing where dry, processed radiographs emerge

Film speed The sensitivity of a film to radiation exposure

Film viewing In dental radiography, the examining of dental radiographs on a light source

Filtration The use of absorbing materials (e.g., aluminum) for removing the low-energy x-rays from the primary beam

Filtration, added Aluminum disks inserted in the dental x-ray machine between the x-ray tube and collimator; absorb low-energy x-rays

Filtration, inherent Filtration placed in the x-ray tube by the manufacturer; includes the glass window of the x-ray tube, insulating oil, and the tube-head seal

Filtration, total The combination of the inherent filtration and added filtration in an x-ray machine

Finger-holding method A method of exposing films in which the patient's finger or thumb stabilizes the film from behind the teeth

Fingernail artifact A film handling error; a fingernail artifact exhibits black, crescent-shaped marks where the film has been damaged by the operator's fingernail during rough handling of the film

Fingerprint artifact A film handling error; a black fingerprint appears on a film wherever the film has been touched by fingers contaminated with fluoride or developer

Fixation A step in film processing; the fixer solution removes the unexposed, undeveloped silver halide crystals from the film emulsion and hardens the film emulsion

Fixer cut-off A film handling error; a straight black border appears on a film as a result of using too low a level of fixer solution during processing

Fixer solution A chemical solution used in film processing; removes the unexposed silver halide crystals and creates white or clear areas on the film

Fixer spots A chemical contamination error; white spots appear on a film as a result of fixer solution contacting the film before processing

Fixing agent One of the four basic ingredients of the fixer solution; contains hypo (sodium thiosulfate or ammonium thiosulfate), which removes or clears all unexposed and undeveloped silver halide crystals from the film emulsion (also known as clearing agent)

Floor of nasal cavity A bony wall formed by the palatal processes of the maxilla and the horizontal processes of the palatine bones; appears radiopaque

Fluoresce To emit visible light in the blue or green spectrum

Fluorescence The emission of a glowing light by certain substances when struck by a particular wavelength (e.g., calcium tungstate screens have phosphors that emit blue light, or fluoresce, when exposed to x-rays)

Focal spot size The size of the tungsten target of the anode; ranges from 0.6 mm^2 to 1.0 mm^2 and is determined by the manufacturer of the x-ray machine

Focal trough A three-dimensional curved zone or image layer in which structures are reasonably well defined; in panoramic radiography, a patient must be positioned so that the dental arches are located within the focal trough area

Foramen An opening or hole in bone; appears radiolucent

Foreshortened images Images of the teeth that appear short with blunted roots; see *Foreshortening*

Foreshortening A term describing images of the teeth that appear too short; foreshortening is the result of excessive vertical angulation

Fossa A broad, shallow, scooped-out or depressed area of bone; appears radiolucent

Fracture The breaking of a part; appears as a thin radiolucent line

Frankfort plane The imaginary plane that intersects the orbital rim of the eye and the opening of the ear

Free radical An uncharged, neutral molecule that exists with a single, unpaired electron in its outermost shell

Frequency The number of wavelengths that pass a given point in a certain amount of time; frequency indicates the energy of a radiation (e.g., high-frequency radiations have more energy than low-frequency radiations)

Furcation area The area between the roots of multi-rooted teeth

Gag reflex Retching evoked by the stimulation of the sensitive tissues of the soft palate (also known as the pharyngeal reflex)

Gagging The strong involuntary effort to vomit (also known as retching)

Gelatin A component of the film emulsion that suspends and disperses silver halide crystals over the film base

Genetic cells Cells that contain genes; reproductive cells (e.g., ova, sperm)

Genetic effects Effects of radiation that are passed on to future generations through genetic cells

Genial tubercles Tiny bumps of bone in the anterior region of the mandible that serve as attachment sites for the genioglossus and geniohyoid muscles; appear radiopaque

Ghost image An artifact on a dental radiograph produced when an area of high density (e.g., earring) is penetrated twice by the x-ray beam; appears radiopaque

Glenoid fossa   A concave, depressed area of the temporal bone on which the mandibular condyle rests

Glossopharyngeal air space   An air space that appears as a radiolucency on a panoramic film posterior to the tongue and oral cavity

Gray (Gy)   A unit for measuring absorbed dose; the SI unit equivalent to the rad; 1 gray = 100 rad

Grid   In extraoral radiography, a device used to prevent scatter radiation from reaching the film during exposure

Half-value layer (HVL)   The thickness of material that, when placed in the path of the x-ray beam, reduces the exposure rate by one-half

Halide   A compound of a halogen (e.g., astatine, bromine, chlorine, fluorine, iodine) and another element; in dental radiography, a halide, such as silver bromide, is suspended in the gelatin of the emulsion

Hamulus   A small, hook-like projection of bone that extends from the medial pterygoid plate of the sphenoid bone; appears radiopaque

Hardening agent   One of the four basic ingredients of the fixer solution; contains the chemical potassium alum that hardens and shrinks the gelatin in the film emulsion

Head positioner   One of the component parts of a panoramic unit consisting of a chin rest, bite stick, forehead rest, and lateral head supports

Hemostat   A small surgical clamp

Herringbone pattern   An image on a dental radiograph that has been placed in the mouth backward and exposed (also known as tire-track pattern)

Humidity level   The amount of moisture in the air

Hydroquinone   A chemical found in the developing agent that generates the black tones and sharp contrast of the radiographic image

Hypercementosis   The excess deposition of cementum on the root surfaces of teeth; appears radiopaque

Hypo   Sodium thiosulfate or ammonium thiosulfate; a common name for these chemicals found in the fixing agent

Hypotenuse   The side of a right triangle opposite the right angle

Identification dot   A small raised dot that appears in one corner of an intraoral film; used to determine film orientation

Image   A picture or likeness of an object

Image receptor   The dental x-ray film; a recording medium; images are recorded on x-ray film when the film is exposed to x-radiation or light

Impulse   In dental radiography, a measure of exposure time; 60 impulses occur in 1 second

Incipient   Small; beginning to exist or appear

Incisive canal   A passageway through bone that extends from the superior foramina of the incisive canal to the incisive foramen

Incisive foramen   An opening or hole in bone located at the midline of the anterior portion of the hard palate directly posterior to the maxillary central incisors; appears radiolucent

Indicator light   A component of the dental x-ray machine control panel; when illuminated, indicates that the dental x-ray machine is turned on

Indirect digital imaging   A method of obtaining a digital image in which an existing radiograph is scanned and converted into digital form using a CCD camera

Indirect theory   A theory suggesting that cell damage results indirectly; x-ray photons are absorbed with the cell, causing the formation of toxins; toxins in turn damage the cell

Infectious waste   Waste that consists of blood, blood products, contaminated sharps, or other microbiologic products

Inferior border of the mandible   A linear prominence of cortical bone that defines the lower border of the mandible

Inferior nasal conchae   Wafer-thin curved plates of bone that extend from the lateral walls of the nasal cavity and appear radiopaque

Informed consent   Permission granted by a patient after the patient has been informed about the particulars of a procedure

Infraorbital foramen   A hole or opening in bone found inferior to the border of the orbit

Instrument, critical   Instruments that are used to penetrate soft tissue or bone

Instrument, noncritical   Instruments that do not come in contact with mucous membranes

Instrument, Rinn XCP   Instruments used with the paralleling technique; these include plastic biteblocks, plastic aiming rings, and metal indicator arms (X = extension, C = cone, P = paralleling)

Instrument, semicritical   Instruments that contact but do not penetrate soft tissue or bone

Insulating oil   Oil that surrounds the x-ray tube and transformers inside the tubehead

Intensity   The total energy of the x-ray beam; the product of the quantity (number of x-ray photons) and quality (energy of each photon) per unit of area per time of exposure

Internal oblique ridge A linear prominence of bone located on the internal surface of the mandible that extends downward and forward from the ramus; appears radiopaque

Interpersonal skills Skills that promote a good relationship between individuals

Interpret To offer an explanation

Interpretation An explanation

Interpretation, radiographic An explanation of what is viewed on a dental radiograph; the ability to read what is revealed by a dental radiograph

Interproximal Between two adjacent surfaces

Interproximal examination A radiographic inspection used to examine the crowns of both the maxillary and mandibular teeth on a single film

Intersecting Cutting across or through

Intraoral Inside the mouth

Intraoral radiographic examination A radiographic inspection of teeth and intraoral adjacent structures

Intraoral radiography See *Intraoral radiographic examination*

Intrusion The abnormal displacement of teeth into bone

Inverse square law A rule that states that "the intensity of radiation is inversely proportional to the square of the distance from the source of radiation"; as distance is increased, radiation intensity at the object is decreased, and vice versa

Inverted Y A radiographic landmark that represents the intersection of the maxillary sinus and the nasal cavity; appears radiopaque

Ion An electrically charged particle; an atom that gains or loses an electron

Ion pair A pair of ions, one positive and one negative, that results when an electron is removed from an atom in the ionization process

Ionization The production of ions; the process of converting an atom into an ion

Isometry Equality of measurement

Isometry, rule of A geometric principle that states that "two triangles are equal if they have two equal angles and share a common side"

Joule (J) The SI unit of measurement equivalent to the work done by the force of 1 newton acting over the distance of 1 meter

Kilo-electron-volt (keV) 1000 electron-volts; the unit of measurement for the binding energies of orbital electrons

Kilogram (kg) 1000 grams; a unit equivalent to 2.205 pounds

Kilovolt (kV) 1000 volts; a unit of electromotive force that drives an electrical current through a circuit

Kilovoltage In radiography, the x-ray tube peak voltage used during an exposure; measured in kilovolts

Kilovoltage peak (kVp) The maximum or peak voltage that is used during an x-ray exposure

Kinetic energy Energy of motion

Label side The outer side of the x-ray film packet that is color coded and contains printed information; the label side of the film faces the tongue

Labial mounting A film mounting method in which radiographs are placed in the film mount with the raised side of the identification dot facing the viewer; the dental radiographer then views the radiographs from the labial aspect

Lamina dura The wall of the tooth socket that surrounds the root of a tooth; appears radiopaque

Latent image The invisible image produced when the film is exposed to x-rays; remains invisible until the film is processed

Latent image centers Aggregates of neutral silver atoms on exposed crystals that collectively become the latent image on the emulsion of the film

Latent period The amount of time that elapses between exposure to ionizing radiation and the appearance of observable clinical signs

Lateral cephalometric projection An extraoral radiographic projection used to determine facial growth in orthodontics and used as a pre- and post-treatment record in oral surgery and orthodontics

Lateral fossa A smooth depressed area of the maxilla located between the canine and lateral incisor; appears radiolucent

Lateral jaw projection—body of mandible An extraoral radiographic projection used to image the posterior body of the mandible

Lateral jaw projection—ramus of mandible An extraoral radiographic projection used to image the ramus of the mandible

Lateral pterygoid plate A wing-shaped bony projection of the sphenoid bone located distal to the maxillary tuberosity region

Lead apron A flexible lead shield used to protect the patient's reproductive and blood-forming tissues from scatter radiation

Lead collimator A lead diaphragm or tubular device used to restrict the size and shape of the x-ray beam

Lead foil sheet One of the four components of the dental x-ray film packet; a single piece of embossed lead foil placed behind the film to shield the film from scattered radiation

Leaded-glass housing The leaded-glass housing of the x-ray tube

Liable Accountable; legally obligated

Light leak (1) Any white light that is seen when all the lights are turned off and the door is closed; (2) an exposure error; a black area appearing on a film as a result of exposure of the film to white light

Light-tight A term used to describe the darkroom, a room that is completely dark and excludes all white light

Lingula A small, tongue-shaped projection of bone seen adjacent to the mandibular foramen

Lingual foramen An opening or hole in bone located on the internal surface of the mandible near the midline; it is surrounded by the genial tubercles and appears radiolucent

Lingual mounting A film mounting method in which radiographs are placed in the film mount with the depressed side of the identification dot facing the viewer; the dental radiographer then views the radiographs from the lingual aspect

Lipline An artifact seen on panoramic radiographs formed by the position of the patient's lips

Localization techniques Radiographic techniques used to determine the buccal or lingual relationship of an object (e.g., foreign bodies, impacted or un-erupted teeth, retained roots, root positions, salivary stones, jaw fractures, broken instruments, or filling materials)

Long axis (tooth) An imaginary line that divides a tooth longitudinally into two equal halves

Long-term effects Effects of radiation that appear years, decades, or generations after exposure; associated with small amounts of radiation absorbed repeatedly over a long period of time

Luxation The abnormal displacement of teeth

Magnification A geometric characteristic; refers to a radiographic image that appears larger than the actual size of the object it represents; influenced by target-film distance and object-film distance

Malpractice Improper or negligent conduct or treatment

Mandibular canal A tube-like passageway through bone in the mandible; appears radiolucent

Mandibular condyle A rounded projection of bone extending from the posterior superior border of the ramus of the mandible

Mandibular foramen An opening or hole in bone on the lingual aspect of the ramus of the mandible

Mass Weight; the physical volume or bulk of a solid body

Mass number See *Atomic weight*

Mastoid process A marked prominence of bone located posterior and inferior to the temporomandibular joint

Matter Something that occupies space and has weight

Maxillary sinus Paired cavities or compartments of bone located within the maxilla; appears radiolucent

Maxillary tuberosity A rounded prominence of bone that extends posterior to the third molar region; appears radiopaque

Maximum accumulated dose (MAD) The maximum radiation dose that may be received by persons who are occupationally exposed to radiation

Maximum permissible dose (MPD) The maximum accumulated dose that may be received during a specific period of time by persons who are occupationally exposed to radiation

Median palatal suture The immovable joint between the two palatine processes of the maxilla; appears radiolucent

Mental foramen An opening or hole in bone located on the external surface of the mandible in the region of the mandibular premolars; appears radiolucent

Mental fossa A scooped-out, depressed area of bone located on the external surface of the anterior mandible; appears radiolucent

Mental ridge A linear prominence of cortical bone located on the external surface of the anterior portion of the mandible; appears radiopaque

Metal housing The metal body of the dental x-ray tubehead that surrounds the x-ray tube and transformers

Midsagittal plane An imaginary line or plane passing through the center of the body that divides it into right and left halves

Milliamperage In radiography, the intensity of the x-ray tube current used during exposure; measured in milliamperes

Milliampere (mA) 1/1000 of an ampere; a unit of measurement used to describe the intensity of an electric current

Milliampere-second (mAs) A unit of radiographic exposure equal to the product of milliamperage and exposure time

Mitotic activity Process of cell division; determines the response of a cell to radiation exposure (e.g., cells that divide frequently are more sensitive to radiation)

Molecule   Two or more atoms joined together by chemical bonds, or the smallest amount of a substance that possesses its characteristic properties

Molybdenum cup   A portion of the cathode in the x-ray tube; focuses the electrons into a narrow beam and directs the beam across the tube toward the tungsten target in the anode

Mount   To place in an appropriate setting, as for display or study

Movement   Movement or motion of the film or patient during radiographic exposure; movement results in a radiographic image with less sharpness

Mylohyoid ridge   A linear prominence of bone located on the internal surface of the mandible; appears radiopaque

Nanometer   A measurement used for wave-length; 1 nanometer equals one-billionth (10^{-9}) of a meter

Nasal cavity   A pear-shaped compartment of bone located superior to the maxilla; appears radiolucent

Nasal septum   A vertical bony wall or partition that divides the nasal cavity into the right and left nasal fossae; appears radiopaque

Nasopharyngeal air space   An air space viewed on a panoramic film that appears as a diagonal radiolucency superior to the soft palate and uvula

Negligence   Omission or failure to provide reasonable precaution, care, or action

Neutron   An electrically neutral or uncharged particle with a mass of one

Nonstochastic effects   Somatic effects that have a threshold and increase in severity with increasing absorbed dose

Normalizing device   A commercially available device used to monitor developer strength and film density

Nucleon   Part of an atomic nucleus (e.g., protons and neutrons)

Nucleus   The central, positively charged core of an atom; composed of protons and neutrons

Nutrient canal(s)   A tiny tube-like passageway through bone that houses nerves and blood vessels; appears radiolucent

Occlusal   The chewing surfaces of the teeth

Occlusal examination   A radiographic examination used to inspect large areas of the maxilla or the mandible on one film

Occlusal projection, mandibular cross-sectional   A type of occlusal projection used to examine the buccal and lingual aspects of the mandible and locate foreign bodies (e.g., salivary stones) in the floor of the mouth

Occlusal projection, mandibular pediatric   A type of occlusal projection used to examine the anterior teeth of the mandible; recommended for children aged 5 years or younger

Occlusal projection, mandibular topographic   A type of occlusal projection used to examine the anterior teeth of the mandible

Occlusal projection, maxillary lateral   A type of occlusal projection used to examine the palatal roots of the molar teeth and locate foreign bodies or lesions in the posterior maxilla

Occlusal projection, maxillary pediatric   A type of occlusal projection used to examine the anterior teeth of the maxilla; recommended for children aged 5 years or younger

Occlusal projection, maxillary topographic   A type of occlusal projection used to examine the palate and anterior teeth of the maxilla

Occlusal surfaces   The chewing surfaces of the posterior teeth

Occlusal technique   A method of radiographic exposure in which large areas of the maxilla or mandible are examined

On-off switch   A component of the control panel on the dental x-ray machine; turns the dental x-ray machine on or off

Operating kilovoltage   See *Kilovoltage*

Orbit   The well-defined path of an electron around the nucleus of an atom (also known as shell)

Outer package wrapping   One of the four components of the dental x-ray film packet; a soft vinyl or paper wrapper that serves to protect the film from exposure to light and saliva

Oxidation   A chemical reaction that occurs when processing solutions are exposed to air; the chemicals break down, resulting in a decreased concentration of solution strength

Packet, film   The intraoral film and its surrounding packaging

Packet, one-film   A film packet containing one film

Packet, two-film   A film packet containing two films

Palate   Roof of the mouth

Palate, hard   The anterior portion of the roof of the mouth

Palate, soft   The posterior portion of the roof of the mouth separating the mouth and pharynx

Palatoglossal air space   An air space on a panoramic film that appears as a horizontal radiolucency between the hard palate and the tongue

Panoramic   A wide view

Panoramic radiography   An extraoral radiographic technique used to examine the upper and lower jaws on a single film (also known as rotational panoramic radiography)

Paper film wrapper   One of the four components of the dental x-ray film packet; a black paper protective sheet covers the film and shields it from light

Parallel   Moving or lying in the same plane; always separated by the same distance and not intersecting

Paralleling technique   An intraoral radiographic technique used to expose periapical films, based on the following concepts: the film is placed parallel to the long axis of the tooth; the central ray is directed perpendicular to the film and long axis of the tooth; a film holder must be used

Pathogen   A microorganism capable of causing disease

Patient relations   The relationship between the patient and the dental professional

Pediatric   A term derived from the Greek word *pedia* meaning child

Pediatric patient   A child patient

Pediatrics   A branch of dentistry dealing with the diagnosis and treatment of dental diseases in children

Penumbra   The unsharpness, or blurring, that surrounds the edges of a radiographic image

Periapical   Around the apex of a tooth

Periapical abscess   A lesion characterized by a localized collection of pus around the apex of a nonvital tooth that results from pulpal death; appears radiolucent

Periapical cyst   A lesion characterized by an epithelial-lined cavity or sac located around the apex of a nonvital tooth that results from pulpal death; appears radiolucent

Periapical examination   A radiographic inspection used to examine the entire tooth and supporting bone

Periapical granuloma   A lesion characterized by a localized mass of granulation tissue, around the apex of a nonvital tooth; appears radiolucent

Periodic table of the elements   A chart that arranges elements in increasing atomic number

Periodontal   Around a tooth

Periodontal disease   A group of diseases that affects the tissues around the teeth

Periodontal ligament space   A space that exists between the root of a tooth and the lamina dura; contains connective tissue fibers, blood vessels, and lymphatics; appears radiolucent

Periodontium   Tissues that invest and support the teeth, such as the gingiva and alveolar bone

Perpendicular   Intersecting at or forming right angles

Phalangioma   An error on a dental radiograph that results from the patient's finger being placed in front of the film; the term refers to the distal phalanx of the finger

Phosphors   Minute crystals that cover intensifying screens and fluoresce, or emit visible light, when exposed to x-rays

Photoelectric effect   One of the interactions of x-radiation with matter; an x-ray photon interacts with an orbital electron, and all of the energy of the photon is absorbed by the displaced electron in the form of kinetic energy

Photon   A bundle of energy with no mass or weight that travels as a wave at the speed of light and moves through space in a straight line

Pixel   A discrete unit of information. In digital electronic images, digital information is contained in, and presented as, discrete units of information (synonym, picture element)

Polychromatic x-ray beam   An x-ray beam containing many different wavelengths of varying intensities

Position-indicating device (PID)   An open-ended, lead-lined cylinder extending from the opening of the metal housing of the tubehead; aims and shapes the x-ray beam (also called the cone)

Posteroanterior projection   An extraoral radiographic projection of the skull used to evaluate facial growth, trauma, diseases, and developmental abnormalities

Potassium alum   The hardening agent in the fixer solution that hardens and shrinks the gelatin in the film emulsion

Potassium bromide   The restrainer in the developing solution; prevents the development of unexposed silver halide crystals; prevents film fogging

Preservative   (1) One of the four basic ingredients of the developer solution; sodium sulfite prevents the developer solution from oxidizing in the presence of air; (2) one of the four basic ingredients of the fixer solution; sodium sulfite prevents the chemical deterioration of the fixing agent

Primary beam   See *Radiation, primary*

Process   A marked prominence of bone; appears radiopaque

Processing, automatic   A method used to process films in which all film processing steps are automated

Processing, film   A series of steps that collectively produce a visible, permanent image on a dental radiograph

Processing, manual   A method used to process films

in which all film processing steps are performed manually (also known as hand processing or tank processing)

Processor, automatic A machine that automates all film processing steps

Processor housing The housing, or protective covering, of the automatic film processor; encases all of the component parts of the automatic processor

Protective barrier A barrier of radiation-absorbing material used to reduce radiation exposure (e.g., a wall)

Protective layer One of the four basic components of x-ray film; a thin, protective coating on top of the emulsion protects the film from manipulation and mechanical and processing damage

Proton A positively charged particle with a mass of one

Pterygomaxillary fissure A narrow space or cleft that separates the lateral pterygoid plate and the maxilla

Pulp cavity A cavity within a tooth that includes both the pulp chamber and the pulp canals; contains blood vessels, nerves, and lymphatics; appears radiolucent

Pulp stones Calcifications found in the pulp chamber or pulp canals of teeth; appear radiopaque

Pulpal obliteration Total calcification of the pulp cavity; appears radiopaque

Pulpal sclerosis A diffuse calcification of the pulp chamber and pulp canals of teeth that results in a pulp cavity of decreased size; appears radiopaque

Quality (of x-ray beam) The mean energy or penetrating ability of the x-ray beam; the quality of the x-ray beam is controlled by kilovoltage

Quality administration The management of the quality assurance plan in the dental office

Quality assurance Special procedures used to ensure the production of high-quality, diagnostic radiographs

Quality control tests Specific tests designed to maintain and monitor dental x-ray equipment, supplies, and film processing

Quality factor (QF) A factor used for radiation protection purposes that accounts for the exposure effects of different types of radiation; for x-rays QF = 1

Quanta See *Photon*

Quantity (of x-ray beam) The number of x-rays produced from the tubehead; the quantity of x-rays produced is controlled by milliamperage

Radiation The emission and propagation of energy through space or a material in the form of waves or stream of particles

Radiation, background A form of ionizing radiation that is ubiquitous in the environment; includes cosmic and terrestrial radiation

Radiation, bremsstrahlung See *Radiation, general*

Radiation, characteristic A form of radiation that occurs when a high-speed electron dislodges an inner shell electron from an atom, causing excitation, or ionization, of the atom

Radiation, electromagnetic The propagation of wave-like energy through space or matter; the propagated energy is accompanied by electric and magnetic fields, hence the term electromagnetic; examples include cosmic rays, gamma rays, x-rays, ultraviolet rays, visible light, infrared light, radar waves, microwaves, and radio waves

Radiation, general A form of radiation that occurs when speeding electrons are slowed because of their interactions with the nuclei of target atoms (also known as bremsstrahlung or braking radiation, referring to the sudden stopping or slowing of high-speed electrons hitting the target)

Radiation, ionizing Radiation capable of producing ions; includes particulate or electromagnetic radiation

Radiation, leakage X-rays that escape from the dental x-ray tubehead, with the exception of the primary beam

Radiation, particulate Tiny particles of matter that possess mass, travel in straight lines, and travel at high speeds (e.g., electrons, beta particles, alpha particles, protons, and neutrons)

Radiation, primary The penetrating x-ray beam produced at the target of the anode (also known as the primary or useful beam)

Radiation, scatter A form of secondary radiation; results from an x-ray beam that has been deflected from its path by the interaction with matter

Radiation, secondary Radiation created when the primary beam interacts with matter; secondary radiation is less penetrating than primary radiation

Radiation absorbed dose (rad) A unit for measuring absorbed dose; the traditional unit of dose equivalent to the gray (Gy); 100 erg of energy per gram of tissue; 100 rad = 1 Gy

Radiation biology The study of the effects of ionizing radiation on living tissues

Radioactivity The process by which certain unstable atoms or elements undergo spontaneous disintegration in an effort to attain a more balanced nuclear state

Radiograph An image produced on photosensitive film by exposing the film to x-rays and then processing the film (also known as x-ray film)

Radiograph, dental Images of teeth and related structures produced on film by exposing the film to x-rays and then processing the film

Radiograph, diagnostic A radiograph that provides a great deal of information with images that have proper density and contrast, sharp outlines, and are of the same shape and size as the object being radiographed

Radiograph, duplicate An identical copy of a radiograph that is made through the process of film duplication

Radiograph, extraoral See *Film, extraoral*

Radiograph, intraoral See *Film, intraoral*

Radiograph, reference A radiograph processed under ideal conditions and then used to compare the film densities of radiographs that are processed daily

Radiographer, dental Any person who positions, exposes, and processes dental x-ray film

Radiography The making of radiographs by the exposure of film to x-rays

Radiography, dental The making of radiographs of the teeth and adjacent structures by the exposure of film to x-rays

Radiology The science or study of radiation as used in medicine

Radiolucent The portion of a processed radiograph that is dark or black; a radiolucent structure readily permits the passage of the x-ray beam and allows more x-rays to reach the film

Radiopaque The portion of a processed radiograph that is light or white; a radiopaque structure is one that resists the passage of the x-ray beam and limits the amount of x-rays that reach the film

Radioresistant cell A cell that is resistant to radiation (e.g., bone, muscle, and nerve)

Radiosensitive cell A cell that is sensitive to radiation (e.g., small lymphocyte, blood cells, immature reproductive cells, young bone cells, epithelial cells)

Rampant Growing or spreading unchecked

Receptor Something that responds to a stimulus

Recovery period The period during which cellular damage is followed by repair

Rectification The conversion of alternating current to direct current

Reduction A chemical reaction during film processing in which the halide portion of the exposed energized silver halide crystal is removed

Reduction, selective A chemical reaction during film processing in which the energized exposed silver halide crystals are changed into black metallic silver, while the unenergized unexposed silver halide crystals are removed from the film

Replenisher A superconcentrated solution added to a processing solution to compensate for the loss of volume and strength that results from oxidation

Replenisher pump A component part of the automatic film processor; automatically maintains proper concentrations and levels of solutions

Replenisher solutions See *Replenisher*

Resorption, external A regressive alteration of tooth structure that occurs along the periphery of the root surface

Resorption, internal A regressive alteration of tooth structure that occurs within the crown or root of a tooth; appears as a radiolucency

Resorption, pathologic Resorption of a tooth not associated with the normal shedding of deciduous teeth

Resorption, physiologic Resorption of the teeth associated with the normal shedding of deciduous teeth

Restrainer One of the four basic ingredients of the developer solution; potassium bromide is used to prevent the development of unexposed silver halide crystals; also prevents film fogging

Reticulation of emulsion A temperature error; a film has a cracked appearance as the result of being subjected to sudden temperature changes

Reverse Towne projection An extraoral radiographic projection used to identify fractures of the condylar neck and ramus area

Ridge A linear prominence of bone; appears radiopaque

Right-angle technique A localization technique in which the orientation of structures can be seen in two radiographs (one periapical and one occlusal)

Rinsing One of the five steps in film processing; a water bath is used to rinse the developer from the film and stop the development process

Risk The likelihood of adverse effects or death resulting from exposure to a hazard

Risk management The policies and procedures that the dental professional should follow to reduce the chance that a patient will take legal action

Roentgen (R) The traditional unit of exposure for x-rays; the quantity of x-radiation or gamma radiation that produces an electrical charge of 2.58×10^{-4} coulombs in 1 kilogram of air at standard pressure and temperature conditions

Roentgen equivalent (in) man (rem)   The traditional unit of the dose equivalent; the product of absorbed dose (rad) and a quality factor (QF) specific for the type of radiation; 100 rem = 1 sievert (Sv)

Roller film transporter   A component part of the automatic film processor; a system of rollers is used to rapidly move the film through the developer, fixer, water, and the drying compartments

Room lighting   One of the two essential types of lighting in a darkroom; room lighting provides adequate illumination for the size of the room to perform tasks such as cleaning, stocking of materials, and mixing of chemicals

Rotation center   In panoramic radiography, the axis on which the film and x-ray tubehead rotate around the patient

Safelight filter   A filter placed over the safelight that is designed to remove the short wavelengths in the blue-green portion of the visible light spectrum that are responsible for exposing and damaging x-ray film

Safelighting   One of the two essential types of lighting in a darkroom; a low-intensity light composed of long wavelengths in the red-orange portion of the visible light spectrum; safelighting provides sufficient illumination in the darkroom to carry out processing activities without exposing or damaging the film

Sclerotic bone   A well-defined radiopacity seen below the apices of vital, noncarious teeth (also known as osteosclerosis, or idiopathic periapical osteosclerosis)

Screen, calcium tungstate   A type of intensifying screen used in extraoral radiography; contains phosphors that emit blue light

Screen, intensifying   A device used in extraoral radiography that converts x-ray energy into visible light; the light, in turn, exposes the screen film

Screen, rare earth   A type of intensifying screen used in extraoral radiography; contains phosphors not commonly found in the earth that emit green light

Self-determination   The legal rights of an individual to make choices about the care he or she receives, including the opportunity to consent to or refuse treatment

Sensitivity speck   An irregularity within the lattice structure of the exposed silver halide crystals that attracts the silver atoms

Sensor   In digital radiography, a small detector that is placed intraorally to capture a radiographic image

Septa   Bony walls that divide a cavity into separate areas; appear radiopaque

Sharp   Any object that can penetrate skin including, but not limited to, needles and scalpels

Sharpness   A geometric characteristic that refers to the capability of x-ray film to reproduce the distinct outlines of an object; influenced by focal spot size, film composition, and movement

Shell   See *Orbit*

Short-term effects   Effects of radiation that appear within minutes, days, or weeks; associated with large amounts of radiation absorbed in a short period of time

Sievert (Sv)   A unit of measurement for dose equivalent; the SI unit of measurement equivalent to the rem; 1 Sv = 100 rem

Silver halide crystals   Crystals that are suspended in the emulsion of the dental x-ray film (e.g., silver bromide, silver iodide); functions to absorb radiation during x-ray exposure and store energy from the radiation

Sinus   A hollow space, cavity, or recess in bone; appears radiolucent

Sodium carbonate   See *Accelerator*

Sodium sulfite   See *Preservative*

Sodium thiosulfate   See *Fixing agent*

Somatic cells   All of the cells in the body, with the exception of the reproductive cells

Somatic effects   Radiation effects that are responsible for poor health (e.g, the induction of cancer, leukemia, and cataracts)

Spine   A sharp projection of bone; appears radiopaque

Standard of care   In dentistry, the quality of care that is provided by dental practitioners in a similar locality under the same or similar conditions

Static electricity   A film handling error; thin, black, branching lines on a film that result from opening a film packet too quickly

Statute of limitations   A period of time during which a patient may bring a malpractice action against a dentist or an auxiliary

Stepwedge   A device constructed of layered aluminum steps used to demonstrate film densities and contrast scales

Sterilization   The act of sterilizing; see *Sterilize*

Sterilize   The use of a physical or chemical procedure to destroy all pathogens, including the highly resistant bacterial and fungal spores

Stimuli, psychogenic   Stimuli originating in the mind

Stimuli, tactile   Stimuli originating from touch

Stirring paddle   A device used in manual processing; agitates the developer and fixer solutions and equalizes the temperature of the solutions prior to processing

Stirring rod   See *Stirring paddle*

Stochastic effects   Occur as a direct function of dose; the probability of occurrence increases with increasing absorbed dose; however, the severity of effects does not depend on the magnitude of the absorbed dose

Storage phosphor imaging   A method of obtaining a digital image in which the image is recorded on phosphor coated plates and then placed into an electronic processor where a laser scans the plate and produces an image on a computer screen

Subject thickness   The thickness of soft tissue and bone in a patient

Submandibular fossa   A depressed area of bone along the lingual surface of the mandible; appears radiolucent

Submentovertex projection   An extraoral radiographic projection used to identify the position of the condyles, demonstrate the base of the skull, and evaluate fractures of the zygomatic arch

Sulfuric acid   See *Acidifier*

Superior foramina of the incisive canal   Two tiny openings in bone located on the floor of the nasal cavity; appear radiolucent

Suture   An immovable joint that represents a line of union between adjoining bones of the skull; appears radiolucent

Tank, insert   In manual processing, a component part of the processing tank; two removable insert tanks are placed in the master tank and hold the developer and fixer solutions

Tank, master   In manual processing, a component part of the processing tank; the master tank is filled with circulating water that surrounds and suspends the two insert tanks

Tank, processing   A tank used in manual processing; divided into compartments for the developer solution, water bath, and fixer solution; a processing tank has two insert tanks and one master tank

Teeth, anterior   Incisors and canines

Teeth, posterior   Premolars and molars

Temporomandibular joint   A joint in the skull that joins the temporal bone and mandible; includes the mandibular condyle, glenoid fossa, articular eminence, and the articular disk (also known as TMJ)

Temporomandibular joint tomography   An extraoral radiographic technique used to examine the temporomandibular joint

Thermionic emission   The release of electrons that occurs when the tungsten filament of the cathode is heated to incandescence; the outer shell electrons of the tungsten atom acquire enough energy to move away from the filament surface and form an electron cloud

Thermometer   A device used to measure temperature

Thyroid collar   A flexible lead shield used to protect the thyroid gland from scatter radiation

Timer   A mechanical device used to measure time intervals

Tomogram   An extraoral radiograph used to examine the bony components of the TMJ

Tomography   A radiographic technique used to image a selected plane of tissue while blurring structures that are outside of the selected plane

Tongue   A muscular organ located on the floor of the mouth

Tooth-bearing areas   Regions of the maxilla and mandible in which the 32 teeth of the human dentition are normally located

Torus (tori, plural)   A bony growth in the oral cavity

Torus, mandibular   A bony growth seen along the lingual aspect of the mandible (also known as the torus mandibularis)

Torus, maxillary   A nodular mass of bone along the midline of the hard palate (also known as the torus palatinus)

Transcranial projection   An extraoral radiographic projection used to evaluate the superior surface of the condyle and the articular eminence; this view can also be used to evaluate the movement of the condyle when the mouth is opened (also called the Lindblom technique)

Transformer   A device used to increase or decrease the voltage of incoming electricity

Transformer, step-down   In dental radiography, a device used to decrease the incoming voltage from 110 or 220 volts to the low voltage required, usually 3 to 5 volts

Transformer, step-up   In dental radiography, a device used to increase the incoming line voltage from 110 or 220 volts to the high voltage required, usually 65,000 to 100,000 volts

Trauma   Injury produced by an external force

Triangle   A figure formed by connecting three points not in a straight line by three straight line segments; the figure has three angles

Triangle, equilateral   A triangle with three equal sides

Triangle, right   A triangle with one 90-degree angle (right angle)

Triangles, congruent   Triangles that are identical and correspond exactly when superimposed

Tube side   The outer side of the x-ray film packet that appears white and exhibits a raised bump in one corner; the tube side of the film faces the teeth and tubehead

Tubehead   The tightly sealed heavy metal housing that contains the dental x-ray tube; includes the metal housing, insulating oil, tubehead seal, x-ray tube, transformers, aluminum disks, lead collimator, and PID

Tubehead seal   The aluminum or leaded glass covering of the tubehead that permits the exit of x-rays from the tubehead; seals the oil in the tubehead and filters the x-ray beam

Tubercle   A tiny bump of bone; appears radiopaque

Tuberosity   A rounded prominence of bone; appears radiopaque

Tungsten filament   A portion of the cathode in the x-ray tube; a coiled wire of tungsten that produces electrons when heated

Tungsten target   A portion of the anode in the x-ray tube; serves as a focal spot and converts bombarding electrons into x-ray photons

Universal precautions   A method of infection control in which all human blood and certain body fluids are treated as if known to be infectious for HIV, hepatitis B virus, and other bloodborne pathogens

Uvula   A small, muscular structure located on the free edge of the soft palate

Vacuum tube   A sealed glass tube from which most of the air has been evacuated

Valve, mixing   In manual processing, a device that mixes the incoming hot and cold water to produce a water bath of optimum temperature (68°F)

Velocity   Speed; in dental radiography, the speed of a wave

Viewbox   A light source used to view dental radiographs (also called the illuminator)

Viewing   Examining or inspecting; see *Film viewing*

Volt (V)   The unit of electromotive force that drives an electrical current through a circuit

Voltage   In dental radiography, electrical pressure or force that drives the electrical current through the circuit of the x-ray machine

Washing   A step in film processing; water is used to wash a film following fixation; removes excess chemicals from the emulsion

Waters projection   An extraoral radiographic projection used to evaluate the maxillary sinus area

Wavelength   The distance between the crest of one wave to the crest of the next wave; determines the energy and penetrating power of the radiation (e.g., the shorter the wavelength, the higher the energy)

X-radiation   A high-energy, ionizing electromagnetic radiation; see *X-rays*

X-ray(s)   A form of ionizing radiation; weightless, neutral bundles of energy (photons) that travel in waves with a specific frequency at the speed of light; a beam of energy that has the power to penetrate substances and record image shadows on photographic film (also known as roentgen rays)

X-ray beam angulation   One of the influencing factors for image distortion; refers to the direction of the x-ray beam; less image distortion results when the x-ray beam is directed perpendicular to the tooth and film

X-ray tube   A component part of the x-ray tubehead that generates x-rays; includes a leaded glass vacuum tube, cathode, and anode

Zygoma   The cheekbone; appears as a diffuse radiopaque band posterior to the zygomatic process of the maxilla (also called the zygomatic or malar bone)

Zygomatic process of the maxilla   A bony projection of the maxilla that articulates with the zygoma; appears as a **J**- or **U**-shaped radiopacity on a maxillary molar periapical film

CHAPTER 1

Matching

1. C	3. A	5. E	7. G	9. B
2. I	4. D	6. H	8. F	

Matching

10. C	12. J	14. G	16. I	18. F
11. H	13. A	15. D	17. B	19. E

Essay

For questions 20 and 21, see discussion in text.

CHAPTER 2

Multiple Choice

1. D	3. C	5. B	7. A	9. A
2. B	4. B	6. D	8. B	10. B

Identification

11. filament	15. copper sleeve	19. aluminum filter	23. x-ray tube
12. molybdenum cup	16. vacuum	20. lead collimator	24. oil
13. electron stream	17. x-ray beam	21. PID	25. unleaded window
14. tungsten target	18. leaded glass	22. tubehead seal	26. metal housing

Multiple Choice

27. B	29. C	31. C	33. B	35. C
28. A	30. B	32. A	34. A	36. A

Identification

37. absorption	39. coherent scatter	41. B	43. C
38. Compton scatter	40. no interaction	42. D	44. A

CHAPTER 3

Multiple Choice

1. A	5. A	9. B	13. A	17. C
2. C	6. D	10. A	14. C	18. C
3. D	7. D	11. A	15. A	19. A
4. B	8. C	12. C	16. B	20. D

CHAPTER 4

Multiple Choice

1. D	6. E	11. C	16. A	21. B
2. E	7. D	12. A	17. A	22. E
3. A	8. B	13. E	18. E	23. B
4. C	9. B	14. C	19. E	24. D
5. C	10. D	15. B	20. C	25. A

CHAPTER 5

True or False

1. true   2. false   3. true   4. false   5. false

Multiple Choice

6. B   8. B   10. B   12. D   14. B
7. C   9. B   11. A   13. A   15. C

Fill in the Blank

16. 1.5; 2.5
17. 90–135

18. $(N - 18) \times 5$ rem/year
    $(N - 18) \times 0.05$ Sv/year
19. 5.0 rem/year (0.05 Sv/year)

20. 0.1 rem/year (0.001 Sv/year)

CHAPTER 6

Multiple Choice

1. C   3. B   5. A   7. C
2. A   4. B   6. B   8. A

CHAPTER 7

Fill in the Blank

1. protective layer
2. film base
3. halides
4. latent image
5. dot on label side of film packet
6. outer package wrapping on label side of film packet
7. lead foil sheet
8. black paper film wrapper
9. identification dot on tube side of film packet
10. intraoral film
11. outer package wrapping on tube side of film packet

Multiple Choice

12. C   16. B   20. A   24. D   28. C
13. D   17. C   21. A   25. B   29. C
14. A   18. A   22. A   26. C   30. A
15. C   19. B   23. B   27. A

CHAPTER 8

Multiple Choice

1. B   8. A   15. A   22. C
2. B   9. D   16. B   23. D
3. D   10. B   17. C   24. B
4. D   11. B   18. A
5. A   12. A   19. D
6. A   13. B   20. C
7. A   14. A   21. A

Fill in the Blank

25. increase   31. increase
26. decrease   32. decrease
27. increase   33. decrease
28. increase   34. decrease
29. decrease   35. increase
30. decrease

CHAPTER 9
Multiple Choice

1. A	8. D	15. D	22. B
2. C	9. D	16. D	23. D
3. C	10. A	17. C	24. J
4. E	11. A	18. D	25. C
5. B	12. D	19. H	26. E
6. C	13. C	20. A	27. F
7. A	14. E	21. G	28. I

Fill in the Blank
29. film duplicator and duplicating film
30. the longer duplicating film is exposed to light, the *lighter* it appears

Matching
31. E   32. D   33. A   34. C   35. B   36. C

Fill in the Blank
37. contamination with developer
38. contamination with fixer; air bubbles
39. exhausted developer or fixer; insufficient fix time; insufficient rinse time
40. reticulation of emulsion
41. developer cut-off
42. fixer cut-off
43. fingernail artifact
44. static electricity
45. scratch marks on film

True or False

46. true	47. false	48. false	49. true	50. true

CHAPTER 10
Multiple Choice

1. B	5. A	9. E	13. D
2. A	6. B	10. C	14. D
3. A	7. D	11. A	15. B
4. B	8. A	12. A	16. A

CHAPTER 11
True or False

1. false	3. true	5. true	7. false	9. true
2. false	4. false	6. true	8. true	10. false

CHAPTER 12
True or False

1. false	5. false	9. false	13. true	17. false
2. false	6. false	10. true	14. true	18. true
3. true	7. false	11. false	15. false	19. true
4. true	8. true	12. true	16. false	20. false

CHAPTER 13
Essay
For questions 1 and 2, see discussion in text.

Short Answer
For questions 3 to 16, see discussion in text.

CHAPTER 14
Multiple Choice

1. C	3. A	5. C	7. B	9. C
2. C	4. A	6. B	8. D	10. A

CHAPTER 15
Matching

1. B	3. J	5. A	7. H	9. D
2. E	4. I	6. G	8. F	10. C

Fill in the Blank
11. to prevent disease transmission
12. direct contact with pathogens, indirect contact with pathogens, and direct contact with airborne contaminants
13. a susceptible host, a pathogen with sufficient infectivity and numbers to cause infection, and a portal of entry through which the pathogen may enter the host

Multiple Choice

14. C	16. D	18. D	20. C
15. B	17. A	19. D	

Essay
For questions 21 to 25, see discussion in text.

CHAPTER 16
Matching

1. F	3. B	5. E	7. G	9. H
2. I	4. J	6. D	8. A	10. C

Short Answer
For questions 11 to 15, see discussion in text.

CHAPTER 17
Matching

1. H	3. F	5. A	7. C
2. G	4. E	6. B	8. D

Fill in the Blank
9. image magnification
   loss of definition
10. film holder
11. X = extension
    C = cone (PID)
    P = parallelling
12. size 1
13. size 2
14. precision film holders; Rinn XCP instruments with snap-on collimators
15. upper arch parallel to the floor; midsagittal plane perpendicular to the floor

Multiple Choice

16. A	18. C	20. B	22. B	24. B
17. B	19. A	21. C	23. B	25. A

Essay
For questions 26 to 33, see discussion in text.

CHAPTER 18

Matching
1. D   2. B   3. C   4. A

Identification
5. C   7. B   9. C
6. B   8. none   10. B

Fill in the Blank
11. magnification results
12. size 2
13. Rinn BAI instruments

14. maxillary arch parallel to the floor; midsagittal plane perpendicular to the floor
15. mandibular arch parallel to the floor; midsagittal plane perpendicular to the floor

Multiple Choice
16. D   17. A   18. D   19. A

Essay
For questions 20 to 30, see discussion in text.

CHAPTER 19

Fill in the Blank
1. patient "bites" on a "wing" (tab) to stabilize film
2. size 2
3. size 0
4. upper arch parallel to the floor; midsagittal plane perpendicular to the floor
5. caries
6. size 3
7. vertical angulation
8. horizontal angulation
9. overlapped contacts
10. if the beam is not centered over the film

Multiple Choice
11. C   12. C   13. A   14. B   15. D

Essay
For questions 16 to 23, see discussion in text.

CHAPTER 20

Identification
1. underexposed film
2. patient movement
3. elongated images
4. reversed film
5. cone-cut
6. overlapped contacts
7. overexposed film
8. incorrect premolar film placement
9. foreshortened images
10. incorrect film placement—no apices

Matching
11. D   12. C   13. B   14. A   15. C

Multiple Choice
16. B   17. A   18. C   19. D   20. A

CHAPTER 21

Fill in the Blank
1. the chewing surfaces of posterior teeth
2. size 4
3. size 2
4. upper arch parallel to the floor
5. see text for uses
6. +65 degrees
7. +60 degrees
8. −55 degrees
9. 90 degrees
10. maxillary = +60 degrees, mandibular = −55 degrees

Short Answer

11. BUCCAL. In the second film, the PID was shifted down, and the amalgam moved up (opposite = buccal).
12. BUCCAL. In the second film, the PID was shifted distally and the fragment moved mesially (opposite = buccal).
13. BUCCAL. In the second film, the PID was shifted down, and the canine moved up (opposite = buccal).
14. LINGUAL. In the second film, the PID was shifted distally, and the gutta percha moved distally (same = lingual).
15. LINGUAL. In the second film, the PID was shifted mesially, and the impacted canine moved mesially (same = lingual).

CHAPTER 22

Multiple Choice

1. C	5. B	9. C	13. A	17. B
2. A	6. A	10. A	14. A	18. A
3. C	7. A	11. B	15. A	19. C
4. A	8. A	12. B	16. A	20. A

Essay

For questions 21 to 25, see discussion in text.

CHAPTER 23

Essay

For questions 1 to 8, see discussion in text.

Multiple Choice

9. C   10. A   11. D   12. B   13. A   14. C   15. D

CHAPTER 24

Matching

1. h	3. i	5. e	7. f	9. b
2. a	4. d	6. g	8. c	

True or False

10. false	12. true	14. false	16. true	18. true
11. false	13. true	15. true	17. true	

Multiple Choice

19. c   20. d   21. b   22. b   23. a   24. d   25. c

CHAPTER 25

True or False

1. false	6. false	11. true	16. false	21. false
2. false	7. false	12. true	17. false	22. false
3. true	8. false	13. true	18. true	23. true
4. true	9. true	14. false	19. false	24. false
5. true	10. false	15. false	20. false	25. true

CHAPTER 26

Matching

1. B	3. A	5. F	7. H
2. D	4. C	6. G	8. E

Identification

9. zygomatic process of the maxilla
10. floor of the maxillary sinus
11. incisive foramen
12. coronoid process
13. lingual foramen
14. internal oblique ridge
15. mandibular canal
16. mental foramen

CHAPTER 27

True or False

1. true	6. true	11. false	16. false
2. false	7. true	12. true	17. true
3. false	8. true	13. false	18. true
4. false	9. false	14. true	19. true
5. true	10. false	15. true	20. false

Short Answer

For questions 21 to 25, see discussion in text.

CHAPTER 28

Question 1

1. glenoid fossa
2. mandibular condyle
3. coronoid process
4. maxillary tuberosity
5. infraorbital foramen
6. mental foramen
7. lingual foramen
8. genial tubercles
9. incisive foramen
10. nasal cavity
11. hard palate
12. zygomatic process of the maxilla
13. mylohyoid ridge
14. internal oblique ridge
15. external oblique ridge

Question 2

1. palatoglossal air space
2. hard palate
3. infraorbital foramen
4. floor of the orbit
5. zygomatic process of the maxilla
6. posterior wall of maxillary sinus
7. zygomaticotemporal suture
8. external auditory meatus
9. lateral pterygoid plate
10. maxillary tuberosity
11. styloid process
12. ear
13. mandibular canal
14. cervical spine
15. hyoid bone
16. mental foramen

CHAPTER 29

Short Answer

For questions 1 to 6, see discussion in text.

True or False

7. true	10. false	13. false
8. true	11. false	14. true
9. true	12. false	15. true

CHAPTER 30

Identification

1. rampant severe caries
2. incipient interproximal caries
3. root surface caries
4. moderate interproximal caries
5. severe interproximal caries

Matching

6. E   7. A   8. B   9. D   10. C   11. G   12. F

Short Answer

For questions 13 to 20, see discussion in text.

CHAPTER 31

Identification

1. horizontal   moderate   ADA case type III
2. horizontal   mild   ADA case type II
3. horizontal   severe   ADA case type IV
4. none   none
5. none   none

Matching

6. C   7. A   8. D   9. B

Fill in the Blank

10. periodontium   14. paralleling technique   18. localized
11. periodontal   15. horizontal   19. generalized
12. furcation   16. vertical   20. calculus
13. periapical   17. periodontal disease

CHAPTER 32

Matching

1. B   2. E   3. A   4. F   5. D   6. C

Identification

7. pulp stone   10. condensing osteitis
8. hypercementosis   11. external resorption
9. pulpal obliteration 12. pulpal sclerosis

Index

Note: Page numbers in *italics* indicate illustrations; t indicates a table; b indicates boxed material; and p indicates a procedure.